# dentEssentials
## High-Yield NBDE® Part I Review

**THIRD EDITION**

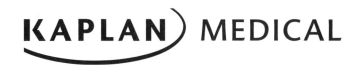

# dentEssentials

## High-Yield NBDE® Part I Review

### THIRD EDITION

**Board Prep for First- and Second-Year Dental Students**

© 2010 by Kaplan, Inc.

Published by Kaplan Publishing, a division of Kaplan, Inc.
1 Liberty Plaza, 24th Floor
New York, NY 10006

Printed in the United States of America

December 2009
10  9  8  7  6  5  4  3  2  1

ISBN-13: 978-1-60714-475-5


Kaplan Publishing books are available at special quantity discounts to use for sales promotions, employee premiums, or educational purposes. Please call the Simon & Schuster special sales department at 866-506-1949.

## LEAD AUTHORS/EDITORS

**Michael S. Manley, M.D.**
*Director, Basic Sciences and Step 1 Curriculum*
*Kaplan Medical*

**Leslie D. Manley, Ph.D.**
*Director, Basic Sciences and Step 1 Curriculum*
*Kaplan Medical*

## EXECUTIVE EDITORS

Sonia Reichert, M.D.
*Hematology/Oncology Fellow*
*Mt. Sinai Medical Center, NY, NY*

Rochelle Rothstein, M.D.
*Chief Medical Officer*

## DENTAL ANATOMY EDITORS

Jeff Linfante, D.D.S.
*Director of Dental Curriculum*
*Kaplan Medical*

Ronald Salyk, D.D.S.
*Morris Heights Health Center*
*Bronx, New York*

## CONTRIBUTORS

Thomas H. Adair, Ph.D.
*Professor*
*Department of Physiology and Biophysics*
*University of Mississippi Medical Center*

Stuart Bentley-Hibbert, M.D., Ph.D.
*New York Presbyterian Hospital*
*Weill Cornell Medical Center*

Steven Daugherty, Ph.D.
*Director of Education and Testing*
*Kaplan Medical*
*Rush Medical College*

Douglas E. Fitzovich, Ph.D.
*Professor of Physiology*
*DeBusk College of Osteopathic Medicine*
*Lincoln Memorial University*

Beth Forshee, Ph.D.
*Assistant Professor of Physiology*
*Lake Erie College of Osteopathic Medicine*

Barbara Hansen, Ph.D.
*Biochemistry Faculty, Kaplan Medical*

Robert F. Kissling III, M.D.

John A. Kriak, Pharm.D.
*Director, Medical Education Conference Archives, Inc.*

Mary J. Ruebush, Ph.D.
*Adjunct Professor of Medical Science, retired*
*Montana State University*
*Microbiology/Immunology Faculty, Kaplan Medical*

Nancy Standler, M.D., Ph.D.
*Pathologist*

James S. White, Ph.D.
*Assistant Professor of Cell Biology*
*School of Osteopathic Medicine*
*University of Medicine and Dentistry of New Jersey*
*Adjunct Assistant Professor of Cell and*
 *Developmental Biology*
*University of Pennsylvania School of Medicine*

Glenn C. Yiu M.D., Ph.D.
*Clinical Fellow in Medicine*
*Harvard Medical School*

# Contents

*(A more comprehensive list appears on the first page of each chapter.)*

## SECTION III: DENTAL ANATOMY, OCCLUSION, AND HISTOLOGY

# Introduction

The completion of the National Board Dental Examination Part I (NBDE Part I) is a milestone for dental students on their way to the practice of dentistry. The exam is one of several forms of evaluation used by the various licensing boards to assess the qualifications of an individual seeking the privilege to practice dentistry. NBDE Part I has been designed to test students' ability to understand both basic and dental science and to integrate this material into a problem-solving context.

## The Examination

NBDE Part I is a comprehensive, computer-based exam that is administered in one day by Prometric, Inc. at Prometric Test Centers in the United States and Canada. It is comprised of 400 multiple-choice items, evenly distributed among the following disciplines:

- Anatomic Sciences
- Biochemistry/Physiology
- Microbiology/Pathology
- Dental Anatomy and Occlusion

Approximately 20% of the total number of questions are grouped into testlets. Testlets are presented in a case-based format, providing some background information on a patient within a given clinical scenario. The questions are developed around this information and have an interdisciplinary and clinical focus.

Candidates are given a total of 7 hours to complete the exam, divided into two sessions—morning and afternoon—with an optional lunch break in between.

The NBDE I score results are reported in standard scores of 49 to 99. The minimum passing score is a standard score of 75. The two factors that affect a candidate's score are (1) the number of correct answers selected by the candidate, and (2) the score scale conversion for the exam.

## dentEssentials: Integrated Basic Science Review Book

The *dentEssentials* review book has been structured by organ system and is presented in a compact and concise manner. It focuses on the most relevant and important basic and dental science information in the form of reference charts and corresponding images. This design allows for a unique level of integration between the disciplines.

This book is divided into three sections. Section I presents the general principles of the basic science disciplines (biochemistry molecular biology, genetics, microbiology, immunology, embryology, and histology). These subjects serve as the fundamental foundation for the organ-specific information, which follows in Section II. Section III focuses on dental anatomy, occlusion, and histology.

## Study Techniques

It is not recommended that you go back to your textbooks and begin the process of preparing for the NBDE by rereading them cover to cover and underlining every word on every page. This is not an efficient use of your time or an effective way to learn. Develop a plan and focus on the material most likely to be on the exam, narrowing down the amount of material you need to cover.

A good way to increase your retention and to help facilitate your recall of information is to be an active user of the material you are learning. Repetition makes memories. Each instance of recall produces a new memory trace, linking concepts and increasing the chance of recall of the information in the future. Recall actually changes the neuronal structures. To make information useful, it needs to be triangulated; it needs to be connected to other concepts and to experiences. It is important to remember that memorization should not be the primary goal during preparation; rather, you should develop the ability to process and apply the material in an integrated manner.

Begin the process of preparation by following the steps listed below:

- Assess your strengths and weaknesses, then rank the order of subjects from weak to strong.
- Start every study session with a list of specific goals.
- Personalize the review book. Use color highlighting, write margin notes, and summarize the topics you have learned.
- After reviewing the topics of the study session, imagine or actually try to teach the material and concepts to someone else.

Every student preparing to take this exam is required to read the *National Dental Board Examination Part I Guide.* This is provided by the ADA and is available online at **ada.org.**

Finally, please let us know what you think by emailing us at **medfeedback@kaplan.com.** Your comments will help us develop future editions of this review book and help future dental students prepare for the National Boards.

On behalf of the Kaplan Medical Team, we wish you good luck and success with your studies and in your dental career.

# General Principles

# Biochemistry

## GLYCOLYSIS

**Glycolysis** is a **cytoplasmic** pathway used by all cells to generate energy from glucose. **One** glucose molecule is converted into **2 pyruvate** molecules, generating a net of **2 ATPs** by substrate-level phosphorylation, and **2 NADHs**. When oxygen is present, NADH delivers electrons to the electron transport chain in mitochondria to generate ATP by oxidative phosphorylation. Under **anaerobic** conditions (e.g., short bursts of intense exercise) or in cells without mitochondria (e.g., RBCs), lactate is generated and the NADH is reoxidized into $NAD^+$.

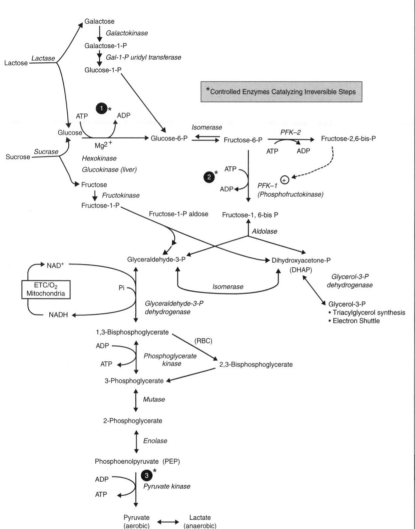

### Regulation

**Three irreversible** steps:

| Hexokinase | Glucokinase* |
|---|---|
| Most tissues | Liver, β-islet cells |
| Low $K_m$ | High $K_m$ |
| ⊖ G-6-P | Induced by insulin in liver |

❷

| PFK-1 | PFK-2 |
|---|---|
| → F-1,6-BP | → F-2,6-BP |
| Rate-limiting step of glycolysis | Glycolysis regulator: ↑ glycolysis ↓ gluconeogenesis |
| ⊕ AMP<br>⊕ F-2,6-BP[†]<br>⊖ ATP<br>⊖ Citrate | ⊕ Insulin<br>⊖ Glucagon |

❸

| Pyruvate kinase | |
|---|---|
| ⊕ F-1,6-BP<br>⊕ Insulin[†] | ⊖ ATP<br>⊖ Acetyl-CoA<br>⊖ Alanine[†]<br>⊖ Glucagon[†] |

*Glukokinase mutations may lead to a form of MODY.
[†]Liver specific

### Glucose Transport

**GLUT-1 and -3:** basal uptake (most cells)

**GLUT-2:** storage (liver); glucose sensor (β-islet)

**GLUT-4:** ↑ by insulin (adipose, skeletal muscle); ↑ by exercise (skeletal muscle)

### Disease Association

| | |
|---|---|
| **Galactokinase deficiency** | Galactosemia/galactosuria, cataracts in childhood (excess galactose is converted to galactitol via aldose reductase); Tx: no galactose in diet |
| **Gal-1-P uridyl transferase deficiency** | Same as above, but more severe with vomiting/diarrhea after milk ingestion, liver disease, lethargy, mental retardation; Tx: no galactose in diet |
| **Fructokinase deficiency** | Fructosuria; benign |
| **Aldolase B deficiency** | Fructosuria, liver and proximal renal tubule disorder; Tx: no fructose in diet |
| **Pyruvate kinase deficiency** | Chronic hemolysis, ↑ 2,3-BPG and other glycolytic intermediates in the RBC, no Heinz bodies, autosomal recessive |

*Definition of abbreviations:* MODY, mature-onset diabetes of the young; PFK, phosphofructokinase; RBC, red blood cell; Tx, treatment.

# THE CITRIC ACID CYCLE

The citric acid cycle (**tricarboxylic acid cycle**) is a **mitochondrial** pathway that occurs **only** under **aerobic conditions**. Each acetyl-CoA generated from pyruvate is used to produce **3 NADH, 1 FADH$_2$, and 1 GTP**. Both the NADH and FADH$_2$ deliver electrons to the electron transport chain (ETC) to generate ATP by oxidative phosphorylation.

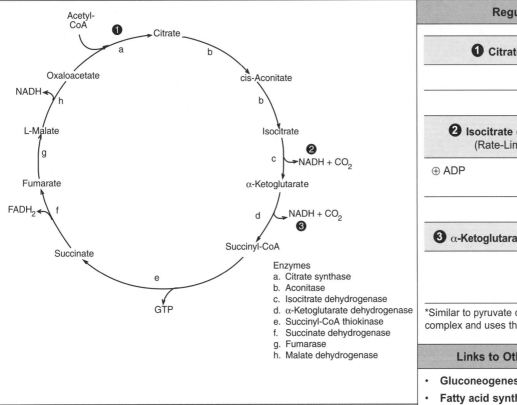

Enzymes
a. Citrate synthase
b. Aconitase
c. Isocitrate dehydrogenase
d. α-Ketoglutarate dehydrogenase
e. Succinyl-CoA thiokinase
f. Succinate dehydrogenase
g. Fumarase
h. Malate dehydrogenase

## Regulation

### ❶ Citrate synthase

| | ⊖ ATP |
|---|---|

### ❷ Isocitrate dehydrogenase
(Rate-Limiting Step)

| ⊕ ADP | ⊖ ATP<br>⊖ NADH |
|---|---|

### ❸ α-Ketoglutarate dehydrogenase*

| | ⊖ Succinyl CoA<br>⊖ ATP<br>⊖ NADH |
|---|---|

*Similar to pyruvate dehydrogenase complex and uses the same cofactors

## Links to Other Pathways

- **Gluconeogenesis** (malate shuttle)
- **Fatty acid synthesis** (citrate shuttle)
- **Amino acid synthesis** (oxaloacetate and α-ketoglutarate)
- **Heme synthesis** (succinyl CoA)

## Stoichiometry of the Citric Acid Cycle

Acetyl-CoA + 3 NAD$^+$ + FAD + GDP + P$_i$ → 2 CO$_2$ + 3 NADH + FADH$_2$ + GTP + CoA

# OXIDATIVE PHOSPHORYLATION

Electron transport and the coupled synthesis of ATP are known as oxidative phosphorylation. The **electron transport chain (ETC)** is a series of carrier enzymes in the **inner mitochondrial membrane** that pass electrons, in a stepwise fashion, from NADH and $FADH_2$ to **oxygen**, the final electron acceptor. These carriers create a proton gradient across the inner membrane, which drives the $F_0/F_1$ ATP synthase, with a net production of **3 ATPs** per **NADH** and **2 ATPs** per **$FADH_2$**.

## Electron Transport Chain

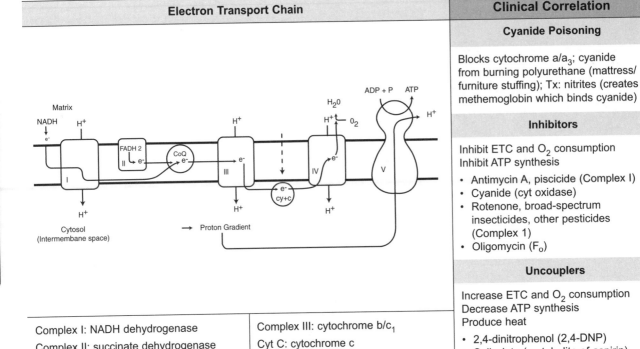

Complex I: NADH dehydrogenase
Complex II: succinate dehydrogenase
CoQ: coenzyme Q

Complex III: cytochrome $b/c_1$
Cyt C: cytochrome c
Complex IV: cytochrome $a/a_3$
Complex V: $F_0F_1$ ATP synthase

## Clinical Correlation

### Cyanide Poisoning

Blocks cytochrome $a/a_3$; cyanide from burning polyurethane (mattress/furniture stuffing); Tx: nitrites (creates methemoglobin which binds cyanide)

### Inhibitors

Inhibit ETC and $O_2$ consumption
Inhibit ATP synthesis

- Antimycin A, piscicide (Complex I)
- Cyanide (cyt oxidase)
- Rotenone, broad-spectrum insecticides, other pesticides (Complex 1)
- Oligomycin ($F_0$)

### Uncouplers

Increase ETC and $O_2$ consumption
Decrease ATP synthesis
Produce heat

- 2,4-dinitrophenol (2,4-DNP)
- Salicylate (metabolite of aspirin)
- Uncoupling proteins (e.g., thermogenin)

## Electron Shuttles

Cytosolic electrons are transported into the mitochondria via the **malate** and **glycerol-3-P** carriers.

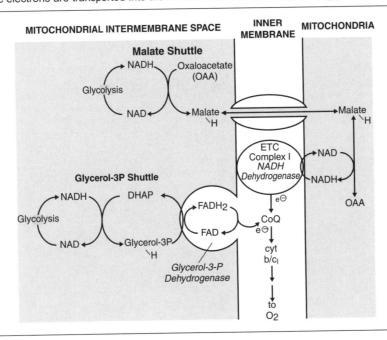

# PYRUVATE METABOLISM

**Lactate dehydrogenase:** *Anaerobic tissues:* converts pyruvate to lactate, reoxidizing cytoplasmic NADH to $NAD^+$. *Liver:* converts lactate to pyruvate for gluconeogenesis or for metabolism to acetyl CoA

**Alanine aminotransferase (ALT, GPT):** *Muscle:* converts pyruvate to alanine to transport amino groups to the liver. *Liver:* converts alanine to pyruvate for gluconeogenesis and delivers the amino group for urea synthesis

**Pyruvate carboxylase:** produces oxaloacetate for gluconeogenesis and the citric acid cycle

**Pyruvate dehydrogenase:** generates acetyl-CoA for fatty acid synthesis and the citric acid cycle; complex of 3 enzymes

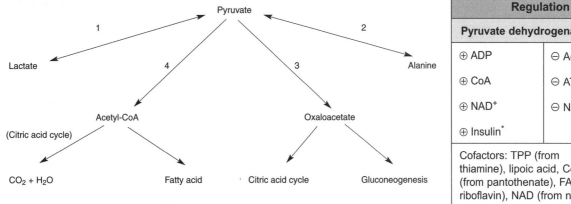

Enzymes: 1. Lactate dehydrogenase; 2. transaminase; 3. pyruvate carboxylase; 4. pyruvate dehydrogenase

| Regulation | |
| --- | --- |
| **Pyruvate dehydrogenase (PDH)** | |
| ⊕ ADP | ⊖ Acetyl-CoA |
| ⊕ CoA | ⊖ ATP |
| ⊕ $NAD^+$ | ⊖ NADH |
| ⊕ Insulin* | |
| Cofactors: TPP (from thiamine), lipoic acid, CoA (from pantothenate), FAD (from riboflavin), NAD (from niacin) | |
| *Liver specific | |

| Stoichiometry of Pyruvate Dehydrogenase |
| --- |
| $Pyruvate + NAD^+ + CoA \rightarrow NADH + CO_2 + acetyl\text{-}CoA$ |

| Disease Association |
| --- |
| **Pyruvate Dehydrogenase Deficiency** |
| Lactic acidosis, seizures, mental retardation, ataxia, spasticity |

## Cori Cycle

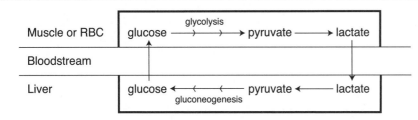

During fasting or exercise, lactate from RBCs or skeletal muscles is sent to the liver to make glucose that can be returned to the RBCs or muscle.

*Definition of abbreviations:* TCA, tricarboxylic acid; TPP, thiamine pyrophosphate.

# HEXOSE MONOPHOSPHATE SHUNT

The **hexose monophosphate (HMP) shunt** (pentose phosphate pathway) is a **cytosolic** pathway that uses **glucose-6-phosphate** to reduce NADP to NADPH, and synthesize **ribose-5-P**. NADPH is important for fatty acid and steroid biosynthesis, maintenance of reduced glutathione to protect against reactive oxygen species (ROS), and for bactericidal activity in polymorphonuclear leukocytes (PMNs). Ribose-5-P is required for nucleotide synthesis.

| Regulation | |
|---|---|
| **Glucose-6-P-dehydrogenase** | |
| ⊕ **NADP⁺** | ⊖ NADPH |

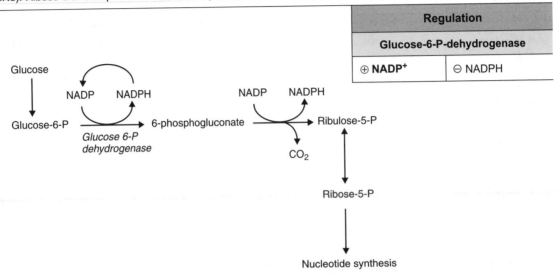

## Disease Association

### Glucose-6-Phosphatase Dehydrogenase Deficiency

Episodic hemolytic anemia induced by infection and drugs (common) or chronic hemolysis (rare); X-linked recessive; female heterozygotes have ↑ resistance to malaria

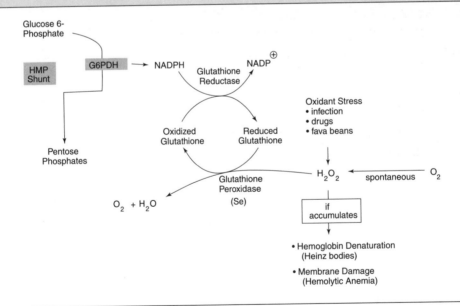

# GLYCOGENESIS AND GLYCOGENOLYSIS

**Glycogen** is a branched polymer of glucose, stored primarily in liver and skeletal muscles, which can be mobilized during hypoglycemia (liver) or muscular contraction (muscles). Synthesis of glycogen (**glycogenesis**) is mediated by **glycogen synthase**, while its breakdown (**glycogenolysis**) is carried out by **glycogen phosphorylase**. Branching of the glycogen polymer occurs via a **branching enzyme**, which breaks an $\alpha$-1,4-bond and transfers a block of glucosyl residues to create a new $\alpha$-1,6-bond. This is reversed by a **debranching enzyme**.

| Glycogen Metabolism | Regulation |
|---|---|

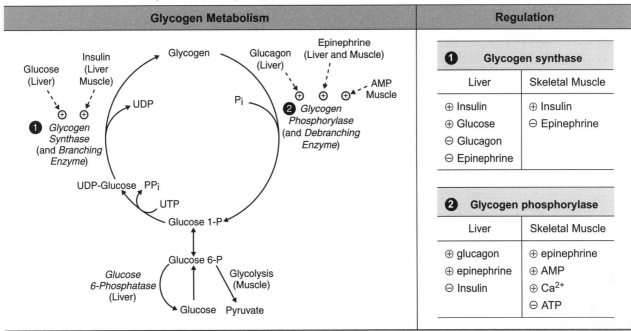

| ❶ | Glycogen synthase | |
|---|---|---|
| Liver | | Skeletal Muscle |
| ⊕ Insulin | | ⊕ Insulin |
| ⊕ Glucose | | ⊖ Epinephrine |
| ⊖ Glucagon | | |
| ⊖ Epinephrine | | |

| ❷ | Glycogen phosphorylase | |
|---|---|---|
| Liver | | Skeletal Muscle |
| ⊕ glucagon | | ⊕ epinephrine |
| ⊕ epinephrine | | ⊕ AMP |
| ⊖ Insulin | | ⊕ $Ca^{2+}$ |
| | | ⊖ ATP |

## Branching and Debranching Steps

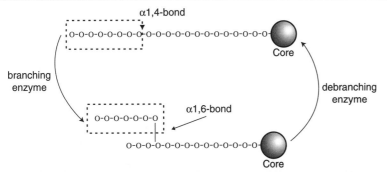

**Branching enzyme** hydrolyzes an $\alpha$-1,4-bond in the growing glycogen chain, then transfers the oligosaccharide unit to a new position and attaches it with an $\alpha$-1,6-bond to create a branch. Glycogen synthase then extends both branches.

**Debranching enzyme** hydrolyzes the $\alpha$-1,4-bond closest to a branch point, transfers the oligosaccharide to the end of another chain, then hydrolyzes the $\alpha$-1,6-bond, releasing the single glucose remaining at the branch point.

## Glycogen Storage Diseases

| | |
|---|---|
| Type I: von Gierke disease ($\downarrow$ glucose-6-phosphatase) | Severe fasting hypoglycemia, lactic acidosis, hepatomegaly, hyperlipidemia, hyperuricemia, short stature |
| Type II: Pompe disease ($\downarrow$ lysosomal-$\alpha$-1,4-glucosidase) | Cardiomegaly, muscle weakness, death by 2 years |
| Type III: Cori disease ($\downarrow$ glycogen debranching enzyme) | Mild hypoglycemia; liver enlargement |
| Type IV: Andersen disease ($\downarrow$ branching enzyme) | Infantile hypotonia, cirrhosis, death by 2 years |
| Type V: McArdle disease ($\downarrow$ muscle glycogen phosphorylase*) | Muscle cramps/weakness during initial phase of exercise, possible rhabdomyolysis and myoglobinuria |
| Type VI: Hers disease ($\downarrow$ hepatic glycogen phosphorylase) | Mild fasting hypoglycemia, hepatomegaly, cirrhosis |

*Also known as myophosphorylase.

# GLUCONEOGENESIS

**Gluconeogenesis** is a pathway for de novo synthesis of **glucose** from **C3 and C4 precursors** using both **mitochondrial** and **cytosolic** enzymes. Occurring only in liver, kidney, and intestinal epithelium, this pathway functions to provide glucose for the body, especially the brain and RBCs, which require glucose for energy (the brain can also use ketone bodies during fasting conditions). Gluconeogenesis occurs during fasting, as glycogen stores become depleted. Important substrates for gluconeogenesis are gluconeogenic **amino acids** (protein from muscle), **lactate** (from RBCs and muscle during anaerobic exercise), and **glycerol-3-P** (from triacylglycerol from adipose tissues).

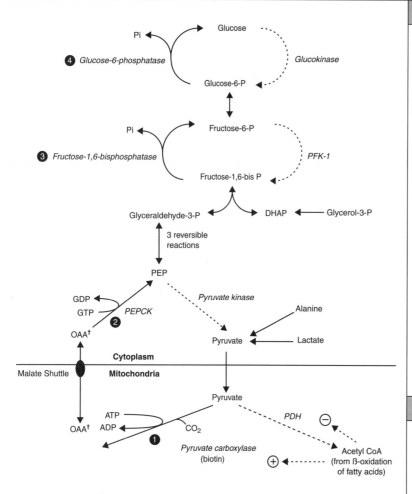

## Regulation

Four **irreversible** steps:

### ❶ Pyruvate carboxylase

Mitochondrial; requires biotin

| ⊕ acetyl CoA | — |
|---|---|

### ❷ PEPCK

Cytosolic; requires GTP

| Induced by glucagon and cortisol | — |
|---|---|

### ❸ Fructose 1,6-bisphosphatase*

Cytosolic

| ⊕ ATP | ⊖ AMP |
|---|---|
|  | ⊖ F-2,6-BP‡ (from PFK2) |

### ❹ Glucose-6-phosphatase*

In endoplasmic reticulum; only in liver

‡Mediates insulin's inhibition and glucagon's stimulation of this enzyme
*Reverse reactions of key glycolytic kinase reactions

## Disease Association

**Glucose-6-Phosphatase Deficiency (von Gierke disease)**

Severe hypoglycemia, lactic acidosis, hepatomegaly, hyperlipidemia, hyperuricemia, short stature

## Alanine Cycle

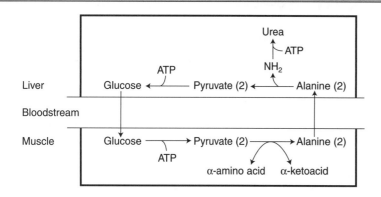

A pathway by which muscles release alanine to the liver, delivering both a gluconeogenic substrate (pyruvate) and an amino group for urea synthesis

*Definition of abbreviations:* PEPCK, phosphoenolpyruvate carboxykinase; PFK2, phosphofructokinase 2; RBC, red blood cell.

† OAA is not transported across the membrane directly. Instead, it is transported as malate in exchange for asparate via the malate shuttle (*see* page 7).

# AMINO ACID STRUCTURES

## Hydrophobic Amino Acids

### Nonpolar, Aliphatic Side Chains

### Aromatic Side Chains

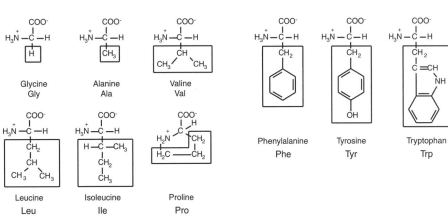

### Hydrophilic Amino Acids

### Positively Charged R Groups

### Polar, Uncharged R Groups

### Negatively Charged R Groups

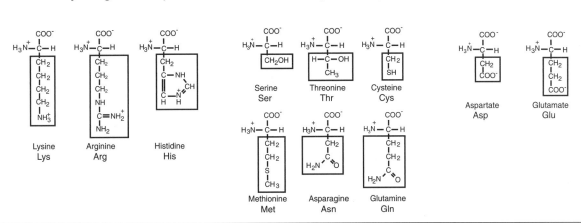

## AMINO ACID DERIVATIVES

Besides being the building blocks of proteins, amino acids are also precursors for various chemicals, such as **hormones**, **neurotransmitters**, and other small molecules.

| Amino Acid | Product | Disease Association |
|---|---|---|
| **Tyrosine** | Thyroid hormones ($T_3$, $T_4$); melanin; catecholamines (dopamine, epinephrine) | **Albinism**<br>Tyrosine hydroxylase (type I) or tyrosine transporter (type II) deficiency; ↓ pigmentation of skin, eyes, and hair, ↑ risk of skin cancer, visual defects |

| **Tryptophan** | Serotonin (5-HT); melatonin; NAD; NADP | **Carcinoid Syndrome**<br>↑ Serotonin excretion from gastrointestinal neuroendocrine tumors (carcinoid tumors); cutaneous flushing, venous telangiectasia, diarrhea, bronchospasm, cardiac valvular lesions |

| **Glycine** | Heme | **Acute Intermittent Porphyria**<br>Porphobilinogen deaminase* deficiency; episodic expression, acute abdominal pain, anxiety, confusion, paranoia, muscle weakness, no photosensitivity, port-wine urine in some patients, urine excretion of ALA and PBG; autosomal dominant; onset at puberty, 15% penetrance, variable expression; more common in women |

**Porphyria Cutanea Tarda**
Uroporphyrinogen decarboxylase† deficiency; photosensitivity, skin inflammation, and blistering; cirrhosis often associated; autosomal dominant; late onset

| **Glutamate** | γ-aminobutyric acid (GABA) | |

**Lead Poisoning**
Inhibits ALA dehydratase and ferrochelatase; microcytic sideroblastic anemia; basophilic stippling of erythrocytes; headache, nausea, memory loss, abdominal pain, diarrhea (lead colic), lead lines in gums, neuropathy (claw hand, wrist-drop), ↑ urine excretion of ALA; Tx: dimercaprol and EDTA

| **Arginine** | Nitric oxide (NO) | |

**Hemolytic Crisis**
Jaundice due to ↑ bilirubin from severe hemolysis; ↓ hemoglobin; ↑ reticulocytes; may result from:
(1) G6PD deficiency hemolysis
(2) Sickle cell crisis
(3) Rh disease of newborn

| **Histidine** | Histamine | |

**UDP-Glucuronyl Transferase Deficiency**
Jaundice due to low bilirubin conjugation; may result from:
(1) Crigler-Najjar syndromes
(2) Gilbert syndrome
(3) Physiologic jaundice of newborn, especially premature infants

| **Methionine** | S-adenosylmethionine (SAM; methylating agent) | |
| **Arginine, glycine, SAM** | Creatine | |

* Also known as hydroxymethylbilane synthase; †an enzyme in the pathway between Uroporphyrinogen-III and Protoporphyrin IX.

# AMINO ACID SYNTHESIS AND METABOLISM

**Amino acids** are required for protein synthesis. Although some amino acids can be synthesized de novo (**nonessential**), others (**essential**) must be obtained from the digestion of dietary proteins. Nonessential amino acids are synthesized from intermediates of glycolysis and the citric acid cycle or from other amino acids. Degradation of amino acids occurs by transamination of the amino group to **glutamate**, while the remaining carbon skeletons of the amino acids may be oxidized to $CO_2 + H_2O$, or reverted to citric acid cycle intermediates for conversion to glucose (**glucogenic**) or ketones (**ketogenic**).

## Genetic Deficiencies of Amino Acid Metabolism

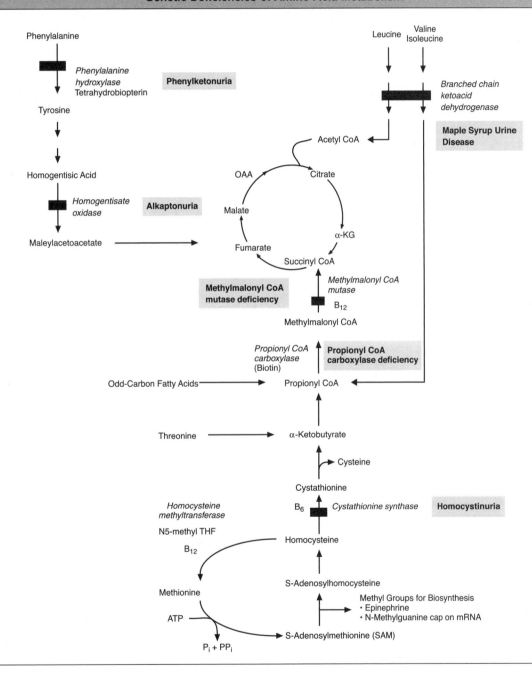

*(Continued)*

### Precursors for Nonessential Amino Acids

Glucose → Phosphoglycerate → Pyruvate → α-Ketoglutarate → Oxaloacetate
       Serine      Alanine      Glutamate      Aspartate
   Glycine  Cysteine        Proline  Glutamine  Asparagine

Glycolysis    TCA cycle

### Essential Amino Acids*

| | |
|---|---|
| Arginine† | Methionine |
| Histidine | Phenylalanine |
| Isoleucine | Threonine |
| Leucine | Tryptophan |
| Lysine | Valine |

*Mnemonic: PVT. TIM HALL; †essential during periods of growth and pregnancy

### Transfer of α-Amino Groups to α-Ketoglutarate

### Glucogenic and Ketogenic Amino Acids

| Ketogenic | Ketogenic and Glucogenic | Glucogenic |
|---|---|---|
| Leucine<br>Lysine | Phenylalanine<br>Tyrosine<br>Tryptophan<br>Isoleucine<br>Threonine | All others |

### Disease Association

| | |
|---|---|
| Hartnup disease | Transport protein defect with ↑ excretion of neutral amino acids; symptoms similar to pellagra; autosomal recessive |
| Phenylketonuria | Phenylalanine hydroxylase or dihydrobiopterin reductase deficiency → buildup of phenylalanine; tyrosine becomes essential; musty body odor, mental retardation, microcephaly, autosomal recessive; Tx: ↓ phenylalanine in diet; avoid aspartame (Nutrasweet®) |
| Alkaptonuria | Homogentisate oxidase deficiency (for tyrosine degradation); ↑ homogentisic acid in blood and urine (darkens when exposed to air), ochronosis (dark pigment in cartilage), arthritis in adulthood |
| Homocystinuria | ↑ homocystine in urine. Classic homocystinuria, caused by a deficiency in cystathionine synthase, is associated with dislocated lens, deep venous thrombosis, stroke, atherosclerosis, mental retardation, and Marfan-like features. Deficiency of pyridoxine, folate, or vitamin $B_{12}$ can produce a mild homocystinemia with elevated risk of atherosclerosis (previously listed symptoms absent). Methionine synthase (homocysteine methyltransferase) deficiency is extremely rare and is associated with megaloblastic anemia and mental retardation. |
| Cystinuria | Transport protein defect with ↑ excretion of lysine, arginine, cystine, and ornithine; excess cystine precipitates as kidney stones; Tx: acetazolamide |
| Maple syrup urine disease | Branched-chain ketoacid dehydrogenase deficiency; branched-chain ketoacidosis from infancy; weight loss, lethargy, alternating hypertonia/hypotonia, maple syrup odor of urine; ketosis/coma/death if untreated; Tx: ↓ valine, leucine, isoleucine in diet |
| Propionyl-CoA carboxylase deficiency<br><br>Methylmalonyl-CoA mutase deficiency | Neonatal ketoacidosis from blocked degradation of valine, isoleucine, methionine, threonine, and odd-carbon fatty acids; Tx: ↓ these amino acids in diet<br>*Propionyl-CoA carboxylase deficiency:* neonatal metabolic acidosis; hyperammonemia; elevated propionic acid, hydroxypropionic acid, and methylcitrate; poor feeding, vomiting, lethargy, coma<br>*Methylmalonyl-CoA mutase deficiency:* symptoms similar to propionyl CoA carboxylase deficiency, but accumulating metabolites differ (↑ methylmalonic acid) |

*Definition of abbreviation:* PLP, pyridoxal-phosphate, formed from vitamin $B_6$.

# UREA CYCLE

Amino acids transported to the liver are transaminated to glutamate, which undergoes deamination to produce $NH_4^+$ or transamination to make **aspartate**. Both of these are used for synthesis of urea in the liver for excretion via the **urea cycle**.

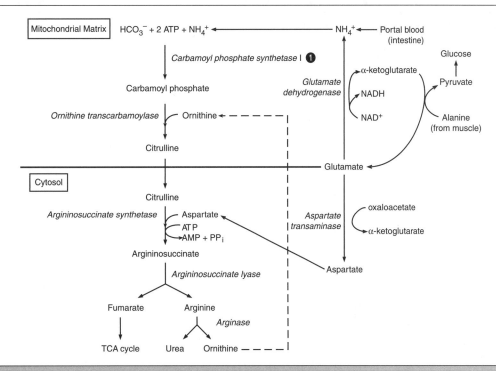

## Regulation

### ❶ Carbamoyl phosphate synthase I

$\oplus$ *N*-acetylglutamate*

*High protein diet → ↑ glutamate in mitochondria → ↑ *N*-acetylglutamate

## Disease Association

| Carbamoyl Phosphate Synthetase Deficiency | Ornithine Transcarbamoylase Deficiency |
|---|---|
| ↑ [$NH_4^+$]; hyperammonemia | ↑ [$NH_4^+$]; hyperammonemia |
| ↑ blood glutamine | ↑ blood glutamine |
| ↓ BUN | ↓ BUN |
| No increase in uracil or orotic acid | Uracil and orotic acid ↑ in blood and urine* |
| Cerebral edema | Cerebral edema |
| Lethargy, convulsions, coma, death | Lethargy, convulsions, coma, death |

*OTC deficiency: ↑ carbamoyl-P stimulates pyrimidine synthesis, causing ↑ orotic acid and uracil

# LIPID SYNTHESIS AND METABOLISM

**Fatty acids** are synthesized from excess glucose in the liver and transported to adipose tissues for storage. Fatty acid **synthesis** occurs in the **cytosol** and involves the transport of **acetyl-CoA** from the mitochondria via the **citrate shuttle**, carboxylation to **malonyl CoA**, and linking together 2 carbons per cycle to form long fatty acid chains. Synthesis stops at $C_{16}$ **palmitoyl-CoA**, requiring **7 ATP** and **14 NADPH**. Metabolism of fatty acids occurs by β-**oxidation**, which takes place in **mitochondria**, and involves transport of fatty acids from the cytosol via the **carnitine shuttle**, then oxidative removal of 2 carbons per cycle to yield **1 NADH**, **1 FADH$_2$**, and **1 acetyl-CoA**.

## Fatty Acid Synthesis and Oxidation

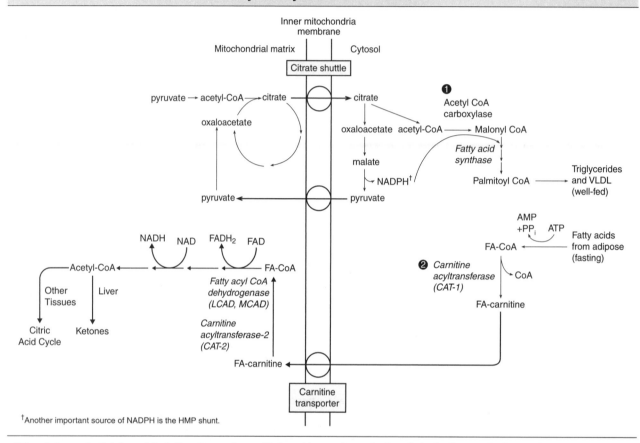

†Another important source of NADPH is the HMP shunt.

**Triacylglycerols (triglycerides)**, the storage form of fatty acids, are formed primarily in the liver and adipose tissues by attaching **3 fatty acids** to a **glycerol-3-P**. Triacylglycerols are transported from liver to adipose as VLDL. Fatty acids from the diet are transported as chylomicrons. Both are digested by lipoprotein lipase (induced by insulin) in the capillaries of adipose and muscle. Fatty acids may be mobilized from triacylglycerols in adipose by hormone-sensitive lipase. Free fatty acids are delivered to tissues for beta oxidation.

| Regulation | | |
|---|---|---|
| **❶ Acetyl-CoA carboxylase** | | **❷ Carnitine acyltransferase-1 (CAT-1)** |
| **Rate-limiting for fatty acid synthesis**; requires biotin | | **Rate-limiting for fatty acid oxidation** |
| ⊕ insulin<br>⊕ citrate | ⊖ glucagon<br>⊖ palmitoyl-CoA | ⊖ malonyl-CoA |

| Disease Association | |
|---|---|
| **Myopathic CAT-2/CPT-2 Deficiency** | **Medium Chain Acyl-Dehydrogenase (MCAD) Deficiency** |
| Muscle aches/weakness, myoglobulinuria provoked by prolonged exercise, ↑ muscle triacylglycerols | Fasting hypoglycemia, no ketone bodies, dicarboxylic acidemia, C8–C10 acyl carnitines in blood, vomiting, coma, death; Tx: give IV glucose, avoid fasting, maintain high carb/low fat diet, including short chain FAs, which can be metabolized |

*(Continued)*

# LIPID SYNTHESIS AND METABOLISM (CONT'D.)

## Triacylglycerol (Triglyceride) Synthesis

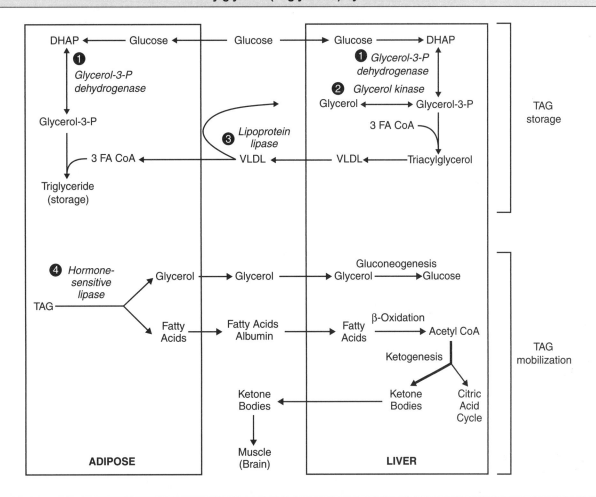

| Notes | |
|---|---|
| ❶ Glycerol-3P-dehydrogenase (adipose, liver) <br> ❷ Glycerol kinase (liver only) | Triacylglycerol synthesis from fatty acids |
| ❸ Lipoprotein lipase | Located on luminal membrane of endothelial cells in adipose tissue |

| Regulation | | | |
|---|---|---|---|
| ❸ Lipoprotein Lipase | | ❹ Hormone sensitive lipase | |
| Digests TGL in VLDL and chylomicrons. Fatty acids enter adipose | | Mobilizes fatty acids from triacylglycerols | |
| Induced by insulin ⊕ ApoC-II | Repressed by ↓ insulin | ⊕ Epinephrine Induced by cortisol | ⊖ insulin |

*Definition of abbreviations:* CAT, carnitine acyltransferase (a.k.a. CPT, carnitine palmitoyl transferase); L/MCAD, long/medium chain acyl-dehydrogenase; TAG, triacylglycerols.

Diabetic ketoacidosis results from overactive hormone-sensitive lipase often in the context of stress, trauma, or infection.

# KETONE BODY METABOLISM

During fasting, the liver converts excess acetyl-CoA from beta-oxidation of fatty acids into ketone bodies, **acetoacetate**, and **β-hydroxybutyrate**, which can be used by muscle and brain tissues. Ketosis represents a normal and advantageous response to fasting/starvation, whereas ketoacidosis is a pathologic condition associated with diabetes and other diseases.

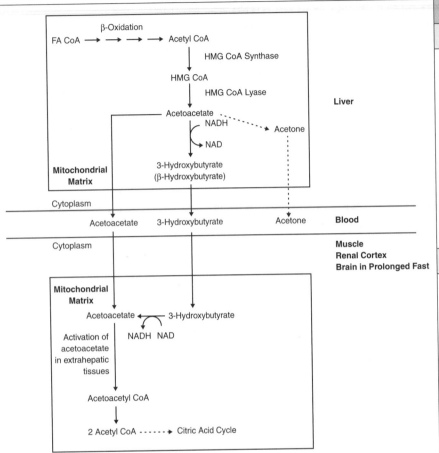

## Disease Association

### Diabetic Ketoacidosis

Excess ketone bodies in blood associated with type 1 diabetes mellitus not adequately managed with insulin, or precipitated by infection or trauma. Characterized by polyuria, dehydration, CNS depression and coma, sweet fruity breath (acetone).

With the prevalence of obesity and stressful environments, ketoacidosis is now becoming more prevalent in type 2 diabetics, e.g., a diabetic in ketoacidosis cannot be assumed to be type 1.

### Alcoholic Ketoacidosis

Excess ketone bodies due to high NADH/NAD ratio in liver; symptoms same as above

*Note:* In either type of ketoacidosis, 3-hydroxybutyrate (β-hydroxybutyrate) is the predominant ketone body formed (not detected by the urine test). Measure 3-hydroxybutyrate to more accurately evaluate ketoacidosis.

# CHOLESTEROL SYNTHESIS

**Cholesterol** is obtained from diet (about 20%) or synthesized de novo (about 80%). Synthesis occurs primarily in the liver for storage and bile acid synthesis, but also in adrenal cortex, ovaries, and testes for steroid hormone synthesis. Cholesterol may also be esterified into **cholesterol esters** by acyl-cholesterol acyl-transferase (**ACAT**) in cells for storage.

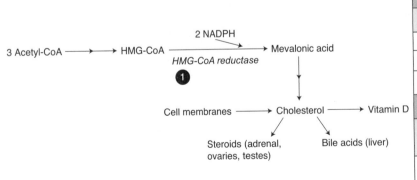

## Regulation

### ❶ HMG-CoA reductase

#### Rate-limiting step

| ⊕ insulin | ⊖ glucagon |
|---|---|
| ⊕ thyroxine | ⊖ cholesterol |

### Pharmacology

#### HMG-CoA Inhibitors ("Statins"), e.g., lovastatin/pravastatin

↓ LDL; used for hypercholesterolemia; side effects: myopathy, liver dysfunction

# LIPOPROTEIN TRANSPORT AND METABOLISM

Free fatty acids are transported by serum albumin, whereas neutral lipids (triacylglycerols and cholesterol esters) are transported by **lipoproteins**. Lipoproteins consist of a hydrophilic shell and a hydrophobic core and are classified by their density into **chylomicrons**, **VLDL**, **LDL**, and **HDL**.

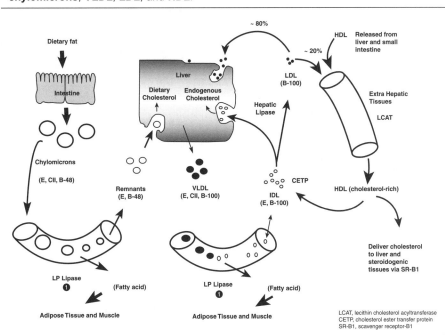

LCAT, lecithin cholesterol acyltransferase
CETP, cholesterol ester transfer protein
SR-B1, scavenger receptor-B1

## Regulation

### ❶ Lipoprotein lipase

Hydrolyzes fatty acids from triacylglycerols from chylomicrons and VLDL

Induced by insulin
⊕ ApoC-II

## Hyperlipidemias

### Type I Hypertriglyceridemia

Lipoprotein lipase deficiency; ↑ triacylglycerols and chylomicrons; orange-red eruptive xanthomas, fatty liver, acute pancreatitis, abdominal pain after fatty meal; autosomal recessive

### Type II Hypercholesterolemia

LDL receptor deficiency; ↑ risk of atherosclerosis and CAD, xanthomas of Achilles tendon, tuberous xanthomas on elbows, xanthelasma (lipid in eyelid), corneal arcus, homozygotes die <20 years; autosomal dominant

## Pharmacology

### Cholestyramine/Colestipol

↑ Elimination of bile salts leads to ↑ LDL receptor expression, leading to ↓ LDL; for hypercholesterolemia; side effect: GI discomfort

### Gemfibrozil/Clofibrate ("Fibrates")

↑ elimination of VLDL leads to ↓ triacylglycerols and ↑ HDL; for hypertriglyceridemia; side effect: muscle toxicity ; acts via PPAR-α to induce LP lipase gene

### Nicotinic Acid

↓ VLDL synthesis leads to ↓ LDL; for hypercholesterolemia and hypertriglyceridemia; side effects: GI irritation; hyperuricemia, hyperglycemia, flushing, pruritus

## CLASSES OF LIPOPROTEINS AND IMPORTANT APOPROTEINS

| Lipoprotein | Functions | Apoproteins | Functions |
|---|---|---|---|
| Chylomicrons | Transport dietary triglyceride and cholesterol from intestine to tissues | apoB-48<br>apoC-II<br>apoE | Secreted by epithelial cells<br>Activates lipoprotein lipase<br>Uptake by liver |
| VLDL | Transports triglyceride from liver to tissues | apoB-100<br>apoC-II<br>apoE | Secreted by liver<br>Activates lipoprotein lipase<br>Uptake of remnants by liver |
| LDL | Delivers cholesterol into cells | apoB-100 | Uptake by liver and other tissues via LDL receptor (apoB-100 receptor) |
| IDL (VLDL remnants) | Picks up cholesterol from HDL to become LDL<br>Picked up by liver | apoE | Uptake by liver |
| HDL | Picks up cholesterol accumulating in blood vessels<br>Delivers cholesterol to liver and steroidogenic tissues via scavenger receptor (SR-B1)<br>Shuttles apoC-II and apoE in blood | apoA-1 | Activates LCAT to produce cholesterol esters |

*Definition of abbreviations:* CAD, coronary artery disease; CETP, cholesterol ester transfer protein; HDL, high-density lipoprotein; LCAT, lecithin-cholesterol acyl transferase; LDL, low-density lipoprotein; PPAR, peroxisome proliferator-activated receptor; SR-B1, scavenger receptor B1; VLDL, very-low-density lipoprotein.

# LIPID DERIVATIVES

Important lipid derivatives include **phospholipids**, **sphingolipids**, and **eicosanoids** (prostaglandins, thromboxanes, and leukotrienes).

## Synthesis of Sphingolipids

## Eicosanoid Metabolism

## Lysosomal Storage Diseases

| Disease | Deficiency and Accumulated Substrate | Features | |
|---|---|---|---|
| Tay-Sachs disease | ↓ Hexosaminidase A <br> ↑ GM$_2$ ganglioside <br> (*whorled membranes in lysosomes*) | • Psychomotor retardation <br> • Cherry red spots in macula <br> • Onset in 1st 6 mos.; death <2 years | AR* |
| Niemann-Pick disease | ↓ Sphingomyelinase <br> ↑ Sphingomyelin <br> (*zebra bodies in lysosomes*) | • Hepatosplenomegaly <br> • Microcephaly <br> • Mental retardation <br> • Foamy macrophages <br> • Neonatal onset | AR |
| Gaucher disease | ↓ β-glucocerebrosidase <br> ↑ Glucocerebroside | • Three clinical subtypes; type 1 is most common <br> • Hepatosplenomegaly <br> • Bone involvement, including fractures and bone pain <br> • Neurologic defects (rare, types 2 and 3) <br> • Mental retardation <br> • Gaucher cells (enlarged macrophages with fibrillary cytoplasm) | AR* |
| Fabry disease | ↓ α-galactosidase A <br> ↑ Ceramide trihexoside | • Renal failure <br> • Telangiectasias <br> • Angiokeratomas <br> • Peripheral neuropathy with pain in extremities | XR |
| Metachromatic leukodystrophy | ↓ arylsulfatase A <br> ↑ sulfatide | • Ataxia <br> • Dementia <br> • Seizures | AR |
| Hurler syndrome (MPSI) | ↓ α-L-iduronidase <br> ↑ dermatan sulfate <br> ↑ heparan sulfate | • Coarse facial features <br> • Corneal clouding <br> • Hepatosplenomegaly <br> • Skeletal deformities <br> • Upper airway obstruction <br> • Recurrent ear infections <br> • Hearing loss <br> • Hydrocephalus <br> • Mental retardation <br> • Death <10 years | AR |
| Hunter syndrome (MPSII) | ↓ L-iduronate-2-sulfatase <br> ↑ dermatan sulfate <br> ↑ heparan sulfate | • Both mild and severe forms <br> • Severe similar to Hurler but retinal degeneration instead of corneal clouding, aggressive behavior, and death <15 years <br> • Mild form compatible with long life | XR |

*Definition of abbreviations:* AR, autosomal recessive; COX, cyclooxygenase; NSAIDs, nonsteroidal anti-inflammatory drugs; XR, X-linked recessive.

*Common in Ashkenazi Jews

# ENZYME KINETICS

Whereas the thermodynamic equilibrium of a chemical reaction is determined by its **free energy** ($\Delta G$), the rate at which the reaction reaches equilibrium is determined by its **activation energy** ($\Delta G^{\ddagger}$). Enzymes increase the rate of a reaction by reducing the energy of activation without affecting the equilibrium constant.

| Michaelis-Menten Equation | Lineweaver-Burk Equation | Classes of Inhibitors |
|---|---|---|
| $$V = \frac{V_{max}[S]}{K_m + [S]}$$ | $$\frac{1}{V} = \frac{K_m}{V_{max}}\frac{1}{[S]} + \frac{1}{V_{max}}$$ | **Competitive, Reversible** |

In the right column:

**Competitive, Reversible**

*(often substrate analogs that compete for the enzyme's binding site)*

$V_{max}$: no effect
$K_m$: ↑

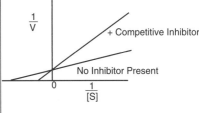

**Noncompetitive, Reversible**

*(bind outside active site but affects enzyme activity, possibly allosterically)*

$V_{max}$: ↓
$K_m$: no effect

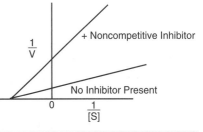

**Irreversible (Inactivator)**

*(binds and inactivates enzyme permanently)*

$V_{max}$: ↓
$K_m$: no effect

V = initial rate or velocity of reaction
[S] = substrate concentration
$V_{max}$ = maximum rate of enzyme
$K_m$ = substrate concentration at $V_{max}/2$

Lineweaver-Burk: Reciprocal form of the Michaelis-Menten equation to achieve a straight line plot

In a typical enzyme-catalyzed reaction, the enzyme (E) is thought to bind reversibly to a substrate (S), forming a complex (ES), from which the product (P) dissociates as the reaction proceeds.

$$E + S \leftrightarrow E - S \rightarrow E + P,$$

where E is the enzyme, S is the substrate and P is the reaction product

The rate of a reaction as determined by both the concentration of enzyme (E) and substrate (S) is described by the **Michaelis-Menten equation**.

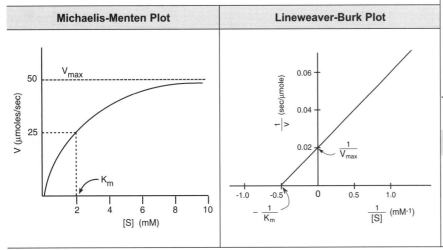

GENERAL PRINCIPLES

BIOCHEMISTRY

**KAPLAN) MEDICAL** 21

## WATER-SOLUBLE VITAMINS

| Vitamin or Coenzyme | Enzyme | Pathway | Deficiency |
|---|---|---|---|
| Biotin | Pyruvate carboxylase<br>Acetyl-CoA carboxylase<br><br>Propionyl-CoA carboxylase | Gluconeogenesis<br>Fatty acid synthesis<br><br>Odd-carbon fatty acids, Val, Met, Ile, Thr | Causes (rare): excessive consumption of raw eggs (contain avidin, a biotin-binding protein)<br><br>Alopecia (hair loss), bowel inflammation, muscle pain |
| Thiamine (B$_1$) | Pyruvate dehydrogenase<br><br>α-Ketoglutarate dehydrogenase<br><br>Transketolase | PDH<br><br>TCA cycle<br><br>HMP shunt | Causes: alcoholism (alcohol interferes with absorption)<br>Wernicke (ataxia, nystagmus, ophthalmoplegia)<br>Korsakoff (confabulation, psychosis)<br>High-output cardiac failure (wet beri-beri) |
| Niacin (B$_3$)<br><br>NAD(H)<br>NADP(H) | Dehydrogenases | Many | Pellagra may also be related to deficiency of tryptophan (corn major dietary staple), which supplies a portion of the niacin requirement<br>Pellagra: diarrhea, dementia, dermatitis, and, if not treated, death |
| Folic acid<br>THF | Thymidylate synthase<br><br>Purine synthesis enzymes | Thymidine (pyrimidine) synthesis<br>Purine synthesis | Causes: alcoholics and pregnancy (body stores depleted in 3 months)<br>Homocystinemia with risk of deep vein thrombosis and atherosclerosis<br>Megaloblastic (macrocytic) anemia<br>Deficiency in early pregnancy causes neural tube defects in fetus |
| Cyanocobalamin (B$_{12}$) | Homocysteine methyltransferase<br>Methylmalonyl-CoA mutase | Methionine, SAM<br>Odd-carbon fatty acids, Val, Met, Ile, Thr | Causes: pernicious anemia. Also in aging, especially with poor nutrition, bacterial overgrowth of terminal ileum, resection of the terminal ileum secondary to Crohn disease, chronic pancreatitis, and, rarely, vegans, or infection with *Diphyllobothrium latum*<br>Megaloblastic (macrocytic) anemia<br>Progressive peripheral neuropathy |
| Pyridoxine (B$_6$)<br>PLP | Aminotransferases (transaminase): AST (SGOT), ALT (SGPT)<br><br>δ-Aminolevulinate synthase | Protein catabolism<br><br>Heme synthesis | Causes: isoniazid therapy<br><br><br>Sideroblastic anemia<br>Cheilosis or stomatitis (cracking or scaling of lip borders and corners of the mouth)<br>Convulsions |
| Riboflavin (B$_2$)<br>FAD(H$_2$) | Dehydrogenases | Many | Corneal neovascularization<br>Cheilosis or stomatitis (cracking or scaling of lip borders and corners of the mouth)<br>Magenta-colored tongue |
| Ascorbate (C) | Prolyl and lysyl hydroxylases<br>Dopamine β-hydroxylase | Collagen synthesis<br>Catecholamine synthesis<br>Absorption of iron in GI tract | Causes: diet deficient in citrus fruits and green vegetables<br>Scurvy: poor wound healing, easy bruising (perifollicular hemorrhage), bleeding gums, increased bleeding time, painful glossitis, anemia |
| Pantothenic acid<br>CoA | Fatty acid synthase<br>Fatty acyl CoA synthetase<br>Pyruvate dehydrogenase<br>α-Ketoglutarate dehydrogenase | Fatty acid metabolism<br><br>PDH<br>TCA cycle | Rare |

*Definition of abbreviations:* ALT, alanine aminotransferase; AST, aspartate aminotransferase; CoA, coenzyme A; FAD(H$_2$), flavin adenine dinucleotide; HMP, hexose monophosphate shunt; NAD(H); nicotinamide adenine dinucleotide; NADP(H), nicotinamide adenine dinucleotide phosphate; PDH, pyruvate dehydrogenase; PLP, pyridoxal phosphate, SAM, S-adenosylmethionine; TCA, tricarboxylic acid cycle; THF, tetrahydrofolate.

| LIPID-SOLUBLE VITAMINS | | |
|---|---|---|
| **Vitamin** | **Important Functions** | **Deficiency** |
| D (cholecalciferol) | In response to hypocalcemia, helps normalize serum calcium levels | Rickets (in childhood): skeletal abnormalities (especially legs), muscle weakness<br>After epiphysial fusion: osteomalacia |
| A (carotene) | Retinoic acid and retinol act as growth regulators, especially in epithelium<br>Retinal is important in rod and cone cells for vision | Night blindness, metaplasia of corneal epithelium, dry eyes, bronchitis, pneumonia, follicular hyperkeratosis |
| K | Carboxylation of glutamic acid residues in many $Ca^{2+}$-binding proteins, importantly coagulation factors II, VII, IX, and X, as well as proteins C and S | Easy bruising, bleeding<br>Increased prothrombin time<br>Associated with fat malabsorption, long-term antibiotic therapy, breast-fed newborns, infants of mothers who took anticonvulsants during pregnancy |
| E ($\alpha$-tocopherol) | Antioxidant in the lipid phase; protects membrane lipids from peroxidation and helps prevent oxidation of LDL particles thought to be involved in atherosclerotic plaque formation | Hemolysis, neurologic problems, retinitis pigmentosa |

# Molecular Biology, Genetics, and Cell Biology

# NUCLEIC ACID STRUCTURE

**Nucleic acids**, including **DNA** and **RNA**, are assembled from **nucleotides**, which contain a five-carbon sugar, a nitrogenous base, and phosphate. The sugar may be **ribose** (RNA) or **deoxyribose** (DNA). The base can be a **purine** (adenine or guanine) or **pyrimidine** (cytosine, uracil, thymidine). Phosphate groups link the 3′ carbon of one sugar to the 5′ carbon of the next, forming phosphodiester bonds. Base sequences are conventionally written in a **5′ → 3′** direction. Nucleotides lacking phosphate groups are called **nucleosides**. In prokaryotes and eukaryotes, RNA is generally single-stranded, while DNA is generally double-stranded in an **antiparallel** orientation, with two hydrogen bonds between base pairs **A and T** and three between **G and C**. Nuclear DNA forms a **double-helix**, which undergoes **supercoiling** via **topoisomerase** activity, and is generally associated with **histones** and other proteins to form **nucleosomes**, the basic packaging unit of **chromatin**.

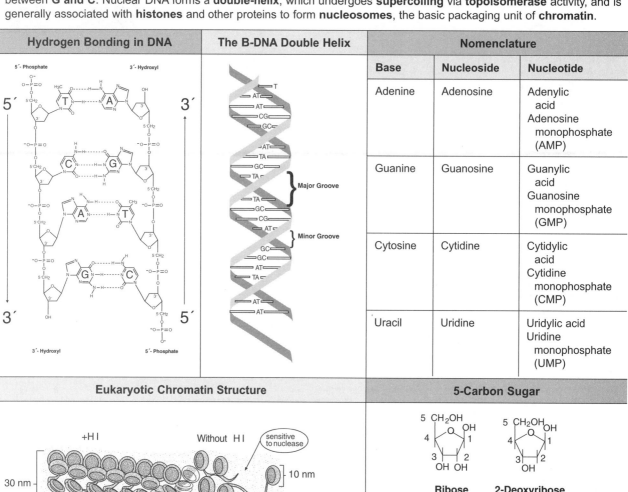

| Hydrogen Bonding in DNA | The B-DNA Double Helix | Nomenclature | | |
|---|---|---|---|---|

### Nomenclature

| Base | Nucleoside | Nucleotide |
|---|---|---|
| Adenine | Adenosine | Adenylic acid<br>Adenosine monophosphate (AMP) |
| Guanine | Guanosine | Guanylic acid<br>Guanosine monophosphate (GMP) |
| Cytosine | Cytidine | Cytidylic acid<br>Cytidine monophosphate (CMP) |
| Uracil | Uridine | Uridylic acid<br>Uridine monophosphate (UMP) |

## Eukaryotic Chromatin Structure

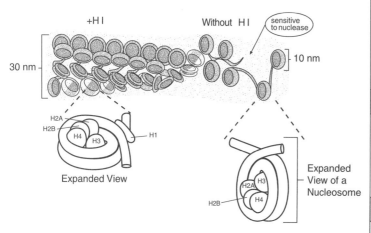

## 5-Carbon Sugar

Ribose    2-Deoxyribose

## Nitrogenous Bases

| Purines | | Pyrimidines | | |
|---|---|---|---|---|
| Adenine | Guanine | Cytosine | Uracil | Thymine |

## Chromatin

| Euchromatin | Heterochromatin |
|---|---|
| Loosely packed | Tightly packed |
| Transcriptionally active | Transcriptionally inactive |

# NUCLEIC ACID SYNTHESIS AND SALVAGE

**Nucleotides** for DNA and RNA synthesis can be generated by de novo synthesis or salvage pathways, both of which require **PRPP** generated from ribose-5-phosphate derived from the HMP shunt. **De novo synthesis** occurs mainly in the liver and generates new purine and pyrimidine bases from precursors. In contrast, **salvage pathways** reuse preformed bases derived from nucleotides during normal RNA turnover or released from dying cells or transported from the liver. Ribonucleotides are converted to deoxyribonucleotides for DNA synthesis by **ribonucleotide reductase**. Antineoplastic drugs that target ribonucleotidase (hydroxyurea), or an enzyme in the dTMP branch of pyrimidine synthesis (5-FU), or reduction of folate (methotrexate) preferentially inhibit DNA synthesis without compromising RNA synthesis and gene expression. Excretion of purine bases occurs in the form of **uric acid** from the kidneys.

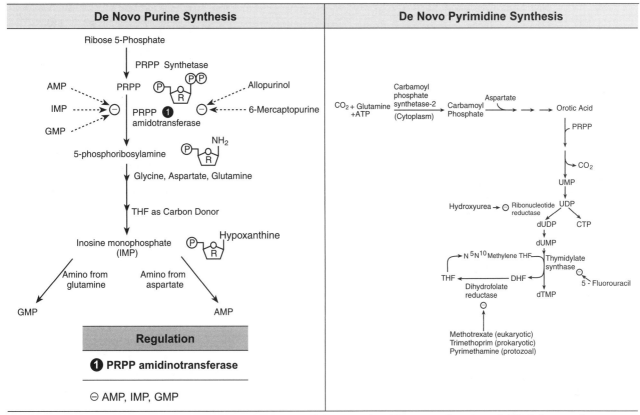

| De Novo Purine Synthesis | De Novo Pyrimidine Synthesis |
|---|---|

**Regulation**

❶ PRPP amidinotransferase

⊖ AMP, IMP, GMP

*Definition of abbreviations:* AMP, adenosine monophosphate; dTMP, deoxythymidine monophosphate; 5-FU, 5-flurouracil; IMP, inosine monophosphate; dUDP, deoxyuridine diphosphate; CTP, cytosine triphosphate; THF, tetrahydrofolate.

## Disease Association

### Adenosine Deaminase Deficiency

- SCID (no B- or T-cell function)
- Multiple infections in children
- Autosomal recessive
- Tx: enzyme replacement, bone marrow transplant

### Gout

↑ production or ↓ excretion of uric acid by kidneys

### Lesch-Nyhan Syndrome

- HGPRT deficiency
- Mental retardation (mild)
- Spastic cerebral palsy
- Self-mutilation
- Hyperuricemia
- X-linked recessive

*(Continued)*

| Purine Salvage Pathway and Excretion | Pharmacology |
|---|---|

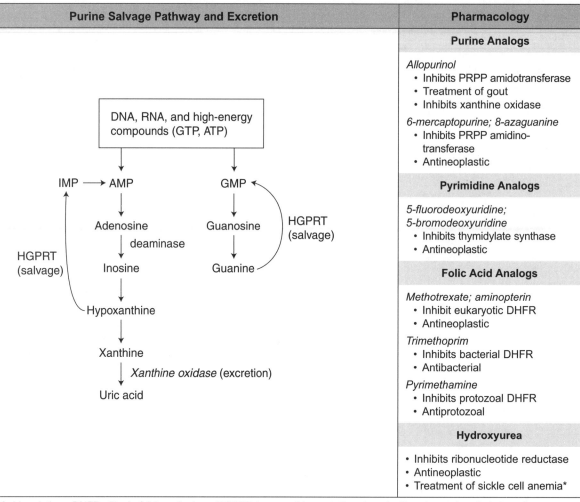

### Purine Analogs

*Allopurinol*
- Inhibits PRPP amidotransferase
- Treatment of gout
- Inhibits xanthine oxidase

*6-mercaptopurine; 8-azaguanine*
- Inhibits PRPP amidino-transferase
- Antineoplastic

### Pyrimidine Analogs

*5-fluorodeoxyuridine; 5-bromodeoxyuridine*
- Inhibits thymidylate synthase
- Antineoplastic

### Folic Acid Analogs

*Methotrexate; aminopterin*
- Inhibit eukaryotic DHFR
- Antineoplastic

*Trimethoprim*
- Inhibits bacterial DHFR
- Antibacterial

*Pyrimethamine*
- Inhibits protozoal DHFR
- Antiprotozoal

### Hydroxyurea

- Inhibits ribonucleotide reductase
- Antineoplastic
- Treatment of sickle cell anemia*

*Definition of abbreviations:* DHFR, dihydrofolate reductase; HGPRT, hypoxanthine-guanine phosphoribosyl pyrophosphate transferase; NSAID, nonsteroidal anti-inflammatory drug; PRPP, phosphoribosylpyrophosphate; THF, tetrahydrofolate; SCID, severe combined immunodeficiency disorder.

*via a different mechanism

# DNA Replication

DNA replication involves the synthesis of new DNA molecules in a 5′ → 3′ direction by **DNA polymerase** using the double-stranded DNA template. One strand (**leading strand**) is made continuously, while the other (**lagging strand**) is synthesized in segments. **Prokaryotic** chromosomes are closed, double-stranded circular DNA molecules with a single origin of replication that separates into two replication forks moving away in opposite directions. **Eukaryotic** chromosomes are double-stranded and linear with multiple origins of replication.

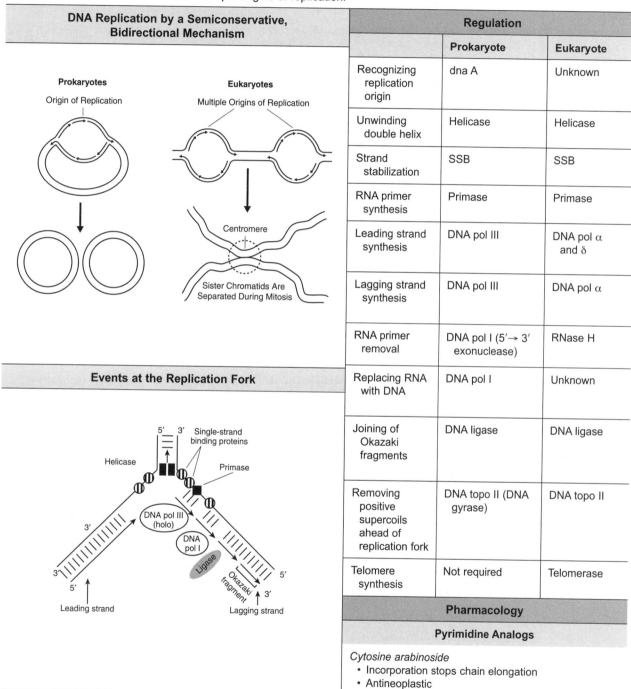

### DNA Replication by a Semiconservative, Bidirectional Mechanism

**Prokaryotes**

Origin of Replication

**Eukaryotes**

Multiple Origins of Replication

Centromere

Sister Chromatids Are Separated During Mitosis

### Events at the Replication Fork

5′  3′  Single-strand binding proteins

Helicase

Primase

DNA pol III (holo)

DNA pol I

Ligase

Okazaki fragment

3′

5′

Leading strand

3′

5′

Lagging strand

### Regulation

| | Prokaryote | Eukaryote |
|---|---|---|
| Recognizing replication origin | dna A | Unknown |
| Unwinding double helix | Helicase | Helicase |
| Strand stabilization | SSB | SSB |
| RNA primer synthesis | Primase | Primase |
| Leading strand synthesis | DNA pol III | DNA pol $\alpha$ and $\delta$ |
| Lagging strand synthesis | DNA pol III | DNA pol $\alpha$ |
| RNA primer removal | DNA pol I (5′→ 3′ exonuclease) | RNase H |
| Replacing RNA with DNA | DNA pol I | Unknown |
| Joining of Okazaki fragments | DNA ligase | DNA ligase |
| Removing positive supercoils ahead of replication fork | DNA topo II (DNA gyrase) | DNA topo II |
| Telomere synthesis | Not required | Telomerase |

### Pharmacology

#### Pyrimidine Analogs

*Cytosine arabinoside*
- Incorporation stops chain elongation
- Antineoplastic

*Definition of abbreviations:* DNA, deoxyribonucleic acid; DNA pol, DNA polymerase; DNA topo, DNA topoisomerase; RNA, ribonucleic acid; SSB, single-stranded DNA-binding protein.

# DNA REPAIR

**DNA** sequence and structure may be altered either during replication or by exposure to chemicals or radiation. Mutations include point mutations such as the **substitution** of one base with another. Substitution mutations in the third position of a codon **(wobble position)** are usually benign because several codons code for the same amino acid. Other types of mutations include (1) deletion or addition of one or two nucleotides (frameshift mutations), (2) large segment deletions (e.g., unequal crossover during meiosis), (3) mutations of 5′ or 3′ splice sites, or (4) triplet repeat expansion, which can lead to a longer, more unstable protein product (e.g., Huntington disease).

| Damage | Cause | Recognition/ Excision Enzyme | Repair Enzymes |
|---|---|---|---|
| Thymine dimers ($G_1$) | UV radiation | Excision endonuclease (deficient in xeroderma pigmentosum) | DNA polymerase DNA ligase |
| Cytosine deamination ($G_1$) | Spontaneous/ chemicals | Uracil glycosylase AP endonuclease | DNA polymerase DNA ligase |
| Apurination or apyrimidination ($G_1$) | Spontaneous/ heat | AP endonuclease | DNA polymerase DNA ligase |
| Mismatched base ($G_2$) | DNA replication errors | A mutation on one of two genes, *hMSH2* or *hMLH1*, initiates defective repair of DNA mismatches, resulting in a condition known as hereditary nonpolyposis colorectal cancer—HNPCC. | DNA polymerase DNA ligase |

## Types of Mutations

**Transition:**   A:T → G:C  or  G:C → A:T
**Transversion:** A:T → T:A  or  G:C → C:G

| Silent | No change in AA | Sub |
|---|---|---|
| **Missense** | Change AA to another | Sub |
| **Nonsense** | Early stop codon | Sub or Ins/Del |
| **Frameshift** | Misreading of all codons downstream | Ins/Del |

### DNA Repair Defects

#### Xeroderma Pigmentosum

*(defect in nucleotide excision-repair)*
- Extreme UV sensitivity
- Excessive freckling
- Multiple skin cancers
- Corneal ulcerations
- Autosomal recessive

#### Ataxia Telangiectasia

*(defect in ATM gene product, a member of PI-3 kinase family involved in mitogenic signal transduction, detection of DNA damage, and cell cycle control)*
- Sensitivity to ionizing radiation
- Degenerative ataxia
- Dilated blood vessels
- Chromosomal aberrations
- Lymphomas
- Autosomal recessive

#### HNPCC

*(defect in mismatch repair; usually hMSH2 or hMLH1 gene)*
- Colorectal cancer
- ⅔ occur in right colon
- Autosomal dominant
- Part of Lynch syndrome (a multi-cancer syndrome)

## Thymine Dimer Repair

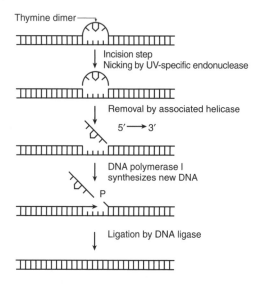

Thymine dimer

Incision step
Nicking by UV-specific endonuclease

Removal by associated helicase
5′ ⟶ 3′

DNA polymerase I synthesizes new DNA
P

Ligation by DNA ligase

*Definition of abbreviations:* AA, amino acid; HNPCC, hereditary nonpolyposis colorectal cancer; Ins/Del, insert or deletion; Sub, substitution

# Transcription and RNA Processing

Transcription involves the synthesis of an RNA in a 5′ → 3′ direction by an RNA polymerase using DNA as a template. An important class of RNA is messenger RNA (mRNA). Initiation of transcription occurs from a promoter region, which is the binding site of RNA polymerase, and stops at a termination signal. In **prokaryotes**, a single mRNA transcript can encode several genes (**polycistronic**), and no RNA processing is required, allowing transcription and translation to proceed simultaneously. In **eukaryotes**, all mRNAs are **monocistronic**, but often include coding segments (**exons**) interrupted by noncoding regions (**introns**). Eukaryotic mRNAs must therefore undergo extensive processing, including a 5′ cap, a 3′ tail, and removal of introns followed by exon splicing. Ribosomal RNA (rRNA) and transfer RNA (tRNA) are also produced by transcription.

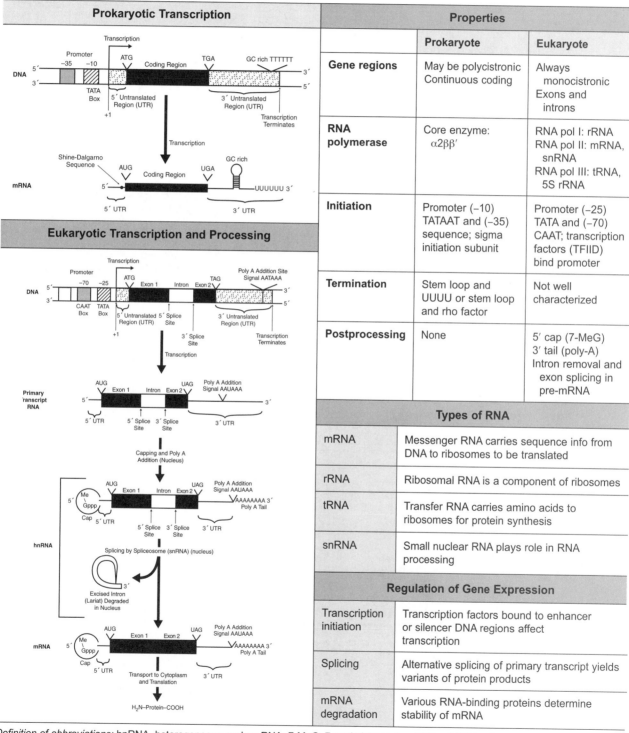

## Properties

| | Prokaryote | Eukaryote |
|---|---|---|
| **Gene regions** | May be polycistronic Continuous coding | Always monocistronic Exons and introns |
| **RNA polymerase** | Core enzyme: α2ββ′ | RNA pol I: rRNA RNA pol II: mRNA, snRNA RNA pol III: tRNA, 5S rRNA |
| **Initiation** | Promoter (−10) TATAAT and (−35) sequence; sigma initiation subunit | Promoter (−25) TATA and (−70) CAAT; transcription factors (TFIID) bind promoter |
| **Termination** | Stem loop and UUUU or stem loop and rho factor | Not well characterized |
| **Postprocessing** | None | 5′ cap (7-MeG) 3′ tail (poly-A) Intron removal and exon splicing in pre-mRNA |

## Types of RNA

| | |
|---|---|
| mRNA | Messenger RNA carries sequence info from DNA to ribosomes to be translated |
| rRNA | Ribosomal RNA is a component of ribosomes |
| tRNA | Transfer RNA carries amino acids to ribosomes for protein synthesis |
| snRNA | Small nuclear RNA plays role in RNA processing |

## Regulation of Gene Expression

| | |
|---|---|
| Transcription initiation | Transcription factors bound to enhancer or silencer DNA regions affect transcription |
| Splicing | Alternative splicing of primary transcript yields variants of protein products |
| mRNA degradation | Various RNA-binding proteins determine stability of mRNA |

*Definition of abbreviations:* hnRNA, heterogeneous nuclear RNA; 7-MeG, 7-methylguanosine; RNA pol, RNA polymerase; UTR, untranslated region.

# PROTEIN TRANSLATION

**Translation** involves the synthesis of protein from mRNA templates in **ribosomes** (complexes of proteins and ribosomal RNAs [**rRNA**]). Protein synthesis begins from an initiation codon (**AUG** = methionine) and ends at a stop codon (**UAA**, **UGA**, or **UAG**). Elongation involves transfer RNAs (**tRNA**), which have an anticodon region at one end to recognize the codon on the mRNA and an amino acid attached at the other end for covalent linkage to the growing polypeptide chain. Several ribosomes can simultaneously transcribe an mRNA, forming a polyribosome, or **polysome**.

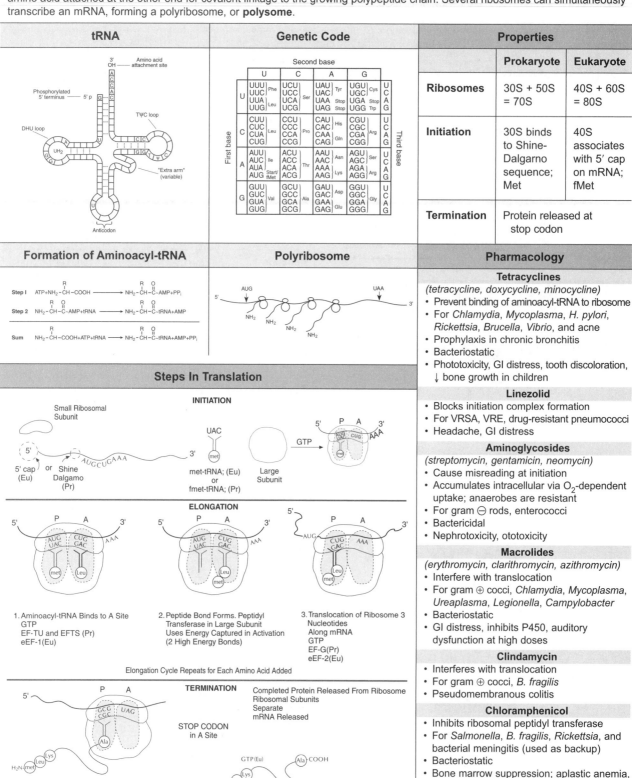

## tRNA

## Genetic Code

## Properties

| | Prokaryote | Eukaryote |
|---|---|---|
| **Ribosomes** | 30S + 50S = 70S | 40S + 60S = 80S |
| **Initiation** | 30S binds to Shine-Dalgarno sequence; Met | 40S associates with 5′ cap on mRNA; fMet |
| **Termination** | Protein released at stop codon | |

## Formation of Aminoacyl-tRNA

## Polyribosome

## Pharmacology

### Tetracyclines
*(tetracycline, doxycycline, minocycline)*
- Prevent binding of aminoacyl-tRNA to ribosome
- For *Chlamydia, Mycoplasma, H. pylori, Rickettsia, Brucella, Vibrio,* and acne
- Prophylaxis in chronic bronchitis
- Bacteriostatic
- Phototoxicity, GI distress, tooth discoloration, ↓ bone growth in children

### Linezolid
- Blocks initiation complex formation
- For VRSA, VRE, drug-resistant pneumococci
- Headache, GI distress

### Aminoglycosides
*(streptomycin, gentamicin, neomycin)*
- Cause misreading at initiation
- Accumulates intracellular via $O_2$-dependent uptake; anaerobes are resistant
- For gram ⊖ rods, enterococci
- Bactericidal
- Nephrotoxicity, ototoxicity

### Macrolides
*(erythromycin, clarithromycin, azithromycin)*
- Interfere with translocation
- For gram ⊕ cocci, *Chlamydia, Mycoplasma, Ureaplasma, Legionella, Campylobacter*
- Bacteriostatic
- GI distress, inhibits P450, auditory dysfunction at high doses

### Clindamycin
- Interferes with translocation
- For gram ⊕ cocci, *B. fragilis*
- Pseudomembranous colitis

### Chloramphenicol
- Inhibits ribosomal peptidyl transferase
- For *Salmonella, B. fragilis, Rickettsia,* and bacterial meningitis (used as backup)
- Bacteriostatic
- Bone marrow suppression; aplastic anemia, "gray baby" syndrome (neonates), optic neuritis (children)

## Steps In Translation

**INITIATION**

**ELONGATION**

1. Aminoacyl-tRNA Binds to A Site
   GTP
   EF-TU and EFTS (Pr)
   eEF-1(Eu)

2. Peptide Bond Forms. Peptidyl Transferase in Large Subunit Uses Energy Captured in Activation (2 High Energy Bonds)

3. Translocation of Ribosome 3 Nucleotides Along mRNA
   GTP
   EF-G(Pr)
   eEF-2(Eu)

Elongation Cycle Repeats for Each Amino Acid Added

**TERMINATION**

STOP CODON in A Site

Completed Protein Released From Ribosome
Ribosomal Subunits Separate
mRNA Released

*Definition of abbreviations:* AA, amino acid; EF-2, elongation factor 2; fMet, formylmethionine; Met, methionine; VRE, vancomycin-resistant enterococci; VRSA, vancomycin-resistant *Staphylococcus aureus*.

# POST-TRANSLATIONAL MODIFICATIONS

Whereas cytoplasmic proteins are translated on free cytoplasmic ribosomes, secreted proteins, membrane proteins, and lysosomal enzymes have an *N*-terminal hydrophobic signal sequence and are translated on ribosomes associated with the rough endoplasmic reticulum (RER). After translation, proteins acquire more complex structures by being folded with the help of molecular **chaperones**. Misfolded proteins are targeted for destruction by **ubiquitin** and digested in cytoplasmic protein-digesting complexes called **proteasomes**.

| Co- and Postranslational Covalent Modifications | | Protein Structure | |
|---|---|---|---|
| **Glycosylation** | Addition of oligosaccharides | **Primary** | Amino acid sequence |
| **Phosphorylation** | Addition of phosphate groups by protein kinases | **Secondary** | $\alpha$-Helix or $\beta$-sheets |
| **$\gamma$-carboxylation (vitamin K dependent)** | Creation of $Ca^{2+}$ binding sites | **Tertiary** | Higher order 3D structure |
| **Prenylation** | Addition of farnesyl/geranyl lipid groups to peripheral membrane proteins | **Quaternary** | Multiple subunits |
| **Mannose phosphorylation** | Addition of phosphates onto mannose residues to target protein to lysosomes | | |

## Synthesis of Secretory, Membrane, and Lysosomal Proteins

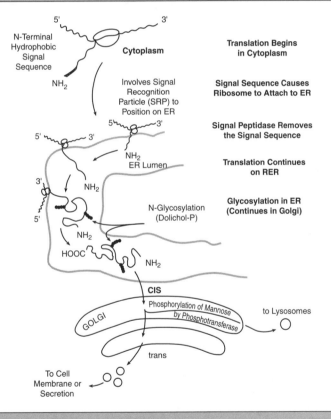

## Disease Association

### I-Cell Disease

*(defect in mannose phosphorylation, causing lysosomal enzyme release into extracellular space)*

- Coarse facial features, gingival hyperplasia, macroglossia
- Craniofacial abnormalities, joint immobility, club-foot, claw-hand, scoliosis
- Psychomotor and growth retardation
- Cardiorespiratory failure
- Death in first decade
- 10–20-fold increase in lysosomal enzyme activity in serum

# COLLAGEN SYNTHESIS

**Collagen** is a structural protein composed of a triple helix of amino acid chains containing a repeating tripeptide Gly-X-Y-Gly-X-Y, where the unique amino acids **hydroxyproline** and **hydroxylysine** are frequently found in the X position. Hydroxylation of proline and lysine requires ascorbate (vitamin C), deficiency of which leads to scurvy.

| Synthesis of Collagen | Disease Association |
|---|---|

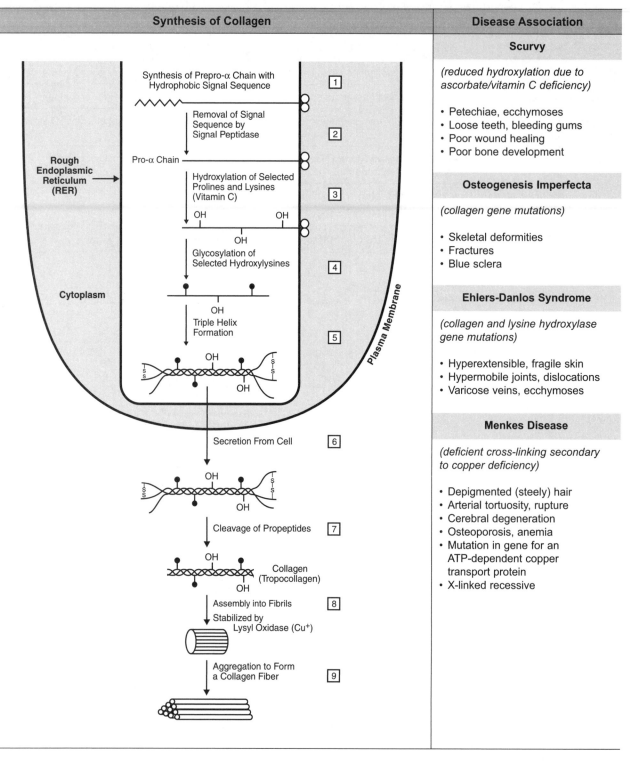

**Synthesis of Collagen**

- Synthesis of Prepro-α Chain with Hydrophobic Signal Sequence  [1]
- Removal of Signal Sequence by Signal Peptidase  [2]
- Pro-α Chain
- Hydroxylation of Selected Prolines and Lysines (Vitamin C)  [3]
- Glycosylation of Selected Hydroxylysines  [4]
- Triple Helix Formation  [5]
- Secretion From Cell  [6]
- Cleavage of Propeptides  [7]
- Collagen (Tropocollagen)
- Assembly into Fibrils  [8]
- Stabilized by Lysyl Oxidase (Cu⁺)
- Aggregation to Form a Collagen Fiber  [9]

Rough Endoplasmic Reticulum (RER)

Cytoplasm

Plasma Membrane

**Disease Association**

## Scurvy

*(reduced hydroxylation due to ascorbate/vitamin C deficiency)*

- Petechiae, ecchymoses
- Loose teeth, bleeding gums
- Poor wound healing
- Poor bone development

## Osteogenesis Imperfecta

*(collagen gene mutations)*

- Skeletal deformities
- Fractures
- Blue sclera

## Ehlers-Danlos Syndrome

*(collagen and lysine hydroxylase gene mutations)*

- Hyperextensible, fragile skin
- Hypermobile joints, dislocations
- Varicose veins, ecchymoses

## Menkes Disease

*(deficient cross-linking secondary to copper deficiency)*

- Depigmented (steely) hair
- Arterial tortuosity, rupture
- Cerebral degeneration
- Osteoporosis, anemia
- Mutation in gene for an ATP-dependent copper transport protein
- X-linked recessive

# RECOMBINANT DNA

**Recombinant DNA** technology allows DNA fragments to be copied, manipulated, and analyzed in vitro. Eukaryotic DNA fragments may be **genomic DNA** containing both introns and exons, or **complementary DNA (cDNA)**, which is reverse-transcribed from mRNA and contains exons only. DNA fragments may be amplified by **polymerase chain reaction (PCR)**, cut with specific **restriction endonucleases**, and ligated into a **DNA vector**. These vectors can then be used for further manipulation or amplification of the DNA to produce genomic DNA or cDNA (expression) libraries, to generate recombinant proteins, or for incorporation into humans (**gene therapy**) or other animals (**transgenic animals**).

| Formation of a Recombinant Plasmid | Polymerase Chain Reaction |
|---|---|

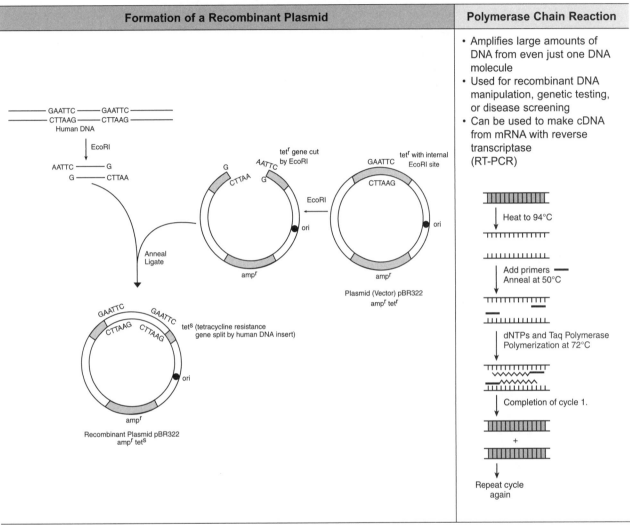

Polymerase Chain Reaction

- Amplifies large amounts of DNA from even just one DNA molecule
- Used for recombinant DNA manipulation, genetic testing, or disease screening
- Can be used to make cDNA from mRNA with reverse transcriptase (RT-PCR)

*(Continued)*

## RECOMBINANT DNA (CONT'D.)

### Screening a DNA Library

① Agar growth plate with bacterial colonies

② Blot

Replica of growth plate on filter

③ Lyse bacteria, denature DNA, and add a $^{32}$P-DNA probe for gene; make autoradiogram

Lyse bacteria, add $^{125}$I-antibody for protein; make autoradiogram

④

Pick positive colony from original plate

Pick positive colony from original plate

### Restriction Endonucleases

- Recognizes palindromes in dsDNA and cuts, leaving sticky or blunt ends
- Used to make restriction maps of DNA or to produce fragments for manipulation

```
           ↓
5'--------GAATTC--------3'
3'--------CTTAAG--------5'
           ↑

          ↓EcoRI

5'-----G          + 5'-AATTC------3'
3'-----CTTAA-5'            G------5'
```

**Sticky Ends**

```
           ↓
5'--------GGCC--------3'
3'--------CCGG--------5'
           ↑

          ↓HaeIII

5'-----GG-3'  +  5'-CC----3'
3'-----CC-5'     3'-GG----5'
```

**Blunt Ends**

### Incorporation of Cloned DNA

Cloned DNA Fragments

Gene Therapy (Somatic)

Cloned gene inserted into DNA of selected somatic cells

Gene not passed to offspring

Vector used to introduce cloned gene into host DNA/nuclei
- retrovirus
- adenovirus
- liposome

Examples
- SCID (severe combined immuno-deficiency); interleukin receptor gene
- Cystic fibrosis; CFTR gene

Transgenic Animals (Germ Line)

Fertilized OVA

Micro-inject cloned DNA

New gene incorporated into germ line DNA

Implant in foster mother

Offspring are transgenic
New gene inserted is a transgene
Design animal model for human disease this way

### DNA Vectors

Circular, self-replicating DNA to carry and amplify DNA fragments in bacteria or yeast

| | |
|---|---|
| ~100–12 kb | **Plasmid** Bacterial; restriction sites, replication origin, selection marker (e.g., antibiotic resistance) |
| ~10–25 kb | **Phage** Packaging virus that infects bacteria; e.g., lambda (λ) |
| Up to 45 kb | **Cosmid** Plasmids with λ cloning sites |
| Up to 10 Mb | **BAC, YAC** Bacterial or yeast artificial chromosomes |

*Definition of abbreviation:* dsDNA, double-stranded DNA.

# GENETIC TESTING

The presence of specific DNA, RNA, and proteins can be identified by first separating these molecules by **gel electrophoresis**, transferring to a membrane by **blotting**, and finally detecting with radioactive nucleic acid probes (for DNA and RNA) or antibodies (for proteins). Direct detection in cells or tissues can also be performed using similar tools to identify mRNA (**in situ hybridization**) or proteins (**immunostaining**). In vitro detection of proteins can also be achieved by enzyme-linked immunosorbent assay (**ELISA**). Using these methods of detection, diversity between individuals or genetic mutations manifested by different restriction endonuclease sites (restriction fragment length polymorphisms [**RFLP**]) or expansion of highly repetitive sequences (e.g., **satellites**, **minisatellites**, and **microsatellites**) may be employed for genetic testing.

|  | DNA | RNA | Protein |  | Repeated Unit | Length of Repeat |
|---|---|---|---|---|---|---|
| **Separation** | Gel electrophoresis | | | **Satellites** | 20–175 bp | 0.1–1 Mb |
| **Blotting (probe)** | Southern ($^{32}$P-DNA) | Northern ($^{32}$P-DNA) | Western ($^{125}$I or antibody) | **Minisatellites** | 20–70 bp | Up to 20 kb |
| **Other detection** | — | In situ hybridization | Immunostaining or ELISA | **Microsatellites** | 2–4 bp | <150 bp |

## Sickle Cell Disease (Southern Blot; RFLP)

*Mst*II restriction digest of patient sample, followed by Southern blotting using a probe against β-globin gene, allows identification of either the normal or sickle allele.

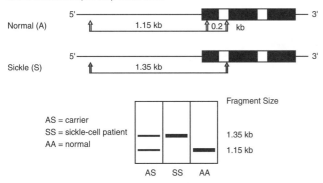

Mst II Restriction Map of the β-Globin Gene

Normal (A): 5'  1.15 kb  0.2 kb  3'

Sickle (S): 5'  1.35 kb  3'

AS = carrier
SS = sickle-cell patient
AA = normal

Fragment Size
1.35 kb
1.15 kb

AS  SS  AA

## Paternity Testing (PCR; STRs or Microsatellites)

PCR amplification of STRs or microsatellite sequences can be used to match the banding pattern to each parent. The child should share one allele with each parent.

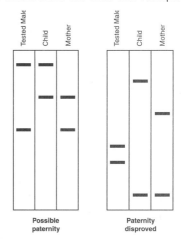

Possible paternity

Paternity disproved

## Cystic Fibrosis (PCR; ASO Dot Blot)

The most common CF mutation, ΔF508, can be detected by comparing PCR product sizes by gel electrophoresis or hybridization with allele-specific oligonucleotide (ASO) probes on a dot blot (a simplified form of Southern blot with no electrophoresis required).

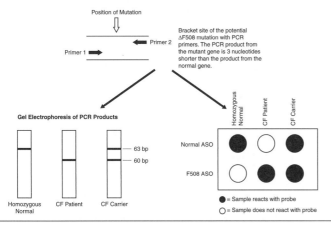

Position of Mutation

Primer 1    Primer 2

Bracket site of the potential ΔF508 mutation with PCR primers. The PCR product from the mutant gene is 3 nucleotides shorter than the product from the normal gene.

Gel Electrophoresis of PCR Products

63 bp
60 bp

Homozygous Normal    CF Patient    CF Carrier

Normal ASO
F508 ASO

Homozygous Normal    CF Patient    CF Carrier

● = Sample reacts with probe
○ = Sample does not react with probe

## HIV Detection (ELISA and Western Blot)

Serum antibodies to HIV are first detected by ELISA and then confirmed by Western blot.

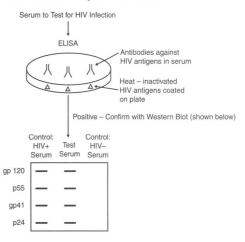

Serum to Test for HIV Infection

ELISA

Antibodies against HIV antigens in serum

Heat – inactivated HIV antigens coated on plate

Positive – Confirm with Western Blot (shown below)

Control: HIV+ Serum    Test Serum    Control: HIV– Serum

gp 120
p55
gp41
p24

*Definition of abbreviation:* STR, short tandem repeats

## Autosomal Dominant

- Affected individuals have an affected parent
- Either sex affected
- Variable to late onset (may be delayed to adulthood)
- Often encode structural proteins

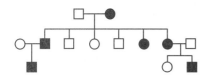

- **Familial hypercholesterolemia**
- **Huntington disease**
- **Neurofibromatosis**
- **Marfan syndrome**
- **von Hippel-Lindau disease**

## Autosomal Recessive

- Affected individuals usually have unaffected (carrier) parents
- Either sex affected
- Early uniform onset (infancy/childhood)
- Often encode catalytic proteins

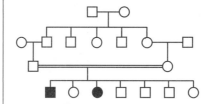

- **Sickle cell anemia**
- **Cystic fibrosis**
- **Phenylketonuria (PKU)**
- **Kartagener syndrome**

## Pedigree Analysis

**Symbols**

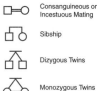

| | | | |
|---|---|---|---|
| □ | Male | ⌀ ⌀ | Dead |
| ○ | Female | □—○ | Mating |
| ◇ | Unknown Sex | □=○ | Consanguineous or Incestuous Mating |
| ● ■ | Affected | | Sibship |
| ◑ ◧ | Carrier of an Autosomal Recessive (Optional) | | Dizygous Twins |
| ⊙ | Carrier of an X-linked Recessive (Optional) | | Monozygous Twins |
| ⌄ | Stillborn or Abortion | | |

## X-Linked Dominant

- Affected individuals have an affected parent
- Either sex affected
- No male-to-male transmission
- Females often have more mild and variable symptoms than males

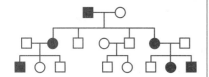

- **Fragile X syndrome**
- **Hypophosphatemic rickets**

## X-Linked Recessive

- Affected individuals usually have unaffected (carrier) parents
- Usually affect males only
- No male-to-male transmission
- Female carriers sometimes show mild symptoms (manifesting heterozygote)

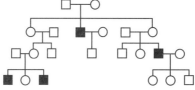

- **Duchenne muscular dystrophy**
- **Lesch-Nyhan syndrome**
- **G6PD deficiency**
- **Hemophilia A and B**

## Mitochondrial Inheritance

- Inherited maternally because only mother contributes mitochondria during conception
- Either sex affected
- Usually neuropathies and myopathies because brain and muscle are highly dependent on oxidative phosphorylation

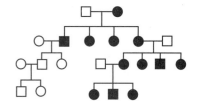

- **Leber hereditary optic neuropathy**
- **MELAS:** **m**itochondrial **e**ncephalomyopathy, **l**actic **a**cidosis, and **s**troke-like episodes
- **Myoclonic epilepsy** with ragged red muscle fiber

## Decision Tree for Determining Mode of Inheritance*

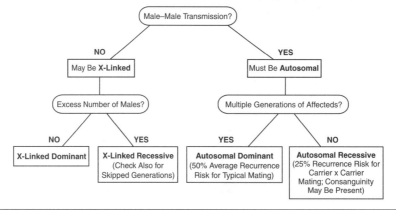

*Definition of abbreviation:* G6PD, glucose-6-phosphate dehydrogenase.

*\*Note:* If transmission occurs only through affected mothers and never through affected sons, the pedigree is likely to reflect mitochondrial inheritance.

## SINGLE-GENE DISORDERS

| Neurofibromatosis (NF) Type 1 (von Recklinghausen Disease) | von Hippel-Lindau Disease | Features |
|---|---|---|
| *(mutation in NF1 tumor-suppressor gene on chromosome 17)*<br><br>• Multiple neurofibromas<br>• Café-au-lait spots (pigmented skin lesions)<br>• Lisch nodules (pigmented iris hamartomas)<br>• Increased risk of meningiomas and pheochromocytoma<br>• 90% of NF cases<br>• Autosomal dominant | *(mutation in tumor-suppressor gene on chromosome 3)*<br><br>• Hemangioblastomas in CNS and retina<br>• Renal cell carcinoma<br>• Cysts in internal organs<br>• Autosomal dominant | **Variable expression—** differences in severity of symptoms for same genotype; allelic heterogeneity can contribute to variable expression<br><br>**Incomplete penetrance—** some individuals with disease genotype do not have disease phenotype |
| **Neurofibromatosis (NF) Type 2 (Bilateral Acoustic Neurofibromatosis)** | **Cystic Fibrosis** | **Delayed age of onset—** individuals do not manifest phenotype until later in life |
| *(mutation in NF2 tumor-suppressor gene on chromosome 22)*<br><br>• Bilateral acoustic neuromas<br>• Neurofibromas and café-au-lait spots<br>• Increased risk of meningiomas and pheochromocytoma<br>• 10% of NF cases<br>• Autosomal dominant | *(mutation in CFTR chloride channel gene on chromosome 7q, leading to thick secretion of mucus plugs)*<br><br>• Recurrent pulmonary infections (*P. aeruginosa* and *S. aureus*)<br>• Pneumonia, bronchitis, bronchiectasis<br>• Pancreatic insufficiency; steatorrhea<br>• Fat-soluble vitamin deficiency<br>• Male infertility<br>• Biliary cirrhosis<br>• Meconium ileus<br>• Most common mutation: $\Delta$F508<br>• Dx: ↑ NaCl in sweat; PCR and ASO probes<br>• Tx: *N*-acetylcysteine, respiratory therapy, enzyme replacement, vitamin supplement<br>• Autosomal recessive | **Pleiotropy—** single disease mutation affects multiple organ systems<br><br>**Locus heterogeneity—** same disease phenotype from mutations in different loci<br><br>**Anticipation—** earlier age of onset and increased disease severity with each generation<br><br>**Imprinting—** symptoms depend on whether mutant gene was inherited from father or mother; due to different DNA methylation patterns of parents (e.g., Prader-Willi versus Angelman syndrome) |
| **Marfan Syndrome** | | |
| *(mutation of fibrillin gene on chromosome 15)*<br><br>• Skeletal abnormalities (tall build with hyperextensible joints)<br>• Subluxation of lens<br>• Cardiovascular defects (cystic medial necrosis, dissecting aortic aneurysm, valvular insufficiency)<br>• Autosomal dominant | | |

*Definition of abbreviations:* ASO, allele-specific oligonucleotides; CFTR, cystic fibrosis transmembrane conductance regulator; CNS, central nervous system; Dx, diagnosis; PCR, polymerase chain reaction; Tx, treatment.

# CHROMOSOMAL ABNORMALITIES

**Aneuploidy** refers to having a chromosome number that is not a multiple of the haploid number. It is the most common type of chromosomal disorder, and its incidence is related to increasing maternal age. Most arise from a **nondisjunction** event, when chromosomes fail to segregate during cell division. Nondisjunction during either phase of meiosis usually leads to spontaneous abortion, but sometimes results in live birth, often with severe physical deformities and mental retardation. Trisomies are the most common genetic cause of pregnancy loss. Nondisjunction during mitosis in the developing embryo can lead to cells in a single individual carrying different karyotypes, a condition known as **mosaicism**. Based on the **Lyon hypothesis**, females are naturally mosaics for genes on the X chromosome because one X chromosome in every cell is randomly inactivated to form a **Barr body**. Fluorescence in situ hybridization (FISH) can detect DNA sequences to identify deletions, translocations, and aneuploidies.

| Nondisjunction During Meiosis I | Autosomal Trisomies |
|---|---|

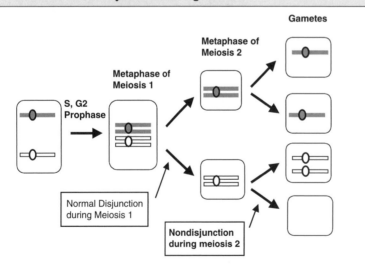

This figure shows the result of nondisjunction of one homologous pair (for example, chromosome 21) during meiosis 1. All other homologs segregate (disjoin) normally in the cell. Two of the gametes are diploid for chromosome 21. When fertilization occurs, the conception will be a trisomy 21 with Down syndrome. The other gametes with no copy of chromosome 21 will result in conceptions that are monosomy 21, a condition incompatible with a live birth.

## Nondisjunction During Meiosis II

This figure shows the result of nondisjunction during meiosis 2. In this case, the sister chromatids of a chromosome (for example, chromosome 21) fail to segregate (disjoin). The sister chromatids of all other chromosomes segregate normally. One of the gametes is diploid for chromosome 21. When fertilization occurs, the conception will be a trisomy 21 with Down syndrome. One gamete has no copy of chromosome 21 and will result in a conception that is a monosomy 21. The remaining two gametes are normal haploid ones.

### Trisomy 21 (Down Syndrome)

- Most common chromosomal disorder
- Epicanthal folds, brachycephaly, flat nasal bridge, low-set ears, and short, broad hands with single transverse palmar crease
- Mental retardation
- Early-onset Alzheimer disease
- Congenital septal defects in heart
- ↑ risk of acute leukemia
- Incidence: 1/800 births (1/25 if age >45 years)
- 95% nondisjunction; 4% Robertsonian translocation

### Trisomy 18 (Edwards Syndrome)

- Intrauterine growth retardation
- Mental retardation
- Failure to thrive
- Short sternum, small pelvis, rocker-bottom feet
- Cardiac, renal, and intestinal defects
- Usually death <1 year
- Incidence: 1/8,000 births

### Trisomy 13 (Patau Syndrome)

- Microcephaly and abnormal brain development
- Cleft lip and palate, polydactyly
- Cardiac dextroposition and septal defects
- Incidence: 1/25,000 births

| Sex Chromosome Aneuploidy |
|---|

### Turner Syndrome (45,XO)

- Short stature, webbed neck, shield chest
- Primary amenorrhea, infertility
- Coarctation of aorta
- Incidence: 1/6,000 female births

### Klinefelter Syndrome (47,XXY)

- Eunuchoid body with lack of male secondary sex characteristics
- Hypogonadism, testicular atrophy
- Incidence: 1/2,000 male births

### XYY Syndrome

- Excessively tall with severe acne
- ↑ risk of behavioral problems
- Incidence: 1/1,000 male births

# OTHER CHROMOSOMAL ABNORMALITIES

In addition to aneuploidy, large segments of chromosomes may also undergo structural aberrations, including deletions, inversions, and translocations. **Deletions** occur when a chromosome loses a segment because of breakage. **Inversions** are rearrangements of the gene order within a single chromosome due to incorrect repair of two breaks. An inversion that includes a centromere is called a **pericentric** inversion, while one that does not involve the centromere is **paracentric**. Finally, **translocations** involve exchange of chromosomal material between nonhomologous chromosomes. **Reciprocal translocations** result when two nonhomologous chromosomes exchange pieces, while **Robertsonian translocations** involve any two acrocentric chromosomes that break near the centromeres and rejoin with a fusion of the q arms at the centromere and loss of the p arms.

## Reciprocal Translocation

When one parent is a reciprocal translocation carrier:
- Adjacent segregation produces unbalanced genetic material and a likely loss of pregnancy
- Alternate segregation produces a normal haploid gamete (and diploid conception) or a liveborn who is a phenotypically normal translocation carrier

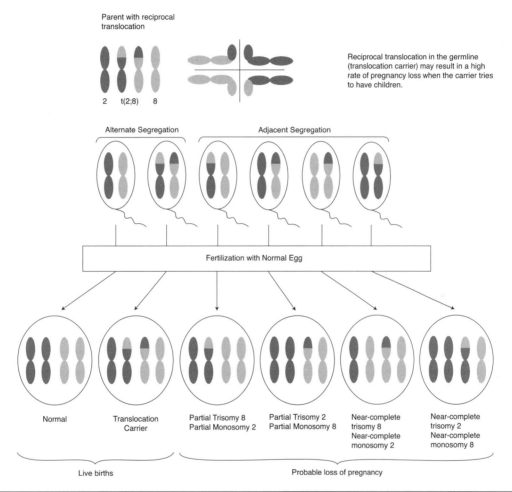

## Reciprocal Translocations in Somatic Cells May Result in Cancer

| | | |
|---|---|---|
| t(9;22) | CML, ALL | *bcr-abl* fusion produces a fusion protein with tyrosine kinase activity. |
| t(8;14) | Burkitt lymphoma | *c-myc* oncogene (chromosome 8) placed near Ig heavy chain locus. Activating Ig heavy chain gene activates *c-myc*. |
| t(11;14) | Mantle cell lymphoma | *bcl-1* (chromosome 11) encodes cyclin D. Translocation places *bcl-1* near Ig heavy chain locus (chromosome 14). |

*Definition of abbreviations:* ALL, acute lymphocytic leukemia; CML, chronic myelogenous leukemia.

*(Continued)*

### Consequences of a Robertsonian Translocation in One Parent

Approximately 5% of Down syndrome cases result from a Robertsonian translocation affecting chromosomes 14 and 21. When a translocation carrier (in this case, a male) produces gametes, the translocation can segregate with the normal 14 or the normal 21. Although adjacent segregation usually results in pregnancy loss, it can result in a **trisomy 21**. Alternate segregation produces a normal haploid gamete (and diploid conception) or a liveborn who is a phenotypically normal translocation carrier.

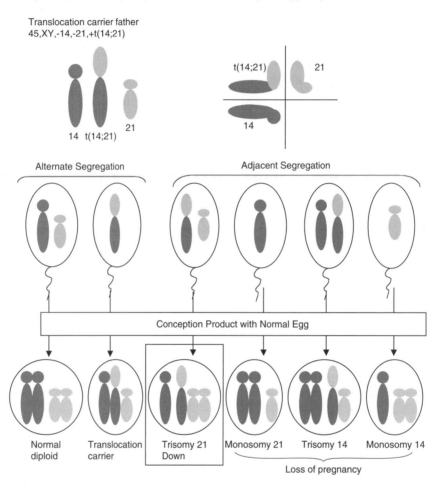

| Down syndrome (nondisjunction during meiosis) | Down syndrome (parent carries a Robertsonian translocation) |
|---|---|
| • 47,XX,+21 or 47,XY,+21 <br> • No association with prior pregnancy loss <br> • Older mother <br> • Very low recurrence rate | • 46,XX,-14,+t(14;21), or 46,XY,-14,+t(14;21) <br> • *May* be associated with prior pregnancy losses <br> • *May* be a young mother <br> • Recurrence rate 10–15% if mom is translocation carrier; 1–2% if dad is translocation carrier |

## ADDITIONAL DISEASES RESULTING FROM CHROMOSOMAL ABNORMALITIES

| Disease | Abnormality | Characteristics |
|---------|-------------|-----------------|
| **Cri-du-chat syndrome** | Terminal or interstitial deletion of 5p | • Mental retardation<br>• **Cat-like cry**<br>• Microcephaly, low-set ears, micrognathia<br>• Epicanthal folds |
| **DiGeorge syndrome** | Deletion of 22q11 | • Hereditary absence of thymus and parathyroid glands due to **abnormal development of 3rd and 4th pharyngeal pouches**<br>• T-cell deficiency<br>• Cardiac outflow tract abnormalities<br>• Abnormal facies<br>• Hypoparathyroidism |
| **Wilms tumor** | Deletion of 11p13 | • Malignant urinary tract tumors<br>• ⅔ diagnosed by age 4<br>• Tx: surgical removal |
| **Angelman syndrome** | Deletion of 15q11-q13 in **mother** | • **"Happy puppet" syndrome**<br>• Always smiling but lacks speech<br>• Hyperactive, hypotonic<br>• Mental retardation, seizures<br>• Dysmorphic facial features<br>• Ataxic, puppet-like gait |
| **Prader-Willi syndrome** | Deletion of 15q11-q13 in **father** | • **Short stature** and **obese** with small hands and feet<br>• **Hyperphagia**<br>• Dysmorphic facial features<br>• Mental retardation<br><br>*NOTE:* **Angelman** and **Prader-Willi** are both examples of the effects of a deletion in an area affected by imprinting. A minority of cases are caused by uniparental disomy. |

## POPULATION GENETICS

The **Hardy-Weinberg equilibrium** states that under certain conditions, if the population is large and randomly mating, the genotypic frequencies of the population will remain stable from generation to generation.

| Hardy-Weinberg Conditions | Factors Affecting Equilibrium |
|---------------------------|-------------------------------|
| 1. No mutations<br>2. No selection against a genotype<br>3. No migration or immigration of the population<br>4. Random mating | **Natural Selection** |
|  | Increases frequencies of genes that promote survival or fertility (e.g., malaria protection in sickle cell heterozygotes) |
|  | **Genetic Drift** |
|  | Gene frequency change due to finite population size |
|  | **Gene Flow** |
|  | Gene exchange between different populations |
|  | **Linkage Disequilibrium** |
|  | Preferential association of an allele at one locus with another allele at a nearby locus more frequently than by chance alone |

If:      frequency of A allele = p

         frequency of a allele = q

Then:    allele frequencies can be expressed as:

$$p + q = 1$$

genotypic frequencies at that locus can be expressed as:

$$p^2 + 2pq + q^2 = 1$$

where $p^2$ = frequency of genotype AA

     $2pq$ = frequency of genotype Aa

     $q^2$ = frequency of genotype aa

## SUBCELLULAR ORGANELLES

In contrast to simple prokaryotic cells that have a cell wall but no membrane-bound nucleus or organelles, eukaryotic cells are, in general, larger and lack a cell wall, but are composed of various subcellular membranous organelles with distinct functions.

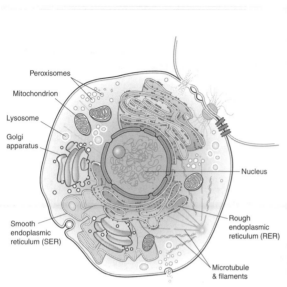

Peroxisomes
Mitochondrion
Lysosome
Golgi apparatus
Nucleus
Smooth endoplasmic reticulum (SER)
Rough endoplasmic reticulum (RER)
Microtubule & filaments

### Nucleus

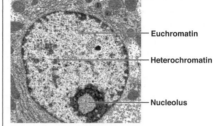

Euchromatin
Heterochromatin
Nucleolus

- Site of **DNA replication and transcription**
- Enclosed by nuclear envelope
- Contains **nucleolus** (site of ribosome synthesis); no membrane surrounds the nucleolus
- Contains DNA packaged with histones to form **chromatin**

### Rough Endoplasmic Reticulum (RER)

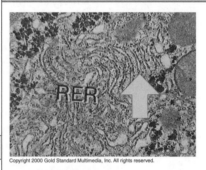

RER

- Contains **ribosomes** for synthesizing proteins destined for RER, SER, Golgi, lysosomes, cell membrane, and secretion
- Cotranslational modifications, including **N-linked glycosylation** (proteins synthesized on free ribosomes are not usually glycosylated)

| Prokaryotic | Eukaryotic |
|---|---|
| Small (1–10 μm) | Large (10–100 μm) |
| Thick, rigid cell wall | No cell wall |
| No membrane-bound organelles | Various subcellular membranous organelles |
| Non-membrane–bound nucleoid region | Nucleus with double-membrane envelope |

### Proteasome

- Small complexes of proteolytic enzymes in cytosol
- Digest (usually misfolded) proteins that are marked with ubiquitin
- Peptides produced are presented along with MHC I at the cell surface

### Ribosomes

- Site of **protein synthesis**
- Composed of ribosomal RNA (rRNA) and proteins forming large 60S + small 40S subunits
- Single mRNA simultaneously translated by several ribosomes is a **polysome**

| Types of Ribosomes | |
|---|---|
| **RER-Bound** | **Free Cytosolic** |
| Proteins for RER, SER, Golgi apparatus, lysosomes, cell membrane, and secretion | Cytosolic, mitochondrial, nuclear, and peroxisomal proteins |

(Continued)

## Golgi Apparatus

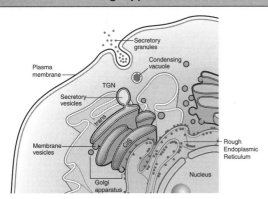

- Site of **post-translational modifications and protein sorting**
- Consists of disk-shaped cisternae in stacks
- *Cis* **(forming) face** associated with RER
- *Trans* **(maturing) face** oriented toward plasma membrane

## Smooth Endoplasmic Reticulum (SER)

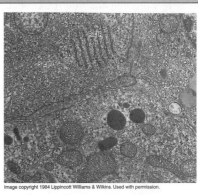

- Involved in detoxification reactions, including **phase I hydroxylation** (via cytochrome P450) and **phase II conjugation** (addition of polar groups)
- Synthesis of phospholipids, lipoproteins, and sterols
- Sequesters $Ca^{2+}$; known as **sarcoplasmic reticulum** in striated and smooth muscle cells

## Mitochondria

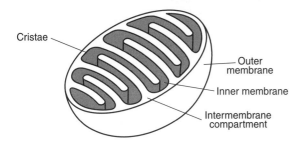

- Major function is ATP synthesis
- Similar to bacteria in size and shape; self-replicating
- Contain their own double-stranded circular DNA
- Smooth, permeable outer membrane; heavily infolded, impermeable inner membrane

## Lysosomes

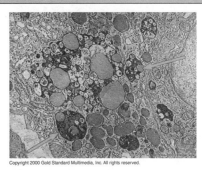

- Enzymatic degradation of extracellular or intracellular macromolecules
- Primary lysosome fuses with phagosomes or cellular organelles to form secondary lysosomes
- Acidic hydrolytic enzymes with optimal activity at pH 5
- Degradation of intracellular organelles known as **autophagy**

## Endosomes

- Formed from endocytosed vesicles acquired by receptor-mediated endocytosis involving **clathrin-coated pits**
- Can fuse with primary lysosomes to form secondary lysosomes to degrade extracellular materials
- Exogenous peptides presented on membrane with MHC II on antigen presenting cells

## Peroxisomes

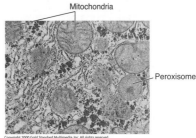

- Synthesis and degradation of hydrogen peroxide
- β-oxidation of very long chain fatty acids ($>C_{24}$)
- Phospholipid exchange reactions
- Bile acid synthesis

# PLASMA MEMBRANE

The **plasma membrane** of a cell is a bilayer of lipids and proteins. The lipids include phospholipids, unesterified cholesterol, and glycolipids and are **amphipathic** (polar head to interact with aqueous environment, and nonpolar tail to interact with the bilayer interior). Proteins may act as adhesion molecules, receptors, transporters, channels, or enzymes. Proteins embedded in the bilayer are **integral proteins**, whereas those loosely associated with the membrane are **peripheral proteins**. In general, **N-glycosylation** of proteins and lipids is associated with location on the external surface, whereas **N-myristoylation**, **prenylation**, and **palmitoylation** of proteins are associated with location on the cytoplasmic face of the plasma membrane.

## Structure of Biologic Membranes

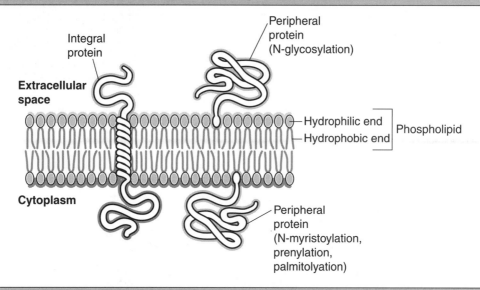

## Types of Integral Membrane Proteins

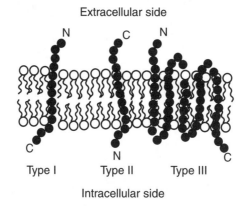

| Types of Transport | | |
|---|---|---|
| **Simple Diffusion** | **Facilitated Diffusion** | **Active Transport** |
| • Movement of highly permeable molecules from a region of higher to lower concentration<br>• e.g., $O_2$, $CO_2$, NO | • Passage of poorly permeable molecules from a region of higher to lower concentration via a carrier<br>• e.g., glucose transporter | • Movement of molecules from a region of lower to higher concentration with *1)* energy expenditure via ATP hydrolysis, or *2)* cotransport using another molecule's chemical gradient<br>• e.g., *1)* $Na^+/K^+$ pump, $Ca^{2+}$-ATPase<br>• e.g., *2)* $Na^+$/glucose symporter |

# CYTOSKELETON

The cytoskeleton consists of a supportive network of tubules and filaments in the cytoplasm of eukaryotic cells. It is a dynamic structure responsible for cellular movement, changes in cell shape, and the contraction of muscle cells. It also provides the machinery for intracellular movement of organelles. The cytoskeleton is composed of three types of supportive structures: **microtubules\***, **intermediate filaments**, and **microfilaments**.

| Microtubules* | Intermediate Filaments | Microfilaments | Disease Association |
|---|---|---|---|
| **Tubulin** (hollow cylindrical polymer of tubulin dimers) | • **Keratin** (epithelium)<br>• **Vimentin** (nonepithelial)<br>• **Neurofilament** (neurons) | **Actin** (double-stranded polymer twisted in helical pattern) | **Chediak-Higashi Syndrome**<br><br>*(defect in microtubule polymerization in leukocytes)* |

| Function | | | |
|---|---|---|---|
| • Movement of chromosomes in mitosis or meiosis<br>• Intracellular transport via motor proteins<br>• Ciliary and flagellar motility | Structural | • Structural<br>• Muscle contraction via interaction with myosin | • Recurrent pyogenic infections of respiratory tract and skin<br>• Partial albinism<br>• Photophobia, nystagmus, peripheral neuropathy, motor dysfunction, seizures<br>• Presents early in childhood |

## Axoneme Structure

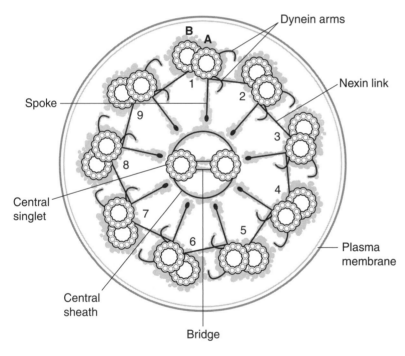

**Kartagener Syndrome**

*(immotile cilia due to defect in axonemal proteins, such as dynein arms)*

• Chronic cough, rhinitis, and sinusitis
• Situs inversus
• Fatigue and headaches
• Male infertility from immotile spermatozoa
• Autosomal recessive

### Pharmacology

**Colchicine**
• Inhibits tubulin polymerization
• Used for gout

**Vincristine/Vinblastine**
• Inhibits tubulin polymerization
• Antineoplastic

**Taxol**
• Promotes tubulin polymerization
• Antineoplastic

## Motor Proteins

**Kinesins** for $\ominus \rightarrow \oplus$ anterograde direction

**Dyneins** for $\oplus \rightarrow \ominus$ retrograde direction

*Microtubules are polarized structures with assembly/disassembly occurring at the $\oplus$ ends, which are oriented toward the cell's periphery.

# CELL ADHESION

A cell must physically interact via cell surface molecules with its external environment, whether it be the extracellular matrix or **basement membrane**. The basement membrane is a sheet-like structure underlying virtually all epithelia, which consists of **basal lamina** (made of type IV collagen, glycoproteins [e.g., laminin], and proteoglycans [e.g., heparin sulfate]), and **reticular lamina** (composed of reticular fibers). Cell junctions anchor cells to each other, seal boundaries between cells, and form channels for direct transport and communication between cells. The three types of junctional complexes include **anchoring, tight,** and **gap junctions**.

| Cell Junctions | Extracellular Matrix |
|---|---|

### Cell Junctions

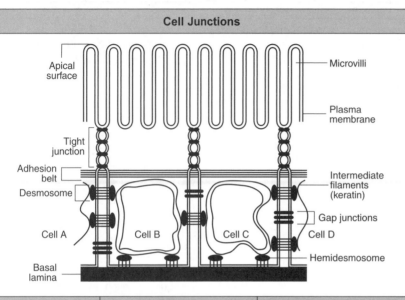

### Extracellular Matrix

**Proteoglycans**
- 90–95% carbohydrate; 5–10% protein
- Forms hydrated gel for embedding fibrous proteins
- Provides shock absorption and lubrication

**Collagen**
- Triple helix of polypeptide chains rich in glycine and proline
- Collagens I–III: fibrous form for structure
- Collagen IV: sheet-like meshwork specific to basal lamina

**Elastin**
- Cross-linked fibers rich in glycine and proline
- Provides elasticity to tissues (e.g., lungs and large arteries)

**Fibronectin**
- Large, fibrous protein with disulfide crosslinks
- Provides adhesion between cells and extracellular matrix

**Laminin**
- Three polypeptide chains in shape of a cross and connected by disulfide bonds
- Major glycoprotein in basal lamina
- Provides adhesion between cells and extracellular matrix

| Anchoring Junctions | Tight Junctions | Gap Junctions |
|---|---|---|
| • **Adherens junction (zonula adherens)**—band-like junction near apical region for attachment to adjacent epithelial cells, forming an "adhesion belt"<br><br>• **Desmosome (macula adherens)**—juxtaposition of two disk-shaped plaques from adjacent cells, with IFs radiating away from the plaques; **hemidesmosomes** anchor cells to the extracellular matrix | **Tight junction (zonula occludens)**—fusion of apposed cell membranes<br><br>_Image copyright 1984 Lippincott Williams & Wilkins. Used with permission._ | **Gap junctions**—direct passage for small particles and ions between cells via **connexon** channel proteins |

### Disease Association

**Pemphigus Vulgaris**
_(autoantibodies against desmosomal proteins in skin cells)_

- Painful flaccid bullae (blisters) in oropharynx and skin that rupture easily
- Postinflammatory hyperpigmentation
- Treatment: corticosteroids

**Bullous Pemphigoid**
_(autoantibodies against basement-membrane hemidesmosomal proteins)_

- Widespread blistering with pruritus
- Less severe than pemphigus vulgaris
- Rarely affects oral mucosa
- Can be drug induced (e.g., middle-aged or elderly patient on multiple medications)
- Treatment: corticosteroids

| Function | | |
|---|---|---|
| For structural integrity of large sheets of tissues (e.g., providing tensile strength of epithelial tissues); adhesion belt also allows epithelial tissue contractions | Provides a tight seal to prevent fluid leak between compartments (e.g., between intestinal lumen and intestinal villi) | Allows direct intercellular communications (e.g., allowing ions to pass for synchronous firing of cardiac pacemaker cells) |

_Definition of abbreviations:_ IF, intermediate filament.

The cell cycle consists of the mitosis phase (M), the presynthetic gap ($G_1$), the DNA synthesis phase (S), and the postsynthetic gap ($G_2$). Mitosis is the shortest phase, consisting of **prophase, metaphase, anaphase**, and **telophase**. Both $G_1$ and $G_2$ phases are variable in duration, with most cells spending much of their time in a stable, nondividing $G_0$ phase. Cells in $G_2$ have twice the amount of DNA as those in $G_1$.

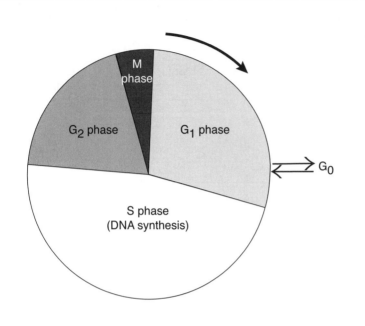

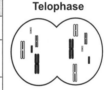

### Phases of Mitosis

| Prophase | |
|---|---|
| | • Chromosomes coil<br>• Nuclear envelope disappears<br>• Spindle apparatus forms |
| **Metaphase** | |
| | Chromosomes align |
| **Anaphase** | |
| | Chromatids separate |
| **Telophase** | |
| | • Chromosomes uncoil<br>• Nuclear envelope reappears<br>• Spindle apparatus disassemble<br>• Cell divides in two (cytokinesis) |

### Regulators of the Cell Cycle

| | |
|---|---|
| **Cyclins** | **Cyclin** levels rise and fall with stages of cell cycle. |
| **CDKs** | **Cyclin-dependent kinases** with various substrates promote cell-cycle progression. |
| **APC** | **Anaphase-promoting complex** triggers chromatid separation; degrades M-phase cyclins. |
| **SPF** | **S-phase promoting factor** includes CDKs and cyclins, which prepare cell for DNA replication. |
| **MPF** | **M-phase/maturation-promoting factor** includes CDKs and cyclins, which promote assembly of mitotic spindle and nuclear envelope breakdown. |
| **p53** | **p53** is a tumor suppressor that blocks cell cycle if DNA is damaged. |
| **RB** | **Retinoblastoma susceptibility protein** is a substrate of CDKs that promotes cell division. |
| **p21** | **p21** is a CDK inhibitor that also blocks cell-cycle progression. |

### Disease Association

#### Retinoblastoma

*(mutation in the RB1 tumor-suppressor gene on chromosome 13)*

• Most common childhood eye tumor
• Leukocoria (white reflex in pupil)
• Strabismus
• "Two-hit model" of carcinogenesis:
  1) inherited mutation of one allele
  2) somatic mutation of second allele

# CELL SIGNALING

In order to act on a cell, external molecules, such as hormones and neurotransmitters, must interact with a **receptor**. In general, small hydrophobic molecules (e.g., cortisol, sex hormones, thyroid hormone, and retinoids) can readily penetrate the plasma membrane to bind **intracellular receptors**, which often act as transcription factors to affect gene expression. Most other molecules bind to cell surface receptors, which include **ion-channel–linked receptors** (e.g., transmitter-gated channels), **G-protein–linked receptors** (the largest family), and **enzyme-linked receptors** (e.g., tyrosine kinase receptors). These cell surface receptors (i.e., the "first messenger") usually transmit their signal via a number of downstream **second messengers**, leading to a **signal transduction cascade**. One exception is the gaseous **nitric oxide** (NO), which readily diffuses across the plasma membrane to activate soluble **guanylate cyclase**, generate **cGMP**, and promote smooth muscle relaxation.

## G-Protein–Coupled Receptor Systems

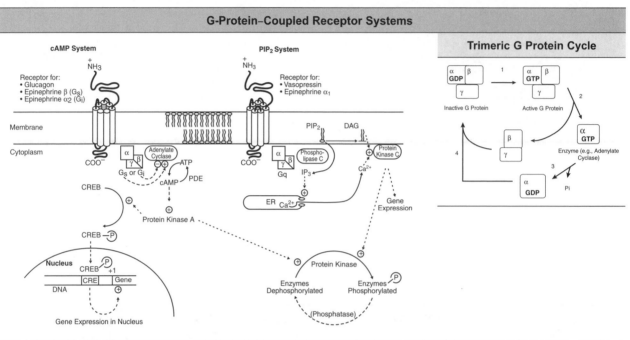

## Tyrosine Kinase Receptor

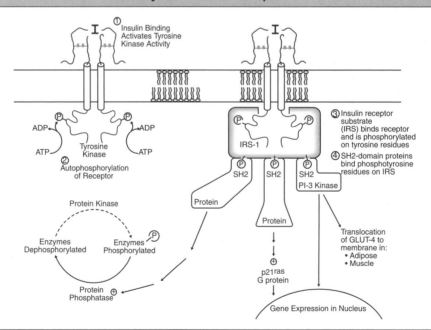

---

*Definition of abbreviations:* See next page.

*(Continued)*

# CELL SIGNALING (CONT'D.)

## Guanylate Cyclase

Receptors for Atrial Natriuretic Factor (ANF)

Produced from Arginine by *Nitric Oxide Synthase* in Vascular Endothelial Cells

Drugs:
• Nitroprusside
• Nitroglycerine
• Isosorbide dinitrate

Nitric Oxide (NO)

Membrane

Cytoplasm

COO⁻

GTP

cGMP

NO ⊕

Soluble Guanylate Cyclase (heme)

GTP

**Vascular Smooth Muscle**

⊕ Protein Kinase G

Relaxation of Smooth Muscle (Vasodilation)

## Pharmacology

| Nitrates | Sildenafil |
|---|---|
| *(nitroglycerin, nitroprusside, isosorbide dinitrate)* <br><br> • Converted to NO, which activates guanylate cyclase, leading to ↑ in cGMP. cGMP causes smooth muscle relaxation of blood vessels. <br><br> • For angina and pulmonary edema <br><br> • Adverse effects: headache, hypotension | • Inhibits cGMP-dependent phosphodiesterase (PDE5), leading to cGMP buildup, causing smooth muscle relaxation and dilation of blood vessels leading to the corpus cavernosum <br><br> • For erectile dysfunction <br><br> • Adverse effects: headache, hypotension |

## Examples of Receptors

### Adrenergic Receptors

• $\alpha_1$ ($G_q$)—smooth muscle contraction
• $\alpha_2$ ($G_{i/o}$)—inhibits NT release
• $\beta_1$ ($G_s$)—↑ heart rate and contractility
• $\beta_2$ ($G_s$)—smooth muscle relaxation

### Muscarinic Acetylcholine Receptors

• $M_1$ ($G_q$)—affects CNS, PNS, gastric parietal cells
• $M_2$ ($G_{i/o}$)—↓ heart rate and contractility
• $M_3$ ($G_q$)—stimulates glandular secretions
• $M_4$ ($G_{i/o}$)—CNS only; role unclear
• $M_5$ ($G_q$)—role unclear

### Dopamine Receptors

• $D_1$ ($G_s$)—smooth muscle relaxation; natriuresis; CNS effects
• $D_2$ ($G_{i/o}$)—inhibits sympathetic transmitter release; CNS effects
• $D_3$ ($G_{i/o}$)—similar to $D_2$
• $D_4$ ($G_{i/o}$)—similar to $D_2$
• $D_5$ ($G_s$)—similar to $D_1$

### Vasopressin Receptors

• $V_1$ ($G_q$)—smooth muscle contraction
• $V_2$ ($G_s$)—↑ $H_2O$ reabsorption in kidney

### Other Receptors

• Insulin (TK)—↑ glycogen synthesis; ↓ glycogenolysis
• Glucagon ($G_s$)—↑ glycogenolysis; ↓ glycogen synthesis
• IGF (TK)—↑ proliferation of various cell types
• PDGF (TK)—↑ proliferation of connective tissue, glial, and smooth muscle cells
• EGF (TK)—↑ proliferation of mesenchymal, glial, and epithelial cells
• ANF (GC)—smooth muscle relaxation; ↑ $Na^+$ and $H_2O$ excretion in kidney
• NO (GC)—smooth muscle relaxation

*Definition of abbreviations:* ANF, atrial natriuretic factor; ATP, adenosine triphosphate; cGMP, cyclic guanosine monophosphate; DAG, diacylglycerol; EGF, epidermal growth factor; ER, endoplasmic reticulum; GC, guanylate cyclase–coupled receptor; $G_{i/o}$, cAMP-inhibiting GPCR; $G_q$, PLC-activating GPCR; $G_s$, cAMP-activating GPCR; IGF, insulin-like growth factor; PDE, phosphodiesterase; PDGF, platelet-derived growth factor; $PIP_2$, phosphoinositol biphosphate; PLC, phospholipase C; NO, nitric oxide; TK, tyrosine kinase receptor.

# Immunology

## Chapter 3

## Overview of the Immune System

## Inflammation

## Clinical Immunology

## Transplantation Immunology

# OVERVIEW OF THE IMMUNE SYSTEM

## CHARACTERISTICS OF INNATE VERSUS ADAPTIVE IMMUNITY

The immune system can be divided into **two** complementary arms: the **innate** (native, natural) immune system and the **adaptive** (acquired, specific) immune system. These two arms work in concert with each other through soluble substances, such as antibodies, complement, and cytokines.

| Characteristics | Innate | Adaptive |
|---|---|---|
| Specificity | For structures shared by groups of microbes | For specific antigens of microbial and nonmicrobial agents |
| Diversity | Limited | **High** |
| Memory | No | **Yes** |
| Self-reactivity | No | No |
| **Components** | **Innate** | **Adaptive** |
| Anatomic and chemical barriers | Skin, mucosa, chemicals (lysozyme, interferons α and β), temperature, pH | Lymph nodes, spleen, mucosal-associated lymphoid tissues |
| Blood proteins | **Complement** | **Antibodies** |
| Cells | **Phagocytes and NK cells** | **Lymphocytes** (other than NK cells) |

## OVERVIEW OF THE IMMUNE RESPONSE

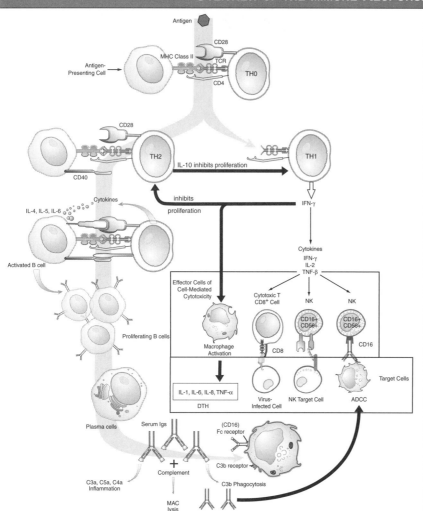

Foreign materials introduced into the body must be processed and presented to TH cells. Processed peptides presented in the MHC class II groove of the antigen-presenting cell are recognized via complementarity with the specific TCR.

Extracellular pathogens stimulate production of TH2 cells, which provide the CD40L costimulatory signal and cytokines to induce B cells to differentiate into plasma cells, which produce antibody. Antibody may assist in phagocytosis (opsonization) or complement-mediated lysis.

Intracellular pathogens stimulate production of TH1 cells, which stimulate the effector cells of cell-mediated immunity. Macrophages are induced to become more effective intracellular killers of the bacteria they ingest. Cytotoxic T cells kill virus-infected cells by recognition of peptides presented in the MHC class I molecule.

Natural killer (NK) cells kill cells devoid of MHC class I that are infected with some viruses or have undergone malignant transformation. In antibody-dependent cell-mediated cytotoxicity (ADCC), abnormal surface molecules on infected or transformed cells are recognized by antibodies and targeted for extracellular lysis by NK cells, eosinophils, neutrophils, or macrophages.

*Definition of abbreviations:* MHC, major histocompatibility complex; TCR, T cell receptor; TH, T helper.

| CELLS OF THE IMMUNE SYSTEM | | | |
|---|---|---|---|
| **Myeloid Cell** | **Location** | **Identifying Features** | **Function** |
| Monocyte | Bloodstream, 0–900/µL | **Kidney bean-shaped nucleus, CD 14 (endotoxin receptor) positive** | **Phagocytic**, differentiate into tissue macrophages |
| Macrophage | Tissues | Ruffled membrane, cytoplasm with vacuoles and vesicles (CD14+) | **Phagocytosis**, secretion of **cytokines** |
| Dendritic cell | Epithelia, tissues | Long, cytoplasmic arms | **Antigen capture**, transport, and presentation<br>(There are also plasmacytoid dendritic cells that look like plasma cells and produce interferon-$\alpha$.) |
| Neutrophil | Bloodstream, 1,800–7,800/µL | **Multilobed** nucleus; **small pink** granules | **Phagocytosis** and activation of bactericidal mechanisms |
| Eosinophil | Bloodstream, 0–450/µL | **Bilobed** nucleus; **large pink** granules | **Killing of antibody-coated parasites** |
| Basophil | Bloodstream, 0–200/µL | **Bilobed** nucleus; **large blue** granules | **Nonphagocytic**, release pharmacologically active substances during **allergy** |
| Mast cell | Tissues, mucosa, and epithelia | **Small** nucleus; **cytoplasm** packed with **large blue** granules | Release of granules containing histamine, etc., during **allergy** |

*(Continued)*

## CELLS OF THE IMMUNE SYSTEM (*CONT'D.*)

| Lymphoid Cell | Location | Identifying Features | Function |
|---|---|---|---|
| Lymphocyte | Bloodstream, 1,000–4,000/μL, lymph nodes, spleen, submucosa, and epithelia | **Large, dark** nucleus, small rim of cytoplasm | **B cells produce antibody** **TH (CD3+CD4+) cells regulate immune responses** **Cytotoxic T cells (CTLs: CD3+CD8+) kill altered or infected cells** |
| Natural killer (NK) lymphocyte | Bloodstream, ≤10% of lymphocytes | **Lymphocytes** with **large cytoplasmic** granules, **CD16+CD56+** | **Kill tumor/virus cell** targets or antibody-coated target cells |
| Plasma cell | Lymph nodes, spleen, mucosal-associated lymphoid tissues, and bone marrow | **Small dark** nucleus, **intensely staining Golgi** apparatus | End cell of B-cell differentiation, **produce antibody** |

## CHARACTERISTICS OF LYMPHOID CELLS
### Comparison of B- and T-lymphocyte Antigen Receptors

| Property | B-Cell Antigen Receptor | T-Cell Antigen Receptor |
|---|---|---|
| Idiotypes/lymphocyte | 1 | 1 |
| Isotypes/lymphocyte | 2 (**IgM and IgD**) | 1 ($\alpha/\beta$) |
| Is secretion possible? | **Yes** | **No** |
| Number of combining sites/molecules | 2 | 1 |
| Mobility | **Flexible** (hinge region) | **Rigid** |
| Signal transduction molecules | Ig-$\alpha$, Ig-$\beta$, **CD19, CD21** | **CD3** |

## GENERATION OF RECEPTOR DIVERSITY IN B AND T LYMPHOCYTES

| Mechanism | Cell in Which Expressed |
|---|---|
| Existence in genome of multiple V, D, J segments | B and T cells |
| **VDJ recombination** (gene segments are selected and recombined randomly to generate unique variable domains) | **B** and **T cells** |
| **N-nucleotide addition** (TdT adds nucleotides randomly where V, D, and J are joined) | **B cells (only heavy chain), T cells (both chains)** |
| Combinatorial association of heavy and light chains | B and T cells |
| **Somatic hypermutation** (mutations in variable domain coding occur during blastogenesis, and natural selection causes affinity maturation) | **B cells only,** after **Ag stimulation** |

*Definition of abbreviation:* Tdt, terminal deoxyribonucleotidyl transferase.

# HUMAN MAJOR HISTOCOMPATIBILITY COMPLEX (MHC) SUMMARY

| MHC Class I | MHC Class II |
|---|---|
| 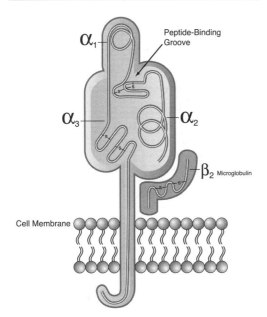 | 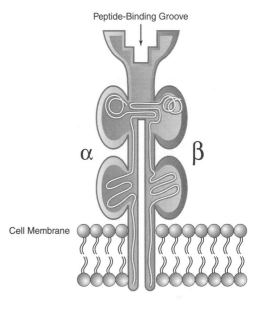 |

| Names | HLA-A, HLA-B, HLA-C | HLA-DP, HLA-DQ, HLA-DR |
|---|---|---|
| **Tissue distribution** | **All nucleated cells**, platelets | **B and T lymphocytes, antigen-presenting cells** |
| **Recognized by** | Cytotoxic T cells **(CD8+)** | Helper T cells **(CD4+)** |
| **Peptides bound** | Endogenously **synthesized** | Exogenously **processed** |
| **Function** | **Elimination of abnormal (infected) host cells** by cytotoxic T cells | **Presentation of foreign antigen** to helper T cells |
| **Invariant chain** | No | **Yes** |
| **$\beta_2$-microglobulin** | **Yes** | No |

## EXAMPLES OF HLA-LINKED IMMUNOLOGIC DISEASES

| Disease | HLA Allele |
|---|---|
| Rheumatoid arthritis | DR4 |
| Insulin-dependent diabetes mellitus | DR3/DR4 |
| Multiple sclerosis, Goodpasture syndrome | DR2 |
| Systemic lupus erythematosus, psoriasis, inflammatory bowel disease, Reiter syndrome | DR2/DR3 |
| Ankylosing spondylitis | B27 |
| Celiac disease | DQ2 or DQ8 |
| Graves disease | B8 |

## SUPERANTIGENS
### (Staphylococcal Enterotoxins, Toxic-Shock Syndrome Toxin-1, and Streptococcal Pyrogenic Exotoxins)

Superantigens act by cross-linking the variable β domain of a T-cell receptor to an α chain of a class II MHC molecule. They activate many clones of T cells in the absence of antigen-specificity and can cause life-threatening **overproduction of inflammatory cytokines (IL-1, IL-6, IFN-γ, and TNF-α)**. **Endotoxin** acts with the same end result, but from a different starting point. Macrophages have CD14 (the receptor for endotoxin) on their surface, and are directly stimulated to produce IL-1, IL-6, and TNF-α in the absence of TH participation.

## T-HELPER CELLS

Naive TH cells (TH0) differentiate into TH1 cells when a strong initial innate immune response leads to production of IL-12 from macrophages or IFN-γ from NK cells. Differentiation of a TH0 cell into a TH2 cell occurs in the absence of an innate immune response. TH1 cells secrete IFN-γ, TNF-β, and IL-2. TH2 cells produce IL-2, IL-4, IL-5, IL-6, and IL-10. IFN-γ, produced by TH1, inhibits TH2. IL4 and IL10, produced by TH2, inhibit TH1. TH17 cells increase inflammation and produce IL-17, and T$_{reg}$ cells decrease inflammation and produce IL-10. These cells have a regulatory role in autoimmune and hypersensitivity diseases. T cells that are exposed to antigen presenting cells in the absence of costimulatory signals will become anergic.

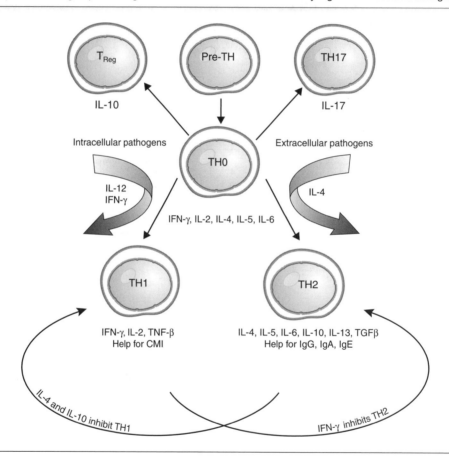

| EFFECTOR CELLS IN CELL-MEDIATED IMMUNITY | | | | |
|---|---|---|---|---|
| **Effector Cell** | **CD Markers** | **Antigen Recognition** | **MHC Recognition Required for Killing** | **Effector Molecules** |
| CTL | TCR, CD3, **CD8**, CD2 | **Specific**, TCR | Yes, **class I** | **Perforin, cytokines** (TNF-β, IFN-γ) |
| NK cell | **CD16, CD56**, CD2 | ADCC: specific by IgG, otherwise recognizes lectins | No, **MHC I recognition inhibits** | **Perforin, cytokines** (TNF-β, IFN-γ) |
| Macrophage | **CD14** | **Nonspecific** | No | **Intracellular** mechanisms |

| KEY CD MARKERS | | |
|---|---|---|
| **CD Designation** | **Cellular Expression** | **Known Functions** |
| CD2 (LFA-2) | T cells, thymocytes, NK cells | Adhesion molecule |
| CD3 | **T cells**, thymocytes | Signal transduction by the TCR |
| **CD4** | **TH cells**, thymocytes, monocytes, and macrophages | Coreceptor for **MHC class II** TH-cell activation, **receptor for HIV** |
| **CD8** | **CTLs**, some thymocytes | Coreceptor for **MHC class I**–restricted T cells |
| CD14 (LPS receptor) | Monocytes, macrophages, granulocytes | Binds LPS |
| **CD16** (Fc receptor) | **NK cells**, macrophages, mast cells | Immune complex-induced cellular activation, ADCC |
| **CD19 and 20** | **B cells** | Coreceptor with CD21 for B-cell activation |
| **CD21** (CR2, C3d receptor) | Mature B cells, follicular dendritic cells | Receptor for complement fragment C3d, forms coreceptor complex with CD19, **Epstein-Barr virus** receptor |
| CD25 | Activated TH cells and T$_{Reg}$ | Alpha chain of IL-2 receptor |
| CD28 | T cells | T-cell receptor for costimulatory molecule B7 |
| **CD40** | B cells, macrophages, dendritic cells, endothelial cells | Binds CD40L, **starts isotype switch** |
| **CD56** | **NK cells** | Not known |

*Definition of abbreviations:* ADCC, antibody-dependent cell-mediated cytotoxicity; CTL, cytotoxic T lymphocytes; LPS, endotoxin (lipopolysaccharide); NK, natural killer; TCR, T-cell receptor.

| CYTOKINES | | |
|---|---|---|
| **Cytokine** | **Source** | **Activity** |
| Interleukin-1 | Monocytes, macrophages | Stimulates cells, **endogenous pyrogen** |
| Interleukin-2 | TH cells | **Induces proliferation**, enhances activity |
| Interleukin-3 | TH cells, NK cells | Supports growth and differentiation of **myeloid cells** |
| Interleukin-4 | TH2 cells | Stimulates activation, differentiation, class switch to IgG1 and **IgE** |
| Interleukin-5 | TH2 cells | Stimulates proliferation and differentiation, class switch to **IgA** |
| Interleukin-6 | Monocytes, macrophages, TH2 cells | Second endogenous pyrogen, promotes differentiation into plasma cells, **induces acute phase response** |
| Interleukin-7 | Primary lymphoid organs | **Stimulates progenitor B- and T-cell production in bone marrow** |
| Interleukin-8 | Macrophages, endothelial cells | **Chemokine** (chemotactic for neutrophils) |
| Interleukin-10 | **TH2 cells** | Suppresses cytokine production of TH1 cells |
| Interleukin-11 | Bone marrow stroma | ↑ platelet count |
| Interleukin-12 | Macrophages | **Stimulates CMI** |
| Interleukin-17 | TH17 cells | ↑ inflammation and tissue damage associated with some autoimmune diseases |
| Interferon-$\alpha$ and -$\beta$ | Leukocytes, fibroblasts | **Inhibits viral protein synthesis** by acting on uninfected cells |
| Interferon-$\gamma$ | **TH1**, CTLs, NK cells | **Stimulates CMI, Inhibits TH2**, increases expression of class I and II MHC |
| Tumor necrosis factor-$\alpha$ and -$\beta$ | CMI cells | Enhances CMI |
| Granulocyte and granulocyte-monocyte colony-stimulating factors (G-CSF and GM-CSF) | Macrophages and TH cells | Induce proliferation in bone marrow; counteract neutropenia following ablative chemotherapy |

*Definition of abbreviation:* CMI, cell-mediated immunity.

| THE BASIC STRUCTURE OF IMMUNOGLOBULIN | |
|---|---|

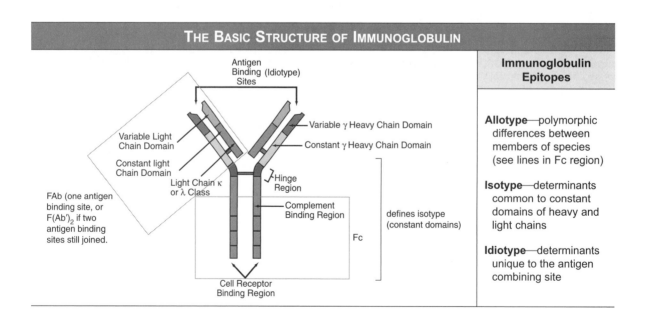

**Immunoglobulin Epitopes**

**Allotype**—polymorphic differences between members of species (see lines in Fc region)

**Isotype**—determinants common to constant domains of heavy and light chains

**Idiotype**—determinants unique to the antigen combining site

## SUMMARY OF THE BIOLOGIC FUNCTIONS OF THE ANTIBODY ISOTYPES

| | IgM | IgG | IgA | IgD | IgE |
|---|---|---|---|---|---|
| Heavy chain | $\mu$ | $\gamma$ | $\alpha$ | $\delta$ | $\varepsilon$ |
| Adult serum levels | 40–345 mg/dL | 650–1,500 mg/dL | 75–390 mg/dL | Trace | Trace |
| **Functions** | | | | | |
| Complement activation, classic pathway | + | + | – | – | – |
| Opsonization | – | + | – | – | – |
| Antibody-dependent, cell-mediated cytotoxicity (ADCC) | – | + | – | – | – |
| Placental transport | – | + | – | – | – |
| Naive B-cell antigen receptor | + | – | – | + | – |
| Memory B-cell antigen receptor (one only) | – | + | + | – | + |
| Trigger mast cell granule release | – | – | – | – | + |

## PRECIPITATION OF AB-AG COMPLEXES

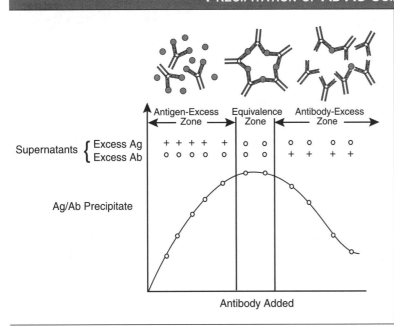

Supernatants { Excess Ag / Excess Ab

Ag/Ab Precipitate

Antibody Added

**Prozone phenomenon**—formation of suboptimal amount of precipitate in antibody excess (secondary syphilis)

**Window period** (hepatitis B)—the equivalence zone for HBsAg/HBsAb combination

# INFLAMMATION

## Acute Inflammation

Acute inflammation is an immediate response to injury, associated with redness, heat, swelling, pain, and loss of function. Understand the sequence of events of acute inflammation (extravasation, chemotaxis, phagocytosis, intracellular killing) and how these events set the stage for the subsequent adaptive immune response.

| Hemodynamic changes | • Transient initial vasoconstriction, followed by massive dilation (mediated by histamine, bradykinin, and prostaglandins) <br> • Increased vascular permeability (due to endothelial cell contraction and/or injury)—histamine, serotonin, bradykinin, leukotrienes (e.g., $LTC_4$, $LTD_4$, $LTE_4$) <br> • Blood stasis due to increased viscosity allows neutrophils to marginate |
|---|---|
| Cellular response | • **Neutrophils:** (segmented) polymorphonuclear leukocytes (PMNs) are important mediators in acute inflammation <br> • Neutrophils have **primary (azurophilic)** and **secondary (specific) granules**: <br>   – **Primary granules contain:** myeloperoxidase, phospholipase A2, lysozyme, acid hydrolases, elastase, defensins, and bactericidal permeability increasing protein (BPI) <br>   – **Secondary granules contain:** phospholipase A2, lysozyme, leukocyte alkaline phosphatase (LAP), collagenase, lactoferrin, vitamin $B_{12}$–binding proteins |

## Neutrophil Margination and Extravasation

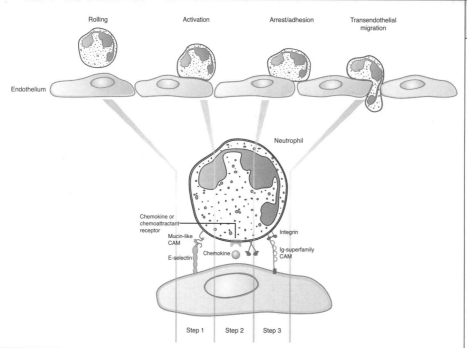

### Neutrophil Margination and Adhesion

At sites of inflammation, the endothelial cells increase expression of **E-selectin** and **P-selectin**, allowing neutrophils to bind weakly to the endothelial selectins and roll along the surface. (1) Then neutrophils are stimulated by chemokines to express their integrins, (2) which mediate firm adherence of the neutrophil to the endothelial cell. (3) Then leukocytes emigrate from the vasculature by moving between the endothelial cells, migrating through the basement membrane toward the inflammatory stimulus (chemotaxis).

GENERAL PRINCIPLES

IMMUNOLOGY

## NEUTROPHIL MIGRATION/CHEMOTAXIS

| Chemoattractive Molecule | Origin |
|---|---|
| Chemokines (**IL-8**) | Tissue mast cells, platelets, neutrophils, monocytes, macrophages, eosinophils, basophils, lymphocytes |
| Complement split product **C5a** | Endothelial damage → activation Hageman factor → plasmin activation |
| Leukotriene B$_4$ | Membrane phospholipids of macrophages, monocytes, neutrophils, mast cells → arachidonic acid cascade → lipoxygenase pathway |
| **Formyl methionyl peptides** | Released from **microorganisms** |

## OTHER CHEMICAL MEDIATORS OF INFLAMMATION

| Monoamine | Sources | Effects | Triggers for Release |
|---|---|---|---|
| Histamine | Basophils, platelets, and mast cells | Vasodilation and increased vascular permeability | • IgE-mediated mast cell reactions<br>• Physical injury<br>• Anaphylatoxins (C3a and C5a)<br>• Cytokines (IL-1) |
| Serotonin | Platelets | | Platelet aggregation |

| Enzyme | Arachidonic Acid Product | Effects | Comments |
|---|---|---|---|
| **Cyclooxygenase** | Thromboxane A$_2$ | Vasoconstriction, platelet aggregation | Produced by platelets |
| | Prostacyclin (PGI$_2$) | **Vasodilation** and inhibits platelet aggregation | Produced by vascular endothelium |
| | PGE$_2$ | Pain | — |
| | PGE$_2$, PGD$_2$, PGF$_2$ | Vasodilation | — |
| **Lipoxygenase** | LTB$_4$ | Neutrophil chemotaxis, **increased vascular permeability, vasoconstriction or vasodilation*** | — |
| | LTC$_4$, LTD$_4$, LTE$_4$ | **Bronchoconstriction, increased vascular permeability, vasoconstriction or vasodilation*** | Slow-reacting substance of anaphylaxis |

### Kinin System

- Bradykinin—vasoactive peptide produced from kininogen by family of enzymes called kallikreins; degraded by different peptidases, including angiotensin-converting enzyme (ACE)
- Activated **Hageman factor (factor XII)** converts prekallikrein → kallikrein
- Kallikrein cleaves high molecular weight kininogen (HMWK) → **bradykinin** (produces increased vascular permeability, pain, vasodilation, bronchoconstriction)

**\*Can be tissue specific (e.g., vasoconstriction in kidneys and heart; vasodilation in skin and nasal mucosa)**

# PHAGOCYTOSIS

There are several steps to phagocytosis: engulfment, fusion of the phagosome and lysosome, and digestion. There are **three** mechanisms of intracellular killing, as shown in the figure: NADPH oxidase-dependent, myeloperoxidase-dependent, and lysosome-dependent. **Opsonization** is the enhancement of phagocytosis with IgG and/or C3b.

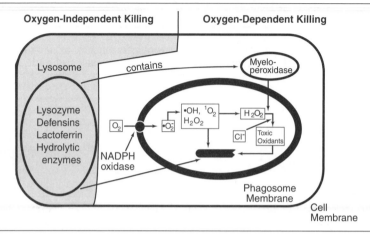

# DEFECTS OF PHAGOCYTIC CELLS

| Disease | Molecular Defect(s) | Symptoms |
|---|---|---|
| **Chronic granulomatous disease (CGD)** | Deficiency of **NADPH oxidase** (any one of four component proteins); failure to generate superoxide anion, other $O_2$ radicals | Recurrent infections with **catalase-positive** bacteria and fungi |
| Chédiak-Higashi syndrome | Granule structural defect | Recurrent infection with bacteria: chemotactic and degranulation defects; **absent NK** activity, **partial albinism** |
| Leukocyte adhesion deficiency | **Absence of CD18**—common β chain of the leukocyte integrins | Recurrent and chronic infections, failure to form pus, **does not reject umbilical cord** stump |

# COMPLEMENT CASCADE

The complement system is a set of interacting serum proteins that enhance inflammation (C3a, C4a, C5a) and opsonization (C3b) and cause lysis of particles (e.g., gram-negative bacteria) via C5b-9. The **alternative** pathway is initiated by **surfaces of pathogens**. The **classical** pathway is activated by **Ag/Ab complexes**.

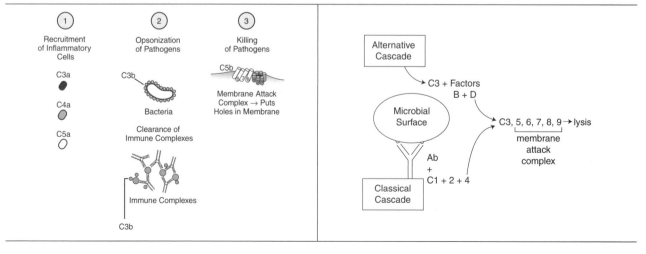

## DEFICIENCIES OF COMPLEMENT OR ITS REGULATION

| Deficiencies in Complement Components | Deficiency | Signs/Diagnosis |
| --- | --- | --- |
| Classical pathway | C1q, C1r, C1s, C2, C4 | Marked increase in immune complex diseases, increased infections with pyogenic bacteria |
| Alternative pathway | Factor B, properdin | Increased neisserial infections |
| Both pathways | C3 | Recurrent bacterial infections, immune complex disease |
| | **C5, C6, C7**, or **C8** | **Recurrent meningococcal and gonococcal infections** |
| Deficiencies in complement regulatory proteins | C1-INH (**hereditary angioedema**) | Overuse of C1, C2, C4 **Edema at mucosal surfaces** |

## SUMMARY OF ACUTE INFLAMMATION

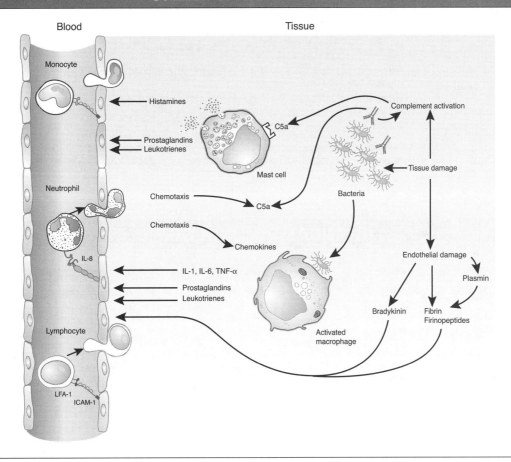

## CHRONIC INFLAMMATION

| Causes | Important Cell Types |
|---|---|

### Macrophages

| | |
|---|---|
| • Following a bout of acute inflammation<br><br>• Persistent infections<br><br>• Infections with certain organisms (viruses, mycobacteria, parasites, fungi)<br><br>• Autoimmune diseases<br><br>• Response to foreign material | Derived from blood monocytes. During inflammation, macrophages are mainly recruited from the blood (circulating monocytes). Macrophages contain acid hydrolases, elastase, and collagenase, secrete monokines.<br>    **Chemotactic factors:** C5a, MCP-1, MIP-1-$\alpha$, PDGF, TGF-$\alpha$<br>    **Tissue-based macrophages:**<br>      • Connective tissue (histiocyte)<br>      • Lung (pulmonary alveolar macrophages)<br>      • Liver (Kupffer cells)<br>      • Bone (osteoclasts)<br>      • Brain (microglia)<br>      • Kidney (mesangial cells) |

### Lymphocytes (e.g., B cells, plasma cells)

• T cells
• Lymphocyte chemokine: lymphotaxin

### Eosinophils

Play an important role in parasitic infections and IgE-mediated allergic reactions
    • Eosinophilic chemokine: eotaxin
    • Granules contain major basic protein, which is toxic to parasites

### Basophils

• Tissue-based basophils are called mast cells, present in high numbers in the lung and skin
• Play an important role in IgE-mediated reactions (allergies and anaphylaxis), release histamine

# CLINICAL IMMUNOLOGY

## COMPARISON OF THE PRIMARY AND SECONDARY IMMUNE RESPONSES

| Feature | Primary Response | Secondary Response |
|---|---|---|
| Time lag after immunization | 5–10 days | 1–3 days |
| Peak response | Small | Large |
| Antibody isotype | IgM then IgG | Increasing IgG, IgA, or IgE |
| Antibody **affinity** | Variable to low | High (**affinity maturation**) |
| Inducing agent | All immunogens | **Protein antigens** |
| Immunization protocol | High dose of antigen (often with adjuvant) | Low dose of antigen (often without adjuvant) |

## TYPES OF IMMUNIZATION USED IN MEDICINE

**Adjuvants** increase immunogenicity nonspecifically. They are given with weak immunogens to enhance the response.

| Type of Immunity | Acquired Through | Examples |
|---|---|---|
| Natural | Passive means | Placental IgG transport, colostrum |
| Natural | Active means | Recovery from infection |
| Artificial | Passive means | Immunoglobulins or immune cells given |
| Artificial | Active means | Vaccination |

## SUMMARY OF BACTERIAL VACCINES

| Organism | Vaccine | Vaccine Type |
|---|---|---|
| C. diphtheriae | **DTP** | Toxoid |
| B. pertussis | DT**P**, DT**aP** | Toxoid plus filamentous hemagglutinin |
| C. tetani | DT**P** | Toxoid |
| H. influenzae | Hib | Capsular polysaccharide and protein |
| S. pneumoniae | PCV Pediatric | 7 capsular serotypes and protein |
| | PPV Adult | 23 capsular serotypes |
| N. meningitidis | MCV | 4 capsular serotypes (Y, W-135, C, A) |

## SUMMARY OF VIRAL VACCINES

| Killed Vaccines | Live Viral Vaccines | Component Vaccines |
|---|---|---|
| **Mnemonic: RIP-A** (Rest In Peace Always—the killed viral vaccines): <br> **R**abies (killed human diploid cell vaccine) <br> **I**nfluenza <br> **P**olio (Salk) <br> **A** Hepatitis | All but adenovirus are attenuated <br> (**mnemonic: Mrr. V.Z. Mapsy**) <br> **M**umps <br> **R**otavirus <br> **R**ubella <br> **V**aricella – **Z**oster <br> **M**easles <br> **A**denovirus (pathogenic [not attenuated] respiratory strains given in enteric coated capsules) <br> **P**olio (Sabin) <br> **S**mall Pox <br> **Y**ellow Fever | Hepatitis B <br> HPV (human papilloma virus) |

## DEFECTS OF HUMORAL IMMUNITY

| Disease | Molecular Defect | Symptoms/Signs |
|---------|------------------|----------------|
| **Bruton X-linked hypogammaglobulinemia** | Deficiency of a tyrosine kinase blocks B-cell maturation | Low immunoglobulin of all classes, **no circulating B cells**, **pre-B cells in bone marrow in normal numbers**, normal cell-mediated immunity |
| **Selective IgA deficiency** | Deficiency of IgA (most common) | Repeated **sinopulmonary and gastrointestinal infections** |
| **X-linked hyper-IgM syndrome** | Deficiency of **CD40L** on activated T cells | **High serum titers of IgM without other isotypes** Normal B- and T-cell numbers, susceptibility to extracellular bacteria and opportunists |
| **Common variable immunodeficiency** | B-cell maturation defect and **hypogammaglobulinemia** | Both sexes affected, childhood onset, recurrent bacterial infections and increased susceptibility to *Giardia* Increased risk later in life to autoimmune disease, lymphoma, or gastric cancer |

## DEFECTS OF T CELLS AND SEVERE COMBINED IMMUNODEFICIENCIES

| Category | Disease | Defect | Clinical Manifestation |
|----------|---------|--------|------------------------|
| Selective T-cell deficiency | **DiGeorge syndrome** | Failure of formation of third and fourth pharyngeal pouches, **thymic aplasia** | Facial abnormalities, hypoparathyroidism, cardiac malformations, depression of T-cell numbers and absence of T-cell responses |
| | **MHC class I deficiency** | Failure of TAP 1 molecules to transport peptides to endoplasmic reticulum | **CD8+ T cells deficient**, CD4+ T cells normal, recurring viral infections, normal DTH, normal Ab production |
| Combined partial B- and T-cell deficiency | **Wiskott-Aldrich syndrome** | Defect in cytoskeletal glycoprotein, X-linked | Defective responses to bacterial polysaccharides and depressed IgM, gradual loss of humoral and cellular responses, **thrombocytopenia and eczema** |
| | **Ataxia telangiectasia** | Defect in kinase involved in the cell cycle | Ataxia (gait abnormalities), telangiectasia (capillary distortions in the eye), deficiency of IgA and IgE production |
| Complete functional B- and T-cell deficiency | Severe combined immunodeficiency (SCID) | Defects in common γ chain of IL-2 receptor (also present in receptors for IL-4, -7, -9, -15) X-linked | Chronic diarrhea; skin, mouth, and throat lesions; opportunistic (**fungal**) infections; low levels of circulating lymphocytes; cells unresponsive to mitogens |
| | | **Adenosine deaminase deficiency** (results in toxic metabolic products in cells) | |
| | | Defect in signal transduction from T-cell IL-2 receptors | |
| | | **Bare lymphocyte syndrome/MHC class II deficiency** | T cells present and responsive to nonspecific mitogens, no GVHD, **deficient in CD4+ T cells,** hypogammaglobulinemia |

# ASSOCIATION BETWEEN IMMUNODEFICIENCY DISEASE AND DEVELOPMENTAL BLOCKS

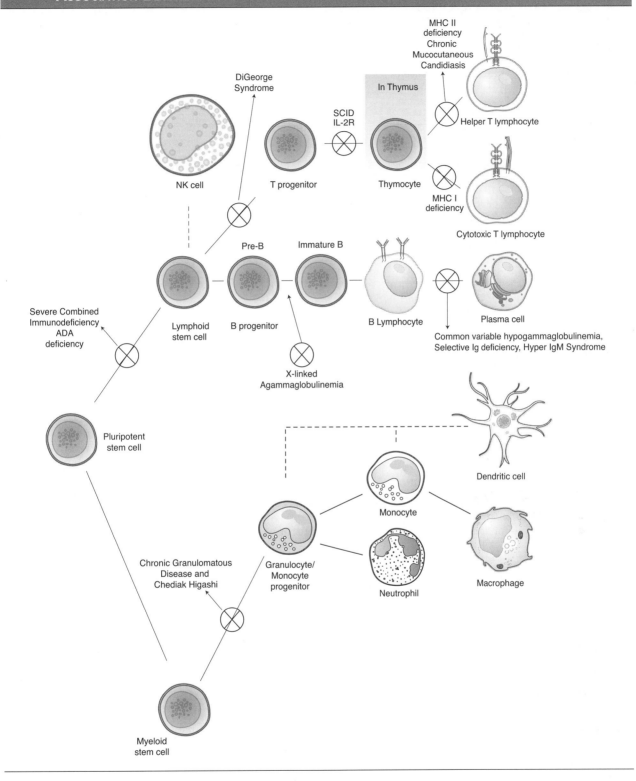

## ACQUIRED IMMUNODEFICIENCY SYNDROME (AIDS)

| | |
|---|---|
| **Definition** | When a patient is HIV-positive with CD4 count less than 200/mm$^3$ *or* HIV-positive with an AIDS-defining disease |
| **Transmission** | • Sexual contact: homosexual > heterosexual in U.S.<br>   – Cofactors: herpes and syphilis<br>• Parenteral transmission:<br>   – Intravenous drug abuse<br>   – Hemophiliacs<br>   – Blood transfusions<br>   – Accidental needle sticks in hospital workers<br>• Vertical transmission (mother to child) |
| **Pathogenesis** | • Human immunodeficiency virus (HIV; an enveloped retrovirus containing reverse transcriptase)<br>• HIV infects CD4+ cells (gp120 binds to CD4)<br>   – CD4+ T cells<br>   – Macrophages<br>   – Lymph node follicular dendritic cells<br>   – Langerhans cells<br>• Entry into cell by fusion requires gp41 and coreceptors<br>   – CCR5 (β-chemokine receptor 5)<br>   – CXCR4 (α-chemokine receptor) |
| **Diagnosis and Monitoring** | • **Initial screening:** Serologic, ELISA<br>• **Confirmation:** Serologic, Western blot<br>• **Detection of virus in blood (evaluate viral load):** RT-PCR<br>• **Detect HIV infection in newborns of HIV+ mother (provirus):** PCR*<br>• **Early marker of infection:** p24 antigen<br>• **Evaluate progression of disease:** CD4:CD8 T-cell ratio |
| **Treatment** | • Combination antiretroviral treatment<br>• Reverse transcriptase inhibitors<br>• Protease inhibitors<br>• Prophylaxis for opportunistic infections based on CD4 count |

*RT-PCR tests for circulating viral RNA and is used to monitor the efficacy of treatment. PCR detects integrated virus (provirus). Viral load has been demonstrated to be the best prognostic indicator during infection.

## OPPORTUNISTIC INFECTION AND COMMON SITES OF INFECTION IN AIDS PATIENTS

| Opportunistic Infection | Common Sites of Infection |
|---|---|
| *Pneumocystis jiroveci (carinii)* | Lung (pneumonia), bone marrow, start prophylaxis at < 200 CD4 |
| *Mycobacterium tuberculosis* | Lung, disseminated |
| *Mycobacterium avium-intracellulare* | Lung, gastrointestinal tract, disseminated |
| *Coccidioides immitis* | Lung, disseminated |
| *Histoplasma capsulatum* | Lung, disseminated, start prophylaxis at < 100 CD4 in endemic area |
| Cytomegalovirus | Lung, retina, adrenals, and gastrointestinal tract, start prophylaxis at < 50 CD4 |
| *Giardia lamblia* | Gastrointestinal tract |
| *Cryptosporidium parvum* | Gastrointestinal tract, start prophylaxis at < 50 CD4 |
| Herpes simplex virus | Esophagus and CNS (encephalitis) |
| *Candida albicans* | Oropharynx and esophagus |
| *Aspergillus* spp. | CNS, lungs, blood vessels |
| *Toxoplasma gondii* | CNS, start prophylaxis at < 100 CD4 |
| *Cryptococcus neoformans* | CNS (meningitis) |
| JC virus | CNS (progressive multifocal leukoencephalopathy) |

## OTHER COMPLICATIONS OF AIDS

| | |
|---|---|
| **Hairy leukoplakia** | Associated with Epstein-Barr virus (EBV) |
| **Kaposi sarcoma** | Associated with human herpes virus 8 (HHV8)<br>Common sites: skin, GI tract, lymph nodes, and lungs |
| **Non-Hodgkin lymphoma** | Tend to be high-grade B-cell lymphomas<br>Extranodal CNS lymphomas common |
| **Miscellaneous** | Cervical cancer<br>HIV wasting syndrome<br>AIDS nephropathy<br>AIDS dementia complex |

## HIV THERAPIES

Anti-HIV therapy usually involves three or more anti-retroviral agents including antimetabolite inhibitors of retroviral reverse transcriptase and viral protease. These aggressive drug combinations (highly active antiretroviral therapy, **HAART**) are typically initiated early after HIV infection and will often reduce viral load, preserve CD-4 counts, and limit opportunistic infections. Drug combinations also slow the development of resistance to drugs as opposed to monotherapy.

| Drug | Mechanism of Action | Side Effects and Comments |
|---|---|---|
| **Nucleoside reverse transcriptase inhibitors (NRTIs)** | | |
| Abacavir (ABC)<br>Didanosine (ddI)<br>Emtricitabine (FTC)<br>Lamivudine (3TC)<br>Stavudine (d4T)<br>Tenofovir (TDF)<br>Zalcitabine (ddC)<br>Zidovudine (ZDV, AZT) | Converted to nucleoside triphosphates, which **inhibit reverse transcriptase**, leading the inhibition of viral replication by chain termination | Dose-limiting pancreatitis (ddI)<br>Dose-limiting peripheral neuropathy (ddC, ddI, d4T)<br>Hypersensitivity reactions (ABC)<br>Lactic acidosis (ddI, d4T)<br>Fanconi syndrome (TDF)<br>Dose-limiting BMS (ZDV)<br>Minimal toxicity (FTC, 3TC)<br>Least toxic and also used for hepatitis B (3TC) |
| **Non-nucleoside reverse transcriptase inhibitors (NNRTIs)** | | |
| Delavirdine (DLV)<br>Efavirenz (EFV)<br>Etravirine (ETR)<br>Nevirapine (NVP) | **Inhibit reverse transcriptase** noncompetitively | Rash (occasional Steven-Johnson syndrome)<br>Adverse CNS effects (EFV)<br>P450 interactions<br>Increased transaminase levels (DLV, EFV) |
| **Protease inhibitors** | | |
| Atazanavir (ATV)<br>Darunavir (DRV)<br>Fosamprenavir (FPV)<br>Indinavir (IDV)<br>Nelfinavir (NFV)<br>Ritonavir (RTV)<br>Saquinavir (SQV)<br><br>Lopinavir + Ritonavir (LPV/r) | **Inhibits aspartate protease** (HIV-1 protease encoded by *pol* gene), blocking structural protein formation of the mature virion core | Inhibit CYP3A4 (especially ritonavir)<br>Crystalluria (indinavir, maintain hydration)<br>Elevated transaminases<br>Lopinavir is only available in combination with ritonavir |
| **Fusion inhibitor** | | |
| Enfuvirtide | **Binds gp41** and **inhibits fusion** of HIV-1 to CD4+ cells | Local injection reactions (100% patients)<br>Hypersensitivity reactions |
| **CCR5 antagonist** | | |
| Maraviroc (MVC) | **Blocks CCR5 receptor**, preventing HIV entry into target cells | Hepatotoxicity, orthostatic hypotension |
| **Integrase inhibitor** | | |
| Raltegravir (RAL) | **Inhibits integrase**, thus blocking viral integration | CPK elevation |

## HYPERSENSITIVITY REACTIONS

| Type | Antibody | Complement | Effector Cells | Examples |
|---|---|---|---|---|
| I (immediate) | **IgE** | No | **Basophil, mast cell** | Hay fever, atopic dermatitis, **insect venom sensitivity**, **anaphylaxis** to drugs, some food allergies, allergy to animals and animal products, **asthma** |
| II (cytotoxic) | IgG, IgM | Yes | PMN, macrophages, NK cells | Autoimmune or drug-induced hemolytic anemia, transfusion reactions, **HDNB**, hyperacute graft rejection, **Goodpasture disease**, **rheumatic fever** |
| II (noncytotoxic) | IgG | **No** | None | Myasthenia gravis, Graves disease, type 2 diabetes mellitus |
| III (immune complex) | IgG, IgM | Yes | PMN, macrophages | **SLE, RA**, polyarteritis nodosa, poststreptococcal glomerulonephritis, Arthus reaction, serum sickness |
| IV (delayed, DTH) | None | No | CTL, TH1, macrophages | **Tuberculin test**, tuberculosis, leprosy, Hashimoto thyroiditis, poison ivy (**contact dermatitis**), acute graft rejection, **GVHD**, IDDM |

*Definition of abbreviations:* GVHD, graft-versus-host disease; HDNB, hemolytic disease of the newborn; IDDM, insulin-dependent diabetes mellitus; RA, rheumatoid arthritis; SLE, systemic lupus erythematosus.

## IMPORTANT AUTOIMMUNE DISEASES

| Autoantibodies | Clinical Features | Comments |
|---|---|---|
| **Systemic lupus erythematosus:** chronic systemic autoimmune disease characterized by a loss of self-tolerance and production of autoantibodies | | |
| Antinuclear antibody (ANA) (>95%): <br><br>**Anti-dsDNA** (40–60%) <br>**Anti-Sm** (20–30%) | • Hemolytic anemia, thrombocytopenia, leukopenia <br>• Arthritis <br>• Skin rashes (including classic "malar" rash) <br>• Renal disease <br>• Libman-Sacks endocarditis <br>• Serositis <br>• Neurologic symptoms | • Females >> Males (M:F = 1:9), peak age 20–45 years, African American > Caucasian <br>• Mechanism of injury: type II and III hypersensitivity reactions <br>• Treatment: steroids and other immunosuppressants |
| **Sjögren syndrome:** an autoimmune disease characterized by destruction of the lacrimal and salivary glands, resulting in the inability to produce saliva or tears | | |
| Antiribonucleoprotein antibodies: <br><br>Anti-SS-A (Ro) <br>Anti-SS-B (La) | • Keratoconjuctivitis sicca (dry eyes) and corneal ulcers <br>• Xerostomia (dry mouth) <br>• Mikulicz syndrome: enlargement of the salivary and lacrimal glands | • Females > males; age range: 30–50 years <br>• Often associated with rheumatoid arthritis and other autoimmune diseases (e.g., SLE) <br>• Increased risk of developing lymphoma |

*(Continued)*

## IMPORTANT AUTOIMMUNE DISEASES (CONT'D.)

| Autoantibodies | Clinical Features | Comments |
|---|---|---|
| **Scleroderma (progressive systemic sclerosis):** characterized by fibroblast stimulation and deposition of collagen in the skin and internal organs; females > males; age range: 20–55 years; activation of fibroblasts by growth factors/cytokines leads to fibrosis | | |
| **Diffuse Scleroderma** | | |
| **Anti-DNA topoisomerase I antibodies (Scl-70)** (70%) | Widespread skin involvement<br>Early involvement of the visceral organs<br>• Esophagus—dysphagia<br>• GI tract—malabsorption<br>• Pulmonary fibrosis—dyspnea on exertion<br>• Cardiac fibrosis—arrhythmias<br>• Kidney fibrosis—renal insufficiency | Raynaud phenomenon is seen in almost all patients and often preceeds other symptoms.<br><br>**Treatment:** vasodilators, ACE inhibitors, NSAIDs, steroids, d-penicillamine |
| **Limited scleroderma (e.g., CREST syndrome)** | | |
| **Anticentromere antibodies** | • Skin involvement of the face and hands<br>• Late involvement of visceral organs (relatively benign clinical course) | (**C**alcinosis, **R**aynaud phenomenon, **E**sophageal dysmotility, **S**clerodactyly, **T**elangiectasia) |

# TRANSPLANTATION IMMUNOLOGY

## GRAFTS USED IN MEDICINE

| Grafts | Definition |
|---|---|
| Autologous (**autografts**) | Tissue is moved from one location to another in the same individual |
| **Isograft** | Transplants between genetically identical individuals (monozygotic twins) |
| **Allograft** | Transplants between genetically different members of the same species |
| **Xenograft** | Transplants between members of different species |

## GRAFT REJECTION REACTIONS

| Type of Rejection | Time Taken | Cause |
|---|---|---|
| Hyperacute | Minutes to hours | Preformed anti-donor antibodies and complement |
| Accelerated | Days | Reactivation of sensitized T cells |
| **Acute** | Days to weeks | Primary activation of T cells |
| **Chronic** | Months to years | Causes are unclear: antibodies, immune complexes, slow cellular reaction, recurrence of disease |
| **Graft versus host** | Weeks to months | Grafted bone marrow T cells attack host |

# Microbiology

## General Principles

## Bacteriology

## Antibacterial Agents

## Parasites

## Virology

## Mycology

# GENERAL PRINCIPLES OF MICROBIOLOGY

## COMPARISON OF MEDICALLY IMPORTANT MICROBIAL GROUPS

| Characteristic | Viruses | Bacteria | Fungi | Parasites |
|---|---|---|---|---|
| Diameter | Minute (0.02–0.3 μ) | Small (0.3–2 μ) | 3–10 μ | 15–25 μ (trophozoites) |
| Cell type | **Acellular**—no nucleus | **Prokaryotic cells** | **Eukaryotic cells** | |
| | • DNA or RNA<br>• 1 nucleocapsid, except in segmented or diploid viruses | • DNA and RNA<br>• 1 chromosome<br>• **No histones** | • DNA and RNA<br>• More than one chromosome | |
| | Replicates in host cells | DNA replicates continuously | G and S phases | |
| | | Exons, **no introns** | Introns and exons | |
| | Some have polycistronic mRNA and post-translational cleavage | **Mono- and polycistronic mRNA** | **Monocistronic RNA** | |
| | Uses host organelles; obligate intracellular parasites | **No membrane-bound organelles** | Mitochondria and other membrane-bound organelles | |
| | No ribosomes | **70S ribosomes (30S+50S)** | **80S** ribosomes (40S+60S) | |
| Replication | Make and assemble viral components | **Binary fission (asexual)** | Cytokinesis with mitosis/meiosis | |
| Cellular membrane | Some are enveloped, but no membrane function | Membranes have **no sterols, except** *Mycoplasma*, which have cholesterol | Membrane **ergosterol** is major sterol | Sterols, such as **cholesterol** |
| Cell wall | No cell wall | **Peptidoglycan** | Complex carbohydrate **cell wall: chitin**, glucans, or mannans | No cell wall |

Note: Prions are infectious proteins (contain no nucleic acids). They are the agents of kuru, mad cow disease, etc.

# BACTERIOLOGY

## BACTERIAL GROWTH CURVE

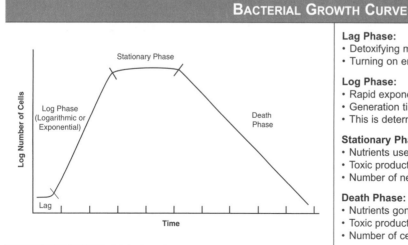

**Lag Phase:**
• Detoxifying medium
• Turning on enzymes to utilize medium

**Log Phase:**
• Rapid exponential growth
• Generation time—time it takes one cell to divide into two
• This is determined during log phase

**Stationary Phase:**
• Nutrients used up
• Toxic products begin to accumulate
• Number of new cells = the number of dying cells

**Death Phase:**
• Nutrients gone
• Toxic products kill cells
• Number of cells dying exceeds the number of cells dividing

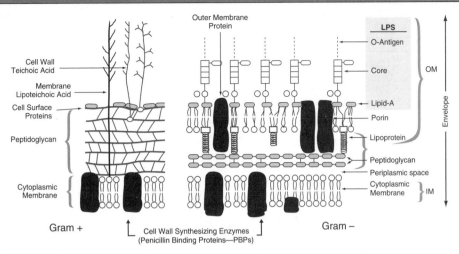

| Envelope Structure | Gram ⊕ or ⊖ | Chemical Composition | Function |
|---|---|---|---|
| **Capsule** (nonessential) = slime = glycocalyx | Both Gram ⊕ and Gram ⊖ | **Polysaccharide gel** (except *B. anthracis*: poly-D-glutamate) | • **Antiphagocytic** <br> • **Immunogenic** (except *S. pyogenes* and *N. meningitidis*, type B) |
| **Outer membrane** | **Gram ⊖ only** | Phospholipid/proteins LPS: <br> • Lipid A <br> • Polysaccharide | Hydrophobic membrane: <br> • **LPS = endotoxin** <br> • **Lipid A = toxic moiety** <br> • PS = immunogenic portion |
| | | Outer membrane proteins | Attachment, virulence, etc. |
| | | Protein porins | Passive transport |
| **Cell wall** = peptidoglycan | Gram ⊕ (thick) Gram ⊖ (thin) | **Peptidoglycan**—open 3-D net of: <br> • *N*-acetyl-glucosamine <br> • *N*-acetyl-muramic acid <br> • Amino acids (including DAP) | • Rigid support, cell shape, and protection from osmotic damage <br> • Synthesis **inhibited by penicillins and** cephalosporins <br> • **Confers Gram reaction** |
| | **Gram ⊕ only** | **Teichoic acids** | • Immunogenic, induces TNF-α, IL-1 <br> • **Attachment** |
| | **Acid-fast** only | **Mycolic acids** | • Acid-fastness <br> • **Resistance to drying and chemicals** |
| Periplasmic space | **Gram ⊖ only** | "Storage space" between the inner and outer membranes | • Enzymes to break down large molecules (β-lactamases) <br> • Aids regulation of osmolarity |
| Cytoplasmic membrane = inner membrane = cell membrane = plasma membrane | Gram ⊕ Gram ⊖ | Phospholipid bilayer with many embedded proteins | • Hydrophobic cell "sac" <br> • Selective permeability and active transport <br> • **Carrier for enzymes** for: <br>   – Oxidative metabolism <br>   – Phosphorylation <br>   – Phospholipid synthesis <br>   – DNA replication <br>   – Peptidoglycan cross linkage <br> • **Penicillin binding proteins** (PBPs) |

*Definition of abbreviation:* DAP, diaminopimelic acid; LPS, lipopolysaccharide.

## NORMAL FLORA ORGANISMS

Most infectious disease vignettes begin with the necessity to rule out the normal flora organisms that are cultured from the patient. Make sure you know those organisms that can confound a simple Gram-stain type of diagnosis, e.g., notice in the oropharynx and vagina, normal flora organisms can be indistinguishable from pathogens by Gram stain alone!

| Site | Common or Medically Important Organisms | Less Common but Notable Organisms |
|---|---|---|
| Blood, internal organs | None, generally sterile | — |
| Cutaneous surfaces | *Staphylococcus epidermidis* | *Staphylococcus aureus, Corynebacteria* (diphtheroids), streptococci, anaerobes, e.g., peptostreptococci, *Candida* spp. |
| Nose | *Staphylococcus aureus* | *S. epidermidis,* diphtheroids, assorted streptococci |
| Oropharynx | **Viridans streptococci**, including *Streptococcus mutans* | Assorted streptococci, **nonpathogenic *Neisseria*, nontypeable *Haemophilus influenzae*,** *Candida albicans* |
| Gingival crevices | Anaerobes: *Bacteroides, Prevotella, Fusobacterium, Streptococcus, Actinomyces* | — |
| Stomach | None | — |
| Colon (microaerophilic/anaerobic) | Adult: ***Bacteroides**/Prevotella* (predominant organism), *Escherichia, Bifidobacterium* | *Eubacterium, Fusobacterium, Lactobacillus*, assorted gram-negative anaerobic rods; *Enterococcus faecalis* and other streptococci |
| Vagina | **Lactobacillus** | Assorted streptococci, gram-negative rods, diphtheroids, yeasts, *Veillonella* (gram-negative diplococcus) |

## BACTERIAL TOXINS

### Endotoxin

**Endotoxin** (lipopolysaccharide = LPS) is part of the gram-negative outer membrane. It is encoded on the chromosome.

- The toxic portion is lipid A. LPS is heat stable and not strongly immunogenic, so it cannot be converted to a toxoid.
- LPS activates macrophages, leading to release of TNF-$\alpha$, IL-1, IL-6, and nitric oxide (NO). IL-1 is a major mediator of fever. Damage to the endothelium from bradykinin-induced vasodilation leads to shock. Coagulation (DIC) is mediated through the activation of Hageman factor. NO production causes hypotension, which contributes to shock.

### Exotoxin

**Exotoxins** are protein toxins, generally quite toxic, and secreted by bacterial cells. They are encoded on plasmids or in lysogenic phage genomes.

- Exotoxins can be modified by chemicals or heat to produce a toxoid that still is immunogenic, but no longer toxic, so it can be used as a vaccine.
- Most are A-B (or "two") component protein toxins. B component binds to specific cell receptors to facilitate the internalization of A (the active [toxic] component)

## MAJOR EXOTOXINS

| | Organism (Gram) | Toxin | Mode of Action | Role in Disease |
|---|---|---|---|---|
| **Protein synthesis inhibitors** | Corynebacterium diphtheriae (⊕) | **Diphtheria toxin** | • ADP ribosyl transferase **inactivates eEF-2**<br>• *Targets:* **heart, nerves, epithelium** | Inhibits eukaryotic cell protein synthesis |
| | Pseudomonas aeruginosa (⊖) | **Exotoxin A** | • ADP ribosyl transferase **inactivates eEF-2**<br>• *Target:* **liver** | Inhibits eukaryotic cell protein synthesis |
| | Shigella dysenteriae (⊖) | **Shiga toxin** | **Interferes with 60S ribosomal subunit** | • Inhibits protein synthesis in eukaryotic cells<br>• Enterotoxic, cytotoxic, and neurotoxic |
| | Enterohemorrhagic E. coli (EHEC) (⊖) | **Verotoxin** (shiga-like) | **Interferes with 60S ribosomal subunit** | Inhibits protein synthesis in eukaryotic cells |
| **Neurotoxins** | Clostridium tetani (⊕) | **Tetanus toxin** | **Blocks release of glycine and GABA** | Inhibits neurotransmission in inhibitory synapses |
| | Clostridium botulinum (⊕) | **Botulinum toxin** | **Blocks release of acetylcholine** | Inhibits cholinergic synapses |
| **Superantigens** | **Staphylococcus aureus** (⊕) | **TSST-1** | • Induces IL-1, IL-6, TNF-α, IFN-γ<br>• Decreases liver clearance of LPS | Fever, increased susceptibility to LPS, rash, shock, capillary leakage |
| | **Streptococcus pyogenes** (⊕) | **Exotoxin A**, also called erythrogenic or pyrogenic toxin | **Similar to TSST-1** | Fever, increased susceptibility to LPS, rash, shock, capillary leakage, cardiotoxicity |
| **cAMP inducers** | Enterotoxigenic Escherichia coli (⊖) | **Heat labile toxin** (LT) | LT stimulates an adenylate cyclase by **ADP ribosylation of GTP-binding protein** | Both LT and ST promote secretion of fluid and electrolytes from intestinal epithelium |
| | Vibrio cholerae (⊖) | **Cholera toxin** | **Similar to E. coli LT** | Profuse, watery diarrhea |
| | Bacillus anthracis (⊕) | **Anthrax toxin (3 proteins** make 2 toxins) | • **EF = edema factor = adenylate cyclase**<br>• **LF = lethal factor**<br>• **PA = protective antigen (B component for both)** | • Decreases phagocytosis<br>• Causes **edema, kills cells** |
| | Bordetella pertussis (⊖) | **Pertussis toxin** | **ADP ribosylates $G_i$,** the negative regulator of adenylate cyclase, leading to increased cAMP | • **Histamine sensitizing**<br>• **Lymphocytosis promotion** (inhibits chemokine receptors)<br>• **Islet activation** |
| **Cytolysins** | **Clostridium perfringens** (⊕) | **Alpha toxin** | **Lecithinase** | • Damages cell membranes<br>• **Myonecrosis** |
| | **Staphylococcus aureus** (⊕) | **Alpha toxin** | **Pore former** | Membrane becomes leaky |

## IMPORTANT PATHOGENIC FACTORS AND DIAGNOSTIC ENZYMES

| Factor | Function | Organisms |
|---|---|---|
| All **capsules** | **Antiphagocytic** | *Streptococcus pneumoniae*, *Klebsiella pneumoniae*, *Haemophilus influenzae*, *Pseudomonas aeruginosa*, *Neisseria meningitidis*, *Cryptococcus neoformans* (mnemonic: **s**ome **k**illers **h**ave **p**retty **n**ice **c**apsules) and many more |
| M protein | Antiphagocytic | Group A streptococci |
| A protein | Binds Fc of IgG to inhibit opsonization and phagocytosis | *Staphylococcus aureus* |
| **Lipoteichoic acid** | Attachment to host cells | All **gram-positive** bacteria |
| All **pili** | Attachment | Many gram-negatives |
| **Pili of *N. gonorrhoeae*** | **Antiphagocytic, antigenic variation** | *N. gonorrhoeae* |
| Hyaluronidase | Hydrolysis of ground substance | Group A streptococci |
| Collagenase | Hydrolysis of collagen | *Clostridium perfringens*, *Prevotella melaninogenica* |
| **Urease** | Increases pH of locale, contributes to kidney stones | ***P**roteus*, ***U**reaplasma*, ***N**ocardia*, ***C**ryptococcus*, ***H**elicobacter* (mnemonic: **PUNCH**) |
| Kinases | Hydrolysis of fibrin | *Streptococcus, Staphylococcus* |
| Lecithinase | Destroys cell membranes | *Clostridium perfringens* |
| Heparinase | Thrombophlebitis | *Bacteroides* |
| **Catalase** | Destroys hydrogen peroxide **(major problem for CGD patients)** | • Most important: *Staphylococcus, Pseudomonas, Aspergillus,* Candida, Enterobacteriaceae<br>• Most anaerobes lack catalase |
| IgA proteases | Destroy IgA, promote colonization of mucosal surfaces | *Neisseria, Haemophilus, Streptococcus pneumoniae* |
| Oxidase | Cytochrome c oxidase is the terminal electron acceptor | *Neisseria* and most gram-negatives, except the *Enterobacteriaceae* |
| **Coagulase** | Produces fibrin clot | ***Staphylococcus aureus*** and *Yersinia pestis* |

## UNUSUAL GROWTH REQUIREMENTS

| Requirements in Culture | Organism |
|---|---|
| Factors **X and V** | ***Haemophilus*** |
| **Cholesterol** | *Mycoplasma* |
| **High salt** | *Staphylococcus aureus*, group D **enterococci** and ***Vibrio*** |
| **Cysteine** | ***Francisella, Legionella, Brucella,* and *Pasteurella*** **(mnemonic:** the 4 Sisters "ELLA" worship in the Cysteine Chapel) |
| **High temperature (42° C)** | ***Campylobacter*** |
| **Lower than atmospheric oxygen pressure (microaerophilic); special CO$_2$ incubator** | ***Campylobacter*** and ***Helicobacter*** |

## BACTERIAL GENETICS

| Recombination | **Homologous**: The one-to-one exchange of linear extrachromosomal DNA for homologous alleles within the chromosome, using recombinase A<br>**Site-specific**: The incorporation of extrachromosomal circles of DNA into another molecule of DNA using restriction endonucleases |
|---|---|
| Conjugation | The donation of chromosomal or plasmid genes from one bacterium to another through a conjugal bridge.<br>• **F+ cells** have a fertility factor plasmid and serve as donors of plasmid DNA<br>• **F− cells** do not have fertility factors and serve as the recipients of DNA in any cross.<br>• **Hfr cells** have incorporated a fertility factor plasmid into their chromosome by site-specific recombination and serve as donors of chromosomal DNA<br>• Conjugation is the most important means of transfer of drug resistance genes in gram-negative bacilli |
| Transduction | The delivery of bacterial genes from one bacterium to another via a virus vector.<br>• **Generalized transduction**: Transfer of any genes from one bacterium to another via an accident in the assembly of a virus with a lytic life cycle.<br>• **Specialized transduction**: The transfer of bacterial chromosomal genes located near the insertion site of a temperate phage from one bacterium to another via an accident of excision.<br>• Transduction has been shown to be the means of transfer of drug resistance to methicillin (MRSA) and imipenem (*Pseudomonas*). |
| Transformation | The uptake and incorporation of free DNA from the environment by competent cells followed by homologous recombination.<br>• Transformation is an important means of transfer of traits in bacteria that are naturally competent (*Streptococcus pneumoniae, Helicobacter, Neisseria,* and *Haemophilus influenzae*) |
| Lysogeny | The stable association of DNA molecules between a bacterium and a temperate phage.<br>• It imparts the important traits: **O** = *Salmonella* O antigen, **B**= Botulinum toxin, **E** = Erythrogenic toxin of *Streptococcus pyogenes,* **D** = Diphtheria toxin; **Mnemonic: OBED** (or a little pregnant with phage).<br>• Bacterial cells with stably integrated temperate phage DNA are said to have undergone **lysogenic conversion**, e.g., cholera toxin and Shiga toxins. |
| Transposon | A mobile genetic element capable of movement within a cell.<br>• They move by a variation of site-specific recombination and are responsible for the formation of multiple drug-resistance plasmids.<br>• VRSA has arisen because *Enterococcus* donated a multi-drug resistance plasmid, produced by transposition, to MRSA. |

# ANTIBACTERIAL AGENTS

## MECHANISMS OF ACTION OF ANTIMICROBIAL AGENTS

| Mechanism of Action | Antimicrobial Agents |
|---|---|
| Inhibition of bacterial cell-wall synthesis | Penicillins, cephalosporins, imipenem/meropenem, aztreonam, vancomycin |
| Inhibition of bacterial protein synthesis | Aminoglycosides, chloramphenicol, macrolides, tetracyclines, streptogramins, linezolid |
| Inhibition of DNA replication or transcription | Fluoroquinolones, rifampin |
| Inhibition of nucleic acid synthesis | Trimethoprim, flucytosine |
| Inhibition of folic acid synthesis | Sulfonamides, trimethoprim, pyrimethamine |
| Disruption of cell membrane function | Azole and polyene antifungal agents |

## CELL WALL SYNTHESIS INHIBITORS

| Class/Example | Mechanism of Action/Resistance | Spectrum | Toxicity/Notes |
|---|---|---|---|
| **Penicillins** | | | |
| **Narrow spectrum, β-lactamase sensitive:** penicillin G, penicillin V | **Mechanism:** inhibit cross-linking of peptidoglycan component of cell wall by transpeptidases; action mediated by binding of penicillin-binding proteins (PBPs) | Gram-positives<br>*N. meningitidis*<br>Clostridia<br>Syphilis<br>*Leptospira*<br>Staph ubiquitously resistant | — |
| **Very narrow spectrum, β-lactamase resistant:** methicillin, nafcillin, oxacillin | **Resistance:** production of β-lactamases, which cleave the β-lactam ring structure; change in PBPs; change in porins | Gram-positives, especially *S. aureus* | Resistant staph emerging "MRSA" |
| **Broad spectrum, aminopenicillins, β-lactamase sensitive:** ampicillin, amoxicillin | | Gram-positives, enterococci,<br>  *H. influenzae*<br>*L monocytogenes*<br>*M. catarrhalis*<br>*E. coli* | Activity may be augmented with penicillinase **β-lactamase inhibitors** (e.g., clavulanic acid, sulbactam, and tazobactam) |
| **Extended spectrum, antipseudomonal, β-lactamase sensitive:** mezlocillin, piperacillin, carbenicillin, ticarcillin | | • Gram-negatives, including **Pseudomonas**<br>• Enterococci (mezlocillin and piperacillin) | — |
| **Cephalosporins** | | | |
| **First generation:** cefazolin, cephalexin | **Mechanism:** inhibition of cell wall formation similar to penicillins | Gram-positives<br>*Proteus mirabilis*<br>*E. coli*<br>*Klebsiella pneumoniae* | • Cross-allergenicity with penicillins occurs in 5%<br>• Anaphylaxis, but not rash, a contraindication in penicillin-sensitive pt.<br>• Disulfiram-like effects (cefotetan) |
| **Second generation:** cefotetan, cefoxitin, cefuroxime, cefaclor | **Resistance:** same as penicillins | Less gram-positive activity and more gram-negative activity than first generation<br>  • *B. fragilis*<br>  • *H. influenzae*<br>  • *M. catarrhalis*<br>  • *P. mirabilis*<br>  • *E. coli*<br>  • *K. pneumoniae*<br>  • *Neisseria, Enterobacter* | |
| **Third generation:** ceftazidime, cefoperazone, cefotaxime, ceftriaxone | | Less gram-positive activity and more gram-negative activity than second generation<br>  • *Serratia* sp.<br>  • *Borrelia burgdorferi*<br>  • *H. influenzae*<br>  • *Neisseria*<br>  • *Enterobacter*<br>Some have anti-*Pseudomonas* activity | • Most penetrate **blood-brain** barrier (not cefoperazone)<br>• Reserved for serious infections<br>• Disulfiram-like effects (cefoperazone) |
| **Fourth generation:** cefepime | | More gram-negative activity while retaining first-generation gram-positive activity | More resistant to β-lactamases |

*(Continued)*

## CELL WALL SYNTHESIS INHIBITORS (CONT'D.)

| Class/Example | Mechanism of Action/Resistance | Spectrum | Toxicity/Notes |
|---|---|---|---|
| **Carbapenems and Monobactams** | | | |
| Carbapenems (meropenem, imipenem) | Similar mechanism to penicillins and cephalosporins | Gram-positives, gram-negative rods, anaerobes | • **Nephrotoxic**<br>• GI distress<br>• Rash<br>• CNS toxicity<br>• **Cilastatin administered concurrently** with imipenem increases the drug's half-life and reduces nephrotoxicity<br>• Beta-lactamase resistant |
| Monobactams (aztreonam) | | Gram-negative rods | • GI distress with superinfection, vertigo, headache<br>• Synergistic with aminoglycosides<br>• Beta-lactamase resistant |
| **Non-Beta Lactam Cell Wall Synthesis Inhibitors** | | | |
| Vancomycin | Binds cell wall precursors (D-ala-D-ala muramyl pentapeptide), preventing polymerization, peptidoglycan elongation | Drug resistant gram-positives, e.g., MRSA sepsis (IV) or *C. difficile* (oral [not absorbed from lumen]) | • Chills, fever, ototoxicity, nephrotoxicity<br>• Flushing or **"red man syndrome"** upon rapid infusion<br>• Resistant strains (VRSA, VRE) emerging |

*Definition of abbreviations:* VRE, vancomycin-resistant enterococcus; VRSA, vancomycin-resistant *Staphylococcus aureus*

## SUMMARY OF MECHANISMS OF PROTEIN SYNTHESIS INHIBITION

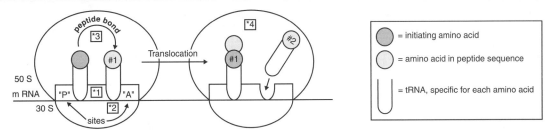

| Event | Antibiotics and Binding Sites | Mechanism |
|---|---|---|
| 1. Formation of initiation complex | Aminoglycosides (30S)<br>Linezolid (50S) | Interfere with initiation codon functions—block association of 50S ribosomal subunit with mRNA-30S (bacteriostatic); misreading of code—incorporation of wrong amino acid (bactericidal) |
| 2. Amino-acid incorporation | Tetracyclines (30S)<br>Dalfopristin/quinupristin (50S) | Block the attachment of aminoacyl tRNA to acceptor site (bacteriostatic) |
| 3. Formation of peptide bond | Chloramphenicol (50S) | Inhibit the activity of peptidyltransferase (bacteriostatic) |
| 4. Translocation | Macrolides and clindamycin (50S) | Inhibit translocation of peptidyl tRNA from acceptor to donor site (bacteriostatic) |

## PROTEIN SYNTHESIS INHIBITORS

| Drug/Class | Site of Inhibition | Spectrum | Mechanisms of Resistance | Toxicities | Notes |
|---|---|---|---|---|---|
| Chloramphenicol | 50S | Wide spectrum, including:<br>• *H. influenzae*<br>• *N. meningitidis*<br>• *Bacteroides*<br>• *Rickettsia*<br>• *Salmonella* | Plasmid-mediated acetyltransferases that inactivate the drug | • **"Gray baby" syndrome** (↓ glucuronyl transferase in neonates)<br>• **Aplastic anemia**/bone marrow suppression<br>• GI irritation | • Toxicity limits clinical use<br>• Reserved for severe *Salmonella* and bacterial meningitis in β-lactam–sensitive patients |
| Tetracyclines:<br>• tetracycline<br>• doxycycline<br>• minocycline | 30S | Gram ⊕ and Gram ⊖:<br>• *Rickettsia*<br>• *Chlamydia*<br>• *Mycoplasma*<br>• *H. pylori*<br>• *Brucella*<br>• *Vibrio* | Plasmid-mediated efflux pumps and reduced uptake via transport systems | • GI irritation<br>• **Tooth enamel dysplasia**<br>• **Bone growth irregularities**<br>• Hepatotoxic<br>• **Photosensitivity**<br>• Vestibular toxicity | • **Fanconi syndrome** with expired tetracycline<br>• Oral absorption limited by multivalent cations |
| Macrolides:<br>• erythromycin,<br>• azithromycin<br>• clarithromycin | 50S | Gram ⊕, some Gram ⊖:<br>• *Chlamydia*<br>• *Mycoplasma*<br>• *Ureaplasma*<br>• *Legionella*<br>• *Campylobacter* | Methylation of binding site on 50S; increased efflux from multidrug exporters | • **GI irritation**<br>• Cholestasis<br>• Hepatitis<br>• Skin rashes<br>• ↓ CYP3A4 (except azithromycin) | Useful in atypical pneumonia |
| Ketolides:<br>• Telithromycin | 50S | Similar spectrum to macrolides | Many macrolide-resistant strains are susceptible to ketolides | • Severe hepatotoxicity<br>• Visual disturbances<br>• Fainting | Its use is limited because of toxicity |
| Clindamycin | 50S | Narrow spectrum: Gram ⊕, anaerobes | Methylation of binding site on 50S | • GI irritation<br>• Skin rash<br>• ***C. difficile* superinfection** | — |
| Aminoglycosides:<br>• gentamicin<br>• neomycin<br>• tobramycin<br>• streptomycin | 30S | Gram ⊖ rods | Plasmid-mediated **group transferases** | Ototoxicity, nephrotoxicity | Neomycin for bowel prep (stays in bowel lumen) |
| Oxazolidinones:<br>• linezolid | 50S | Gram ⊕ cocci | Resistance rare | • Thrombocytopenia, neutropenia, esp. in immunocompromised<br>• MAO inhibition (dietary and drug restrictions) | No cross-resistance with other protein synthesis inhibitors, so often reserved for resistant infections |

## FOLIC ACID SYNTHESIS INHIBITORS

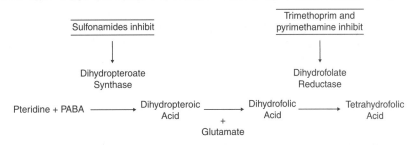

| Class/Drug | Mechanism of Action | Spectrum | Mechanism of Resistance | Toxicity | Notes |
|---|---|---|---|---|---|
| Sulfonamides | PABA antimetabolite inhibits bacterial dihydropteroate synthase, thus curbing folate synthesis | Gram ⊖, gram ⊕, *Chlamydia*, *Nocardia* | Decreased accumulation of drugs, decreased affinity of drug for **dihydropteroate synthase** | • Hypersensitivity<br>• Hemolytic anemia in G6PD-deficient<br>• Nephrotoxicity<br>• Kernicterus in newborns | Combined with trimethoprim for increased efficacy |
| Trimethoprim | Inhibits bacterial dihydrofolate reductase, thus inhibiting folate synthesis | *H. influenzae*<br>*M. catarrhalis* | Production of bacterial **dihydrofolate reductase** with decreased affinity for drug | • Megaloblastic anemia<br>• Leukopenia<br>• Granulocytopenia | • Adverse effects may be reduced by concurrent **folinic acid**<br>• Good for UTIs because it is excreted in urine unchanged |

## DNA REPLICATION INHIBITORS

| Class/Drug | Mechanism of Action | Spectrum | Mechanism of Resistance | Toxicity | Notes |
|---|---|---|---|---|---|
| **Fluoroquinolones:**<br>• ciprofloxacin<br>• ofloxacin<br>• levofloxacin | Interfere with bacterial DNA topoisomerase II and IV (DNA gyrase), resulting in inhibition of DNA synthesis | Gram ⊖ rods, *Neisseria*, occasional gram ⊕ | • Decreased intracellular drug concentrations through efflux pumps and altered porins<br>• Alteration of drug's binding site | • **GI distress**<br>• Skin rash<br>• Superinfection | Contraindicated in pregnancy due to cartilage formation abnormalities in animal studies |

## MISCELLANEOUS

| Class/Drug | Mechanism of Action | Spectrum | Mechanism of Resistance | Toxicity | Notes |
|---|---|---|---|---|---|
| Metronidazole | When reduced, interferes with nucleic acid synthesis (bactericidal) | Anaerobes (except *Actinomyces*) | Rare plasma-mediated resistance | • GI distress<br>• Disulfiram-like reaction with alcohol<br>• Peripheral neuropathy, ataxia | • Strong metallic taste<br>• DOC in pseudomembranous colitis |

*Definition of abbreviations:* DOC, drug of choice; G6PD, glucose-6-phosphate dehydrogenase; PABA, para-aminobenzoic acid; UTI, urinary tract Infection.

# PARASITES

## OBLIGATE INTRACELLULAR PARASITES

- Cannot be cultured on inert media. Intracellular organisms (both obligate and facultative) protected from antibody and complement. Intracellular pathogens tend to elicit cell-mediated immune responses, so end pathologic lesion frequently a granuloma
- **All rickettsiae, chlamydiae, *Mycobacterium leprae***
- **All viruses**
- ***Plasmodium, Toxoplasma gondii, Babesia*,** *Leishmania, Trypanosoma cruzi* (amastigotes in cardiac muscle)

## FACULTATIVE INTRACELLULAR PARASITES

- Live inside phagocytic cells in the body, but can be cultured on inert media
- *Francisella tularensis,* **Listeria monocytogenes, Mycobacterium tuberculosis**, *Brucella* species, nontuberculous mycobacteria, *Salmonella typhi, Legionella pneumophila, Yersinia pestis, Nocardia, Borrelia burgdorferi,* **Histoplasma capsulatum**

## PROTOZOANS

| Common Name | Amebae | Flagellates | Apicomplexa (Intracellular) |
|---|---|---|---|
| Important genera | ***Entamoeba***<br>*Naegleria*<br>*Acanthamoeba* | LUMINAL (GUT, UG)<br>**Trichomonas**<br>**Giardia**<br>HEMOFLAGELLATES<br>*Leishmania*<br>*Trypanosoma* | BLOOD/TISSUE<br>**Plasmodium**<br>**Toxoplasma**<br>*Babesia*<br>INTESTINAL<br>**Cryptosporidium**<br>*Isospora* |

| PROTOZOAN PARASITES | | | | |
|---|---|---|---|---|
| **Species** | **Disease/ Organs Most Affected** | **Form/Transmission** | **Diagnosis** | **Treatment** |
| *Entamoeba histolytica* | • **Amebiasis:** dysentery<br>• **Inverted, flask-shaped lesions** in large intestine with extension to peritoneum and liver, lungs, brain, and heart<br>• Blood and pus in stool<br>• Liver abscesses | • Cysts<br>• Fecal-oral transmission: water, fresh fruits, and vegetables<br>• Travel to tropics | • Trophozoites or cysts (with 4 nuclei) in stool<br><br>• Nuclei have sharp central karyosome and fine chromatin "spokes"<br><br>• Serology | Metronidazole followed by iodoquinol |
| *Giardia lamblia* | **Giardiasis:** Ventral sucking disk attaches to lining of duodenal wall, causing a **fatty**, foul-smelling diarrhea (diarrhea → *malabsorption* in duodenum, jejunum) | • Cysts<br>• Fecal (human, beaver, muskrat, etc.), oral transmission: water, food, day care, oral-anal sex<br>• Campers and hikers | • Trophozoites or cysts in stool or fecal antigen test (replaces "string" test)<br><br>• "Falling leaf" motility | Metronidazole |
| *Cryptosporidium* **spp.** | Cryptosporidiosis: transient diarrhea in healthy; severe in immunocompromised hosts | • Cysts<br>• Undercooked meat, water; not killed by chlorination | Acid fast oocysts in stool: biopsy shows dots (cysts) in intestinal glands | Nitazoxanide, puromycin, azithromycin |
| *Trichomonas vaginalis* (urogenital) | Trichomoniasis: frothy green, unpleasant smelling vaginal discharge, itching, burning vaginitis | • Trophozoites<br>• **Sexual** | Motile trophozoites in methylene blue wet mount | Metronidazole |

| FREE-LIVING AMEBAE THAT OCCASIONALLY INFECT HUMANS | | | | |
|---|---|---|---|---|
| **Species** | **Disease/Locale** | **Form/Transmission** | **Diagnosis** | **Treatment** |
| *Naegleria* | **Primary amebic meningoencephalitis** (PAM): severe prefrontal headache, nausea, high fever, often an altered sense of smell; often fatal | • Free-living amebae picked up while swimming or **diving in very warm fresh water**<br>• Penetrates cribriform plate | • Motile trophozoites in CSF<br>• Culture on plates seeded with gram ⊖ bacteria; amebae will leave trails | Amphotericin B (rarely successful) |
| *Acanthamoeba* | **Keratitis; GAE** in immunocompromised patients; insidious onset but progressive to death | • Free-living amebae in contaminated **contact lens solution (airborne cysts)**<br>• Not certain for GAE; inhalation or contact with contaminated soil or water | • Star-shaped cysts on biopsy; rarely seen in CSF<br>• Culture as above | Keratitis: topical miconazole and propamidine isethionate<br>GAE: sulfadiazine (rarely successful) |

*Definition of abbreviations:* CSF, cerebrospinal fluid; GAE, granulomatous amaebic encephalitis.

# PLASMODIUM LIFE CYCLE

Each *Plasmodium* has two distinct hosts:

- A vertebrate, such as the human (intermediate host), where asexual phase (schizogony) takes place in the liver and red blood cells
- An arthropod (definitive) host (*Anopheles* mosquito), where gametogony (sexual phase) and sporogony take place

Disease is caused by a variety of mechanisms, including metabolism of hemoglobin and lysis of infected cells, leading to anemia and to agglutination of the infected RBCs. Paroxysms (chills, fever spike, and malarial rigors) occur when the infected RBCs are lysed, liberating a new crop of merozoites.

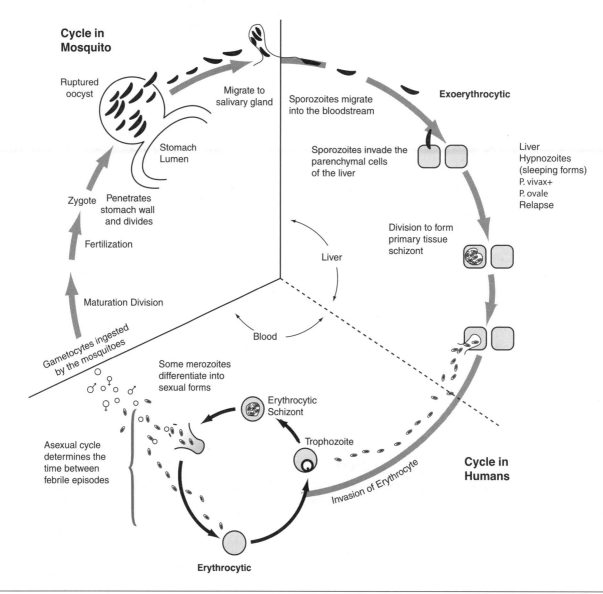

*Definition of abbreviation:* RBCs, red blood cells.

## PLASMODIUM SPECIES

| Species | Disease | Important Features | Blood Smears | Liver Stages | Treatment |
|---|---|---|---|---|---|
| *Plasmodium vivax* | Benign tertian | 48-hour fever spikes | Enlarged host cells; ameboid trophozoites | Persistent hypnozoites Relapse* | Chloroquine PO$_4$ then primaquine |
| *Plasmodium ovale* | Benign tertian | 48-hour fever spikes | Oval, jagged, infected RBCs | Persistent hypnozoites Relapse | Chloroquine PO$_4$ then primaquine |
| *Plasmodium malariae* | Quartan or malarial | 72-hour fever spikes; recrudescence* | Bar and band forms; rosette schizonts | No persistent stage* | Chloroquine PO$_4$ (no radical cure necessary) |
| *Plasmodium falciparum* | Malignant tertian | Irregular fever spikes; causes cerebral malaria; most dangerous | Multiple ring forms crescent-shaped gametes | No persistent stage* | Chloroquine resistance a problem† |

*Definition of abbreviations:* PO, by mouth; RBCs, red blood cells.

*Recrudescence is a recurrence of symptoms from low levels of organisms remaining in **red** cells. Relapse is an exacerbation from liver stages (hypnozoites).

†Use quinine sulfate plus pyrimethamine-sulfadoxine.

## ANTIMALARIAL DRUGS

1. Suppressive (to avoid infection)
2. Therapeutic (eliminate erythrocytic)
3. Radical cure (eliminate exoerythrocytic)
4. Gametocidal (destruction of gametocytes)

Successful treatment is accomplished with chloroquine followed by primaquine. Chloroquine therapy is suppressive, therapeutic, and gametocidal, whereas primaquine eliminates the exoerythrocytic form.

### Chloroquine-Sensitive Malaria

| | |
|---|---|
| P. falciparum | Chloroquine |
| P. malariae | Chloroquine |
| P. vivax | Chloroquine plus primaquine |
| P. ovale | Chloroquine plus primaquine |

### Chloroquine-Resistant Malaria

**Prophylaxis:** mefloquine; backup drugs: doxycycline, atovaquone-proguanil
**Treatment:** quinine ± either doxycycline, clindamycin, or pyrimethamine

## ADVERSE EFFECTS OF ANTIMALARIAL DRUGS

| Drug | Side Effects | Contraindications and Cautions |
|---|---|---|
| Chloroquine, hydroxychloroquine | GI distress, pruritus, headache, dizziness, hemolysis, retinopathy | Avoid in psoriasis |
| Mefloquine | NVD, dizziness, syncope, extrasystoles, CNS effects (rare) | Avoid in seizures, psychiatric disorders, and in cardiac conduction defects |
| Primaquine | GI distress, headache, dizziness, neutropenia, hemolysis | Avoid in pregnancy, G6PD deficiency, and autoimmune disorders |
| Quinine | GI distress, cinchonism, CNS effects, hemolysis, hematotoxicity | Avoid in pregnancy |

*Definition of abbreviations:* CNS, central nervous system; GI, gastrointestinal; G6PD, glucose-6-phosphate dehydrogenase; NVD, nausea, vomiting, diarrhea.

## HEMOFLAGELLATES

Hemoflagellates (Trypanosomes and *Leishmania*) infect blood and tissues. They are found in:

- Human blood as **trypomastigotes** with flagellum and an undulating membrane.
- Tissues as **amastigotes (oval cells having neither the flagellum nor undulating membrane)**. *Leishmania* spp. have only amastigotes in the human.

| Trypomastigote | Amastigote |
|---|---|
| 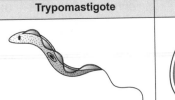 | Flagellar pocket / Nucleus |

| Species | Disease | Vector/Form/ Transmission | Reservoirs | Diagnosis | Treatment |
|---|---|---|---|---|---|
| *Trypanosoma cruzi* * | • **Chagas' disease** (American trypanosomiasis)<br>• Latin America<br>• Swelling around eye (**Romaña's sign**): common early sign<br>• Cardiac muscle (dilated cardiomyopathy), liver, brain often involved | **Reduviid bug (kissing or cone bug**; genus *Triatoma*) passes trypomastigote (flagellated form) **in feces** as it bites; scratching implants in bite site | • Cats, dogs, armadillos, opossums<br>• Poverty housing | Blood films, **trypomastigotes** | Nifurtimox |
| *Trypanosoma brucei gambiense* *Trypanosoma b. rhodesiense* | • **African sleeping sickness** (African trypanosomiasis)<br>• **Antigenic variation** | Trypomastigote in saliva of **tsetse fly** contaminates bite | Humans, some wild animals | • **Trypomastigotes in blood films**, CSF<br>• High immunoglobulin levels in CSF | • Acute: suramin<br>• Chronic: melarsoprol |
| *Leishmania donovani*† complex | • **Visceral leishmaniasis**<br>• Kala-azar | **Sandfly** bite | • Urban: humans<br>• Rural: rodents and wild animals | **Amastigotes in macrophages** in bone marrow, liver, spleen | **Stibogluconate sodium** (from CDC) |
| *Leishmania* (about 15 different species) | Cutaneous leishmaniasis (Oriental sore, etc.) | **Sandfly** bite | • Urban: humans<br>• Rural: rodents and wild animals | **Amastigotes in macrophages** in cutaneous lesions | Stibogluconate sodium |
| *Leishmania braziliensis* complex | Mucocutaneous leishmaniasis | **Sandfly** bite | • Urban: humans<br>• Rural: rodents and wild animals | Same | Stibogluconate sodium |

*Definition of abbreviations:* CDC, Centers for Disease Control and Prevention; CSF, cerebrospinal fluid.

*\*T. cruzi*: An estimated 0.5 million Americans are infected, creating some risk of transfusion transmission in the United States. In babies, acute infections are often serious and involve the CNS. In older children and adults, mild acute infections may become chronic with the risk of development of cardiomyopathy and heart failure.

† All *Leishmania*: intracellular, sandfly vector, stibogluconate

## MISCELLANEOUS APICOMPLEXA INFECTING BLOOD OR TISSUES

| Species | Disease/Locale of Origin | Transmission | Diagnosis | Treatment |
|---------|-------------------------|--------------|-----------|-----------|
| **Babesia** (primarily a disease of cattle) Humans: *Babesia microti*, WA1 and MO1 strains | Babesiosis (hemolytic, **malaria-like**) Same range as Lyme: N.E., N. Central, California, and N.W. United States | • **Ixodes tick** • Coinfections with **Borrelia** | Giemsa stain of blood smear or hamster inoculation | Clindamycin plus quinine |
| **Toxoplasma gondii** | • Most common parasitic disease • Infections **after birth are most commonly asymptomatic** or mild; may mimic mononucleosis • Produces **severe disease in AIDS** or other immunocompromised **(ring-enhancing lesions in brain)** • **Primary maternal infection during pregnancy may infect fetus:** – **Severe** congenital infections (intracerebral calcifications, chorioretinitis, hydro- or microcephaly, seizures) if *Toxoplasma* **crosses the placenta early** – **Later term congenital infection** may produce **progressive blindness** | **Cat** is **essential definitive** host; many other animals are intermediate hosts Mode: • Raw meat in U.S.; pork is #1 • Contact with cat feces | Serology: High IgM or rising IgM acute infection | Pyrimethamine plus sulfadiazine |

## MAJOR PROTOZOAL INFECTIONS AND DRUGS OF CHOICE

| Infection | Drug of Choice | Comments |
|-----------|---------------|----------|
| Amebiasis | Metronidazole | Diloxanide for noninvasive intestinal amebiasis |
| Giardiasis | Metronidazole or furazolidone | "Backpacker's diarrhea" from contaminated water or food |
| Trichomoniasis | Metronidazole | Treat both partners |
| Pneumocystosis | TMP-SMX | Atovaquone or pentamidine IV are backups |
| Toxoplasmosis | Pyrimethamine and sulfadiazine | TMP-SMX is also prophylactic against *Pneumocystis carinii* in AIDS |
| Leishmaniasis | Stibogluconate | — |
| Trypanosomiasis | • Nifurtimox (Chagas disease) • Arsenicals, pentamidine, suramin (African sleeping sickness) | — |

## METAZOANS: WORMS*

| Phylum | Flat worms (Platyhelminthes) | | Roundworms (Nemathelminthes) |
|--------|------------------------------|--|------------------------------|
| **Class** (common name) | **Trematodes** (flukes) | **Cestodes** (tapeworms) | **Nematodes**[†] (roundworms) |
| Genera | *Fasciola* *Fasciolopsis* *Paragonimus* *Clonorchis* **Schistosoma** | **Diphyllobothrium** *Hymenolepis* *Taenia* *Echinococcus* | **Necator** **Enterobius** Ⓦ*uchereria/Brugia* **Ascaris** and **Ancylostoma** *Toxocara, Trichuris,* and *Trichinella* Onchocerca Dracunculus Eyeworm (*Loa loa*) Strongyloides |

*Metazoans also include the Arthropoda, which serve mainly as intermediate hosts (the crustaceans) or as vectors of disease (the Arachnida and Insecta).

†Nematodes **mnemonic** (turn the "W" upsidedown)

Trematodes:
- Are commonly called flukes, which are generally flat and fleshy, leaf-shaped worms
- Are hermaphroditic, except for *Schistosoma*, which has separate males and females
- Have complicated life cycles occurring in two or more hosts
- Have operculated eggs (except for *Schistosoma*), which contaminate water, perpetuating the life cycle, and which are also used to diagnose infections
- **The first intermediate hosts are snails**

| Organism | Common Name | Acquisition | Progression in Humans | Important Ova | Treatment |
|---|---|---|---|---|---|
| *Schistosoma mansoni* <br><br> *S. japonicum* | **Intestinal schistosomiasis** | Contact with water; skin penetration | Skin penetration (itching) → mature in veins of mesentery → eggs cause granulomas in liver (**portal hypertension** and liver fibrosis in chronic cases) | | Praziquantel |
| *Schistosoma haematobium* | **Vesicular schistosomiasis** | Contact with water; skin penetration | Skin penetration (itching) → mature in bladder veins; chronic infection has high association with **bladder carcinoma in Egypt and Africa** | | Praziquantel |
| Nonhuman schistosomes | **Swimmer's itch** | Contact with water; skin penetration | Penetrate skin, producing **dermatitis** without further development in humans; itching is most intense at 2 to 3 days | — | Trimeprazine, calamine, sedatives |
| *Clonorchis sinensis* | **Chinese liver fluke** | Raw fish ingestion | Inflammation of **biliary tract**, pigmented gallstones, cholangiocarcinoma | Operculated eggs | Praziquantel |
| *Paragonimus westermani* | **Lung fluke** | Raw crabs, crayfish | **Hemoptysis**, secondary bacterial infection of lung | Operculated eggs | Praziquantel |

# GASTROINTESTINAL CESTODES (TAPEWORMS)

- Consist of three basic portions: the head or scolex; a "neck" section, which produces the proglottids; and the segments or proglottids, which mature as they move away from the scolex
- Are diagnosed by finding eggs or proglottids in the feces
- Have complex life cycles involving extraintestinal larval forms in intermediate hosts; when humans are intermediate host, these infections are generally more serious than intestinal infections with adult tapeworms

| Cestode (Common Name) | Form/ Transmission | Human Host Type | Disease/Organ Involvement/Symptoms (Sx) | Diagnosis | Treatment |
|---|---|---|---|---|---|
| *Taenia solium* (pork tapeworm)<br>IH: swine; rare: humans<br>DH: humans, developing and Slavic countries | Water, vegetation, food contaminated with **eggs** Autoinfection | IH | **Cysticercosis**/eggs → larva develop in brain, eye, heart, lung, etc. **Epilepsy** with onset after age 20 | Biopsy | Praziquantel; surgery in some sites |
| | Rare/raw pork containing the **cysticerci** ingested by humans | DH | • **Intestinal tapeworm**<br>• Sx: same as for *Taenia saginata* | **Proglottids** or **eggs** in feces | Praziquantel |
| *Diphyllobothrium latum* (fish tapeworm)<br>2 IHs: crustaceans → fish; rare: humans<br>DH: humans/mammals; cool lake regions | Drinking pond water containing copepods (crustaceans) carrying the **larval** forms or frog/snake poultices | IH | **Sparganosis**/larvae penetrate intestinal wall and encyst | Biopsy | Praziquantel |
| | Rare, raw pickled fish containing a **sparganum** | DH | **Intestinal tapeworm** (up to 10 meters)/small intestine, **megaloblastic anemia** | Proglottids or eggs in feces | Praziquantel |
| *Echinococcus granulosus*<br>IH: herbivores; rare: humans<br>DH: carnivores in sheep-raising areas | Ingestion of eggs | IH | **Hydatid cyst disease**; liver and lung, where cysts containing blood capsules develop | Imaging, serology | Surgery, albendazole |

*Definition of abbreviations:* IH, intermediate host; DH, definitive host.

## ROUNDWORMS (NEMATODES)

Roundworms are transmitted by:

- Ingestion of eggs (*Enterobius*, *Ascaris*, or *Trichuris*)
- Direct invasion of skin by larval forms (*Necator*, *Ancylostoma*, or *Strongyloides*)
- Ingestion of meat containing larvae (*Trichinella*)
- Infection involving insects transmitting the larvae with bites (*Wuchereria*, *Loa loa*, *Mansonella*, *Onchocerca*, and *Dracunculus*)

| | ROUNDWORMS (NEMATODES) TRANSMITTED BY EGGS | | | |
|---|---|---|---|---|
| **Species** | **Disease/Organs Most Affected** | **Form/ Transmission** | **Diagnosis** | **Treatment** |
| *Enterobius vermicularis* <br><br> (Most frequent helminth parasite in U.S.) | **Pinworms**, large intestine, perianal itching | • **Eggs**/person to person <br> • **Autoinfection** | • Sticky swab of perianal area <br> • Ova have flattened side with larvae inside <br><br> | Mebendazole <br> Treat entire family |
| *Trichuris trichiura* | **Whipworm** cecum, appendicitis, and rectal prolapse | **Eggs** ingested | **Barrel-shaped eggs with bipolar plugs** in stools <br><br> | Mebendazole |
| *Ascaris lumbricoides* <br><br> (Most common helminth worldwide; largest roundworm) | **Ascariasis** <br> Ingest egg → larvae migrate through lungs (cough) and mature in small intestine; may obstruct intestine or bile duct | **Eggs** ingested | **Bile stained, knobby eggs** <br><br> <br><br> Adult 35 to 40 cm | • Supportive therapy during pneumonitis <br> • Surgery for ectopic migrations <br> • Mebendazole |
| *Toxocara canis or cati* <br><br> (Dog/cat ascarids) | **Visceral larva migrans** <br> Larvae wander aimlessly until they die, cause inflammation | **Eggs** ingested/from handling puppies or from eating dirt in yard (pica) | Clinical findings and serology | Mebendazole; self-limiting in most cases |

## ROUNDWORMS (NEMATODES) TRANSMITTED BY LARVAE

| Species | Disease/Organs | Form/Transmission | Diagnosis | Treatment |
|---|---|---|---|---|
| *Necator americanus* (New World hookworm) | **Hookworm** infection Lung migration → pneumonitis Bloodsucking → anemia | Filariform **larva penetrates intact skin of bare feet** | Fecal larvae (up to 13 mm) and ova: oval, transparent with 2–8 cell-stage visible inside Fecal occult blood may be present | Mebendazole and iron therapy |
| *Ancylostoma braziliense* *Ancylostoma caninum* (dog and cat hookworms) | **Cutaneous larva migrans**/intense skin itching, snake-like tracks | Filariform larva penetrates intact skin but cannot mature in humans | Usually a presumptive diagnosis; exposure | Thiabendazole |
| *Strongyloides stercoralis* | **Threadworm** strongyloidiasis: *Early:* pneumonitis, abdominal pain, diarrhea *Later:* malabsorption, ulcers, bloody stools | Filariform **larva penetrates intact skin; autoinfection** leads to indefinite infections unless treated | Larvae in stool, serology | Thiabendazole |
| *Trichinella spiralis* | Trichinosis: larvae encyst in muscle → pain | **Viable encysted larvae in meat** are consumed: wildgame meat | Muscle biopsy; clinical findings: **fever, myalgia, splinter hemorrhages, eosinophilia** | Steroids for severe symptoms and mebendazole |

## FILARIAL NEMATODES

| Species | Disease | Transmission/Vector | Diagnosis | Treatment |
|---|---|---|---|---|
| *Wuchereria bancrofti; Brugia malayi* | Elephantiasis | Mosquito | Microfilariae in blood, eosinophilia | Surgery, ivermectin and diethylcarbamazine (DEC) |
| *Loa loa* (African eye worm) | Pruritus, calabar swellings | Chrysops, mango flies | Microfilariae in blood, eosinophilia | Surgical removal of worms; DEC |
| *Onchocerca volvulus* | River blindness, itchy "leopard" rash | Blackflies | Skin snips from calabar swellings | Surgical removal of worms; DEC or ivermectin |
| *Dracunculus medinensis* (Guinea worm, fiery serpent) | Creeping eruptions, ulcerations, rash | Drinking water with infected copepods | Increased IgE; worm eruption from skin | Slow, cautious worm removal with stick; metronidazole |

# VIROLOGY

## VIRAL STRUCTURE AND MORPHOLOGY

| The Basic Virion | Viral Structure |
|---|---|
| DNA or RNA + Structural proteins = Nucleocapsid (Naked Capsid Virus)<br><br>Nucleocapsid + Host Membrane with Viral Specified Glycoproteins* = Enveloped Virus<br><br>*critical for infectiousness of viral progeny | 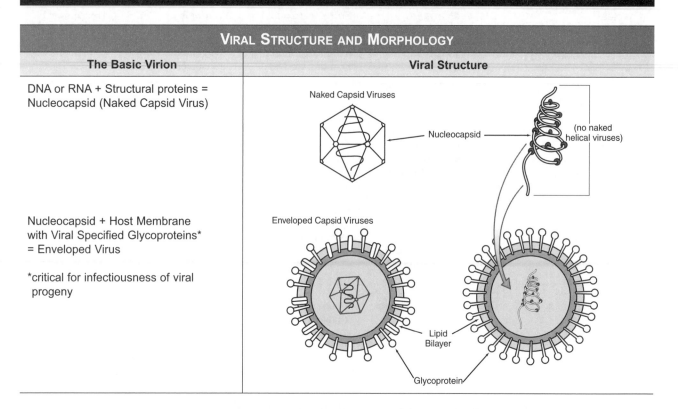 |

## DNA VIRUSES

**General Comments About DNA Viruses:**
- All are double-stranded except Parvo
- All are icosahedral except Pox, which are brick-shaped complex
- All replicate in the nucleus except Pox

| Virus Family | DNA Type | Polymerase | Envelope | Area of Replication | Major Viruses |
|---|---|---|---|---|---|
| Parvovirus | **ssDNA** | No | **Naked** | Nucleus | **B19** |
| Papilloma | dsDNA Circular | No | **Naked** | Nucleus | Papilloma |
| Polyomavirus | dsDNA Circular | No | **Naked** | Nucleus | Polyoma |
| Adenovirus | dsDNA Linear | No | **Naked** | Nucleus | Adenovirus |
| Hepadnavirus | Partially dsDNA Circular | **Yes** | Enveloped | Nucleus via RNA intermediate | HBV |
| Herpesvirus | dsDNA Linear | No | Enveloped **Nuclear** | Nucleus, assembled in nucleus | **HSV, VZV, EBV, CMV** |
| Poxvirus | dsDNA Linear | **Yes** | Enveloped | **Cytoplasm** | Variola, vaccinia Molluscum contagiosum |

*Definition of abbreviations:* CMV, cytomegalovirus; ds, double-stranded; EBV, Epstein-Barr virus; HBV, hepatitis B virus; HSV, herpes simplex virus; ss, single-stranded; VZV, varicella-zoster virus.

*Note:* Viruses are listed from top to bottom in order of increasing size. If you know them in this order, then you can remember that the smallest 4 are naked (wearing more clothing makes you larger).

**Mnemonic:  P**ardon **PaPa A**s **H**e **H**as **P**ox

# RNA VIRUSES

**General Comments About RNA Viruses:**

- All are single-stranded except Reo
- Most are enveloped. Only naked ones are **H**epe, **C**alici, **P**ico, and **R**eo (**Mnemonic: H**elp! **CPR!**)
- Some are segmented (**ROBA: R**eo, **O**rthomyxo, **B**unya, and **A**rena)
- Positive sense RNA = (+)RNA (can be used itself as mRNA)
- Negative sense RNA = (−)RNA
  - Complementary to mRNA
  - Cannot be used as mRNA
  - Requires virion-associated, RNA-dependent RNA polymerase (as part of mature virus)
- Others that carry a polymerase are Reo, Arena, and Retro

## DOUBLE-STRANDED RNA VIRUSES: REOVIRIDAE

| | RNA Structure | Polymerase | Envelope | Shape | Major viruses |
|---|---|---|---|---|---|
| **Reovirus** | • Linear dsRNA<br>• **10–11 segments** | Yes | **Naked** | • Icosahedral<br>• **Double shelled** | • Reovirus<br>• **Rotavirus** |

## POSITIVE-SENSE RNA VIRUSES

| Family | RNA Structure | Polymerase | Envelope | Shape | Area of Replication | Major Viruses |
|---|---|---|---|---|---|---|
| Calicivirus | • ss⊕RNA, linear<br>• Nonsegmented | No | **Naked** | Icosahedral | Cytoplasm | • Norwalk<br>• **Cruise ship agent** |
| Hepevirus | • ss⊕RNA, linear<br>• Nonsegmented | No | **Naked** | Icosahedral | Cytoplasm | Hepatitis E |
| Picornavirus | • ss⊕RNA, linear<br>• Nonsegmented | No | **Naked** | Icosahedral | Cytoplasm | • Polio, ECHO, Entero<br>• Rhino, coxsackie<br>• Hepatitis A |
| Flavivirus | • ss⊕RNA, linear<br>• Nonsegmented | No | Enveloped | Icosahedral | Cytoplasm | Yellow fever, dengue, SLE, hepatitis C, **West Nile virus** |
| Togavirus | • ss⊕RNA, linear<br>• Nonsegmented | No | Enveloped | Icosahedral | Cytoplasm | Rubella<br>WEE, EEE, VEE |
| Coronavirus | • ss⊕RNA, linear<br>• Nonsegmented | No | Enveloped | **Helical** | Cytoplasm | Coronaviruses<br>**SARS agent** |
| **Retrovirus** | • **Diploid**<br>• ss⊕RNA, linear<br>• Nonsegmented | **RNA-dependent DNA polymerase** | Enveloped | Icosahedral or truncated conical | **Nucleus** | HIV<br>HTLV<br>Sarcoma |

*Definition of abbreviations:* EEE, eastern equine encephalitis; HIV, human immunodeficiency virus; HTLV, human T-cell lymphocytotropic virus; VEE, Venezuelan equine encephalitis; WEE, Western equine encephalitis.

**Mnemonic:** Again from smallest (top) to largest (bottom): **C**all **P**ico and **F**lo **T**o **C**ome **R**ightaway
**Mnemonic:** Picornaviruses: **PEE C**o **R**n **A** viruses (**P**olio, **E**ntero, **E**cho, **C**oxsackie, **R**hino, Hep **A**)

## NEGATIVE-SENSE RNA VIRUSES

| Virus | RNA | Polymerase | Envelope | Shape | Area Where Multiplies | Major Viruses |
|---|---|---|---|---|---|---|
| Paramyxovirus | • ssΘRNA, linear<br>• Nonsegmented | Yes | Yes | Helical | Cytoplasm | Mumps, measles RSV, parainfluenza |
| Rhabdovirus | • ssΘRNA, linear<br>• Nonsegmented | Yes | Yes | **Bullet-shaped,** helical | Cytoplasm | Rabies, VSV |
| Filovirus | • ssΘRNA, linear<br>• Nonsegmented | Yes | Yes | Helical | Cytoplasm | Marburg, Ebola |
| Orthomyxovirus | • ssΘRNA, linear<br>• **8 segments** | Yes | Yes | Helical | **Cytoplasm and nucleus** | Influenza |
| Bunyavirus | • ssΘRNA, linear to circular<br>• 3 segments, ambisense | Yes | Yes | Helical | Cytoplasm | California and LaCrosse encephalitis, Hantavirus |
| Arenavirus | • ssΘRNA, circular,<br>• 2 segments: 1 Θ sense, 1 ambisense | Yes | Yes | Helical | Cytoplasm | Lymphocytic choriomeningitis virus, Lassa fever |

*Definition of abbreviations:* ds, double-stranded; RSV, respiratory syncytial virus; ss, single-stranded; VSV, vesicular stomatitis virus.

**Mnemonic** (in order of increasing size): **P**ain **R**esults **F**rom **O**ur **B**unions **A**lways (Pain is a negative thing!)
Or, to remind you of life-cycle: **B**ring **A** **P**olymerase **O**r **F**ail **R**eplication

## VIRAL GENETICS

| | |
|---|---|
| **Phenotypic mixing** | • Related viruses coinfect cell (virus A and virus B)<br>• Resulting proteins on the surface are a mixture capsid of AB around nucleic acid of either A or B |
| **Phenotypic masking** | • Related viruses coinfect cell (virus A and virus B)<br>• Capsid of proteins of virus A form around nucleic acid of B |
| **Complementation** | • Two related defective viruses infect the same cell; if they are defective in different genes, viral progeny (still with mutated DNA) will be formed<br>• If they are defective in the same gene, no progeny will be formed<br>• Coinfection of hepatitis B and D is a clinical example of complementation where HBV supplies the needed surface antigen for hepatitis D |
| **Genetic reassortment (genetic shift)** | • Two different strains of a segmented RNA virus infect the same cell.<br>• Major new genetic combinations are produced through "shuffling," resulting in stable and dramatic changes<br>• This results in **pandemics** of disease |
| **Genetic drift** | • Minor antigenic changes from mutation<br>• Occurs in many viruses, particularly RNA types<br>• Most noted in HIV and influenza |
| **Viral vectors** | • Recombinant viruses are produced that have combinations of human replacement genes with the defective viral nucleic acid |

# ANTIVIRAL AGENTS

As viruses rely on host machinery to produce viral products, selectivity must be achieved by targeting minute differences in viral enzymes. This may be accomplished at any stage in the viral "life cycle" including adsorption, penetration, nucleic acid synthesis, late protein synthesis, protein processing, viral product packaging, and viral release.

| Class/Agent | Mechanism of Action | Spectrum/Clinical Applications | Mechanism(s) of Resistance | Toxicity/Notes |
|---|---|---|---|---|
| **ANTIHERPETICS**<br>Acyclovir<br>Famciclovir<br>Valacyclovir | **Inhibit viral DNA polymerases**<br>Activated by viral thymidine kinase (TK);<br>• Famciclovir is oral prodrug converted to penciclovir<br>• Valacyclovir is oral prodrug of acyclovir<br>• Mechanism of penciclovir same as acyclovir | HSV, VZV (esp. famciclovir, valacyclovir) | Decreased activity or loss of thymidine kinase/ DNA polymerase | • Fairly well-tolerated (esp. oral), some nausea/vomiting<br>• IV use associated with seizure, delirium, crystalluria (maintain hydration)<br>• Famciclovir and valacyclovir have much greater oral bioavailability and longer $t_{1/2}$ than acyclovir |
| Ganciclovir | Similar to acyclovir | CMV (e.g., CMV retinitis), HSV, VZV | Similar to acyclovir | Dose-limiting leukopenia, thrombocytopenia; crystalluria (maintain hydration) |
| Foscarnet | **Inhibits DNA and RNA polymerases**; does not require activation by kinases (may be effective in acyclovir-, ganciclovir-resistant strains) | • CMV retinitis in AIDS patients<br>• Acyclovir-resistant mucocutaneous HSV in immuno-compromised patients | | • Dose limiting nephrotoxicity<br>• Electrolyte imbalance (can lead to seizures) |
| **ANTI-INFLUENZA DRUGS**<br>Amantadine<br>Rimantadine | Block viral penetration/ uncoating of influenza A virus via interaction with viral M2 protein | • Influenza A (prophylaxis)<br>• Amantadine also used in Parkinson disease to stimulate dopamine release | Resistance due to mutations in M2 protein (no cross resistance to neuraminidase inhibitors) | • Ataxia<br>• Increased seizure activity<br>• Dizziness & hypotension<br>• Rimantadine better tolerated in elderly |
| Oseltamivir<br>Zanamivir | **Inhibit neuraminidases** made by influenza A and B (enzymes that promote virion release and prevent clumping of these virions), decreasing viral spread | Prophylaxis, but may ↓ duration of flu symptoms by 2-3 days | Mutations to viral neuraminidase | Oseltamivir: oral prodrug; GI discomfort<br>Zanamivir: inhalational drug; cough, bronchospasm in asthmatics |
| Ribavirin | Inhibits viral RNA synthesis by altering the nucleotide pools and normal messenger RNA formation | Influenza A & B, Parainfluenza, RSV, paramyxoviruses HCV (combined with α–interferon), HIV | Unknown | Dose-dependent hemolytic anemia |

*(Continued)*

## ANTIVIRAL AGENTS *(CONT'D.)*

| Class/Agent | Mechanism of Action | Spectrum/Clinical Applications | Mechanism(s) of Resistance | Toxicity/Notes |
|---|---|---|---|---|
| **HIV THERAPY:** For details on HIV therapy, see Ch. 4, General Principles of Immunology | | | | |
| Interferons[†] | Interferons are a class of related proteins with antiviral, antiproliferative, and immune regulating activity. They induce the synthesis of a number of antiviral proteins (e.g., RNAse and a protein kinase) that protect the cell against subsequent challenges by a variety of viruses. | • Hepatitis B & C<br>• Kaposi sarcoma<br>• Leukemias<br>• Malignant melanoma | Anti-interferon antibodies are seen with prolonged use | • Interferons can cause influenza-like symptoms, especially in the first week of therapy<br>• Bone marrow suppression<br>• Profound fatigue, myalgia, weight loss, and increased susceptibility to bacterial infections<br>• Depression is seen in up to 20% of patients |

*Definition of abbreviations:* CMV, cytomegalovirus; HCV, hepatitis C virus; HSV, herpes simplex virus; RSV, respiratory syncytial virus; VZV, varicella zoster virus.

[†]For more information on interferons and other immunosuppressants, see Chapter 4, General Principles of Immunology

# MYCOLOGY

## MYCOLOGY: OVERVIEW

Fungi are eukaryotic organisms with complex carbohydrate cell walls (the reason they frequently calcify in chronic infections) and ergosterol as their major membrane sterol (which is targeted with nystatin and the imidazoles). Morphologic and geographic clues are very important in determining the identity of the organism.

| Fungi come in two basic forms | • **Hyphae**—filamentous forms may either have cross walls (septate) or lack them (aseptate)<br>• **Yeasts**—single-celled oval/round forms<br>• **Dimorphic fungi**—may convert from hyphal to yeast forms (key examples: *Histoplasma*, *Blastomyces*, *Coccidioides*, and *Sporothrix*).<br>**Mnemonic:** **H**eat **C**hanges **B**ody **S**hape: yeast in the heat, mold in the cold |
|---|---|
| **Pseudohyphae** | • Hyphae formed by budding off yeasts; formed by **Candida albicans**; the basis of the germ tube test for diagnosis of invasive *C. albicans* |
| **Spores** are used for reproduction and dissemination | • **Conidia**—asexual spores form off hyphae<br>• **Blastoconidia**—asexual spores like buds on yeasts<br>• **Arthroconidia**—asexual spores formed with joints between<br>• **Spherules** with **endospores**—sexual spores in tissues (*Coccidioides*) |

## NONSYSTEMIC FUNGAL INFECTIONS

| Organism | Disease | Notes |
|---|---|---|
| *Malassezia furfur* | **Pityriasis** or **tinea versicolor** | • Superficial infection of keratinized cells<br>• **Hypopigmented spots on the chest/back** (blotchy suntan)<br>• KOH mount of skin scales: "spaghetti and meatballs," yeast clusters and short, curved septate hyphae<br>• Treatment is topical selenium sulfide; recurs. |
| | **Fungemia** | • In **premature infants** |
| *Candida albicans, Candida* spp. | **Cutaneous or mucocutaneous candidiasis** | • Causes oral thrush and vulvovaginitis in immunocompetent individuals<br>• Source of opportunistic infections in hospitalized and immunocompromised (*see* Opportunistic Mycoses)<br><br><br>Pseudohyphae    Budding Yeasts    Germ Tubes    True Hyphae |
| *Trichophyton, Microsporum, Epidermophyton* | **Tinea** (capitis, barbae, corporis, cruris, pedis) | • Infects **skin, hair, and nails**<br>• **Monomorphic** filamentous fungi<br>• KOH mount shows **arthroconidia, hyphae**<br>• **Pruritic lesions with serpiginous borders and central clearing** |
| *Sporothrix schenckii* <br>Hyphae with sleeves<br><br>or rosettes of conidia | • **Sporotrichosis (rose gardener's disease)**<br><br>• **Pulmonary sporotrichosis** (in alcoholics/ homeless) | Dimorphic fungus:<br>• Environmental form: hyphae with rosettes and sleeves of conidia<br>• Tissue form: cigar-shaped yeast |

## SYSTEMIC FUNGAL INFECTIONS

| Organism | Disease | Notes |
|---|---|---|
| **General Comments** | | |
| *Histoplasma* *Coccidioides* *Blastomyces* | • Acute pulmonary (asymptomatic or self-resolving in about 95% of the cases) <br> • Chronic pulmonary <br> • Disseminated infections | **Diagnosis** (most people never see doctor): <br> • Sputum cytology (calcofluor white staining helpful) <br> • **Sputum cultures** on blood agar and **special fungal media** (inhibitory mold agar, Sabouraud's agar) <br> • **Peripheral blood cultures are useful for** *Histoplasma* **because it circulates in RES cells** |
| **Specific Organisms** | | |
| *Histoplasma capsulatum* | Fungus flu (a pneumonia) <br> • Asymptomatic or flu-like <br> • **Hepatosplenomegaly** may be present <br> • May **disseminate in AIDS patient** <br> | **Dimorphic fungus:** <br> • **Environmental form: hyphae** with **microconidia** and **tuberculate macroconidia** <br>   – Endemic region: **Eastern Great Lakes, Ohio, Mississippi,** and **Missouri River beds** <br>   – Found in **soil (dust) enriched with bird or bat feces** (caves, chicken coops) <br> • **Tissue form: small intracellular yeasts** with narrow neck on bud; **no capsule** <br> • **Facultative intracellular parasite** found in **RES cells** (tiny; can get 30 or so in a human cell) |
| *Coccidioides immitis* (endospores/spherules) (arthroconidia) | Coccidioidomycosis (San Joaquin Valley fever) <br> | • Dimorphic fungus <br> • Asymptomatic to **self-resolving pneumonia** <br> • Desert bumps (erythema nodosum) <br> • **Pulmonary lesions may calcify** <br> • **May disseminate in AIDS and immunocompromised** (meningitis, mucocutaneous lesions) <br> • Has a tendency to **disseminate in third trimester of pregnancy** |
| *Blastomyces dermatitidis* | Blastomycosis <br> | • Dimorphic fungus <br> • Environmental form: hyphae with conidia <br> • Tissue form: broad-based budding yeast <br> • Pulmonary disease <br> • Disseminated disease |

*Definition of abbreviations:* RES, reticuloendothelial.

## OPPORTUNISTIC FUNGI

| | | |
|---|---|---|
| *Aspergillus fumigatus*<br> | • **Allergic bronchopulmonary aspergillosis**/asthma, allergies<br>• **Fungus ball:** free in preformed lung cavities<br>• **Invasive aspergillosis**/severe neutropenia, CGD, CF, burns<br>  – Invades tissues, causing infarcts and hemorrhage<br>  – Nasal colonization →**pneumonia or meningitis**<br>  – **Cellulitis**/in burn patients; may also disseminate | • **Dichotomously branching**<br>• **Generally acute angles**<br>• **Septate**<br>• Compost pits, moldy marijuana<br>• May cause disease in immunocompromised patients |
| *Candida albicans* (and other spp. of *Candida*) | • Involvement of the oral cavity and digestive tract<br>• Septicemia, endocarditis in IV drug abusers<br>• Mucocutaneous candidiasis | **Diagnosis:**<br>• KOH: pseudohyphae, true hyphae, budding yeasts<br>• Septicemia: culture lab identification: biochemical tests/formation of germ tubes<br>**Treatment:**<br>• Topical imidazoles or oral imidazoles; nystatin<br>• Disseminated: amphotericin B or fluconazole |
| *Cryptococcus neoformans*<br>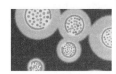 | • **Meningitis/Hodgkin, AIDS (the dominant meningitis)**<br>• **Acute pulmonary** (usually asymptomatic)/**pigeon breeders** | • **Encapsulated yeast (monomorphic)**<br>• **Environmental source:** Soil enriched with pigeon droppings<br>• **Diagnosis of meningitis: CSF**<br>  – Detect capsular antigen in CSF (by latex particle agglutination or counter immunoelectrophoresis)<br>  – **India ink mount** (misses 50%) of CSF sediment to find budding yeasts with capsular "halos"<br>  – Cultures (urease ⊕ yeast)<br>• **Treatment:** amphotericin B plus flucytosine until afebrile and culture ⊖, then fluconazole |
| *Mucor, Rhizopus, Absidia* (Zygomycophyta family)<br>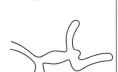 | **Rhinocerebral infection** (mucormycosis) caused by *Mucor* (or other Zygomycophyta) | • Nonseptate, filamentous fungi<br>• Characterized by paranasal swelling, necrotic tissues, hemorrhagic exudates from nose and eyes, mental lethargy<br>• Occurs in **ketoacidotic diabetic patients** and **leukemic patients**<br>• These fungi penetrate without respect to anatomic barriers, progressing rapidly from sinuses into brain tissue<br>• **Diagnosis:** KOH of tissue; broad, ribbon-like nonseptate hyphae with about 90° angles on branches<br>• **Treatment:** débride necrotic tissue and start amphotericin B fast; high fatality rate because of rapid growth and invasion |
| *Pneumocystis jiroveci* (formerly *carinii*)<br> | Pneumonia in AIDS patients, malnourished babies, premature neonates, other immunocompromised | • An exudate with foamy or **honeycomb appearance on H & E stain**<br>• **Patchy infiltrative (ground-glass appearance) on x-ray**<br>• **Diagnosis: silver-staining cysts** in bronchial alveolar lavage fluids or biopsy<br>• Treatment: trimethoprim/sulfamethoxazole |

*Definition of abbreviations:* CF, cystic fibrosis; CSF, cerebrospinal fluid; CGD, chronic granulomatous disease; KOH, potassium hydroxide.

# ANTIFUNGAL AGENTS

Because fungi are eukaryotic, finding selectively toxic antifungal agents is difficult. Consequently, treating fungal infections poses a clinical challenge, especially in immunocompromised patients. Fungal cell membranes contain ergosterol, a sterol not found in mammalian tissue. Thus, this difference provides the basis for most systemically administered antifungal agents.

| Class/Agent | Mechanism of Action | Spectrum/Clinical Use | Mechanism(s) of Resistance | Toxicity/Notes |
|---|---|---|---|---|
| **Agents for Systemic Infections** | | | | |
| Amphotericin B | Binds ergosterol, causing formation of artificial pores, thus altering membrane permeability, killing the cell | Widest antifungal spectrum: *Aspergillus* *Coccidioides* *Blastomyces* *Candida albicans* *Cryptococcus* *Histoplasma* *Mucor* *Sporothrix schenckii* | Very uncommon; ↓ or structurally altered ergosterol | • Fever and chills ("cytokine storm") <br>• **Nephrotoxicity** limits dosing (cumulative over lifetime) <br>• Reversible anemia (secondary to ↓ erythropoietin) <br>• Arrhythmias <br>• IV only |
| Flucytosine | Permease allows entry, deaminated to 5-FU, then converted to 5-FdUMP (thymidylate synthase inhibitor) | Narrow spectrum: *Cryptococcus* *Candida albicans* (systemic) | Rapid if used as a single agent; ↓ activity of fungal permeases and deaminases | • Reversible **bone marrow suppression** <br>• Alopecia <br>• Typically **combined with amphotericin B** or fluconazole |
| Azoles: fluconazole, itraconazole, voriconazole, ketoconazole | Inhibit synthesis of ergosterol, leading to altered membrane permeability | Varies: *Candida* *Coccidioides* *Cryptococcus* *Aspergillus* *Histoplasma* | ↓ sensitivity of target enzymes | • Vomiting and diarrhea <br>• Skin rash <br>• Hepatotoxicity (rare) <br>• **Gynecomastia** <br>• ↓ P450 |
| Echinocandin/ caspofungin | Inhibits synthesis of β-1,2 glycan, a component of fungal cell walls | *Candida* *Aspergillus* | — | • Not very toxic <br>• Headache <br>• Infusion-related reactions |
| **Systemic Agents for Superficial Infections** | | | | |
| Griseofulvin | • Uptake by energy-dependent transport <br>• Interferes with microtubule formation in dermatophytes <br>• May inhibit polymerization of nucleic acids | • Dermatophytes of the hair and scalp <br>• Accumulates in keratin | ↓ in transport/uptake | • Confusion and vertigo <br>• Headache <br>• Blurred vision <br>• Nausea/vomiting <br>• ↑ P450 <br>• GI irritation <br>• **Disulfiram-like reaction** with ethanol |
| Terbinafine | Inhibits squalene epoxidase (for sterol biosynthesis) | Accumulates in keratin, used in onychomycosis | | • GI irritation <br>• Rash <br>• Headache <br>• Taste disturbance |
| Azoles (*see* above) | — | — | — | — |
| **Topical Antifungals †** | | | | |
| Nystatin | Disrupts membrane by binding ergosterol | *Candida*, especially in oral candidiasis (thrush) | Same as amphotericin B | • Contact dermatitis <br>• Stevens-Johnson syndrome |

† Topical azoles, such as miconazole and clotrimazole are also widely used.

# Embryology

## Chapter 5

**General Principles of Embryology**

## EARLY EMBRYOLOGY

### Week 1

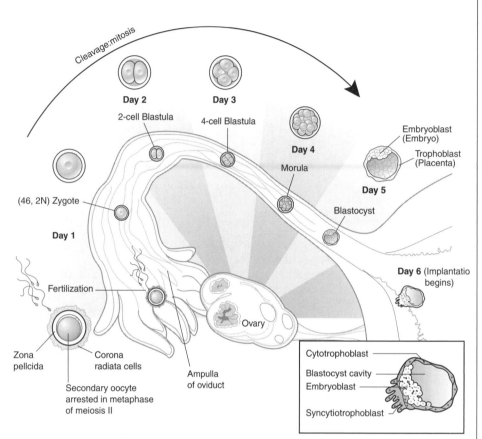

Fertilization occurs in the **ampulla of the uterine tube** when the male and female pronuclei fuse to form a **zygote**. At fertilization, the secondary oocyte rapidly completes meiosis II.

During the first 4 to 5 days of the first week, the zygote undergoes rapid mitotic division (**cleavage**) in the oviduct to form a **blastula**, consisting of increasingly smaller **blastomeres**. This becomes the **morula** (32-cell stage).

A **blastocyst** forms as fluid develops in the morula. The blastocyst consists of an inner cell mass known as the **embryoblast**, and the outer cell mass known as the **trophoblast** becomes the placenta.

At the end of the first week, the trophoblast differentiates into the **cytotrophoblast** and **syncytiotrophoblast** and then implantation begins. Implantation usually occurs in the **posterior superior wall** of the uterus.

| Clinical Correlation: Ectopic Pregnancy | |
|---|---|
| **Tubal** | The **most common form** of ectopic pregnancy |
| | Usually occurs when the blastocyst **implants within the ampulla** of the uterine tube because of delayed transport |
| | **Risk factors:** endometriosis, pelvic inflammatory disease (PID), tubular pelvic surgery, or exposure to diethylstilbestrol (DES) |
| | **Clinical signs:** abnormal or brisk uterine bleeding, sudden onset of abdominal pain that may be confused with appendicitis, missed menstrual period (e.g., LMP 60 days ago), positive human chorionic gonadotropin (hCG) test, culdocentesis showing intraperitoneal blood, positive sonogram |
| **Abdominal** | Most commonly occurs in the **rectouterine pouch** (pouch of Douglas) |

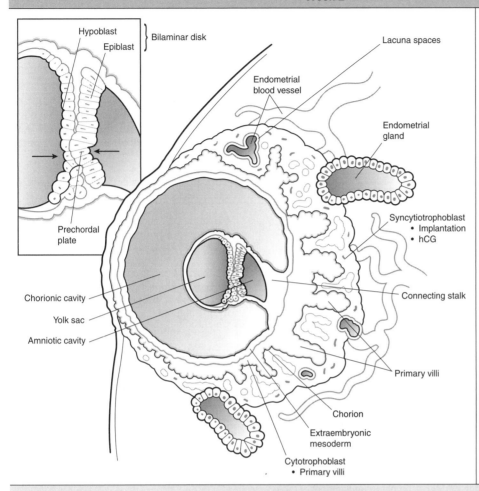

The embryoblast differentiates into the **epiblast** and **hypoblast**, forming a **bilaminar embryonic disk**.

The epiblast forms the **amniotic cavity**, and hypoblast cells migrate from the **primary yolk sac**.

The **prechordal plate**, formed from fusion of epiblast and hypoblast cells, is the site of the future **mouth**.

**Extraembryonic mesoderm** is derived from the epiblast. **Extraembryonic somatic mesoderm** lines the cytotrophoblast, forms the connecting stalk, and covers the amnion. **Extraembryonic visceral mesoderm** covers the yolk sac.

The connecting stalk suspends the conceptus within the chorionic cavity. The wall of the chorionic cavity is called the **chorion**, consisting of extraembryonic somatic mesoderm, the cytotrophoblast, and the syncytiotrophoblast.

**Clinical Correlation**

**Human chorionic gonadotropin (hCG)** is a glycoprotein produced by the syncytiotrophoblast. It stimulates progesterone production by the corpus luteum. hCG can be assayed in maternal blood or urine and is the basis for early pregnancy testing. hCG is detectable throughout pregnancy. **Low hCG** levels may predict a spontaneous abortion or ectopic pregnancy. **High hCG** levels may predict a multiple pregnancy, hydatidiform mole, or gestational trophoblastic disease.

## Weeks 3 Through 8

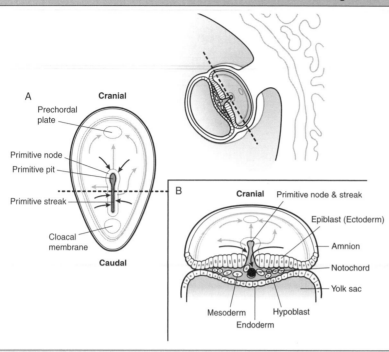

**Third week:** gastrulation and early development of nervous and cardiovascular systems; corresponds to first missed period

**Gastrulation**—a process that produces the three primary germ layers: **ectoderm, mesoderm**, and **endoderm**; begins with the formation of the **primitive streak** within the epiblast

Ectoderm → **neuroectoderm** and **neural crest** cells

Mesoderm → **paraxial mesoderm** (35 pairs of somites), **intermediate mesoderm**, and **lateral mesoderm**

All major organ systems begin to develop during the **embryonic period (Weeks 3–8)**. By the end of this period, the embryo begins to look human.

### Clinical Correlation

**Sacrococcygeal teratoma:** a tumor that arises from remnants of the primitive streak; often contains various types of tissue (bone, nerve, hair, etc.).

**Chordoma:** a tumor that arises from remnants of the notochord, found either intracranially or in the sacral region

**Caudal dysplasia (sirenomelia):** a constellation of syndromes ranging from minor lesions of the lower vertebrae to complete fusion of lower limbs. Occurs as a result of abnormal gastrulation, in which migration of mesoderm is disturbed. Associated with VATER (vertebral defects, anal atresia, tracheoesophageal fistula, and renal defects) or VACTERL (vertebral defects, anal atresia, cardiovascular defects, tracheoesophageal fistula, renal defects, and upper limb defects)

**Hydatidiform mole:** results from the partial or complete replacement of the trophoblast by dilated villi

- **In a complete mole, there is no embryo;** a haploid sperm fertilizes a blighted ovum and reduplicates so that the karyotype is 46,XX, with all chromosomes of paternal origin. In a **partial mole**, there is a haploid set of maternal chromosomes and usually two sets of paternal chromosomes so that the typical karyotype is 69,XXY.
- **Molar pregnancies have high levels of hCG, and 20% develop into a malignant trophoblastic disease, including choriocarcinoma.**

### GERM LAYER DERIVATIVES

| Ectoderm | |
| --- | --- |
| Surface ectoderm | Epidermis, hair, nails, inner and external ear, tooth enamel, lens of eye, anterior pituitary (from Rathke pouch), major salivary, sweat, and mammary glands; epithelial lining of nasal and oral cavities and ear |
| Neuroectoderm | CNS (brain and spinal cord), retina and optic nerve, pineal gland, neurohypophysis, astrocytes, oligodendrocytes, ependymal cells |
| Neural crest | Adrenal medulla, ganglia (sensory, autonomic), melanocytes, Schwann cells, meninges (pia, arachnoid), pharyngeal arch cartilage, bones of the skull, odontoblasts, parafollicular (C) cells, laryngeal cartilage, aorticopulmonary septum, endocardial cushions (abnormal development can lead to many congenital defects) |
| **Mesoderm** | Muscle (smooth, cardiac, skeletal), connective tissue, serous membranes, bone and cartilage, blood and blood vessels, lymphatics, cardiovascular organs, adrenal cortex, gonads and internal reproductive organs, spleen, kidney and ureter, dura mater |
| **Endoderm** | Epithelial parts: GI tract, tonsils, thymus, pharynx, larynx, trachea, bronchi, lungs, urinary bladder, urethra, tympanic cavity, auditory tube and other pharyngeal pouches<br>Parenchyma: liver, pancreas, tonsils, thyroid, parathyroids, glands of GI tract, submandibular and sublingual glands |

## PLACENTA

The placenta permits exchange of nutrients and waste products between maternal and fetal circulations.

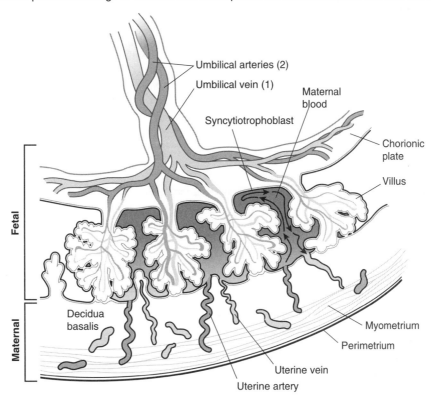

| Fetal component | Chorionic plate and villi<br>**Syncytiotrophoblast:** outer layer of chorionic villi; secretes hCG<br>**Cytotrophoblast:** inner layer of chorionic villi |
|---|---|
| **Maternal component** | **Decidua basalis:** Maternal blood vessels from the decidua conduct blood into the intervillous spaces of the placenta, where floating villi are present |
| **Placental barrier** | The syncytiotrophoblast, cytotrophoblast, basement membrane, fetal capillary endothelium separate the maternal and fetal blood |
| **Umbilical cord** | 1 **umbilical vein** supplies **oxygenated** blood from the placenta to the fetus<br>2 **umbilical arteries** carries **deoxygenated** blood back from the fetus to the placenta<br>**Urachus:** Removes nitrogenous waste from the fetal bladder |

## TWINNING

The type of twinning depends on the point in time in which cleavage occurs. If the twinning occurs very early on (before the chorion forms), two separate chorions will form (dichorionic). All other possible types of twins are monochorionic because the chorion has already formed. Fraternal twins are **dizygotic** and identical twins are **monozygotic**.

| Placental morphology | Time of cleavage | Type of twin |
|---|---|---|
| Dichorionic diamniotic | Very early (Days 1–3) | Fraternal or identical |
| Monochorionic diamniotic | Early (Days 4–8) | Identical |
| Monochorionic monoamniotic | Later (Days 8–13): identical<br>Even later (Days 13–15): conjoined | Identical, conjoined |

| TERATOGENS | |
|---|---|
| ACE inhibitors; ARBS | Renal damage |
| Aminoglycosides | CN VIII toxicity |
| Androgens | Masculinization of female fetus |
| Anticonvulsants | Neural tube defects (carbamazepine, valproic acid), phenytoin (fetal hydantoin syndrome); multiple congenital defects |
| Antithyroid drugs | Congenital goiter, hypothyroidism |
| Diethylstilbestrol (DES) | Vaginal clear cell adenocarcinoma; vaginal adenosis |
| Ethanol | Fetal alcohol syndrome (e.g., growth retardation, facial abnormalities, microcephaly, cardiac defects) |
| Folate antagonists | Multiple congenital anomalies |
| Lithium | Ebstein anomaly |
| Radiation | Multiple abnormalities |
| Tetracyclines | Discoloration of teeth |
| Thalidomide | Phocomelia (limb reduction defects) |
| Warfarin | Bone and cartilage abnormalities, hemorrhage, etc. |
| Vitamin A excess; vitamin A derivatives | Multiple abnormalities, e.g., cleft palate, cardiac abnormalities, mental retardation |

# Physiology

## PHYSIOLOGIC TERMINOLOGY

| Equilibrium | Equilibrium occurs when the balance of opposing forces has reached the **lowest free energy state**, and as a result, a given variable has reached a constant value. |
|---|---|
| Steady state | Steady state is a condition in which a variable is maintained within narrow limits by regulating an opposing activity. This process requires energy. |
| Negative feedback | This is a common system that acts to oppose changes in the internal environment. Negative feedback systems promote stability and act to restore steady-state function after a perturbation. |
| Positive feedback | This is a less common system (also called a vicious cycle) that acts to magnify a change in the internal environment; the initial change in a system is increased as a result of feedback activity. In a viable organism, any positive feedback system is ultimately overridden by one or more negative feedback systems. |

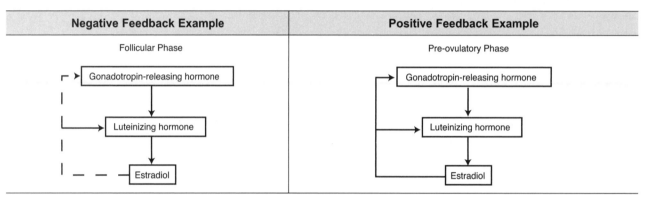

| Negative Feedback Example | Positive Feedback Example |
|---|---|
| Follicular Phase | Pre-ovulatory Phase |

The figures above show the negative feedback relationship between estrogens and the gonadotropins that dominates during the follicular phase, which transforms into a positive feedback relationship, producing the LH surge prior to ovulation.

## TRANSPORT

| Type of Transport | Energy Source | Example | Other Characteristics | Clinical Correlation |
|---|---|---|---|---|
| Simple diffusion | Passive | Pulmonary gases | — | Pulmonary edema decreases diffusion |
| Carrier-mediated or facilitated diffusion | Passive | Glucose uptake by muscle | • Insulin controls carrier population<br>• Chemical specificity | Insulin-dependent glucose uptake impaired in diabetes mellitus |
| Primary active transport | Direct use of ATP | $Na^+/K^+$-ATPase<br><br>$H^+/K^+$-ATPase | Antiport (countertransport) | Inhibition by cardiac glycosides |
| Secondary active transport | Electrochemical gradient for sodium is most common driving force | $Na^+$-glucose in kidney<br><br>$Na^+$-$H^+$ exchange | Symport (cotransport)<br><br>Antiport (countertransport) | Osmotic diuresis results when transporters saturated<br><br>Renal tubular acidosis |

### Key Points

- Passive processes are directly related to concentration gradients.
- Active processes create or increase a concentration gradient and thus depend upon metabolic energy.
- Both carrier-mediated facilitated diffusion and active transport can be saturated; maximum transport rate depends on population and activity of transport molecules.
- Primary active transport proteins have an ATPase as part of their structure.
- Most secondary active transport depends upon the electrochemical gradient of sodium ions, which in turn depends on the activity of the primary active transporter, sodium-potassium ATPase.

## DIFFUSION KINETICS

| Simple diffusion | The rate is estimated by **Fick's law of diffusion**: J = –DA($\Delta$C/$\Delta$X)<br>J = net flux, D = diffusion coefficient, A = surface area, $\Delta$C = concentration or pressure gradient, $\Delta$X = diffusion distance<br><br>Changes in surface area or diffusion distance are most important in disease states (e.g., the decrease in surface area caused by destruction of alveoli in emphysema or the decreased diffusion of oxygen during pulmonary edema related to increased diffusion distance). |
|---|---|
| Carrier-mediated transport | 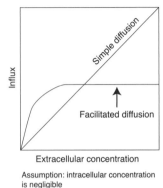 Assumption: intracellular concentration is negligible  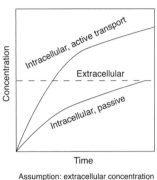 Assumption: extracellular concentration does not change  **Facilitated diffusion** increases transport rate above that capable with **simple diffusion**, but has saturation kinetics (*left*).<br><br>**Active transport** can produce a concentration gradient, and **passive processes** will lead to an equilibrium state (*right*). |

## FLUID VOLUME COMPARTMENTS AND DISTRIBUTION

| | % of Body Weight | Fraction of TBW | Markers Used to Measure Volume | Primary Cations | Primary Anions |
|---|---|---|---|---|---|
| **Total body water (TBW)** | 60 | 1.0 | Tritiated $H_2O$<br>$D_2O$ | — | — |
| **Intracellular fluid volume (ICF)** | 40 | ⅔ | TBW – ECF* | $K^+$ | Organic phosphates; protein |
| **Extracellular fluid volume (ECF)** | 20 | ⅓ | Inulin<br>Mannitol | $Na^+$ | $Cl^-$<br>$HCO_3^-$ |
| **Plasma** | 5 | ¹⁄₁₂ (¼ of ECF) | RISA<br>Evans blue | $Na^+$ | $Cl^-$<br>$HCO_3^-$<br>Plasma proteins |
| **Interstitial fluid** | 15 | ¼ (¾ of ECF) | ECF-plasma volume* | $Na^+$ | $Cl^-$<br>$HCO_3^-$ |

### Principles of Fluid Distribution

1. Osmolarity of the ICF and ECF are equal.
2. Intracellular volume changes only when extracellular osmolarity changes.
3. All substances enter or leave the body by passing through the extracellular compartment.

### Measurement of Fluid Volumes

$$\text{Volume} = \frac{\text{Mass}}{\text{Concentration}}$$

*Example:* 100 mg of inulin is infused. After equilibration, its concentration = 0.01 mg/mL. What is patient's ECF volume?

*Answer:* ECF = 100 mg/0.01 mg/mL = 10,000 mL, or 10 L

### Osmolarity and Mass

1. Plasma osmolarity in mOsm/L can be quickly estimated as twice the plasma sodium concentration in mmol/L. More rigorously, plasma osmolarity (mOsm/L) = (2 × serum sodium [mEq/L]) + (BUN [mg/dL]/2.8) + (glucose [mg/dL]/18).
2. Mass of solutes in the TBW, ICF, or ECF in mOsm is calculated by the relevant volume multiplied by the osmolarity.

*Definition of abbreviation:* RISA, radio-iodinated serum albumin.
*Indirect measurement

## SUMMARY OF VOLUME AND OSMOLARITY CHANGES OF BODY FLUIDS

Body osmolarity and intracellular and extracellular fluid volumes change in clinically relevant situations. The **Darrow-Yannet diagram** *(right)* represents this information. The *y*-axis is solute concentration or osmolarity. The *x*-axis is the volume of ICF and ECF. The *solid line* represents the control state, and the *dashed line* represents changes in volume or osmolarity. In this example, osmolarity ↓, ICF volume ↑, and ECF volume ↓.

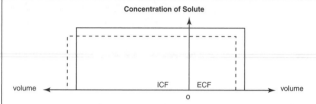

| Type | Examples | ECF Volume | Body Osmolarity | ICF Volume | D-Y Diagram |
|---|---|---|---|---|---|
| **Isosmotic volume contraction** (loss of isotonic fluid) | Diarrhea, hemorrhage, vomiting | ↓ | No change | No change | |
| **Isosmotic volume expansion** (gain of isotonic fluid) | Isotonic saline infusion | ↑ | No change | No change | |
| **Hyperosmotic volume contraction** (loss of water) | Dehydration, diabetes insipidus | ↓ | ↑ | ↓ | |
| **Hyperosmotic volume expansion** (gain of NaCl) | Excessive NaCl intake, hypertonic mannitol | ↑ | ↑ | ↓ | |
| **Hyposmotic volume contraction** (loss of NaCl) | Adrenal insufficiency | ↓ | ↓ | ↑ | |
| **Hyposmotic volume expansion** (gain of water) | SIADH, water intoxication | ↑ | ↓ | ↑ | |

*Definiton of abbreviation:* SIADH, syndrome of inappropriate antidiuretic hormone.

## MEMBRANE POTENTIALS

| | |
|---|---|
| **Equilibrium potential** | Amount of voltage needed to balance the chemical force due to its concentration gradient<br>The **Nernst equation** can determine this. For a monovalent cation:<br><br>$$E_x = \frac{60 \text{ mV}}{Z} \log_{10} \frac{[X]_o}{[X]_i}; \; E_x = \text{equilibrium potential}, [X] = \text{ion concentration (out and in)}, Z = \text{charge}$$<br>$(Na^+ = 1, Cl^- = -1, Ca^{2+} = 2)$ |
| **Resting membrane (RM) potential** | • RM is the potential difference across a cell membrane in millivolts (mV); –70 mV is typical.<br>• RM occurs because of an **unequal distribution of ions** between the ICF and ECF and the **selective permeability** of the membrane to ions. **Proteins (anions)** in cells that do not diffuse help establish the electrical potential across the membrane.<br>• The relative effect of an ion on the membrane potential is in proportion to the conductance or permeability of that ion. The **greater the conductance**, the closer the membrane will approach the **equilibrium potential** of that ion.<br>• The resting potential of cells is negative inside. **Hyperpolarization** occurs when the membrane potential becomes more negative. **Depolarization** occurs when the membrane potential becomes less negative or even positive. |
| **Chord conductance equation** | $E_m = (g_K/\Sigma g \times E_K) + (g_{Na}/\Sigma g \times E_{Na}) + (g_{Cl}/\Sigma g \times E_{Cl})$<br>$E_m$ = membrane potential in mV; g = conductance of individual ion; $\Sigma g$ = total conductance of cell membrane; E = equilibrium potential of individual ion from Nernst equation<br><br>• Used to calculate membrane potential; useful to evaluate effects of ion conductance and concentrations; explains action potential, synaptic potentials, and electrolyte disorders |

| **Properties of ions in a typical neuron** | Ion | Extracellular (mM) | Intracellular (mM) | Equilibrium Potential (mV) | Conductance |
|---|---|---|---|---|---|
| | $Na^+$ | 150.0 | 15.0 | +60 | Very low |
| | $K^+$ | 5.5 | 150.0 | –90 | High |
| | $Cl^-$ | 125.0 | 9.0 | –70 | High |

- Because potassium and chloride have a high conductance, their equilibrium potentials dominate the membrane potential, so the inside of the cell is negative.
- Changes in EC $K^+$ can produce large changes in the membrane potential:

$$\uparrow \text{EC } K^+ \rightarrow \text{depolarization}; \downarrow \text{EC } K^+ \rightarrow \text{hyperpolarization}.$$

- Changes in EC $Na^+$ have little effect on membrane potential, but an increase in $Na^+$ conductance → depolarization.

*Definition of abbreviation*: EC, extracellular.

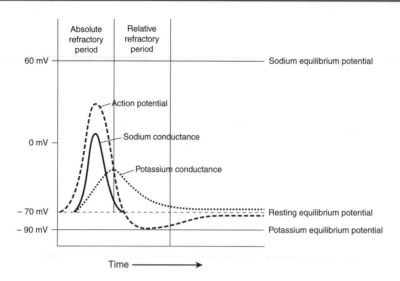

The action potentials (AP) of excitable cells involve the opening and closing of voltage-gated channels for sodium, potassium, and in some cells, calcium. The figure above shows a neuronal AP. The opening of a channel increases conductance. Steps are shown below.

- Inward currents depolarize the membrane potential to **threshold**.
- **Voltage-gated Na⁺ channels open**, causing an **inward Na⁺ current**. The membrane potential approaches the Na⁺ equilibrium potential. These channels can be blocked by **tetrodotoxin**.
- These Na⁺ channels close rapidly **(inactivation)**, even though the membrane is still depolarized.
- Depolarization slowly opens K⁺ channels, **increasing K⁺ conductance (outward current)**, leading to **repolarization**.
- **Absolute refractory period:** An AP cannot be elicited because Na⁺ channels are closed.
- **Relative refractory period:** Only a greater than normal stimulus can produce an AP because the K⁺ conductance is still higher than at rest.
- The **Na⁺-K⁺ pump** restores ion concentrations. It is **electrogenic** (3 Na⁺ pumped out for every 2 K⁺ pumped in).

## Clinical Correlations

**Calcium** has a low resting conductance and does not contribute to the resting potential. It has a very positive equilibrium potential, so when conductance increases (e.g., cardiac and smooth muscle cells), **depolarization** occurs. Calcium concentration affects the action potentials and force of contraction of **cardiac and smooth muscle**.

**Hypercalcemia** stabilizes excitable membranes, leading to flaccid paralysis of skeletal muscle. **Hypocalcemia** destabilizes membranes, leading to spontaneous action potentials and spasms.

Abnormal increases and decreases of **extracellular potassium** have severe consequences for cardiac conduction and rhythm.

Renal and gastrointestinal disorders are likely to cause abnormalities of electrolytes and alteration of resting potentials and action potentials.

# Pathology

# CELLULAR INJURY AND ADAPTATION

Changing conditions in the cell's environment can produce changes from adaptation to injury or even cell death. The cellular response to injury depends on the *type, duration,* and *severity* of injury, the *type of cell* injured, *metabolic state,* and *ability to adapt.*

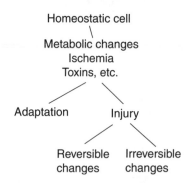

| CAUSES | EXAMPLES |
|---|---|
| **Hypoxia (most common)** | • Ischemia (e.g., arteriosclerosis, thromboembolus)<br>• Cardiopulmonary failure<br>• Severe anemia |
| **Infections** | Viruses, bacteria, parasites, rickettsiae, fungi, prions |
| **Immunologic reactions** | • Hypersensitivity reactions<br>• Autoimmune |
| **Congenital/metabolic disorders** | • Inborn errors of metabolism (e.g., phenylketonuria, galactosemia, glycogen storage diseases) |
| **Chemical injury** | • Drugs (e.g., therapeutic, drugs of abuse)<br>• Poisons<br>• Pollution<br>• Occupational exposure (e.g., $CCl_4$, CO, asbestos) |
| **Physical injury** | Trauma, burns, frostbite, radiation |
| **Nutritional or vitamin imbalance** | • Inadequate calorie/protein intake (e.g., marasmus, kwashiorkor, anorexia nervosa)<br>• Excess caloric intake (e.g., obesity, atherosclerosis)<br>• Vitamin deficiencies<br>• Hypervitaminosis |

## Important Mechanisms of Cell Injury

- Oxygen-free radicals (superoxide [$O_2^-$], hydroxyl radical [$OH\cdot$], hydrogen peroxide [$H_2O_2$]) damage DNA, proteins, lipid membranes, and circulating lipids (LDL) by peroxidation
- ATP depletion
- Increased cell-membrane permeability
- Influx of calcium—activates a wide spectrum of enzymes: proteases, ATPases, phospholipases, endonucleases
- Mitochondrial dysfunction, formation of mitochondrial permeability transition (MPT) channels
- Decreased oxidative phosphorylation
- Release of cytochrome c is a trigger for apoptosis

## Protective Factors Against Free Radicals

1. *Antioxidants*—vitamins A, E, and C
2. *Superoxide dismutase*—superoxide → hydrogen peroxide
3. *Glutathione peroxidase*—hydroxyl ions or hydrogen peroxide → water
4. *Catalase*—hydrogen peroxide → oxygen and water

## DIRECT AND INDIRECT RESULTS OF REVERSIBLE CELL INJURY

| Direct Result | Consequences | Pathophysiologic Correlates |
|---|---|---|
| Decreased synthesis of ATP by oxidative phosphorylation | Decreased function of $Na^+/K^+$ ATPase → influx of $Na^+$ and water, efflux of $K^+$, and swelling of the ER | Cellular swelling (hydropic swelling), swelling of endoplasmic reticulum, membrane blebs, myelin figures |
| Increased glycolysis → glycogen depletion | Increased lactic acid production → decreased intracellular pH | Tissue acidosis |
| Ribosomes detach from rough ER | Decreased protein synthesis | Lipid deposition (fatty change) |

### AS THE DEGREE OF CELLULAR INJURY WORSENS...

| | | |
|---|---|---|
| Severe plasma membrane damage | Massive influx of calcium, efflux of intracellular enzymes and proteins into the circulation | Markers of cellular damage detectable in serum (LDH, CK, ALT, AST, troponin, etc.) |
| Calcium influx into mitochondria | Irreparable damage to oxidative phosphorylation | Mitochondrial densities |
| Lysosomal contents leak out | Lysosomal hydrolases are activated intracellularly | Autolysis, heterolysis, nuclear changes (pyknosis, karyorrhexis, karyolysis) |

## IRREVERSIBLE INJURY AND CELL DEATH

| Morphologic Pattern | Characteristics |
|---|---|
| **Coagulative** necrosis | **Most common** (e.g., heart, liver, kidney)<br>Proteins denatured, nucleus is lost, but cellular shape is maintained |
| **Liquefactive** necrosis | **Abscesses**, **brain infarcts**, pancreatic necrosis<br>Cellular destruction by hydrolytic enzymes |
| **Caseous** necrosis | Seen in **tuberculosis**<br>Combination of coagulation and liquefaction necrosis → soft, friable, and "cottage-cheese–like" appearance |
| **Fat** necrosis | Caused by the action of lipases on fatty tissue (e.g., with **pancreatic damage**)<br>Chalky white appearance |
| **Fibrinoid** necrosis | Eosinophilic homogeneous appearance—resembles fibrin |
| **Gangrenous** necrosis | *Common sites:* lower limbs, gallbladder, GI tract, and testes<br>    Dry gangrene—coagulative necrosis<br>    Wet gangrene—liquefactive necrosis |
| **Apoptosis** | A specialized form of **programmed cell death**, an active process under genetic control<br>Mediated by a cascade of **caspases** (digest nuclear and cytoskeletal proteins and activate endonucleases)<br>Often affects only single cells or small groups of cells |

**Myocardial ischemia** is a good example of cellular injury and death.

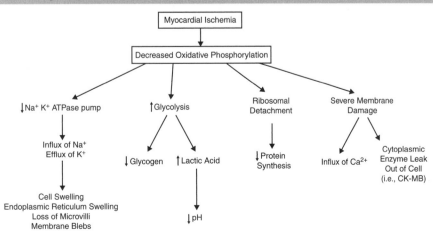

| APOSTOSIS | | | | |
|---|---|---|---|---|
| Morphology | Stimuli for Apoptosis | Genetic Regulation | Physiologic Examples | Pathologic Examples |
| • Cells shrink, cytoplasm is dense and eosinophilic<br>• Nuclear chromatin condenses, then fragments<br>• Cell membrane blebs<br>• Cell fragments (apoptotic bodies) are phagocytized by adjacent cells or macrophages<br>• **Lack of inflammatory response** | • Cell injury and DNA damage<br>• Lack of hormones, cytokines, or growth factors<br>• Receptor-ligand signals:<br>  – **Fas** binding to Fas ligand<br>  – Tumor necrosis factor (**TNF**) binding to TNF receptor 1 (TNFR1) | • *bcl-2* (inhibits apoptosis)<br>• *p-53* (stimulates apoptosis) | • Embryogenesis— organogenesis and development<br>• Hormone-dependent apoptosis (menstrual cycle)<br>• Selective death of lymphocytes in thymus | • Viral hepatitis (Councilman body)<br>• Graft versus host disease<br>• Cystic fibrosis (CF)— duct obstruction and pancreatic atrophy |

| ADAPTIVE CELLULAR RESPONSES TO INJURY (POTENTIALLY REVERSIBLE) | | |
|---|---|---|
| Types | Definitions | Causes |
| Atrophy | **Decrease in cell size and functional ability.** Cells shrink; lipofuscin granules can be seen microscopically. EM—autophagosomes | • Deceased workload/disuse<br>• Ischemia<br>• Lack of hormonal or neural stimulation<br>• Malnutrition<br>• Aging |
| Hypertrophy | **An increase in cell size and functional ability** mediated by growth factors, cytokines, and other trophic stimuli, leading to increased expression of genes and increased protein synthesis. May coexist with hyperplasia. | • Increased mechanical demand, e.g., striated muscle of weight lifters, cardiac muscle in hypertension<br>• Increased endocrine stimulation, e.g., puberty, pregnancy, lactation |
| Hyperplasia | **An increase in the number of cells** in a tissue or organ, mediated by growth factors, cytokines, and other trophic stimuli. Increased expression of growth-promoting genes (proto-oncogenes), increased DNA synthesis, and cell division | **Physiologic causes:**<br>• Compensatory (e.g., after partial hepatectomy)<br>• Hormonal stimulation (e.g., breast development at puberty)<br>• Antigenic stimulation (e.g., lymphoid hyperplasia)<br>**Pathologic causes:**<br>• Endometrial hyperplasia<br>• Prostatic hyperplasia of aging |
| Metaplasia | **A reversible change of one cell type to another** | Irritation |
| Dysplasia | **An abnormal proliferation of cells** characterized by changes in cell size, shape, and loss of cellular organization; premalignant, e.g., cervical dysplasia | Similar to stimuli that produce cancer (e.g., HPV, esophageal reflux) |

Wound healing involves **regeneration** of cells in a damaged tissue, along with repair of the connective tissue matrix.

## CAPACITY OF CELLS TO REGENERATE

| Cell Type | Properties | Examples |
|---|---|---|
| Labile | Regenerate throughout life | Skin and mucosal lining cells<br>Hematopoietic cells<br>Stem cells |
| Stable | Replicate at a low level throughout life<br>Have the capacity to divide if stimulated by some initiating event | Hepatocytes<br>Proximal tubule cells<br>Endothelium |
| Permanent | Cannot replicate | Neurons and cardiac muscle |

### Growth Factors and Cytokines Involved in Growth Repair

- Transforming growth factor $\alpha$ (TGF-$\alpha$)
- Platelet-derived growth factor (PDGF)
- Fibroblast growth factor (FGF)
- Vascular endothelial growth factor (VEGF)
- Epidermal growth factor (EGF)
- Tumor necrosis factor $\alpha$ (TNF-$\alpha$) and IL-1

## CONNECTIVE TISSUE COMPONENTS

**Collagen** production requires vitamin C (wound healing impaired in scurvy) and copper. Different types of collagen are found in different body sites.

- Type I collagen is the most common form.
- Type II collagen is found in cartilage.
- Type III collagen is an immature form found in granulation tissue.
- Type IV collage is found in basement membranes.

Other extracellular matrix components include:

- adhesion molecules
- proteoglycans
- glycosaminoglycans

## WOUND HEALING

### Primary Union (healing by first intention)

Occurs with clean wounds when there has been little tissue damage and wound edges are closely approximated, e.g., a surgical incision

### Secondary Union (healing by second intention)

Occurs in wounds that have large tissue defects (the two skin edges are not in contact):

- Granulation tissue fills in the defects
- Often accompanied by significant wound contraction; may produce large residual scar

### Keloids

Occur as result of excessive scar collagen deposition/hypertrophy, especially in dark-skinned people

### Connective Tissue Diseases

#### Scurvy

Vitamin C deficiency first affecting collagen with highest hydroxyproline content, such as that found in blood vessels. Thus, an early symptom is bleeding gums.

#### Ehlers-Danlos (ED) Syndrome

Defect in collagen synthesis or structure. There are many types. ED type IV is a defect in type III collagen.

#### Osteogenesis Imperfecta

Defect in collagen type I

# STAINING METHODS

| Stain | Cell Type/Component |
|---|---|
| Hematoxylin (stains blue to purple) | Nuclei, nucleoli, bacteria, calcium |
| Eosin (stains pink to red) | Cytoplasm, collagen, fibrin, RBCs, thyroid colloid |
| Prussian blue | Iron |
| Congo red | Amyloid |
| Periodic acid-Schiff (PAS) | Glycogen, mucin, mucoprotein, glycoprotein, as well as fungi |
| Gram stain | Microorganisms |
| Trichrome | Collagen |
| Reticulin | Reticular fibers in loose connective tissue |
| Immunohistochemical (antibody) stains:<br><br>• Cytokeratin<br>• Vimentin<br>• Desmin<br>• Prostate-specific antigen (PSA)<br>• S-100, neuron specific enolase, neurofilament<br>• GFAP | <br><br>• Epithelial cells<br>• Connective tissue<br>• Muscle<br>• Prostate<br>• Neurons, neuronally derived, neural crest–derived growths<br>• Glial cells (including astrocytes) |

*Definition of abbreviations:* GFAP, glial fibrillary acidic protein.

# AMYLOIDOSIS

An accumulation of various insoluble fibrillar in various tissues. It stains with **Congo red** and shows **apple-green birefringence** with polarized light.

| Disease | Amyloid Type |
|---|---|
| Primary amyloidosis (e.g., plasma cell disorders) | AL (kappa or lambda chains) |
| Secondary amyloidosis (e.g., neoplasia, rheumatoid arthritis, SLE, TB, Crohn disease, osteomyelitis, familial Mediterranean fever) | AA (from serum amyloid A [SAA]) |
| Renal hemodialysis | Amyloid protein $A\beta_2M$ and fibrillary protein $\beta_2$ microglobulin |
| Senile cerebral amyloidosis | Amyloid protein $A\beta$ and fibrillary protein $\beta$-amyloid precursor protein ($\beta$APP) |
| Cardiac amyloidosis | Amyloid protein ATTR and fibrillary protein transthyretin |
| Medullary carcinoma of thyroid | Procalcitonin |
| Type 2 diabetes, pancreatic islet-cell tumors | Amylin |

*Definition of abbreviations:* ATTR, amyloid transthyretin; SLE, systemic lupus erythematosus; TB, tuberculosis.

# NEOPLASIA

**Carcinogenesis** is a multistep process involving multiple genetic changes from inherited germ-line mutations or acquired mutations, leading to monoclonal expansion of a mutated cell.

**Progression of epithelial cancer:** normal epithelium → atypical hyperplasia → dysplasia → carcinoma in situ → invasion, metastasis (collagenases, hydrolases aid in penetration of barriers, such as basement membrane)

| BASIC TERMS | |
|---|---|
| **Anaplasia** | Loss of cell differentiation and tissue organization |
| **Atypical hyperplasia** | Increased cell number with morphologic abnormalities |
| **Carcinoma** | Malignant tumor of epithelium |
| **Carcinoma in situ** | Malignant tumor of epithelium that does not penetrate basement membrane to underlying tissue |
| **Desmoplasia** | Excessive fibrous tissue formation in tumor stroma |
| **Dysplasia** | Abnormal atypical cellular proliferation |
| **Metaplasia** | Replacement of one type of adult cell or tissue by another (within the same germ cell line) that is not normally present in that site |
| **Metastasis** | Secondary, discontinuous malignant growth (spread), such as a lung metastasis of a colon carcinoma |
| **Sarcoma** | A nonepithelial (mesenchymal) malignant tumor |

| SELECTED RISK FACTORS FOR CANCER | | |
|---|---|---|
| **Geographic/Racial** | Stomach cancer (Japan); hepatocellular carcinoma (Asia) | |
| **Occupational/Environmental exposures** | **Aflatoxin:** hepatocellular carcinoma<br>**Alkylating agents:** leukemia, lymphoma, other cancers<br>**Aromatic "–amines" and "azo–" dyes:** hepatocellular carcinoma<br>**Arsenic:** squamous cell carcinomas of skin and lung, angiosarcoma of liver<br>**Asbestos:** bronchogenic carcinoma, mesothelioma<br>**Benzene:** leukemia | **Chromium and nickel:** bronchogenic carcinoma<br>**Cigarette smoke:** multiple malignancies<br>**CCl$_4$:** fatty change and centrilobular necrosis of the liver<br>**Ionizing radiation:** thyroid cancer, leukemia<br>**Naphthylamine:** bladder cancer<br>**Nitrosamines:** gastric cancer<br>**Polycyclic aromatic hydrocarbons:** bronchogenic carcinoma<br>**Ultraviolet exposure:** skin cancers<br>**Vinyl chloride:** angiosarcoma of liver |
| **Age** | Increases risk of most cancers (exceptions: Wilms, etc.) | |
| **Hereditary predisposition** | Familial retinoblastoma; multiple endocrine neoplasia, familial polyposis coli | |
| **Acquired risk factors** | Cervical dysplasia, endometrial hyperplasia, cirrhosis, ulcerative colitis, chronic atrophic gastritis | |

There are many proposed mechanisms of carcinogenesis. The most important mutations involve growth-promoting genes (proto-oncogenes), growth-inhibiting tumor suppressor genes, and genes regulating apoptosis.

### Clinically Important Oncogenes

**Proto-oncogenes** are normal cellular genes involved with growth and cellular differentiation. **Oncogenes** are derived from proto-oncogenes by changing the gene sequence (resulting in a new gene product, oncoprotein) or a loss of gene regulation → overexpression of the normal gene product. Oncogenes lack regulatory control and are overexpressed → unregulated cellular proliferation.

| Oncogene | Tumor | Gene Product | Mechanism of Activation |
|---|---|---|---|
| hst-1/int-2 | Cancer of the stomach, breast, bladder, and melanoma | **Growth factor** Fibroblast growth factor | Overexpression |
| sis | Astrocytoma | Platelet-derived growth factor | Overexpression |
| erb-B1 | SCC of lung | **Growth factor receptor** Epidermal growth factor receptor | Overexpression |
| erb-B2 | Breast, ovary, lung | Epidermal growth factor receptor | Amplification |
| erb-B3 | Breast | Epidermal growth factor receptor | Overexpression |
| ret | MEN II and III, familial thyroid (medullary) cancer | Glial neurotrophic factor receptor | Point mutation |
| abl | CML, ALL | **Signal transduction proteins** bcr-abl fusion protein with tyrosine kinase activity | Translocation t(9;22) |
| Ki-ras | Lung, pancreas, and colon | GTP-binding protein | Point mutation |
| c-myc | Burkitt lymphoma | Nuclear regulatory protein | Translocation t(8;14) |
| L-myc | Small cell lung carcinoma | Nuclear regulatory protein | Amplification |
| N-myc | Neuroblastoma | Nuclear regulatory protein | Amplification |
| bcl-1 | Mantle cell lymphoma | **Cell-cycle regulatory proteins** Cyclin D protein | Translocation t(11;14) |
| CDK4 | Melanoma, glioblastoma multiforme | Cyclin-dependent kinase | Amplification |
| c-kit | Gastrointestinal stromal tumor (GIST) | KIT (also called CD117) is a stem cell factor receptor, a receptor tyrosine kinase | Overexpression or mutation |

*Definition of abbreviations:* ALL, acute lymphocytic leukemia; CML, chronic myelogenous leukemia; MEN, multiple endocrine neoplasia; SCC, squamous cell carcinoma.

## Inactivation of Tumor Suppressor Genes

**Tumor suppressor genes** encode proteins that regulate and suppress cell proliferation by inhibiting progression through the cell cycle. Inactivation of these genes → uncontrolled cellular proliferation.

| Gene | Chromosome | Tumors |
|------|-----------|--------|
| VHL | 3p25 | Von Hippel-Lindau disease, renal cell carcinoma |
| WT-1 | 11p13 | Wilms tumor |
| WT-2 | 11p15 | Wilms tumor |
| Rb | 13q14 | Retinoblastoma, osteosarcoma |
| p53 | 17p13.1 | Lung, breast, colon, etc. |
| BRCA-1 | 17q12-21 | Hereditary breast and ovary cancers |
| BRCA-2 | 13q12-13 | Hereditary breast cancer |
| APC | 5q21 | Adenomatous polyps and colon cancer |
| DCC | 18q21 | Colon cancer |
| NF-1 | 17q11.2 | Neurofibromas |
| NF-2 | 22q12 | Acoustic neuromas, meningiomas |
| p16 | 9p | Melanoma |
| DPC4 | 18q21 | Pancreatic cancer |

## Failure of Apoptosis Is Another Cause of Cancer

### bcl-2

- **Prevents apoptosis**
- Overexpressed in follicular lymphomas t(14:18) (chromosome 14 [immunoglobulin heavy chain gene]; chromosome 18 [bcl-2])

### bax, bad, bcl-xS, bid

- **Promote apoptosis**
- *p53* promotes apoptosis in mutated cells by stimulating *bax* synthesis; inactivation → failure of apoptosis

### c-myc

- Promotes cellular proliferation
- When associated with *p53* → promotes apoptosis; when associated with *bcl-2* → inhibits apoptosis

## ONCOGENIC VIRUSES

| Specific virus | Human T-cell leukemia virus (HTLV-1)* | Hepatitis B (HBV) Hepatitis C (HCV)* | Epstein-Barr | Human papilloma virus (types 16, 18 in genital sites) | Human herpesvirus 8 (HHV-8) |
|---|---|---|---|---|---|
| Associated disease | Adult T-cell leukemia/lymphoma | Hepatocellular carcinoma | Burkitt lymphoma, B-cell lymphoma, nasopharyngeal carcinoma | Cervical, vulvar, vaginal, penile, and anal carcinoma; some head and neck cancers | Kaposi sarcoma |

*RNA oncogenic viruses

## SERUM TUMOR MARKERS

These are usually normal cellular components that are increased in neoplasms but may also be elevated in non-neoplastic conditions. Can be used for screening, monitoring of treatment efficacy, and detecting recurrence.

| Marker | Associated Cancers |
|---|---|
| α-fetoprotein (AFP) | Hepatocellular carcinoma, nonseminomatous testicular germ-cell tumors |
| β-human chorionic gonadotropin (hCG) | Trophoblastic tumors, choriocarcinoma |
| Calcitonin | Medullary carcinoma of the thyroid |
| Carcinoembryonic antigen (CEA) | Carcinomas of the lung, pancreas, stomach, breast, colon |
| CA-125 | Ovarian epithelial carcinoma |
| CA19-9 | Pancreatic adenocarcinoma |
| Placental alkaline phosphatase | Seminoma |
| Prostatic acid phosphatase | Prostate cancer |
| Prostate-specific antigen (PSA) | Prostate cancer |
| S-100 | Melanoma, neural-derived tumors, astrocytoma |
| Tartrate-resistant acid phosphatase (TRAP) | Hairy cell leukemia |
| Bombesin | Small cell lung cancer, carotid body tumor |

## PARANEOPLASTIC SYNDROMES

| Syndrome | Neoplasm | Mechanism |
|---|---|---|
| Carcinoid syndrome | Carcinoid tumor (metastatic, bronchial, ovarian) | Serotonin, bradykinin |
| Cushing syndrome | Small cell carcinoma of the lung, neural tumors | ACTH, ACTH-like peptide |
| Hypercalcemia | Squamous cell carcinoma of the lung; breast, renal, and ovarian carcinomas | PTH-related peptide, TGF-α, TNF, IL-1 |
| Lambert-Eaton myasthenic syndrome | Small cell carcinoma of the lung | Antibodies against presynaptic voltage-gated $Ca^{2+}$ channels at the neuromuscular junction |
| Polycythemia | Renal cell carcinoma, hepatocellular carcinoma, cerebellar hemangioblastoma | Erythropoietin |
| SIADH | Small cell carcinoma of the lung; intracranial neoplasms | ADH |

*Definition of abbreviations:* ACTH, adrenocorticotropic hormone; IL, interleukin; TGF, transforming growth factor; TNF, tumor necrosis factor; PTH, parathyroid hormone; SIADH, syndrome of inappropriate antidiuretic hormone

| GRADING AND STAGING | |
|---|---|
| Grade | • An estimate of the cytologic malignancy of a tumor, including the degree of anaplasia and number of mitoses.<br>• Nuclear size, chromatin content, nucleoli, and nuclear-to-cytoplasmic ratio are all used. |
| Stage | • The clinical estimate of the extent of spread of a malignant tumor. Low stage means a localized tumor. Stage rises as tumors spread locally then metastasize.<br>• **TNM** is typically used; **T** = size of **t**umor; **N** = **n**ode involvement; **M** = **m**etastases |

| CANCER INCIDENCE AND MORTALITY | | |
|---|---|---|
| **Incidence** | **Males** | **Females** |
| | Prostate: 25% | Breast: 26% |
| | Lung and bronchus: 15% | Lung and bronchus: 14% |
| | Colon and rectum: 10% | Colon and rectum: 10% |
| **Mortality** | **Males** | **Females** |
| | Lung and bronchus: 31% | Lung and bronchus: 26% |
| | Prostate: 10% | Breast: 15% |
| | Colon and rectum: 8% | Colon and rectum: 9% |

# Organ Systems

# The Nervous System

## Development of the Nervous System

## Peripheral Nervous System

## Meninges, Ventricular System, and Venous Drainage

## Neurohistology and Pathologic Correlates

## Spinal Cord

## Cranial Nerves and Brain Stem

## Visual System

## Brain Stem Lesions

## Cerebellum

## Diencephalon

## Basal Ganglia

## Limbic System

## Cerebral Cortex

## Blood Supply

## Seizures and Anticonvulsants

## Opioid Analgesics and Related Drugs

## Local Anesthetics

# DEVELOPMENT OF THE NERVOUS SYSTEM

## Neurulation

- **Neurulation** begins in the third week.
- The **notochord** induces the overlying ectoderm to form the neural plate.
- By end of the third week, **neural folds** grow over midline and fuse to form **neural tube**.
- During closure, **neural crest** cells form from neuroectoderm.

- **Neural tube** → brain and spinal cord (plus lower motoneurons, preganglionic neurons)
- Brain stem and spinal cord have an **alar** plate (**sensory**) and a **basal** plate (**motor**); plates are separated by the **sulcus limitans**.
- **Neural tube** → 3 primary vesicles → 5 primary vesicles

- **Neural crest** → sensory and postganglionic neurons

- **Peripheral NS (PNS):** cranial nerves (12 pairs) and spinal nerves (31 pairs)

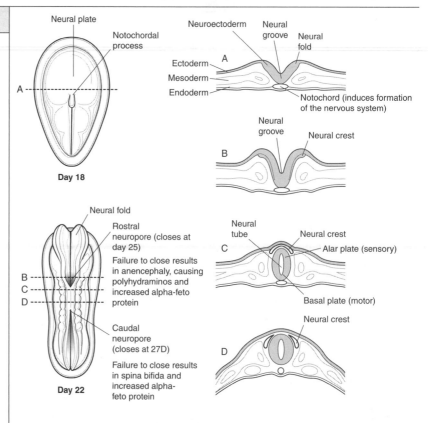

## CENTRAL NERVOUS SYSTEM

| | Adult Derivatives | |
|---|---|---|
| | **Structures** | **Ventricles** |
| Telencephalon | Cerebral hemispheres, most of basal ganglia | Lateral ventricle |
| Diencephalon | Thalamus, hypothalamus, subthalamus, epithalamus (pineal gland), retina | Third ventricle |
| Mesencephalon | Midbrain | Cerebral aqueduct |
| Metencephalon | Pons, cerebellum | Fourth ventricle |
| Myelencephalon | Medulla | |

ORGAN SYSTEMS

NERVOUS

## CONGENITAL MALFORMATIONS OF THE NERVOUS SYSTEM

| Condition | Types | Description |
|---|---|---|
| Anencephaly | — | Failure of **anterior neuropore** to close<br>Brain does not develop<br>Incompatible with life<br>Increased AFP |
| Spina bifida | Failure of **posterior neuropore** to close ||
| | Spina bifida occulta **(Figure A)** | Mildest form<br>**Vertebrae** fail to form around spinal cord<br>**No** increase in **AFP**<br>Asymptomatic |
| | Spina bifida with meningocele **(Figure B)** | **Meninges** protrude through vertebral defect<br>Increase in AFP |
| | Spina bifida with meningomyelocele **(Figure C)** | **Meninges** and **spinal cord** protrude through vertebral defect<br>Increase in AFP |
| | Spina bifida with myeloschisis **(Figure D)** | Most severe<br>**Spinal cord** can be seen **externally**<br>Increase in AFP |

A
- Vertebral arch
- Muscle
- Skin
- Dura and arachnoid
- Subarachnoid space
- Spinal cord
- Vertebral body

B  C  D

| Condition | Types | Description |
|---|---|---|
| Arnold-Chiari malformation | Type I | Most common<br>Mostly **asymptomatic**<br>Downward displacement of cerebellar tonsils through foramen magnum |
| | Type II | More often **symptomatic**<br>Downward displacement of **cerebellar vermis** and **medulla** through foramen magnum<br>Compression of IV ventricle → obstructive **hydrocephaly**<br>Frequent lumbar **meningomyelocele**<br>Frequent association with **syringomyelia** |
| Dandy-Walker malformation | | Failure of foramina of Luschka and Magendie to open → **dilation of IV ventricle**<br>Agenesis of cerebellar vermis and splenium of the corpus callosum |
| Hydrocephalus | | Most often caused by stenosis of cerebral aqueduct<br>CSF accumulates in ventricles and subarachnoid space<br>Increased head circumference |
| Holoprosencephaly | | Incomplete separation of cerebral hemispheres<br>One ventricle in telencephalon<br>Seen in trisomy 13 (Patau) |

*Definition of abbreviation:* AFP, α-fetoprotein.

## AUTONOMIC AND SOMATIC NERVOUS SYSTEMS

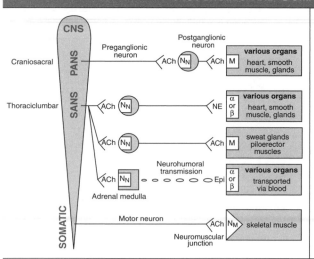

- **Somatic NS:** 1 neuron (from spinal cord → effector organ)

- **Autonomic NS:** 2 neurons (from spinal cord → effector organ)

  - **Preganglionic** neuron: cell body in CNS
  - **Postganglionic** neuron: cell body in ganglia in PNS

  - **Parasympathetic:** long preganglionic, short postganglionic
  - **Sympathetic:** short preganglionic, long postganglionic (except adrenal medulla)

*Definition of abbreviations:* $N_N$, neuronal nicotinic receptor; $N_M$, muscle nicotinic receptor; NE, norepinephrine; M, muscarinic receptor; ACh, acetylcholine.

*Note:* Arrows indicate lesion sites that result in Horner syndrome.

## PARASYMPATHETIC NERVOUS SYSTEM

1. Ciliary ganglion
Pupillary sphincter
Ciliary m.
III
2. Submandibular VI ganglion
Submandibular gland
Sublingual gland
IV
V
Midbrain
3. Pterygopalatine ganglion
Lacrimal gland
Nasal mucosa
Oral mucosa
VII
a
VIII
IX
Pons
Parotid gland
X
4. Otic ganglion
XI
Medulla
C1
Viscera of the thorax and abdomen (foregut and midgut)
Terminal ganglia

Preganglionic ○——⊢
Postganglionic ○------⊰

T1

L1

Terminal ganglia
Hindgut and pelvic viscera (including the bladder, erectile tissue, and rectum)
S2
S3
S4
Pelvic splanchnics

## SYMPATHETIC NERVOUS SYSTEM

Hypothalamus
III
IV
V
VII VI
VIII
IX
X
XI
X

Head (sweat glands, dilator pupillae *m.*, superior tarsal *m.*)

Internal carotid *a.*
External carotid *a.*

Descending hypothalamic fibers (drive all preganglionic sympathetic neurons)

Superior cervical ganglion
Middle cervical ganglion
Vertebral ganglion
Cervicothoracic ganglion

T1
Heart, trachea, bronchi, lungs (Thorax)

Smooth muscle and glands of the foregut and midgut

Thoracic splanchnic nerves
*
*
*
Prevertebral ganglia

L1
L2
Smooth muscle and glands of the hindgut and pelvic viscera

Lumbar splanchnic nerves
Prevertebral ganglia

Sympathetic chain

Gray rami
*Rejoin branches of spinal nerve

*Note:* Arrows indicate lesion sites that result in Horner syndrome.

| PARASYMPATHETIC = CRANIOSACRAL OUTFLOW | | | SYMPATHETIC = THORACOLUMBAR OUTFLOW | | |
|---|---|---|---|---|---|
| **Origin** | **Site of Synapse** | **Innervation** | **Origin** | **Site of Synapse** | **Innervation** |
| Cranial nerves III, VII, IX | 4 cranial ganglia | Glands and smooth muscle of the head | Spinal cord levels T1–L2 | Sympathetic chain ganglia (paravertebral ganglia) | Smooth and cardiac muscle and glands of body wall and limbs; head and thoracic viscera |
| Cranial nerve X | Terminal ganglia (in or near the walls of viscera) | Viscera of the neck, thorax, foregut, and midgut | Thoracic splanchnic nerves T5–T12 | Prevertebral ganglia (collateral; e.g., celiac, aorticorenal superior mesenteric ganglia) | Smooth muscle and glands of the foregut and midgut |
| Pelvic splanchnic nerves (S2, S3, S4) | Terminal ganglia (in or near the walls of viscera) | Hindgut and pelvic viscera (including bladder and erectile tissue) | Lumbar splanchnic nerves L1, L2 | Prevertebral ganglia (collateral; e.g., inferior mesenteric and pelvic ganglia) | Smooth muscle and glands of the pelvic viscera and hindgut |

## AUTONOMIC EFFECTS ON ORGAN SYSTEMS

As a general rule, the **sympathetic autonomic nervous system (SANS)** mediates **"fight or flight"** responses, such as increasing heart rate and contractility, dilating airways and pupils, inhibiting GI and GU functions, and directing blood flow away from skin and GI tract and toward skeletal muscles. In contrast, the **parasympathetic autonomic nervous system (PANS)** causes the body to **"rest and digest,"** reducing heart rate and contractility, contracting airways and pupils, inducing secretion from lacrimal and salivary glands, and promoting GI and GU motility. Blood vessels are solely innervated by SANS nerve fibers.

| | Sympathetic "Fight or Flight" | | Parasympathetic "Rest and Digest" | |
|---|---|---|---|---|
| **Organ** | **Action** | **Receptor** | **Action** | **Receptor** |
| **Cardiovascular** | | | | |
| Heart | | | | |
| SA node | ↑ heart rate | $\beta_1$, $(\beta_2)$ | ↓ heart rate | $M_2$ |
| Atria | ↑ contractility | | ↓ contractility | |
| AV node | ↑ conduction velocity and automaticity[1] | | ↓ conduction velocity and automaticity[1] | |
| Ventricles | ↑ contractility | | ↓ contractility (slight) | |
| Arterioles[2] | Contract: ↑ resistance | $\alpha_1$ | — | $(M_3)$[3] |
| Veins | Contract: ↑ venous pressure | $\alpha_1$ | — | — |
| Kidney | Renin release | $\beta_1$ | — | — |
| **Respiratory** | | | | |
| Bronchiolar smooth muscle | Relax: ↓ resistance | $\beta_2$ | Contract: ↑ resistance | $M_3$ |

*(Continued)*

[1] When acting as a pacemaker; otherwise, the SA node suppresses automaticity in these cells

[2] $\beta_2$ receptors that mediate relaxation and decrease resistance are also present on coronary arteries and arterioles. Low doses of epinephrine (or $\beta_2$ agonists) act selectively on $\beta_2$ receptors and can decrease systemic vascular resistance, but increased sympathetic tone increases systemic vascular resistance because vasoconstriction dominates.

[3] $M_3$ receptors are on vascular endothelium (not smooth muscle, like the adrenergic receptors) and cause vasodilation via nitric oxide (NO) generation; this has little physiologic significance because vasculature is not innervated by PANS, but is more important with muscarinic agonist administration.

| AUTONOMIC EFFECTS ON ORGAN SYSTEMS (*CONT'D.*) | | | | |
|---|---|---|---|---|
| | Sympathetic "Fight or Flight" | | Parasympathetic "Rest and Digest" | |
| Organ | Action | Receptor | Action | Receptor |
| **Gastrointestinal** | | | | |
| GI smooth muscle | | | | |
|   Walls | ↓ GI motility | $\alpha_2,^4 \beta_2$ | ↑ GI motility | $M_3$ |
|   Sphincters | Contracts | $\alpha_1$ | Relaxes | $M_3$ |
| Glandular secretion | — | — | Increases | $M_3$ |
| Liver | Gluconeogenesis | $\beta_2, \alpha$ | — | — |
| | Glycogenolysis | $\beta_2, \alpha$ | — | — |
| Fat cells | Lipolysis | $\beta_3$ | — | — |
| **Genitourinary** | | | | |
| Bladder | | | | |
|   Walls | Relaxes | $\beta_2$ | Contracts | $M_3$ |
|   Sphincters | Contracts | $\alpha_1$ | Relaxes | $M_3$ |
| Uterus, pregnant | Relaxes | $\beta_2$ | — | — |
| | Contracts | $\alpha$ | Contracts | $M_3$ |
| Penis, seminal vesicles | Ejaculation | $\alpha$ | Erection | M |
| **Skin** | | | | |
| Sweat glands | Secretion | $M,^5 \alpha^6$ | — | — |
| **Eye** | | | | |
|   Radial dilator muscle | Contracts (dilates pupil) | $\alpha_1$ | — | — |
|   Pupillary sphincter muscle | — | — | Contracts (constricts pupil). | $M_3$ |
|   Ciliary muscle | Relaxes—far vision | $\beta$ | Contracts—near vision | $M_3$ |

[4] Probably via inhibition of cholinergic nerve terminals

[5] Generalized

[6] Localized (e.g., palms of hands)

## CHOLINERGIC TRANSMISSION

**Acetylcholine (ACh)** is synthesized from acetate and choline in synaptic nerve terminals via **choline acetyltransferase (ChAT)** and stored in synaptic vesicles and released by $Ca^{2+}$ influx upon depolarization. The **uptake of choline** into the nerve terminal is the **rate-limiting step** of ACh synthesis and can be blocked by **hemicholinium**. ACh then binds to postsynaptic receptors to elicit somatic ($N_M$) or autonomic ($N_N$ and M) effects. Signal termination occurs by degradation of ACh by **acetylcholinesterase (AChE)**.

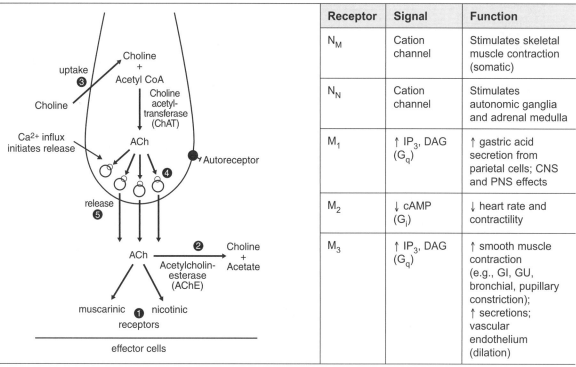

| Receptor | Signal | Function |
|---|---|---|
| $N_M$ | Cation channel | Stimulates skeletal muscle contraction (somatic) |
| $N_N$ | Cation channel | Stimulates autonomic ganglia and adrenal medulla |
| $M_1$ | ↑ $IP_3$, DAG ($G_q$) | ↑ gastric acid secretion from parietal cells; CNS and PNS effects |
| $M_2$ | ↓ cAMP ($G_i$) | ↓ heart rate and contractility |
| $M_3$ | ↑ $IP_3$, DAG ($G_q$) | ↑ smooth muscle contraction (e.g., GI, GU, bronchial, pupillary constriction); ↑ secretions; vascular endothelium (dilation) |

*Definition of abbreviations:* DAG, diacylglycerol; GI, gastrointestinal; GU, genitourinary; $IP_3$, inositol triphosphate.

*Note:* The numbers in the figure correspond to the numbers in the table below.

## CHOLINERGIC PHARMACOLOGY

| Mechanism of Action | Agent | Clinical Uses | Other Notes and Toxicity |
|---|---|---|---|
| **❶ ACh receptor** | | | |
| **Nicotinic ($N_M$) agonist/antagonists** (skeletal muscle) | | | |
| **Nicotinic ($N_N$) antagonists** (ganglion blockers) | Hexamethonium Trimethaphan Mecamylamine | Rarely used due to toxicities | Blocks both SANS and PANS; effectively reduces predominant tone (*see table below*) |
| **Cholinergic agonists** M = muscarinic N = nicotinic B = both | Bethanechol (M) | Ileus (postop/neurogenic) Urinary retention | Heart block, cardiac arrest Syncope |
| | Methacholine (M) | Diagnosis of bronchial hyperreactivity in asthma | Partially sensitive to cholinesterase (others listed here are resistant) |
| | Pilocarpine (M) | Glaucoma (topical) Xerostomia | — |
| | Carbachol (B) | Glaucoma (topical) | — |
| | Nicotine (N) | Smoking deterrence | — |

*(Continued)*

| CHOLINERGIC PHARMACOLOGY (*CONT'D.*) | | | |
|---|---|---|---|
| **Mechanism of Action** | **Agent** | **Clinical Uses** | **Other Notes and Toxicity** |
| **Muscarinic antagonists**<br><br>Class known as "Belladonna" alkaloids (meaning "beautiful lady") from their origin from *Atropa belladonna*, which was used to dilate pupils (believed to make women look more attractive).<br><br>Other drugs with anti-muscarinic effects:<br><br>• Antihistamines<br>• Tricyclics<br>• Antipsychotics<br>• Quinidine<br>• Amantadine<br>• Meperidine | Atropine | Counteracts cholinergic toxicity<br>Antidiarrheal<br>Mydriatic agent for eye exams<br>Reversal of sinus bradycardia and heart block | Mydriasis and cycloplegia **(blind as a bat)**<br>Decreased secretions **(dry as a bone)**<br>Vasodilation **(red as a beet)**<br>Delirium and hallucinations **(mad as a hatter)**<br>Hyperthermia<br>Tachycardia<br>Urinary retention and constipation<br>Sedation, amnesia |
| | Homatropine<br>Cyclopentolate<br>Tropicamide | Ophthalmology (topical), for mydriasis | — |
| | Ipratropium | Asthma and COPD | Localized effect because is a quaternary amine; few antimuscarinic side effects |
| | Scopolamine | Motion-sickness<br>Antiemetic | (*See side effects for atropine.*) |
| | Benztropine<br>Trihexyphenidyl<br>Biperiden | Parkinsonism<br>Acute extrapyramidal symptoms from neuroleptics | |
| | Glycopyrrolate<br>Dicyclomine | Reduces hypermotility in GI and GU tracts | |
| **❷ Metabolism (AChE inhibitors)** | | | |
| *Short-acting:* | Edrophonium | Diagnosis of myasthenia gravis | Seizures |
| *Tertiary amines:* | Physostigmine | Glaucoma<br>Reversal of anticholinergic toxicity | Carbamylating inhibitor<br>Seizures |
| *Quaternary amines:* | Neostigmine<br>Pyridostigmine<br>Ambenonium | Ileus, urinary retention<br>Myasthenia gravis<br>Reversal of nondepolarizing neuromuscular blockers | Carbamylating inhibitors |
| *Lipid-soluble:* | Donepezil<br>Tacrine<br>Rivastigmine<br>Galantamine | Alzheimer disease | Hepatotoxicity<br>GI bleeding |

(Continued)

## CHOLINERGIC PHARMACOLOGY (CONT'D.)

| Mechanism of Action | Agent | Clinical Uses | Other Notes and Toxicity |
|---|---|---|---|
| **Organophosphates:**<br><br>(long-acting and irreversible)<br><br>(causes time-dependent **aging**, which permanently inactivates AChE) | Echothiophate<br><br>Malathion<br>Parathion<br><br>Sarin<br>VX | Glaucoma<br><br>Insecticide<br><br><br>Nerve agents<br>(chemical warfare) | **D**iarrhea<br>**U**rination<br>**M**iosis<br>**B**radycardia<br>**B**ronchoconstriction<br>**E**xcitation (CNS and muscle)<br>**L**acrimation, **s**alivation, **s**weating<br>**Mnemonic: DUMBBELSS**<br>Acute treatment with **atropine** and **pralidoxime (2-PAM)** to regenerate AChE before aging occurs |
| ❸ **Reuptake inhibitors** | Hemicholinium | Only used in research settings | Blocks choline reuptake, slowing ACh synthesis |
| ❹ **Vesicular transport inhibitors** | Vesamicol | Only used in research settings | Blocks ACh uptake into vesicles, preventing storage and leading to ACh depletion |
| ❺ **Vesicle release inhibitors** | Botulinum toxin | Blepharospasm<br>Strabismus/Hyperhydrosis<br>Cervical dystonia<br>Cosmetics | Prevents fusion of cholinergic vesicles to membrane, thereby inhibiting ACh release |

*Definition of abbreviations:* ACh, acetylcholine; AChE, acetylcholinesterase; ChAT, choline acetyltransferase; COPD, chronic obstructive pulmonary disorder.

## PREDOMINANT TONE AND THE EFFECT OF GANGLIONIC BLOCKERS

The effects of ganglionic blockers can be easily predicted if you know the predominant autonomic tone to a particular effector organ. The effect of the blockade will be the opposite of what the predominant tone causes. In general, the predominant tone to vessels is sympathetic, and most everything else is parasympathetic.

| Site | Predominant Tone | Effect of Ganglionic Blockade |
|---|---|---|
| Arterioles | Sympathetic | Dilation (↓ blood pressure) |
| Veins | Sympathetic | Dilation (↓ venous return) |
| Heart | Parasympathetic | ↑ heart rate |
| GI tract | Parasympathetic | ↓ motility and secretions |
| Eye | Parasympathetic | Pupillary dilation, focus to far vision |
| Urinary bladder | Parasympathetic | Urinary retention |
| Salivary glands | Parasympathetic | Dry mouth |
| Sweat glands | Sympathetic (cholinergic) | Anhidrosis |

**Norepinephrine (NE)**, **epinephrine (EPI)**, and dopamine are part of the **catecholamine** family, which are synthesized from **tyrosine**. The first step of the synthetic pathway is carried out by **tyrosine hydroxylase**; it is also the **rate-limiting** step. NE levels inside the presynaptic terminal may also be regulated by metabolism by **monoamine oxidase (MAO)**. Once released, NE binds to various adrenergic receptors to transmit its signal. NE primarily binds $\alpha_1$, $\alpha_2$, and $\beta_1$ receptors, whereas EPI (released by the adrenal medulla) binds $\alpha_1$, $\alpha_2$, $\beta_1$, and $\beta_2$ receptors. **Reuptake** (especially uptake-1) and diffusion are most important in the termination of action of NE (and DA). Metabolism occurs via **catechol-O-methyltransferase ([COMT]** extracellular) and **MAO** (intracellular). Metabolites such as **metanephrine**, **normetanephrine**, **vanillylmandelic acid (VMA)** can be measured in the urine and are used in diagnosis diseases such as pheochromocytoma.

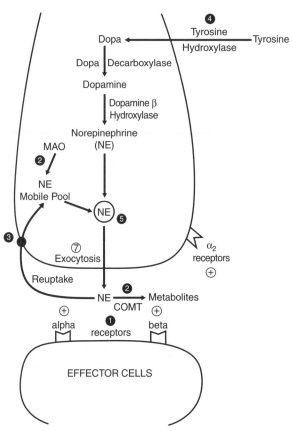

| Receptor | Signal | Function |
|---|---|---|
| $\alpha_1$ | ↑ IP$_3$, DAG (G$_q$) | ↑ smooth muscle contraction (in vascular walls, radial dilator muscle [eye], and GI and bladder sphincters); ↑ glycogenolysis in liver |
| $\alpha_2$ | ↓ cAMP (G$_i$) | Inhibits neurotransmitter release; inhibits insulin release and lipolysis |
| $\beta_1$ | ↑ cAMP (G$_s$) | ↑ heart rate and contractility; ↑ AV conduction velocity; ↑ renin secretion |
| $\beta_2$ | | ↑ smooth muscle relaxation (in vascular, bronchial, GI, and bladder walls); ↑ glycogenolysis in liver, ↑ insulin release |
| $\beta_3$ | | ↑ lipolysis from adipose tissues |

**Mnemonic:** You can get an adrenaline rush from a **QISSS** ($G_qG_iG_sG_sG_s$).

*Definition of abbreviations:* DAG, diacylglycerol; GI, gastrointestinal; GU, genitourinary; IP$_3$, inositol triphosphate.

*Note:* The numbers in the figure correspond to the numbers in the table below.

| | ADRENERGIC PHARMACOLOGY | | |
|---|---|---|---|
| **Mechanism of Action** | **Agent** | **Clinical Uses** | **Other Notes and Toxicity** |
| ❶ Adrenergic receptor | | | |
| α-adrenergic agonists | $\alpha_1$: Phenylephrine | Nasal congestion<br>Vasoconstriction<br>Mydriasis (topical) | — |
| | $\alpha_1$: Methoxamine | Paroxysmal supra-ventricular tachycardia | Bradycardia (vagal reflex) |
| | $\alpha_2$: Clonidine<br>Methyldopa | Hypertension | Decreases sympathetic outflow<br>Methyldopa: prodrug converted to methylnorepinephrine |
| α-adrenergic antagonists | **Nonselective:**<br>Phentolamine | Pheochromocytoma | **Reversible**, competitive inhibitor<br>Postural hypotension, reflex tachycardia |
| | **Nonselective:**<br>Phenoxybenzamine | Pheochromocytoma | **Irreversible** inhibitor<br>Postural hypotension, reflex tachycardia |
| | $\alpha_1$: Prazosin<br>Doxazosin<br>Terazosin<br>Tamsulosin | Hypertension<br>Benign prostatic hypertrophy | Postural hypotension on first dose |
| | $\alpha_2$: Yohimbine | Impotence<br>Postural hypotension | Clinical use limited |
| | $\alpha_2$: Mirtazapine | Depression | May also block 5HT receptors |
| β-adrenergic agonists | $\beta_1 = \beta_2$: Isoproterenol | Bronchospasm<br>Heart block and bradyarrhythmias | Clinical use limited<br>↓ BP, ↑ HR<br>Arrhythmias |
| | $\beta_1 > \beta_2$: Dobutamine | Acute heart failure | — |
| | $\beta_2$: Albuterol<br>Terbutaline<br>Metaproterenol<br>Salmeterol | Asthma | Tachycardia, skeletal muscle tremor<br>Pulmonary delivery to minimize side effects<br>Salmeterol is long-acting<br>Suppress premature labor (terbutaline) |
| | $\beta_2$: Ritodrine | Premature labor | — |
| β-adrenergic antagonists | $\beta_1$: Acebutolol<br>Atenolol<br>Esmolol<br>Metoprolol | Hypertension<br>Angina<br>Chronic heart failure (carvedilol, labetalol, metoprolol)<br>Arrhythmia (propanolol, acebutolol, esmolol)<br>Glaucoma (timolol)<br>Migraine, tremor, thyrotoxicosis (propanolol) | Sedation<br>Decreases libido<br>Bradycardia<br>$\beta_1$ selectivity safer in asthma, diabetes, and vascular diseases<br>Pindolol and acebutolol have **intrinsic sympathomimetic activity** (useful in asthmatics); should not be used in patients with recent MI |
| | **Nonselective:**<br>Pindolol<br>Propranolol<br>Nadolol<br>Timolol | | |
| | α **and** β:<br>Labetalol<br>Carvedilol | CHF | Similar to above<br>Liver damage (labetalol) |

*Definition of abbreviation:* CHF, congestive heart failure.

*(Continued)*

ORGAN SYSTEMS

NERVOUS

# ADRENERGIC PHARMACOLOGY (CONT'D.)

| Mechanism of Action | Agent | Clinical Uses | Other Notes and Toxicity |
|---|---|---|---|
| **❷ Metabolism** | | | |
| **MAO inhibitors**<br><br>MAO-A: mainly liver but <u>A</u>nywhere<br>MAO-B: mainly in <u>B</u>rain | Phenelzine<br>Tranylcypromine<br>Isocarboxazid | Depression | Nonselective MAO-A/B inhibitors<br>Tyramine (red wine, cheese) ingestion → hypertensive crisis<br>Insomnia<br>Postural hypotension<br>MAO-AIs: moclobemide (reversible), clorgyline available in Europe |
| | Selegiline<br>Rasagiline | Parkinson disease | Selective MAO-B inhibitor |
| **COMT inhibitors** | Entacapone<br>Tolcapone | Parkinson disease | — |
| **❸ Reuptake inhibitors** | Cocaine | Local anesthesia<br>Abuse | Inhibits monoamine reuptake<br>Addiction |
| **Tricyclic antidepressants** | Amitriptyline<br>Imipramine<br>Desipramine<br>Nortriptyline | Depression | Inhibits monoamine reuptake<br>Sedation<br>Postural hypotension<br>Tachycardia<br>Atropine-like effects |
| **❹ Synthesis inhibitors** | α-Methyltyrosine (metyrosine) | Hypertension | Inhibits tyrosine hydroxylase<br>Only for hypertension associated with pheochromocytoma |
| **❺ Drugs affecting release** | | | |
| **Adrenergic neuron blockers** | Reserpine | Hypertension | Inhibits monoamine vesicular uptake, leading to neurotransmitter depletion<br>Sedation, depression |
| | Guanethidine | Hypertension | Inhibits NE release from sympathetic nerve endings<br>Requires neuronal uptake to work, so interferes with other drugs that require uptake carrier (e.g., cocaine, amphetamine, cyclic antidepressants) |
| **Indirect-acting sympathomimetics** | Amphetamine<br>Methylphenidate | Narcolepsy and ADHD | Displaces NE from mobile pool<br>Addiction<br>Restlessness and rebound fatigue |
| | Ephedrine<br>Pseudoephedrine | For vasoconstriction | Displaces NE from mobile pool<br>Pseudoephedrine: OTC for nasal congestion |

*Definition of abbreviations:* ADHD, attention deficit and hyperactivity disorder; COMT, catechol-O-methyltransferase; MAO, monoamine oxidase; NE, norepinephrine; OTC, over the counter.

# MENINGES, VENTRICULAR SYSTEM, AND VENOUS DRAINAGE

## MENINGES AND MENINGEAL SPACES

Meninges consist of three connective tissue membranes that surround the brain and spinal cord. Meningeal spaces are spaces or potential spaces adjacent to the meninges.

| Meninges | Meningeal Space | Anatomic Description | Clinical Correlate |
|---|---|---|---|
| | Epidural space | Tight potential space between dura and skull<br>Contains **middle meningeal artery** | **Epidural hematoma**<br>Temporal bone fracture → rupture of **middle meningeal artery**<br>**Lens-shaped biconvex** hematoma |
| **Dura** | | Tough outer layer; dense connective tissue | |
| | Subdural space | Contains **bridging veins** | **Subdural hematoma**<br>Rupture of bridging veins<br>**Crescent-shaped** hematoma |
| **Arachnoid** | | Delicate, nonvascular connective tissue | |
| | Subarachnoid space | Contains **CSF**<br>Ends at S2 vertebra | **Subarachnoid hemorrhage**<br>**"Worst headache of my life"**<br>Often caused by **berry aneurysms**<br>**Lumbar puncture** between L4, L5 discs |
| **Pia** | | Thin, highly vascular connective tissue<br>Adheres to brain and spinal cord | |

## MENINGITIS (INFECTION OF THE MENINGES, ESPECIALLY THE PIA AND ARACHNOID)

| | |
|---|---|
| **Acute purulent (bacterial) meningitis** | • **Headache, fever, nuchal rigidity**, obtundation; coma may occur<br>• Meninges opaque; neutrophilic exudate present<br>• Sequelae: hydrocephalus, herniation, cranial nerve impairment |
| **Acute aseptic (viral) meningitis** | • Leptomeningeal inflammation (lymphomonocytic infiltrates) due to viruses (Enterovirus most frequent)<br>• Fever, signs of meningeal irritation, depressed consciousness, but low mortality |
| **Mycobacterial meningoencephalitis** | • Can be caused by *Mycobacterium tuberculosis* or atypical mycobacteria<br>• Usually involves the **basal surface** of the brain with tuberculomas within the brain and dura mater<br>• Frequent in AIDS patients, particularly by *Mycobacterium avium-intracellulare* (MAI) |
| **Fungal meningoencephalitis** | • *Candida, Aspergillus, Cryptococcus*, and *Mucor* species most frequent agents<br>• *Aspergillus* and *Mucor* attack blood vessels → vasculitis, rupture of blood vessels, and hemorrhage<br>• *Cryptococcus* causes diffuse meningoencephalitis |

## ORGANISMS CAUSING BACTERIAL MENINGITIS BY AGE GROUP

| Neonates | Infants/Children | Adolescents/Young Adults | Elderly |
|---|---|---|---|
| **Group B streptococci**<br>***Escherichia coli***<br>Listeria monocytogenes | ***Haemophilus influenzae* B**<br>(if not vaccinated)<br>Streptococcus pneumoniae<br>Neisseria meningitidis | ***Neisseria meningitidis*** | ***Streptococcus pneumoniae***<br>Listeria monocytogenes |

## CSF Parameters in Meningitis

| Condition | Cells/μl | Glucose (mg/dL) | Proteins (mg/dL) | Pressure (mm H$_2$O) |
|---|---|---|---|---|
| **Normal values** | <5 lymphocytes | 45–85 (50–70% of blood glucose) | 15–45 | 70–180 |
| **Purulent (bacterial)** | Up to 90,000 neutrophils | Decreased (<45) | Increased (>50) | Markedly elevated |
| **Aseptic (viral)** | 100–1,000 most lymphocytes | Normal | Increased (>50) | Slightly elevated |
| **Granulomatous (mycobacterial/fungal)** | 100–1,000 most lymphocytes | Decreased (<45) | Increased (>50) | Moderately elevated |

## Viral Encephalitis

*Pathology:* perivascular cuffs, microglial nodules, neuron loss, and neuronophagia
*Clinical:* fever, headache, mental status changes, often progressing to coma

| Arthropod-Borne | Herpes Simplex | Rabies | HIV |
|---|---|---|---|
| St. Louis, California, Eastern equine, Western equine, Venezuelan | Characteristic **hemorrhagic necrosis of temporal lobes** | **Negri bodies** in hippocampal and Purkinje neurons of the cerebellum | **Microglial nodules, multinucleated giant cells** |

## Ventricular System and Venous Drainage

The brain and spinal cord float within a protective bath of cerebrospinal fluid (CSF), which is produced by the lining of the ventricles, the choroid plexus. CSF circulation begins in the ventricles and then enters the subarachnoid space to surround the brain and spinal cord.

### Ventricles and CSF Circulation

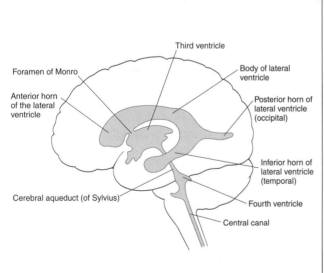
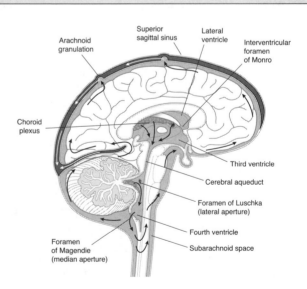

Lateral ventricles $\xrightarrow{A}$ third ventricle $\xrightarrow{B}$ fourth ventricle → subarachnoid space (via foramina of Luschka and foramen of Magendie)
(**A,** interventricular foramen of Monro; **B,** cerebral aqueduct.)

*(Continued)*

### CSF Production and Barriers

**Choroid plexus**—contains **ependymal cells** and is in the lateral, third, and fourth ventricles. **Secretes CSF.** Tight junctions form **blood-CSF barrier**.

**Blood-brain barrier**—formed by capillary endothelium with tight junctions; astrocyte foot processes contribute.

Once CSF is in the subarachnoid space, it goes up over convexity of the brain and enters the venous circulation by passing through **arachnoid granulations** into the **superior sagittal sinus**.

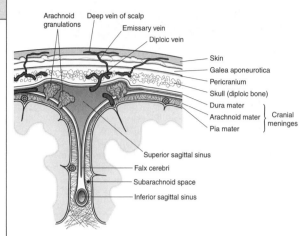

### Sinuses

**Superior sagittal sinus** (in superior margin of falx cerebri)—drains into two **transverse sinuses**. Each of these drains blood from the **confluence of sinuses** into **sigmoid sinuses**. Each sigmoid sinus exits the skull (via **jugular foramen**) as the **internal jugular veins**.

**Inferior sagittal sinus** (in inferior margin of falx cerebri)—terminates by joining with the great cerebral vein of Galen to form the **straight sinus** at the falx cerebri and tentorium cerebelli junction. This drains into the confluence of sinuses.

**Cavernous sinus**—a plexus of veins on either side of the **sella turcica**. Surrounds internal carotid artery and cranial nerves III, IV, V, and VI. It drains into the transverse sinus (via the **superior petrosal sinus**) and the internal jugular vein (via the **inferior petrosal sinus**).

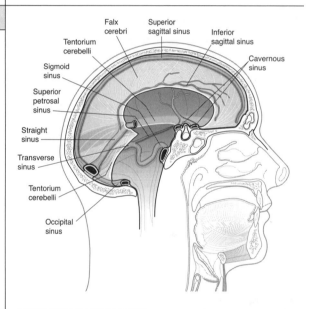

| HYDROCEPHALUS | |
|---|---|
| Excess Volume or Pressure of CSF, Leading to Dilated Ventricles | |
| Noncommunicating | **Obstruction of flow within ventricles**; most commonly occurs at narrow points, e.g., foramen of Monro, cerebral aqueduct, fourth ventricle |
| Communicating | **Impaired CSF reabsorption** in arachnoid granulations or obstruction of flow in subarachnoid space |
| Normal pressure | CSF is not absorbed by arachnoid villi (a form of communicating hydrocephalus). CSF pressure is usually normal. Ventricles chronically dilated. Produces **triad** of **dementia, ataxic gait,** and **urinary incontinence**. |
| Hydrocephalus ex vacuo | Descriptive term referring to excess CSF in regions where brain tissue is lost due to atrophy, stroke, surgery, trauma, etc. |

# NEUROHISTOLOGY AND PATHOLOGIC CORRELATES

## CELL TYPES OF THE NERVOUS SYSTEM

| Neuron | Glia (non-neuronal cells of the nervous system) |
|---|---|
| *Composed of:*<br><br>• **Dendrites:** receive info and transmit to the cell body<br>• **Cell body:** contains organelles<br>• **Axon:** transmits electrical impulse down to the nerve terminals<br>• **Nerve terminals:** contain synaptic vesicles and release neurotransmitter into the synapse | • **Oligodendrocytes:** form **myelin** in the **CNS** (one cell myelinates many axons)<br>• **Astrocytes:** control microenvironment of neurons and help maintain the blood/brain barrier with foot processes<br>• **Schwann cells:** form **myelin** in the **PNS** (one cell myelinates one internode)<br>• **Ependymal cells:** ciliated neurons that line the ventricles and central canal of the spinal cord<br>• **Microglia:** are **phagocytic** and are part of the **mononuclear phagocyte system** |

## DISORDERS OF MYELINATION

Demyelinating diseases are acquired conditions involving selective damage to myelin. Other diseases (e.g., infectious, metabolic, inherited) can also affect myelin and are generally called **leukodystrophies**.

| Disease | Symptoms | Notes |
|---|---|---|
| Multiple sclerosis (MS) | **Symptoms separated in space and time**<br>Vision loss (**optic neuritis**)<br>**Internuclear ophthalmoplegia** (MLF degeneration)<br>Motor and sensory deficits<br>Vertigo<br>Neuropsychiatric | Occurs twice as often in **women**<br>Onset often in **third or fourth decade**<br>Higher prevalence in **temperate zones**<br>**Relapsing–remitting course** is most common<br>Well-circumscribed **demyelinated plaques** often in periventricular areas<br>Chronic inflammation; axons initially preserved<br>Increased IgG (**oligoclonal bands**) in CSF<br>**Treatment:** high-dose steroids, interferon-beta, glatiramer (Copaxone®), natalizumab |
| Metachromatic leukodystrophy | Varied neurologic and psychiatric symptoms | **Arylsulfatase A deficiency** |
| Progressive multifocal leukoencephalopathy (PML) | Varied neurologic symptoms, dementia | Caused by **JC virus**<br>Affects **immunocompromised, especially AIDS**<br>Demyelination, astrogliosis, lymphohistiocytosis |
| Central pontine myelinolysis (CPM) | **Pseudobulbar palsy**<br>**Spastic quadriparesis**<br>Mental changes<br>May produce the "locked-in" syndrome<br>Often fatal | Focal demyelination of central area of basis pontis (affects corticospinal, corticobulbar tracts)<br>Seen in **severely malnourished, alcoholics, liver disease**<br>Probably **caused by overly aggressive correction of hyponatremia** |
| Guillain-Barré syndrome | Acute symmetric ascending inflammatory neuropathy<br>**Weakness begins in lower limbs and ascends; respiratory failure can occur** in severe cases<br>Autonomic dysfunction may be prominent<br>Cranial nerve involvement is common<br>Sensory loss, pain, and paresthesias occur<br>**Reflexes invariably decreased or absent** | Two-thirds of patients have **history of respiratory or GI illness 1–3 weeks prior to onset**<br>Elevated CSF protein with normal cell count (**albuminocytologic dissociation**) |
| Charcot-Marie-Tooth disease | Slowly progressing weakness in distal limbs; usually lower extremities before upper extremities<br>Abnormal proprioception/vibration sensation | Most common inherited neurologic disorder<br>Onset usually in 1st two decades of life<br>Different constellation of symptoms can occur, demyelination or axonal disease, depending on type |

*(Continued)*

ORGAN SYSTEMS

NERVOUS

## DISORDERS OF MYELINATION (CONT'D.)

| | | |
|---|---|---|
| Acute disseminated (postinfectious) encephalomyelitis | Symptoms can be similar to MS, but is associated with constitutional symptoms, mental status changes, seizures, and fewer dorsal column abnormalities | Nonvasculitic inflammatory demyelinating disease<br>History of preceding infectious illness or immunization<br>Most often in prepubertal children |

*Definition of abbreviation:* MLF, medial longitudinal fasciculus.

## TUMORS OF THE CNS AND PNS

One half of brain and spinal cord tumors are metastatic. Some differences between primary and metastatic tumors are listed below:

| Primary | Metastatic |
|---|---|
| Poorly circumscribed | Well circumscribed |
| Usually single | Often multiple |
| Location varies by specific type | Usually located at the junction between gray and white matter |

## PRIMARY TUMORS

| Tumor | Features | Pathology |
|---|---|---|
| Glioblastoma multiforme (grade IV astrocytoma) | • **Most common primary brain tumor**<br>• **Highly malignant**<br>• Usually lethal in 8–12 months | • Can cross the midline via the corpus callosum ("**butterfly glioma**")<br>• Areas of necrosis surrounded by rows of neoplastic cells (**pseudopalisading necrosis**) |
| Astrocytoma (pilocytic) | • Benign tumor of children and young adults<br>• Usually in **posterior fossa in children** | • **Rosenthal fibers**<br>• Immunostaining with **GFAP** |
| Oligodendroglia | • Slow growing<br>• Long survival (average 5–10 years) | **"Fried-egg" appearance**—perinuclear halo |
| Ependymoma | • Ependymal origin<br>• Can arise in IV ventricle and lead to **hydrocephalus** | Rosettes and pseudorosettes |
| Medulloblastoma | • Highly malignant cerebellar tumor<br>• A type of primitive neuroectodermal tumors (PNET) | Blue, small, round cells with pseudorosettes |
| Meningioma | • Second most common primary brain tumor<br>• Dural convexities; parasagittal region | • Attaches to the dura, compresses underlying brain without invasion<br>• Microscopic—**psammoma bodies** |
| Schwannoma | • Third most common primary brain tumor<br>• Most frequent location: **CN VIII at cerebellopontine angle**<br>• **Hearing loss, tinnitus**<br>• Good prognosis after surgical resection | • Antoni A (hypercellular) and B (hypocellular) areas<br>• **Bilateral acoustic schwannomas—pathognomonic for neurofibromatosis type 2** |
| Retinoblastoma | • Sporadic—unilateral<br>• **Familial—bilateral; associated with osteosarcoma** | Small, round, blue cells; may have rosettes |
| Craniopharyngioma | • Derived from odontogenic epithelium (remnants of **Rathke pouch**)<br>• Usually children and young adults<br>• Often calcified<br>• Symptoms due to encroachment on pituitary stalk or optic chiasm<br>• Benign but may recur | Histology resembles **adamantinoma** (most common tumor of tooth) |

*Definition of abbreviation:* GFAP, glial fibrillary acidic protein.

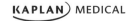

# SPINAL CORD

The spinal cord is divided internally into 31 segments that give rise to **31 pairs of spinal nerves** (from rostral to caudal): **8 cervical**, **12 thoracic**, **5 lumbar**, **5 sacral**, and **1 coccygeal**. Each segment is divided into an inner butterfly-like gray matter containing neuronal cell bodies and a surrounding area of white matter. The ventral horn contains alpha and gamma motoneurons; the intermediate horn contains preganglionic neurons and Clarke's nucleus; and the dorsal horn contains sensory neurons. The outer covering of the spinal cord is the white matter containing ascending and descending axons that form tracts located within funiculi.

ORGAN SYSTEMS

NERVOUS

| GENERAL SPINAL CORD FEATURES | |
|---|---|
| **Conus medullaris** | Caudal end of the spinal cord (S3–S5). In adult, ends at the L2 vertebra |
| **Cauda equina** | Nerve roots of the lumbar, sacral, and coccygeal spinal nerves |
| **Filum terminale** | Slender pial extension that tethers the spinal cord to the bottom of the vertebral column |
| **Doral root ganglia** | Cell bodies of primary sensory neurons |
| **Dorsal and ventral roots** | Each segment has a pair |
| **Dorsal** | **In (sensory)** |
| **Ventral** | **Out (motor)** |
| **Spinal nerve** | Formed from dorsal and ventral roots (mixed nerve) |
| **Cervical enlargement** | (C4–T1) → branchial plexus → upper limbs |
| **Lumbar enlargement** | (L2–S3) → lumbar and sacral plexuses → lower limbs |

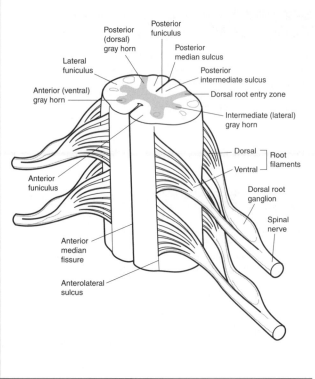

The following figure shows additional features of the spinal cord, such as the gray and white communicating rami, which are part of the autonomic nervous system.

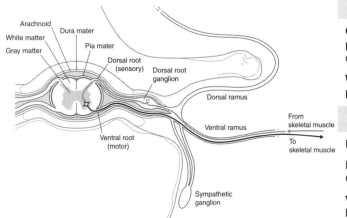

## Communicating Rami

**Gray** communicating rami contain **unmyelinated postganglionic sympathetic** fibers at all levels of spinal cord.

**White** communicating rami contain **myelinated preganglionic sympathetic** fibers from T1–L3.

## Gray Matter

**Dorsal horn:** sensory comes in

**Intermediate zone:** has preganglionic nerve cell bodies; Clarke's column (C8–L3)

**Ventral horn:** has alpha and gamma motoneuron cell bodies; motor goes out

## White Matter

**Tract:** a collection of axons with the same origin, function, and termination; are named by stating site of origin followed by site of termination, e.g., corticospinal (cortex → spinal cord)
**Fasciculi:** bundle of axons
**Funiculi:** a region of white matter (dorsal, lateral, ventral) that may have functionally different fasciculi

The most essential descending pathway is that which mediates voluntary skilled motor activity. This is formed by the **upper motor neuron (UMN; corticospinal tract)** and the **lower motor neuron (LMN)**.

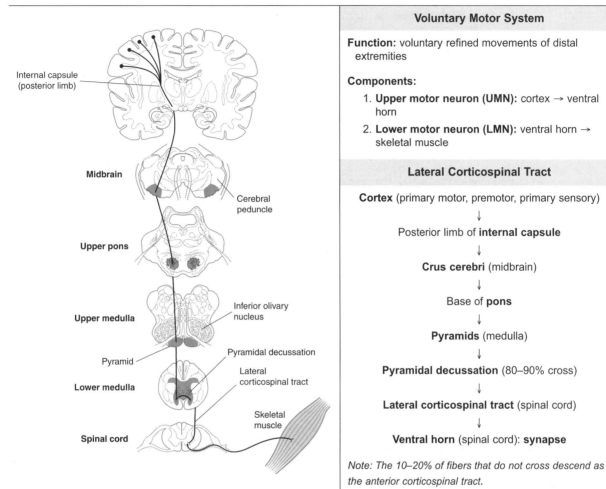

### Voluntary Motor System

**Function:** voluntary refined movements of distal extremities

**Components:**

1. **Upper motor neuron (UMN):** cortex → ventral horn
2. **Lower motor neuron (LMN):** ventral horn → skeletal muscle

### Lateral Corticospinal Tract

**Cortex** (primary motor, premotor, primary sensory)
↓
Posterior limb of **internal capsule**
↓
**Crus cerebri** (midbrain)
↓
Base of **pons**
↓
**Pyramids** (medulla)
↓
**Pyramidal decussation** (80–90% cross)
↓
**Lateral corticospinal tract** (spinal cord)
↓
**Ventral horn** (spinal cord): **synapse**

*Note: The 10–20% of fibers that do not cross descend as the anterior corticospinal tract.*

| UPPER VERSUS LOWER MOTOR NEURON LESIONS | | |
|---|---|---|
| **Clinical Signs** | **Upper Motor Neuron** | **Lower Motor Neuron** |
| Paralysis | Spastic | Flaccid |
| Muscle tone | Hypertonia | Hypotonia |
| Muscle bulk | Disuse atrophy | Atrophy, fasciculations |
| Deep tendon reflexes | Hyperreflexia | Hyporeflexia |
| Pathologic reflexes | Babinski | None |
| *Area of body involved:* | | |
| Size: | Large | Small |
| Side: | Contralateral if above decussation; ipsilateral if below decussation | Ipsilateral |

ORGAN SYSTEMS

NERVOUS

## COMMONLY TESTED MUSCLE STRETCH REFLEXES

The **deep tendon (stretch, myotatic) reflex** is monosynaptic and ipsilateral. The **afferent limb** consists of a **muscle spindle receptor, Ia sensory neuron,** and **efferent limb (lower motor neuron)**. These reflexes are useful in the clinical exam.

| Reflex | Cord Segment Involved | Muscle Tested |
|---|---|---|
| Knee (patellar) | L2–L4 | Quadriceps |
| Ankle | S1 | Gastrocnemius |
| Biceps | C5–C6 | Biceps |
| Triceps | C7–C8 | Triceps |
| Forearm | C5–C6 | Brachioradialis |

## ASCENDING PATHWAYS

The two most important ascending pathways use a three-neuron system to convey sensory information to the cortex. Key general features are listed below.

| Pathway | Function | Overview |
|---|---|---|
| Dorsal column–medial lemniscus | Discriminative touch, conscious proprioception, vibration, pressure | **3 neuron system:**<br>1° neuron: cell body in **DRG**<br>2° neuron: **decussates**<br>3° neuron: **thalamus (VPL) → cortex** |
| Anterolateral (spinothalamic) | Pain and temperature | |

*Definition of abbreviations:* DRG, dorsal root ganglia; VPL, ventral posterolateral nucleus.

## DORSAL COLUMN–MEDIAL LEMNISCUS

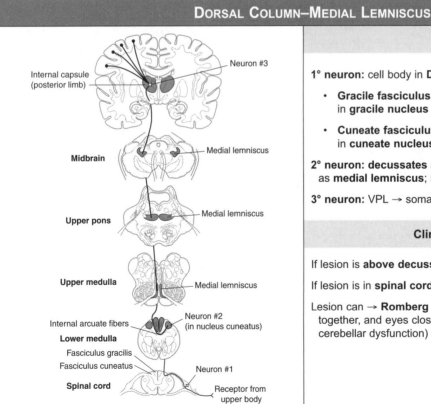

### Pathway

**1° neuron:** cell body in **DRG**, synapses in **lower medulla**

- **Gracile fasciculus** from **lower** extremities; terminates in **gracile nucleus**

- **Cuneate fasciculus** from **upper** extremities; terminates in **cuneate nucleus**

**2° neuron: decussates** as **internal arcuate fibers**; ascends as **medial lemniscus**; synapses in **VPL** of the thalamus

**3° neuron:** VPL → somatosensory cortex

### Clinical Correlation

If lesion is **above decussation** → **contralateral** loss of function

If lesion is in **spinal cord** → **ipsilateral** loss of function

Lesion can → **Romberg sign** (sways when standing, feet together, and eyes closed; swaying with eyes open indicates cerebellar dysfunction)

## ANTEROLATERAL (SPINOTHALAMIC)

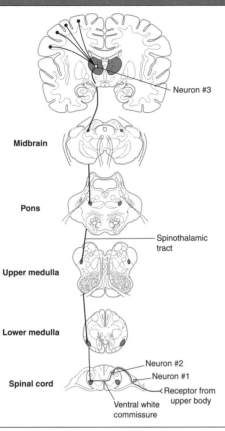

Neuron #3

Midbrain

Pons

Spinothalamic tract

Upper medulla

Lower medulla

Spinal cord

Neuron #2
Neuron #1
Receptor from upper body
Ventral white commissure

### Pathway

**1° neuron:** cell body in **DRG**, enters cord via dorsolateral tract of Lissauer (ascends or descends one or two segments), **synapses in dorsal horn** of spinal cord. Fibers are **A-δ** (fast) or **C** (slow).

**2° neuron:** decussates as **ventral white commissure**; ascends in **lateral spinothalamic tract**; synapses in **VPL**

**3° neuron:** VPL → somatosensory cortex

### Clinical Correlation

Lesion of lateral spinothalamic tract → loss of pain and temperature sensation on **contralateral** body, starting one or two segments below lesion

## CLASSIC SPINAL CORD LESIONS

There are several classic and very testable spinal cord syndromes. An understanding of basic spinal cord anatomy makes the symptoms easy to predict.

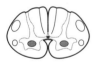

**Polio**
a. Flaccid paralysis
b. Muscle atrophy
c. Fasciculations
d. Areflexive

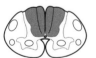

**Tabes dorsalis**
a. Bilateral dorsal column signs below lesions
b. Associated with late stage syphilis, plus Romberg sign: sways with eyes closed; Argyll Robertson pupils

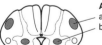

**Amyotrophic lateral sclerosis (ALS)**
a. Progressive spinal muscular atrophy (ventral horn)
b. Primary lateral sclerosis (corticospinal tract)
 • Spastic paralysis in lower limbs
 • Increased tone and reflexes
 • Flaccid paralysis in upper limbs

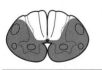

**Anterior spinal artery (ASA) occlusion**
a. DC spared
b. All else bilateral signs

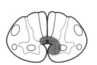

**Subacute combined degeneration**
a. Vitamin B$_{12}$, pernicious anemia; AIDS
b. Demyelination of the:
 • Dorsal columns
 • Corticospinal tracts (CST)

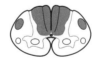

**Syringomyelia**
a. Cavitation of the cord (usually cervical)
b. Bilateral loss of pain and temperature at the level of the lesion
c. As the disease progresses, there is muscle weakness; eventually flaccid paralysis and atrophy of the upper limb muscles due to destruction of ventral horn cells

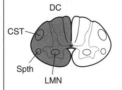

DC
CST
Spth
LMN

**Hemisection: Brown-Séquard syndrome**
a. DC: Ipsilateral loss of position and vibratory senses at and below level of the lesion
b. Spinothalamic tract: Contralateral loss of P&T below lesion and bilateral loss at the level of the lesion
c. CST: Ipsilateral paresis below the level of the lesion
d. LMN: Flaccid paralysis at the level of the lesion
e. Descending hypothalamics: Ipsilateral Horner syndrome (if cord lesion is above T$_1$)
 • Facial hemianhydrosis
 • Ptosis (slight)
 • Miosis

*Definition of abbreviations:* DC, dorsal column; LMN, lower motor neuron.

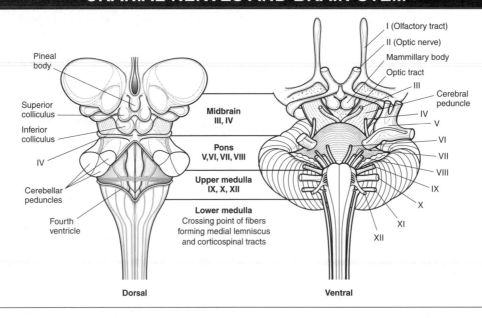

| Dorsal | | Ventral |
|---|---|---|

(Labels on diagram: Pineal body, Superior colliculus, Inferior colliculus, IV, Cerebellar peduncles, Fourth ventricle, Midbrain III, IV, Pons V,VI, VII, VIII, Upper medulla IX, X, XII, Lower medulla Crossing point of fibers forming medial lemniscus and corticospinal tracts, I (Olfactory tract), II (Optic nerve), Mammillary body, Optic tract, III, Cerebral peduncle, IV, V, VI, VII, VIII, IX, X, XI, XII)

| CRANIAL NERVES: FUNCTIONAL FEATURES | | | | |
|---|---|---|---|---|
| **CN** | **Name** | **Type** | **Function** | **Results of Lesions** |
| I | Olfactory | Sensory | Smells | Anosmia |
| II | Optic | Sensory | Sees | Visual field deficits (anopsia)<br>Loss of light reflex with III<br>Only nerve to be affected by MS |
| III | Oculomotor | Motor | Innervates SR, IR, MR, IO extraocular muscles: adduction (MR) most important action<br>Raises eyelid (levator palpebrae superioris)<br><br>Constricts pupil (sphincter pupillae)<br>Accommodates (ciliary muscle) | Diplopia, external strabismus<br>Loss of parallel gaze<br>Ptosis<br><br><br>Dilated pupil, loss of light reflex with II<br>Loss of near response |
| IV | Trochlear | Motor | Superior oblique—depresses and abducts eyeball (makes eyeball look down and out)<br>Intorts | Weakness looking down with adducted eye<br>Trouble going down stairs<br>Head tilts away from lesioned side |
| V | Trigeminal<br><br>Ophthalmic (V1)<br><br>Maxillary (V2)<br><br>Mandibular (V3) | Mixed | General sensation (touch, pain, temperature) of forehead/scalp/cornea<br><br>General sensation of palate, nasal cavity, maxillary face, maxillary teeth<br><br>General sensation of anterior two thirds of tongue, mandibular face, mandibular teeth<br><br>Motor to muscles of mastication (temporalis, masseter, medial and lateral pterygoids) and anterior belly of digastric, mylohyoid, tensor tympani, tensor palati | V1—loss of general sensation in skin of forehead/scalp<br>Loss of blink reflex with VII<br><br>V2—loss of general sensation in skin over maxilla, maxillary teeth<br><br>V3—loss of general sensation in skin over mandible, mandibular teeth, tongue, weakness in chewing<br><br>Jaw deviation toward weak side<br><br>Trigeminal neuralgia—intractable pain in V2 or V3 territory |

*Definition of abbreviations:* IO, inferior oblique; MR, medial rectus; IR, inferior rectus; MS, multiple sclerosis; SR, superior rectus.

*(Continued)*

## CRANIAL NERVES: FUNCTIONAL FEATURES (CONT'D.)

| CN | Name | Type | Function | Results of Lesions |
|----|------|------|----------|--------------------|
| VI | Abducens | Motor | Lateral rectus—abducts eyeball | Diplopia, internal strabismus<br>Loss of parallel gaze, "pseudoptosis" |
| VII | Facial | Mixed | To muscles of facial expression, posterior belly of digastric, stylohyoid, stapedius<br>Salivation (submandibular, sublingual glands)<br><br>Taste in anterior two thirds of tongue/palate<br>Tears (lacrimal gland) | Corner of mouth droops, cannot close eye, cannot wrinkle forehead, loss of blink reflex, hyperacusis; Bell palsy—lesion of nerve in facial canal<br>Alteration or loss of taste (ageusia)<br>Eye dry and red |
| VIII | Vestibulocochlear | Sensory | Hearing<br>Angular acceleration (head turning)<br>Linear acceleration (gravity) | Sensorineural hearing loss<br>Loss of balance, nystagmus |
| IX | Glossopharyngeal | Mixed | Sense of pharynx, carotid sinus/body<br>Salivation (parotid gland)<br>Taste and somatosensation of posterior one third of tongue<br>Motor to one muscle—stylopharyngeus | Loss of gag reflex with X |
| X | Vagus | Mixed | To muscles of palate and pharynx for swallowing except tensor palati (V) and stylopharyngeus (IX)<br>To all muscles of larynx (phonates)<br>Sensory of larynx and laryngopharynx<br><br>Sensory of GI tract<br>To GI tract smooth muscle and glands in foregut and midgut | Nasal speech, nasal regurgitation<br>Dysphagia, palate droop<br>Uvula pointing away from affected side<br>Hoarseness/fixed vocal cord<br>Loss of gag reflex with IX<br>Loss of cough reflex |
| XI | Accessory | Motor | Head rotation to opposite side (sternocleidomastoid)<br>Elevates and rotates scapula (trapezius) | Weakness turning head to opposite side<br><br>Shoulder droop |
| XII | Hypoglossal | Motor | Tongue movement (styloglossus, hyoglossus, genioglossus, and intrinsic tongue muscles—palatoglossus is by X) | Tongue pointing toward same (affected) side on protrusion |

## SKULL BASE ANATOMY

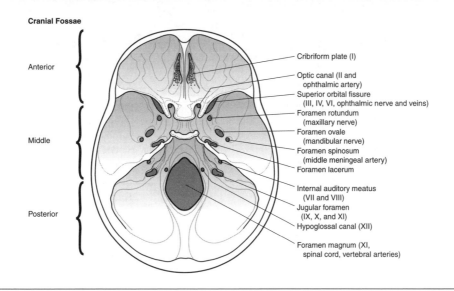

Cranial Fossae

Anterior

Middle

Posterior

Cribriform plate (I)
Optic canal (II and ophthalmic artery)
Superior orbital fissure (III, IV, VI, ophthalmic nerve and veins)
Foramen rotundum (maxillary nerve)
Foramen ovale (mandibular nerve)
Foramen spinosum (middle meningeal artery)
Foramen lacerum
Internal auditory meatus (VII and VIII)
Jugular foramen (IX, X, and XI)
Hypoglossal canal (XII)
Foramen magnum (XI, spinal cord, vertebral arteries)

# VISUAL SYSTEM

## VISUAL FIELD DEFECTS

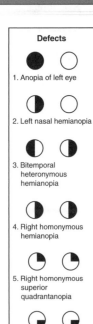

**Defects**

1. Anopia of left eye
2. Left nasal hemianopia
3. Bitemporal heteronymous hemianopia
4. Right homonymous hemianopia
5. Right homonymous superior quadrantanopia
6. Right homonymous inferior quadrantanopia
7. Right homonymous hemianopia with macular sparing

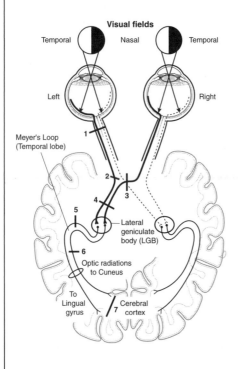

**Visual fields**

Temporal — Nasal — Temporal

Left — Right

Meyer's Loop (Temporal lobe)

Lateral geniculate body (LGB)

Optic radiations to Cuneus

To Lingual gyrus — Cerebral cortex

### Notes

Like a camera, the lens inverts the image of the visual field, so the nasal retina receives information from the temporal visual field, and the temporal retina receives information from the nasal visual field.

At the **optic chiasm**, optic nerve fibers from the nasal half of each retina cross and project to the contralateral optic tract.

Most fibers from the **optic tract** project to the **lateral geniculate body (LGB)**; some also project to the pretectal area (light reflex), the superior colliculi (reflex gaze), and the suprachiasmatic nuclei (circadian rhythm). The LGB projects to the **primary visual cortex** (striate cortex, Brodmann area 17) of the occipital lobe via the optic radiations.

- Visual information from the lower retina (upper contralateral visual field) → temporal lobe **(Meyer loop)** → **lingual gyrus**
- Visual information from the upper retina (lower contralateral visual field) → parietal lobe → **cuneus gyrus**

### Clinical Correlate (Some Causes of Lesions)

1. Optic neuritis, central retinal artery occlusion
2. Internal carotid artery aneurysm
3. Pituitary adenoma, craniopharyngioma

5. Middle cerebral artery (MCA) occlusion
6, 7. Posterior cerebral artery occlusion
Macula is spared in 7 due to collateral blood supply from MCA.

## ANATOMY OF THE EYE AND GLAUCOMA

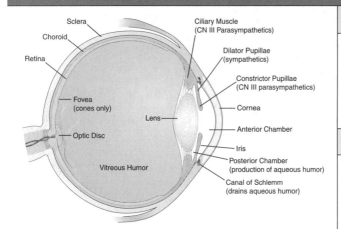

Sclera
Choroid
Retina
Fovea (cones only)
Optic Disc
Vitreous Humor
Lens
Ciliary Muscle (CN III Parasympathetics)
Dilator Pupillae (sympathetics)
Constrictor Pupillae (CN III parasympathetics)
Cornea
Anterior Chamber
Iris
Posterior Chamber (production of aqueous humor)
Canal of Schlemm (drains aqueous humor)

### Open-Angle Glaucoma

A chronic condition (often with increased intraocular pressure [IOP]) due to decreased reabsorption of aqueous humor, leading to progressive (painless) visual loss and, if left untreated, blindness. IOP is a balance between fluid formation and its drainage from the globe.

### Narrow-Angle Glaucoma

An acute (painful) or chronic (genetic) condition with increased IOP due to blockade of the canal of Schlemm. Emergency treatment prior to surgery often involves cholinomimetics, carbonic anhydrase inhibitors, and/or mannitol.

ORGAN SYSTEMS

NERVOUS

The eye is predominantly innervated by the parasympathetic nervous system. Therefore, application of muscarinic antagonists or ganglionic blockers has a large effect by blocking the parasympathetic nervous system.

| Structure | Predominant Receptor | Receptor Stimulation | Receptor Blockade |
|---|---|---|---|
| Pupillary sphincter ms. (iris) | $M_3$ receptor (PANS) | Contraction → miosis | Relaxation → mydriasis |
| Radial dilator ms. (iris) | $\alpha$ receptor (SANS) | Contraction → mydriasis | Relaxation → miosis |
| Ciliary ms. | $M_3$ receptor (PANS) | Contraction → accommodation for near vision | Relaxation → focus for far vision |
| Ciliary body epithelium | $\beta$ receptor (SANS) | Secretion of aqueous humor | Decreased aqueous humor production |

*Definition of abbreviations:* ms., muscle; PANS, parasympathetic nervous system; SANS, sympathetic nervous system.

## DRUGS USED TO TREAT GLAUCOMA

| Drug Class | Drug | Mechanism |
|---|---|---|
| Cholinomimetics (miotics) | Pilocarpine (mAChR agonist) Carbachol (mAChR agonist) Physostigmine (AChEI) Echothiophate (AChEI) | Contracts ciliary muscle and opens trabecular meshwork, increasing the outflow of aqueous humor through the canal of Schlemm |
| Beta blockers | Timolol (nonselective) Betaxolol ($\beta_1$) | Blocks actions of NE at ciliary epithelium to ↓ aqueous humor secretion |
| Prostaglandins | Latanoprost ($PGF_{2\alpha}$ analog) | ↑ aqueous humor outflow; can darken the iris |
| Alpha agonists | Epinephrine Dipivefrin | ↑ aqueous humor outflow |
| Alpha-2 agonists | Apraclonidine Brimonidine | ↓ aqueous humor secretion |
| Diuretics | Acetazolamide (oral; CAI) Dorzolamide, brinzolamide (topical; CAI) Mannitol (for narrow-angle; osmotic) | CAI: ↓ $HCO_3^-$ → ↓ aqueous humor secretion |

*Definition of abbreviations:* AChEI, acetylcholinesterase inhibitor; CAI, carbonic anhydrase inhibitor; mAChR, muscarinic cholinergic receptor.

## PUPILLARY LIGHT REFLEX PATHWAY

| Afferent Limb: CN II |
|---|
| Light stimulates ganglion retinal cells → impulses travel up **CNII**, which projects **bilaterally** to the **pretectal nuclei** (midbrain) |
| The pretectal nucleus projects **bilaterally** → **Edinger-Westphal nuclei (CN III)** |

| Efferent Limb: CN III |
|---|
| Edinger-Westphal nucleus (preganglionic parasympathetic) → **ciliary ganglion** (postganglionic parasympathetic) → **pupillary sphincter ms.** → **miosis** |
| *Note:* This is a simplified diagram; the ciliary ganglion is not shown. |

Because cells in the pretectal area supply the Edinger-Westphal nuclei bilaterally, shining light in one eye → constriction in the ipsilateral pupil (direct light reflex) and the contralateral pupil (consensual light reflex).

Because this reflex does not involve the visual cortex, a person who is cortically blind can still have this reflex.

## ACCOMMODATION–CONVERGENCE REACTION

When an individual focuses on a nearby object after looking at a distant object, three events occur:

1. **Accommodation**
2. **Convergence**
3. **Pupillary constriction (miosis)**

In general, stimuli from light → visual cortex → superior colliculus and pretectal nucleus → Edinger-Westphal nucleus (1, 3) and oculomotor nucleus (2).

**Accommodation:** Parasympathetic fibers contract the ciliary muscle, which relaxes suspensory ligaments, allowing the lens to increase its convexity (become more round). This increases the refractive index of the lens, thereby focusing a nearby object on the retina.

**Convergence:** Both medial rectus muscles contract, adducting both eyes.

**Pupillary constriction:** Parasympathetic fibers contract the pupillary sphincter muscle → miosis.

## CLINICAL CORRELATIONS

### Pupillary Abnormalities

| | |
|---|---|
| **Argyll Robertson pupil** (pupillary light-near dissociation) | No direct or consensual light reflex; accommodation-convergence intact<br>Seen in **neurosyphilis**, diabetes |
| **Relative afferent (Marcus Gunn) pupil** | Lesion of afferent limb of pupillary light reflex; diagnosis made with swinging flashlight<br>Shine light in Marcus Gunn pupil → pupils do not constrict fully<br>Shine light in normal eye → pupils constrict fully<br>Shine light immediately again in affected eye → apparent dilation of both pupils because stimulus carried through that CN II is weaker; seen in multiple sclerosis |
| **Horner syndrome** | Caused by a lesion of the oculosympathetic pathway; syndrome consists of miosis, ptosis, apparent enophthalmos, and hemianhidrosis |
| **Adie pupil** | Dilated pupil that reacts sluggishly to light, but better to accommodation; often seen in women and often associated with loss of knee jerks |
| **Transentorial (uncal) herniation** | Increased intracranial pressure → leads to uncal herniation → CN III compression → fixed and dilated pupil, "down-and-out" eye, ptosis |

# EYE MOVEMENT CONTROL SYSTEMS

## Extraocular Muscles: Function and Innervation

| CN III | **Medial rectus:** adducts eye<br>**Superior rectus:** elevates, intorts, adducts eye<br>**Inferior rectus:** depresses, extorts, adducts eye<br>**Inferior oblique:** elevates, extorts, abducts eye | CN IV | **Superior oblique:** depresses, intorts, abducts eye |
| | | CN VI | **Lateral rectus:** Abducts eye |

Two important eye movements are **abduction** (away from nose, **CN VI**) and **adduction** (toward nose, **CN III**).

For the eyes to move together **(conjugate gaze)**, the oculomotor nuclei and abducens nuclei are interconnected by the **medial longitudinal fasciculus (MLF)**.

Horizontal gaze is controlled by two gaze centers:

1. **Frontal eye field** (contralateral gaze)
2. **PPRF** (paramedial pontine reticular formation, ipsilateral gaze)

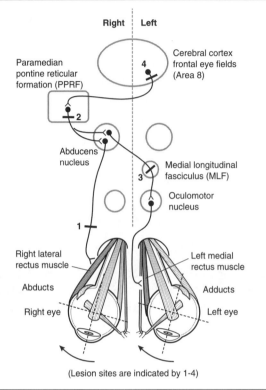

(Lesion sites are indicated by 1-4)

## Clinical Correlation

| Lesion Examples | Symptoms |
|---|---|
| 1. Right CN VI | Right eye cannot look right |
| 2. Right PPRF | Neither eye can look right |
| 3. Left MLF | **Internuclear ophthalmoplegia (INO)**<br>Left eye cannot look right; convergence is intact (this is how to distinguish an INO from an oculomotor lesion); right eye has nystagmus; seen in multiple sclerosis |
| 4. Left frontal eye field | Neither eye can look right; but slow drift to left |

## TRIGEMINAL NERVE (V)

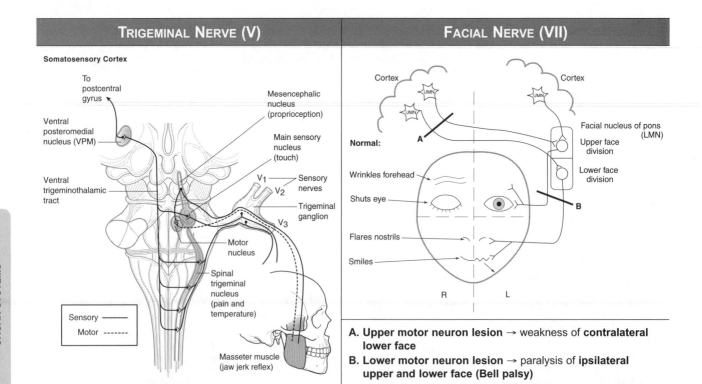

Somatosensory Cortex

To postcentral gyrus

Ventral posteromedial nucleus (VPM)

Ventral trigeminothalamic tract

Mesencephalic nucleus (proprioception)

Main sensory nucleus (touch)

V₁ → Sensory nerves
V₂
Trigeminal ganglion
V₃

Motor nucleus

Spinal trigeminal nucleus (pain and temperature)

Sensory ———
Motor --------

Masseter muscle (jaw jerk reflex)

## FACIAL NERVE (VII)

Cortex          Cortex

UMN     UMN     UMN

Normal:

Facial nucleus of pons (LMN)
Upper face division
Lower face division

Wrinkles forehead

Shuts eye

Flares nostrils

Smiles

R          L

A. **Upper motor neuron lesion** → weakness of **contralateral lower face**
B. **Lower motor neuron lesion** → paralysis of **ipsilateral upper and lower face (Bell palsy)**

## VESTIBULAR SYSTEM (VIII)

Three **semicircular** ducts respond to **angular acceleration and deceleration** of the head. The **utricle** and **saccule** respond to **linear acceleration** and the pull of **gravity**. There are four **vestibular nuclei** in the medulla and pons, which receive information from CN VIII. Fibers from the vestibular nuclei join the MLF and supply the motor nuclei of CNs III, IV, and VI, thereby regulating conjugate eye movements. Vestibular nuclei also receive and send information to the **flocculonodular lobe** of the cerebellum.

| Vestibulo-Ocular Reflex | Caloric Test |
|---|---|

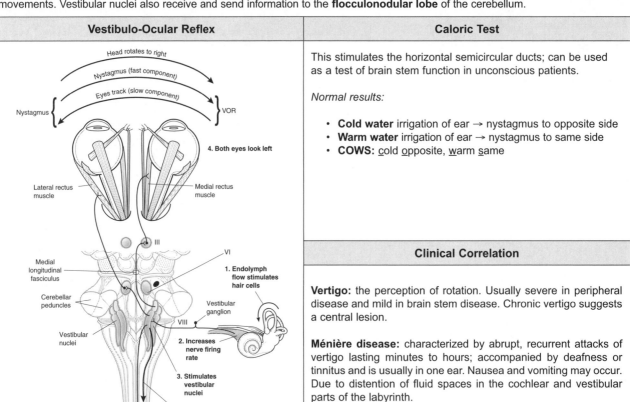

Head rotates to right
Nystagmus (fast component)
Eyes track (slow component)
Nystagmus          VOR

4. Both eyes look left

Lateral rectus muscle
Medial rectus muscle

III

VI

Medial longitudinal fasciculus

Cerebellar peduncles

Vestibular nuclei

VIII

1. Endolymph flow stimulates hair cells

Vestibular ganglion

2. Increases nerve firing rate

3. Stimulates vestibular nuclei

Lateral vestibulospinal tract (to antigravity muscles)

This stimulates the horizontal semicircular ducts; can be used as a test of brain stem function in unconscious patients.

*Normal results:*

- **Cold water** irrigation of ear → nystagmus to opposite side
- **Warm water** irrigation of ear → nystagmus to same side
- **COWS:** cold opposite, warm same

### Clinical Correlation

**Vertigo:** the perception of rotation. Usually severe in peripheral disease and mild in brain stem disease. Chronic vertigo suggests a central lesion.

**Ménière disease:** characterized by abrupt, recurrent attacks of vertigo lasting minutes to hours; accompanied by deafness or tinnitus and is usually in one ear. Nausea and vomiting may occur. Due to distention of fluid spaces in the cochlear and vestibular parts of the labyrinth.

# AUDITORY SYSTEM (VIII)

## Inner Ear

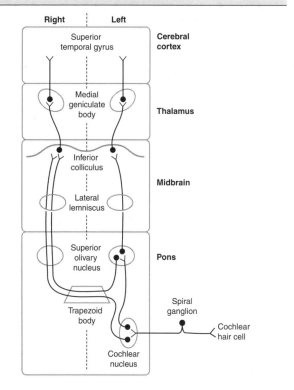

Semicircular duct
Ampulla
Ossicles
Semicircular canal

**Cross section through one turn of the cochlea**

Tympanic membrane
Oval window
Round window
Eustachian tube

Scala media (endolymph)
Stria vascularis (endolymph production)
Tectorial membrane
Basilar membrane
Organ of Corti
Spiral ganglion
VIII nerve (cochlear division)

Scala vestibuli (perilymph)
Scala tympani (perilymph)

## Auditory Pathways

Right    Left

Superior temporal gyrus — **Cerebral cortex**
Medial geniculate body — **Thalamus**
Inferior colliculus — **Midbrain**
Lateral lemniscus
Superior olivary nucleus — **Pons**
Trapezoid body
Spiral ganglion
Cochlear hair cell
Cochlear nucleus

- Lesions to CN VIII or cochlear nuclei → **ipsilateral** sensorineural hearing loss
- Lesions to all other auditory structures in brainstem, thalamus, or cortex → **bilateral** ↓ in hearing and ↓ ability to localize sound

## Deafness

**Conduction deafness:** passage of sound waves through external or middle ear is interrupted
Causes: obstruction, otosclerosis, otitis media
**Sensorineural deafness:** damage to cochlea, CN VIII, or central auditory connections

## Auditory Tests

**Weber test:** place tuning fork on vertex of skull. If **unilateral conduction deafness** → vibration is louder in affected ear; if **unilateral sensorineural deafness** → vibration is louder in normal ear

**Rinne test:** place tuning fork on mastoid process (bone conduction) until vibration is not heard, then place fork in front of ear (air conduction). If **unilateral conduction deafness** → no air conduction after bone conduction is gone; if **unilateral sensorineural deafness** → air conduction present after bone conduction is gone

# BRAIN STEM LESIONS

## MEDULLA

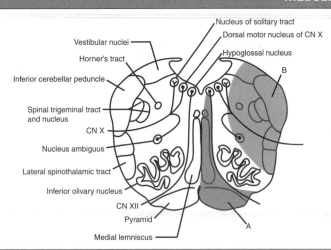

Nucleus of solitary tract
Dorsal motor nucleus of CN X
Hypoglossal nucleus
Vestibular nuclei
Horner's tract
Inferior cerebellar peduncle
Spinal trigeminal tract and nucleus
CN X
Nucleus ambiguus
Lateral spinothalamic tract
Inferior olivary nucleus
CN XII
Pyramid
Medial lemniscus
B
A

### Medial Medullary Syndrome (A)
Anterior Spinal Artery

**Pyramid:** contralateral spastic paresis (body)

**Medial lemniscus:** contralateral loss of tactile, vibration, conscious proprioception (body)

**XII nucleus/fibers:** ipsilateral flaccid paralysis of tongue

### Lateral Medullary Syndrome (B)
PICA, Wallenberg Syndrome

**Inferior cerebellar peduncle:** ipsilateral limb ataxia
**Vestibular nuclei:** vertigo, nausea/vomiting, nystagmus (away from lesion)
**Nucleus ambiguus (CN IX, X, XI):** ipsilateral paralysis of larynx, pharynx, palate → dysarthria, dysphagia, loss of gag reflex
**Spinal V:** ipsilateral pain/temperature loss (face)
**Spinothalamic tract:** Contralateral pain/temperature loss (body)
**Descending hypothalamics:** ipsilateral Horner syndrome

## PONS

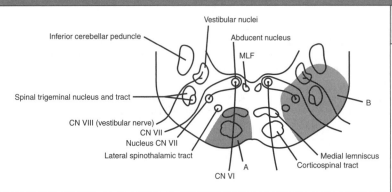

Vestibular nuclei
Abducent nucleus
MLF
Inferior cerebellar peduncle
Spinal trigeminal nucleus and tract
CN VIII (vestibular nerve)
CN VII
Nucleus CN VII
Lateral spinothalamic tract
CN VI
Medial lemniscus
Corticospinal tract
A
B

### Medial Pontine Syndrome (A)
Paramedian Branches of Basilar Artery

**Corticospinal tract:** contralateral spastic hemiparesis

**Medial lemniscus:** contralateral loss of tactile/position/vibration sensation on body

**Fibers of VI:** medial strabismus

### Lateral Pontine Syndrome (B)
AICA

**Middle cerebellar peduncle:** ipsilateral ataxia
**Vestibular nuclei:** vertigo, nausea and vomiting, nystagmus
**Facial nucleus and fibers:** ipsilateral facial paralysis; ipsilateral loss of taste (anterior 2/3 tongue), lacrimation, salivation, and corneal reflex; hyperacusis
**Spinal trigeminal nucleus/tract:** ipsilateral pain/temperature loss (face)
**Spinothalamic tract:** contralateral pain/temperature loss (body)
**Cochlear nucleus/VIII fibers:** ipsilateral hearing loss
**Descending sympathetics:** ipsilateral Horner syndrome

# MIDBRAIN

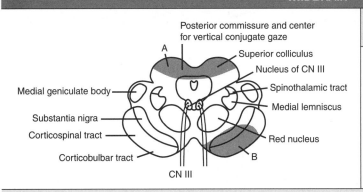

Posterior commissure and center for vertical conjugate gaze
A
Superior colliculus
Nucleus of CN III
Medial geniculate body
Spinothalamic tract
Medial lemniscus
Substantia nigra
Corticospinal tract
Red nucleus
Corticobulbar tract
B
CN III

## Dorsal Midbrain (Parinaud) Syndrome (A)
### Tumor in Pineal Region

**Superior colliculus/pretectal area:** paralysis of upward gaze, various pupillary abnormalities

**Cerebral aqueduct:** noncommunicating hydrocephalus

## Medial Midbrain (Weber) Syndrome (B)
### Branches of PCA

**Fibers of III:** ipsilateral oculomotor palsy (lateral strabismus, dilated pupil, ptosis)
**Corticospinal tract:** contralateral spastic hemiparesis
**Corticobulbar tract:** contralateral spastic hemiparesis of lower face

# CEREBELLUM

The cerebellum controls posture, muscle tone, learning of repeated motor functions, and coordinates voluntary motor activity. Diseases of the cerebellum result in disturbances of gait, balance, and coordinated motor actions, but there is no paralysis or inability to start or stop movement.

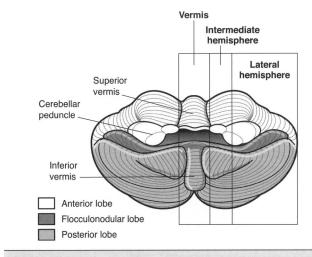

Vermis
Intermediate hemisphere
Lateral hemisphere
Superior vermis
Cerebellar peduncle
Inferior vermis
☐ Anterior lobe
■ Flocculonodular lobe
■ Posterior lobe

| Input |
|---|
| **Climbing fibers** (from inferior olivary nucleus of medulla), **mossy fibers** (from vestibular nucleus, spinal cord, pons); most input via **ICP** and **MCP** |

| Output |
|---|
| From deep cerebellar nucleus (fastigial, interpositus, dentate); most output via **SCP** |

| Three Layers |
|---|
| Molecular, Purkinje, granule cell |

| Major Pathway | Dysfunction |
|---|---|
| Purkinje cells → deep cerebellar nucleus; dentate nucleus → contralateral VL → 1° motor cortex → pontine nuclei → contralateral cerebellar cortex | • **Hemisphere lesions** → ipsilateral symptoms; **intention** tremor, dysmetria, dysdiadochokinesia, scanning dysarthria, nystagmus, hypotonia<br>• **Vermal lesions** → truncal ataxia |

*Definition of abbreviations:* ICP, inferior cerebellar peduncle; MCP, middle cerebellar peduncle; SCP, superior cerebellar peduncle; VL, ventral lateral nucleus.

# DIENCEPHALON
## Thalamus, Hypothalamus, Epithalamus, Subthalamus

**Thalamus**—serves as a major sensory relay for information that ultimately reaches the neocortex. Motor control areas (basal ganglia, cerebellum) also synapse in the thalamus before reaching the cortex. Other nuclei regulate states of consciousness.

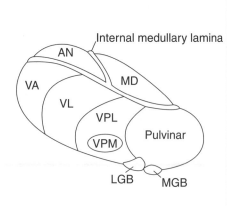

Internal medullary lamina

| THALAMIC NUCLEI | INPUT | OUTPUT |
|---|---|---|
| VPL | Sensory from **body and limbs** | Somatosensory cortex |
| VPM | Sensory from **face** | Somatosensory cortex |
| VA/VL | **Motor** info from BG, cerebellum | Motor cortices |
| LGB | **Visual** from optic tract | 1° visual cortex |
| MGB | **Auditory** from inferior colliculus | 1° auditory cortex |
| AN | Mammillary nucleus (via mamillothalamic tract) | Cingulate gyrus (part of **Papez** circuit) |
| MD | (Dorsomedial nucleus). Involved in **memory** Damaged in **Wernicke-Korsakoff** syndrome | |
| Pulvinar | Helps integrate somesthetic, visual, and auditory input | |
| Midline/intralaminar | Involved in **arousal** | |

**Hypothalamus**—helps maintain homeostasis; has roles in the autonomic, endocrine, and limbic systems

| HYPOTHALAMIC NUCLEI | FUNCTIONS AND LESIONS |
|---|---|
| Lateral hypothalamic | **Feeding center;** lesion → starvation |
| Ventromedial | **Satiety center;** lesion → hyperphagia, obesity, savage behavior |
| Suprachiasmatic | Regulates circadian rhythms |
| Supraoptic and paraventricular | Synthesizes **ADH** and **oxytocin; regulates water balance** Lesion → **diabetes insipidus**, characterized by polydipsia and polyuria |
| Mammillary body | Input from hippocampus; damaged in Wernicke encephalopathy |
| Arcuate | Produces hypothalamic releasing and inhibiting factors and gives rise to tuberohypophysial tract Has neurons that produce dopamine (prolactin-inhibiting factor) |
| Anterior | **Temperature regulation;** lesion → hyperthermia Stimulates the parasympathetic nervous system |
| Posterior | **Temperature regulation;** lesion → poikilothermia (inability to thermoregulate) Stimulates sympathetic nervous system |
| Preoptic area | Regulates release of gonotrophic hormones; contains sexually dimorphic nucleus Lesion before puberty → arrested sexual development; lesion after puberty → amenorrhea or impotence |
| Dorsomedial | Stimulation → savage behavior |

**Epithalamus**—Consists of pineal body and habenular nuclei. The **pineal body** aids in the regulation of **circadian rhythms**.

**Subthalamus**—The **subthalamic nucleus** is involved in **basal ganglia** circuitry. Lesion → **hemiballismus** (contralateral flinging movements of one or both extremities)

*Definition of abbreviations:* ADH, antidiuretic hormone; AN, anterior nuclear group; BG, basal ganglia; LBG, lateral geniculate body; MD, mediodorsal nucleus; MGB, medial geniculate body; VA, ventral anterior nucleus; VL, ventral lateral nucleus; VLP, ventroposterolateral nucleus; VPM, ventroposteromedial nucleus.

ORGAN SYSTEMS

NERVOUS

# BASAL GANGLIA

The basal ganglia initiate and provide gross control over skeletal muscle movements. The basal ganglia are sometimes called the **extrapyramidal** nervous system because they modulate the pyramidal (corticospinal) nervous system.

| BASAL GANGLIA COMPONENTS | |
|---|---|
| **Striatum (caudate and putamen)** | **Subthalamic nucleus** (diencephalon) |
| **Globus pallidus** (external and internal segments) | **Lentiform nucleus** (globus pallidus and putamen) |
| **Substantia nigra** (midbrain) | **Corpus striatum** (lentiform nucleus and caudate) |

Together with the cerebral cortex and **VA/VL** thalamic nuclei, these structures form two parallel but antagonistic circuits known as the **direct** and **indirect pathways**. The direct pathway increases cortical excitation and promotes movement, and the indirect pathway decreases cortical excitation and inhibits movement. Hypokinetic movement disorders (e.g., Parkinson disease) result in a lesion of the direct pathway, and hyperkinetic movement disorders (e.g., Huntington disease, hemiballismus) result from indirect pathway lesions.

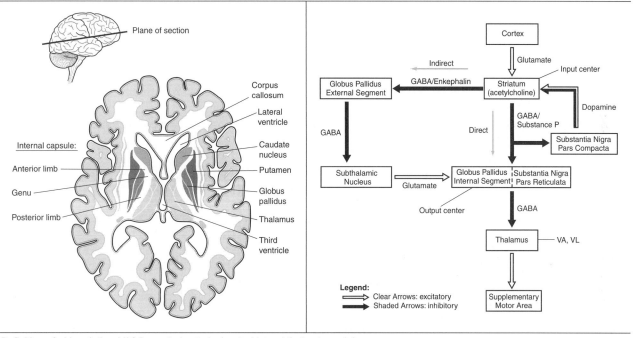

*Definition of abbreviation:* VA/VL, ventral anterior/ventral lateral thalamic nuclei.

## DISEASES OF THE BASAL GANGLIA

| Disease | Clinical Manifestations | Notes |
|---------|------------------------|-------|
| Parkinson disease | Bradykinesia, cogwheel rigidity, pill rolling (resting) tremor, shuffling gate, stooped posture, masked facies, depression, dementia | **Loss of pigmented dopaminergic neurons from substantia nigra** **Lewy bodies:** intracytoplasmic eosinophilic inclusions, contain α-synuclein Known causes of parkinsonism: infections, vascular, and toxic insults (e.g., **MPTP**) |
| Huntington disease | Chorea (multiple, rapid, random movements), athetosis (slow writhing, movements), personality changes, dementia Onset: 20–40 years | **Degeneration** of GABAergic neurons in **neostriatum**, causing atrophy of neostriatum (and ventricular dilatation) **Autosomal dominant** **Unstable nucleotide repeat** on gene in chromosome 4, which codes for huntingtin protein Disease shows **anticipation** and **genomic imprinting** **Treatment:** antipsychotic agents, benzodiazepines, anticonvulsants |
| Wilson disease (hepatolenticular degeneration) | Tremor, asterixis, parkinsonian symptoms, chorea, neuropsychiatric symptoms; fatty change, hepatitis, or cirrhosis of liver | **Autosomal recessive defect in copper transport** Accumulation of copper in liver, brain, and eye (Descemet membrane, producing **Kayser-Fleischer ring**) Lesions in basal ganglia (especially putamen) **Treatment: penicillamine** (a chelator), zinc acetate (blocks absorption) |
| Hemiballism | Wild flinging movements of half the body | Hemorrhagic destruction of **contralateral subthalamic nucleus** Hypertensive patients |
| Tourette syndrome | Motor tics and vocal tics (e.g., snorting, sniffing, uncontrolled and often obscene vocalizations), commonly associated with OCD and ADHD | **Treatment:** Antipsychotic agents |

*Definition of abbreviations:* ADHD, attention deficit hyperactivity disorder; MPTP, 1-methyl-4-phenyl-1,2,3,6-tetrahydropyridine; OCD, obsessive-compulsive disorder.

## TREATMENT FOR PARKINSON DISEASE

The pharmacologic goal in the treatment of Parkinson disease is to **increase DA and/or decrease ACh** activity in the striatum, thereby correcting the DA/ACh imbalance. Additional treatment strategies include surgical intervention, such as pallidotomy, thalamotomy, deep brain stimulation, and transplantation.

| Agents | Mechanism | Notes |
|--------|-----------|-------|
| **Dopamine precursor:** L-dopa | Dopamine precursor that crosses the blood–brain barrier (BBB) Converted to DA by DOPA decarboxylase (L-aromatic amino acid decarboxylase) | Side effects include on/off phenomena, dyskinesias, psychosis, postural hypotension, nausea/vomiting |
| **DOPA decarboxylase inhibitor:** carbidopa | Inhibits DOPA decarboxylase in the periphery, preventing L-dopa from being converted to dopamine in the periphery; instead, L-dopa crosses the BBB and is converted to dopamine in the brain | Often given in combination with L-dopa (Sinemet®) |
| **DA agonists:** bromocriptine pergolide pramipexole ropinirole | Stimulates $D_2$ receptors in the striatum; pramipexole and ropinirole are also $D_3$ agonists | Pramipexole and ropinirole now considered first-line drugs in the initial management of PD; pramipexole and ropinirole are also used in **restless legs syndrome** |
| **MAO B inhibitor:** selegiline rasagiline | Inhibits MAO type B, which preferentially metabolizes dopamine | Not to be taken with SSRIs (serotonin syndrome) or meperidine |
| **Antimuscarinics:** benztropine trihexyphenidyl biperiden | Blocks muscarinic receptors in the striatum | ↓ tremor and rigidity, have little effect on bradykinesia Antimuscarinic side effects |
| **COMT inhibitors:** entacapone tolcapone | COMT inhibitors increase the efficacy of L-dopa. COMT metabolizes L-dopa to 3-O-methyldopa (3OMD), which competes with L-dopa for active transport into the CNS | Used as an adjunct to L-dopa/carbidopa, increases the "on" time |
| **Amantadine** | Increases dopaminergic neurotransmission, antimuscarinic; also an antiviral | Antimuscarinic effects, livedo reticularis |

ORGAN SYSTEMS

NERVOUS

# LIMBIC SYSTEM

The limbic system is involved in emotion, memory, attention, feeding, and mating behaviors. It consists of a core of cortical and diencephalic structures found on the medial aspect of the hemisphere. The limbic system modulates feelings, such as fear, anxiety, sadness, happiness, sexual pleasure, and familiarity.

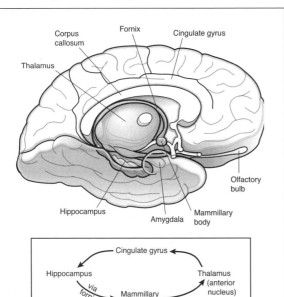

## Limbic Structures and Function

- Hippocampal formation (hippocampus, dentate gyrus, the subiculum, and entorhinal cortex)
- Amygdala
- Septal nuclei
- The hippocampus is important in learning and memory. The amygdala attaches an emotional significance to a stimulus and helps imprint the emotional response in memory.

## Limbic Connections

- The limbic system is interconnected with anterior and dorsomedial nuclei of the thalamus and the mammillary bodies.
- The cingulate gyrus is the main limbic cortical area.
- Limbic-related structures also project to wide areas of the prefrontal cortex.
- Central projections of olfactory structures reach parts of the temporal lobe and the amygdala.

## Papez Circuit

Axons of hippocampal pyramidal cells converge to form the fimbria and, finally, the fornix. The fornix projects mainly to the mammillary bodies in the hypothalamus. The mammillary bodies project to the anterior nucleus of the thalamus (mammillothalamic tract). The anterior nuclei project to the cingulate gyrus, and the cingulate gyrus projects to the entorhinal cortex (via the cingulum). The entorhinal cortex projects to the hippocampus (via the perforant pathway).

## CLINICAL CORRELATIONS

### Anterograde Amnesia

Bilateral damage to the medial temporal lobes, including the **hippocampus**, results in a profound loss of the ability to acquire new information.

### Wernicke Encephalopathy and Korsakoff Syndrome

**Wernicke encephalopathy** typically occurs in alcoholics who have a **thiamine deficiency**. Patients present with ocular palsies, confusion, and gait ataxia. If the thiamine deficiency is not corrected in time, patients can develop **Korsakoff syndrome**, characterized by **anterograde amnesia**, retrograde amnesia, and confabulation. Lesions are found in the **mammillary bodies** and the **dorsomedial nuclei of the thalamus**. Wernicke encephalopathy is reversible; Korsakoff syndrome is not.

### Klüver-Bucy Syndrome

Klüver-Bucy syndrome results from bilateral lesions of the anterior temporal lobes, including the **amygdala**. Symptoms include placidity (decrease in aggressive behavior), psychic blindness (visual agnosia), increased oral exploratory behavior, hypersexuality and loss of sexual preference, hypermetamorphosis (visual stimuli are repeatedly approached as if they were new), and anterograde amnesia.

# CEREBRAL CORTEX

The cerebral cortex is highly convoluted with bulges (**gyri**) separated by spaces (**sulci**). Several prominent sulci separate the cortex into four lobes: **frontal**, **parietal**, **temporal**, and **occipital**. The figures below show the lateral and medial views of the right cerebral hemispheres.

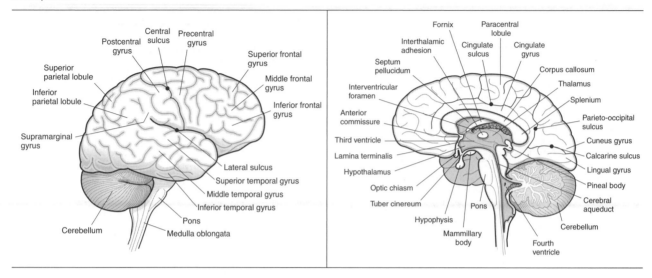

Most of the cortex has **six layers** (**neocortex**). The olfactory cortex and hippocampus have **three layers** (**allocortex**). The figure below shows the six-layered cortex:

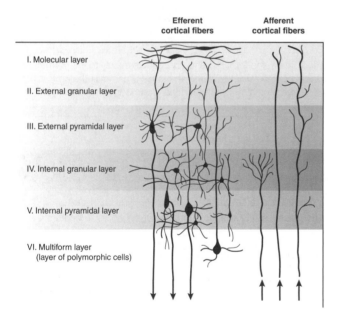

### Key Afferents/Efferents

**Layer IV** receives thalamocortical inputs.

**Layer V** gives rise to corticospinal and corticobulbar tracts.

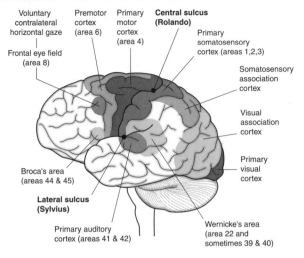

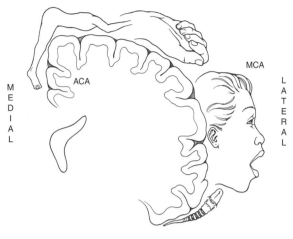

| Lobes | Important Regions | Deficit After Lesion |
|---|---|---|
| **Frontal** | Primary motor and premotor cortex | Contralateral spastic paresis (region depends on area of homunculus affected; see figure above) |
| | Frontal eye fields | Eyes deviate to ipsilateral side |
| | Broca speech area* | **Broca aphasia (expressive, nonfluent aphasia):** patient can understand written and spoken language, but speech and writing are slow and effortful; patients are aware of their problem; often associated with contralateral facial and arm weakness |
| | Prefrontal cortex | **Frontal lobe syndrome:** symptoms can include poor judgment, difficulty concentrating and problem solving, apathy, inappropriate social behavior |
| **Parietal** | Primary somatosensory cortex | Contralateral hemihypesthesia (region depends on area of homunculus affected) |
| | Superior parietal lobule | Contralateral astereognosis and sensory neglect, apraxia |
| | Inferior parietal lobule | **Gerstmann syndrome** (if dominant hemisphere): right/left confusion, dyscalculia and dysgraphia, finger agnosia, contralateral hemianopia or lower quadrantanopia |
| **Temporal** | Primary auditory cortex | Bilateral damage → deafness<br>Unilateral leads to slight hearing loss |
| | Wernicke area* | **Wernicke aphasia (receptive, fluent aphasia):** patient cannot understand any form of language; speech is fast and fluent, but not comprehensible |
| | Hippocampus | Bilateral lesions lead to inability to consolidate short-term to long-term memory |
| | Amygdala | **Klüver-Bucy syndrome:** hyperphagia, hypersexuality, visual agnosia |
| | Olfactory bulb, tract, primary cortex | Ipsilateral anosmia |
| | Meyer loop (visual radiations) | Contralateral upper quadrantanopia ("pie in the sky") |
| **Occipital** | Primary visual cortex | Blindness |

*In the dominant hemisphere. Eighty percent of people are left-hemisphere dominant.

ORGAN SYSTEMS

NERVOUS

# ALZHEIMER DISEASE

- Alzheimer disease accounts for 60% of all cases of dementia. The incidence increases with age.
- **Clinical:** insidious onset, progressive memory impairment, mood alterations, disorientation, aphasia, apraxia, and progression to a bedridden state with eventual death
- Five to 10% of AD cases are hereditary, early onset, and transmitted as an autosomal dominant trait.

## GENETICS OF ALZHEIMER DISEASE

| Gene | Location | Notes |
|------|----------|-------|
| Amyloid precursor protein (*APP*) gene | Chromosome 21 | Virtually all Down syndrome patients are destined to develop AD in their forties. Down patients have triple copies of the *APP* gene. |
| Presenilin-1 gene | Chromosome 14 | Majority of hereditary AD cases—early onset |
| Presenilin-2 gene | Chromosome 1 | Early onset |
| Apolipoprotein E gene | Chromosome 19 | Three allelic forms of this gene: epsilon 2, epsilon 3, and epsilon 4<br>The allele epsilon 4 of apolipoprotein E (*ApoE*) increases the risk for AD, epsilon 2 confers relative protection |

## PATHOLOGY OF ALZHEIMER DISEASE

Lesions involve the neocortex, hippocampus, and subcortical nuclei, including forebrain cholinergic nuclei (i.e., basal nucleus of Meynert). These areas show atrophy, as well as characteristic microscopic changes. The earliest and most severely affected areas are the hippocampus and temporal lobe, which are involved in learning and memory.

| | |
|---|---|
| **Intra- and extracellular accumulation of abnormal proteins** | **Aβ amyloid:** 42-residue peptide from a normal transmembrane protein, the amyloid precursor protein (APP)<br>**Abnormal *tau*** (a microtubule-associated protein) |
| **Senile plaques** | Core of Aβ amyloid surrounded by dystrophic neuritic processes associated with microglia and astrocytes |
| **Neurofibrillary tangles (NFT)** | Intraneuronal aggregates of insoluble cytoskeletal elements, mainly composed of abnormally phosphorylated tau forming **paired helical filaments** (PHF) |
| **Cerebral amyloid angiopathy (CAA)** | Accumulation of Aβ amyloid within the media of small and medium-sized intracortical and leptomeningeal arteries; associated with intracerebral hemorrhage |
| **Granulovacuolar degeneration (GVD) and Hirano bodies (HBs)** | GVD and HBs develop in the hippocampus and are less significant diagnostically |

## TREATMENT OF ALZHEIMER DISEASE

### AChE Inhibitors
(rivastigmine, donepezil, galantamine, tacrine)

These agents prevent the metabolism of ACh to counteract the depletion in ACh in the cerebral cortex and hippocampus. Rivastigmine and tacrine also inhibit BuChE. Indicated for mild to moderate AD.

### NMDA Antagonist
(memantine)

This is the newest class of agents used for the treatment of AD. It is hypothesized that overstimulation of NMDA receptors contributes to the symptomatology of AD. Indicated for moderate to severe AD. Often used in combination with the AChEIs.

*Definition of abbreviations:* AChE, acetylcholinesterase; BuChE, butyrylcholinesterase; NMDA, *N*-methyl-D-aspartate.

## CREUTZFELDT-JAKOB DISEASE (CJD)

### Mechanism of Disease

Caused by a **prion protein** (PrP = 30-kD protein normally present in neurons encoded by gene on chromosome 20); PrP$^c$ = normal conformation = alpha-helix; PrP$^{sc}$ = abnormal conformation = beta-pleated sheet. PrP$^{sc}$ facilitates conformational change of other PrP$^c$ molecules into PrP$^{sc}$.

Spontaneous change from one form to another → sporadic cases (85% of total) of CJD

Mutations of PrP → hereditary cases (15% of total) of CJD

### Pathology

**Spongiform change:** vacuolization of the neuropil in gray matter (especially cortex) due to large membrane-bound vacuoles within neuronal processes
- Associated with neuronal loss and astrogliosis
- **Kuru plaques** are deposits of amyloid of altered PrP protein

### Clinical Manifestations

Rapidly progressive dementia, memory loss, startle myoclonus or other involuntary movements. EEG changes. Death within 6–12 months.

### Variant CJD (vCJD)

Affects young adults. May be related to bovine spongiform encephalopathy (BSE; mad cow disease). Pathologically similar to CJD.

## PICK DISEASE (LOBAR ATROPHY)

- Rare cause of dementia
- Striking **atrophy of frontal and temporal lobes** with sparing of posterior structures
- Microscopic: swollen neurons (Pick cells) or neurons containing **Pick bodies** (round to oval inclusions that stain with silver stains)

## CNS TRAUMA

| | |
|---|---|
| **Concussion** | Occurs with a change in momentum of the head (impact against a rigid surface)<br>Loss of consciousness and reflexes, temporary respiratory arrest, and amnesia for the event |
| **Contusion** | Bruising to the brain resulting from impact of the brain against inner calvarial surfaces, especially along crests of orbital gyri (frontal lobe) and temporal poles<br>Coup (site of injury) and contrecoup (site diametrically opposite) develop when the head is **mobile** at the time of impact. |
| **Diffuse axonal injury** | Injury to white matter due to acceleration/deceleration produces damage to axons at nodes of Ranvier with impairment of axoplasmic flow<br>Poor prognosis, related to duration of coma |

## CEREBRAL HERNIATIONS

| | | |
|---|---|---|
| **Subfalcine (cingulate)** | Cingulate gyrus displaced underneath the falx to the opposite side with compression of anterior cerebral artery | |
| **Transtentorial (uncal)** | The uncus of the temporal lobe displaced over the free edge of the tentorium<br>Compression of the third nerve, with pupillary dilatation on the same side<br>Infarct in dependent territory<br>Advanced stages: **Duret hemorrhage** within the central pons and midbrain | |
| **Cerebellar tonsillar** | Displacement of cerebellar tonsils through the foramen magnum<br>Compression of medulla leads to cardiorespiratory arrest | |

# BLOOD SUPPLY

The blood supply of the cortex is supplied by branches of the **two internal carotid arteries** and **two vertebral arteries**.

- On the ventral surface of the brain, the anterior cerebral and middle cerebral branches of the internal carotid arteries connect with the posterior cerebral artery (derived from the basilar artery) and form the **circle of Willis**. This circle of vessels is completed by the anterior and posterior communicating arteries.

- The **middle cerebral artery** mainly supplies the lateral surface of the frontal, parietal, and upper aspect of the temporal lobe. Deep branches also supply part of the basal ganglia and internal capsule.

- The **anterior cerebral artery** supplies the medial aspect of the frontal and parietal lobes.

- The entire occipital lobe, lower aspect of temporal lobe, and the midbrain are supplied by the **posterior cerebral artery**.

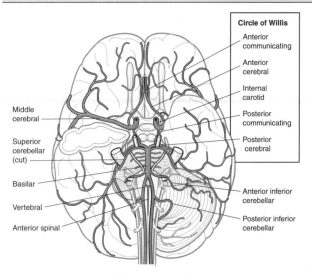

Circle of Willis
- Anterior communicating
- Anterior cerebral
- Internal carotid
- Posterior communicating
- Posterior cerebral

Middle cerebral
Superior cerebellar (cut)
Basilar
Vertebral
Anterior spinal
Anterior inferior cerebellar
Posterior inferior cerebellar

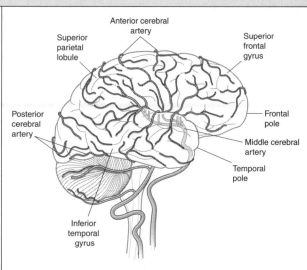

Anterior cerebral artery
Superior parietal lobule
Superior frontal gyrus
Posterior cerebral artery
Frontal pole
Middle cerebral artery
Temporal pole
Inferior temporal gyrus

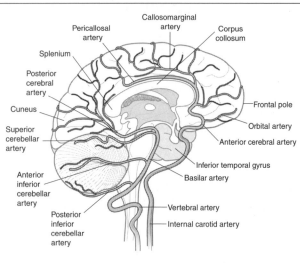

Pericallosal artery
Callosomarginal artery
Corpus collosum
Splenium
Posterior cerebral artery
Cuneus
Superior cerebellar artery
Anterior inferior cerebellar artery
Posterior inferior cerebellar artery
Frontal pole
Orbital artery
Anterior cerebral artery
Inferior temporal gyrus
Basilar artery
Vertebral artery
Internal carotid artery

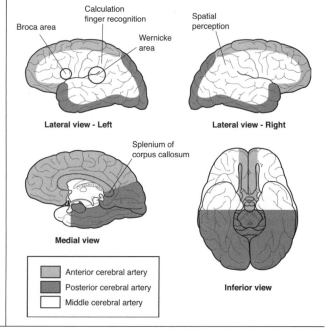

Calculation finger recognition
Broca area
Wernicke area
Spatial perception

**Lateral view - Left**   **Lateral view - Right**

Splenium of corpus callosum

**Medial view**

Anterior cerebral artery
Posterior cerebral artery
Middle cerebral artery

**Inferior view**

## BLOOD SUPPLY (CONT'D.)

| System | Primary Arteries | Branches | Supplies | Deficits after Stroke |
|---|---|---|---|---|
| Vertebrobasilar (posterior circulation) | Vertebral arteries | **Anterior spinal artery** | Anterior 2/3 of spinal cord | Dorsal columns spared; all else bilateral |
| | | **Posterior cerebellar (PICA)** | Dorsolateral medulla | See brain stem lesions on pages 160–161. |
| | Basilar artery | Pontine arteries | Base of pons | |
| | | **Anterior inferior cerebral (AICA)** | Inferior cerebellum, cerebellar nuclei | |
| | | Superior cerebellar artery | Dorsal cerebellar hemispheres; superior cerebellar peduncle | |
| | | Labyrinthine artery (sometimes arises from AICA) | Inner ear | |
| | Posterior cerebral arteries | — | Midbrain, thalamus, occipital lobe | **Contralateral hemianopia with macular sparing** Alexia without agraphia* |
| Internal carotid (anterior circulation) | Ophthalmic artery | Central artery of retina | Retina | Blindness |
| | Posterior communicating artery | — | — | Second most common **aneurysm** site (often with CN III palsy) |
| | Anterior cerebral artery | — | Primary motor and sensory cortex (leg/foot) | Contralateral spastic paralysis and anesthesia of **lower limb** Frontal lobe abnormalities |
| | Anterior communicating artery | — | — | Most common site of **aneurysm** |
| | Middle cerebral artery | Outer cortical | Lateral convexity of hemispheres | Contralateral spastic paralysis and anesthesia of **upper limb/face** **Gaze palsy** **Aphasia*** Gerstmann syndrome* Hemi inattention and neglect of contralateral body† |
| | | Lenticulostriate | Internal capsule, caudate, putamen, globus pallidus | |

*If dominant hemisphere is affected (usually the left).
†Right parietal lobe lesion

| CEREBROVASCULAR DISORDERS | | |
|---|---|---|
| **Disorder** | **Types** | **Key Concepts** |
| **Cerebral infarcts** | Thrombotic | **Anemic/pale** infarct; usually atherosclerotic complication |
| | Embolic | **Hemorrhagic/red** infarct; from heart or atherosclerotic plaques; **middle cerebral artery** most vulnerable to emboli |
| | Hypotension | **"Watershed"** areas and **deep cortical layers** most affected |
| | Hypertension | **Lacunar** infarcts; **basal ganglia** most affected |
| **Hemorrhages** | Epidural hematoma | Almost always traumatic<br>Rupture of **middle meningeal artery** after skull fracture<br>Lucid interval before loss of consciousness ("talk and die" syndrome) |
| | Subdural hematoma | Usually caused by trauma<br>Rupture of **bridging veins** (connect brain and sagittal sinus) |
| | Subarachnoid hemorrhage | **Ruptured berry aneurysm** is most frequent cause<br>Predisposing factors: Marfan syndrome, Ehlers-Danlos<br>  type 4, adult polycystic kidney disease, hypertension, smoking |
| | Intracerebral hemorrhage | Common causes: hypertension, trauma, infarction |

# SEIZURES AND ANTICONVULSANTS

| SEIZURES | |
|---|---|
| **Partial** | Occur in localized region of brain; can become secondarily generalized<br>**Drugs of choice:** carbamazepine, phenytoin, valproic acid<br>**Backup and adjuvants:** most newer drugs are also effective |
| **Simple** | • **Consciousness unaffected**<br>• Can be motor, somatosensory or special sensory, autonomic, psychic |
| **Complex** | • Consciousness is impaired<br>• The four "A"s: aura, alteration of consciousness, automatisms, amnesia<br>• Often called "psychomotor" or "temporal lobe seizures" |
| **Generalized** | Affects **entire brain** |
| **Absence** | • Impaired consciousness (usually abrupt onset and brief); automatisms sometimes occur<br>• Begin in childhood, often end by age 20<br>• Also called **petit mal**<br>• **Drugs of choice:** ethosuximide (1st line if only absence is present), valproic acid<br>• **Backup and adjuvants:** clonazepam, lamotrigine, topiramate |
| **Tonic-clonic** | • Alternating tonic (stiffening) and clonic (movements); loss of consciousness<br>• Also called grand mal<br>• **Drugs of choice:** valproic acid, carbamazepine, phenytoin, phenobarbital<br>• **Backup and adjuvants:** lamotrigine, topiramate, levetiracetam, phenobarbital, others |
| **Myoclonic** | Single or multiple myoclonic jerks<br>• **Drug of choice:** valproic acid<br>• **Backup and adjuvants:** clonazepam, topiramate, lamotrigine, levetiracetam |
| **Status epilepticus** | • Seizure activity (often tonic-clonic), continuous or intermittent (without recovery of consciousness) for at least 30 minutes; life-threatening<br>• **Drugs of choice:** diazepam, lorazepam, phenytoin, fosphenytoin<br>• **Backup and adjuvants:** phenobarbital, general anesthesia |

| ANTICONVULSANTS | | |
|---|---|---|
| **Drug** | **Mechanism** | **Notes** |
| Benzodiazepines | ↑ frequency of $GABA_A$ ($Cl^-$) receptor opening | Sedation, dependence, tolerance |
| Carbamazepine | Blocks $Na^+$ channels | Diplopia, ataxia, blood dyscrasias (agranulocytosis, aplastic anemia), P450 induction, teratogenic |
| Ethosuximide | Blocks T-type $Ca^{2+}$ channels (thalamus) | GI distress, headache, lethargy, hematotoxicity, Stevens-Johnson syndrome |
| Phenobarbital | ↑ duration of $GABA_A$ ($Cl^-$) receptor opening | Induction of cytochrome P450, sedation, dependence, tolerance |
| Phenytoin | Blocks $Na^+$ channels | Gingival hyperplasia, hirsutism, sedation, anemia, nystagmus, diplopia, ataxia, teratogenic (fetal hydantoin syndrome), P450 induction, zero-order kinetics |
| Valproic acid | Blocks $Na^+$ channels, inhibits GABA transaminase | GI distress, hepatotoxic (rare but can be fatal), inhibits drug metabolism, neural tube defects |

| NEWER AGENTS | |
|---|---|
| **Drug** | **Side Effects** |
| Felbamate | Aplastic anemia, hepatoxicity |
| Gabapentin | Sedation, dizziness |
| Lamotrigine | Life-threatening rash, Stevens-Johnson syndrome |
| Levetiracetam | Neuropsychiatric effects, sedation |
| Tiagabine | Sedation, dizziness |
| Topiramate | Sedation, dizziness, ataxia, anomia, renal stones, weight loss |
| Vigabatrin | Sedation, dizziness, visual field defects, psychosis |

# OPIOID ANALGESICS AND RELATED DRUGS

Opioid analgesics act by stimulating receptors for endogenous opioid peptides (e.g., enkephalins, β-endorphin, dynorphins). Opioid receptors are G-protein coupled, and the three major classes are μ **(mu),** κ **(kappa),** and δ **(delta).** β-Endorphin has the greatest affinity for the μ receptor, dynorphins for the κ receptor, and enkephalins for the δ receptor. The effects of specific drugs depend on the receptor subtype with which they interact, and whether they act as full agonists, partial agonists, or antagonists. The μ receptor is primarily responsible for analgesia, respiratory depression, euphoria, and physical dependence.

## INDIVIDUAL AGENTS

### Strong Agonists

| | | |
|---|---|---|
| **Morphine** | Full μ agonist | Prototype of this class; poor oral bioavailability; histamine release |
| **Methadone** | | Orally active; long duration; useful in maintenance |
| **Meperidine** | | Muscarinic antagonist (no miosis or smooth muscle contraction); forms normeperidine → possible seizures; do not combine with MAO inhibitors or SSRIs |

Additional strong agonists: fentanyl, heroin (schedule I), levorphanol

### Moderate Agonists

| | | |
|---|---|---|
| **Codeine** | Partial μ agonist | Antitussive, often given in combination with NSAIDs |

Additional moderate agonists: oxycodone, hydrocodone

### Weak Agonists

| | | |
|---|---|---|
| **Propoxyphene** | Partial μ agonist | Analgesia weaker than codeine; toxic in overdose; large doses → drug dependence |

### Mixed Agonist–Antagonists

| | | |
|---|---|---|
| **Pentazocine** <br> **Nalbuphine** <br> **Butorphanol** | κ agonist/weak μ agonist | In general, less analgesia than morphine <br> Can cause hallucinations and nightmares <br> Has less respiratory depression and abuse liability than the pure agonists |
| **Buprenorphine** | Partial μ agonist/ weak κ and δ antagonist | Binds tightly to receptor, so is more resistant to naloxone reversal |

### Antitussives

| | |
|---|---|
| **Codeine** <br> **Dextromethorphan** | Codeine is by prescription; dextromethorphan is available OTC |

### Antidiarrheals

| | |
|---|---|
| **Diphenoxylate** <br> **Loperamide** | Diphenoxylate used in combination with atropine to prevent abuse <br> Loperamide available OTC |

### Antagonists

| | |
|---|---|
| **Naloxone (IV)** <br> **Naltrexone (PO)** <br> **Nalmefene (IV)** | All are used in the management of acute opioid overdose. Naloxone has a short half-life and may require multiple doses. Naltrexone ↓ craving for ethanol and is used in alcohol dependency programs. |

## CHARACTERISTICS OF OPIOID ANALGESICS

### Effects and Side Effects

- Analgesia
- Sedation
- Respiratory depression
- Constipation
- Smooth muscle: (except meperidine)
  - ↑ tone: biliary tract (biliary colic), bladder, ureter
  - ↓ tone: uterus (prolongs labor), vascular

- Euphoria
- Cough suppression
- Nausea and vomiting
- Pupillary miosis (except meperidine)
- Cardiovascular:
  Cerebrovascular dilation (esp. with ↑ $P_{CO_2}$) leads to ↑ intracranial pressure
  ↓ BP may occur; bradycardia

### Clinical Uses

Analgesia, cough suppression, treatment of diarrhea, preoperative medications and adjunct to anesthesia, management of pulmonary edema

### Chronic Effects

- Pharmacodynamic tolerance (tolerance does not develop to constipation or miosis)
- **Dependence:** Psychological and physical
- **Abstinence syndrome (withdrawal):** anxiety, hostility, GI distress (cramps and diarrhea) gooseflesh ("cold turkey"), muscle cramps and spasms ("kicking the habit"), rhinorrhea, lacrimation, sweating, yawning
- Abstinence syndrome can be precipitated in tolerant individuals by administering an opioid antagonist

### Overdose

- **Classic triad:** Respiratory depression, miosis (pinpoint pupils), coma
- Diagnosis confirmed with naloxone (short duration, may need repeat dosing); give supportive care

### Contraindications and Cautions

- Use of full agonists with weak partial agonists. Weak agonists can precipitate withdrawal from the full agonist.
- Use in patients with pulmonary dysfunction (acute respiratory failure). Exception: pulmonary edema
- Use in patients with head injuries (possible increased intracranial pressure)

- Use in patients with hepatic/renal dysfunction (drug accumulation)
- Use in patients with adrenal or thyroid deficiencies (prolonged and exaggerated responses)
- Use in pregnant patients (possible neonatal depression or dependence)

# LOCAL ANESTHETICS

Local anesthetics **block voltage-gated sodium channels**, preventing sensory information from being transmitted from a local area to the brain. These agents are initially uncharged and diffuse across the axonal membrane to enter the cytoplasm. Once inside, they become ionized and block the $Na^+$ channels from the **inside**. These agents bind best to channels that are open or recently inactivated, rather than resting, and therefore work better in rapidly firing fibers (**use-dependence**). Infection leads to a more acidic environment, making the basic local anesthetic more likely to be ionized, therefore higher doses may be required. **Order of blockade:** small fibers > larger fibers; myelinated fibers > unmyelinated fibers. **Modality blocked:** autonomic and pain > touch/pressure > motor. There are two main classes: **amides** and **esters**.

| Amides<br>(metabolized in **liver**) | | Esters<br>(metabolized by<br>**plasma cholinesterases**) | | Side Effects |
|---|---|---|---|---|
| Bupivacaine | (L) | Tetracaine | (L) | 1. **Neurotoxicity:** lightheadedness, nystagmus, restlessness, convulsions |
| Etidocaine | (L) | Cocaine | (M)† | |
| Ropivacaine | (L) | Procaine | (S) | |
| Lidocaine | (M)* | Benzocaine‡ | | 2. **Cardiovascular toxicity**: ↓ CV parameters (except cocaine which ↑ HR and BP); bupivacaine especially notable for CV toxicity |
| Mepivacaine | (M) | | | |
| Prilocaine | (M) | | | |
| **Notes** | | | | 3. **Allergic reaction:** esters via PABA formation; switch to amides if allergic to esters |
| Duration of action can be increased by coadministration of a vasoconstrictor (e.g., epinephrine) to limit blood flow | | | | |
| **Hint:** Amide drugs have two "i"s, and ester drugs have one "i" in their names. | | | | |

*Definition of abbreviations:* L, long acting; M, medium acting; S, short acting.
*Also a IB antiarrhythmic
†Primarily used topically; sympathomimetic; drug of abuse (schedule II)
‡Topical only

# The Cardiovascular System

## Embryology

## Cardiovascular Anatomy

## Cardiovascular Physiology

## Cardiovascular Pathology

## DEVELOPMENT OF THE HEART TUBE

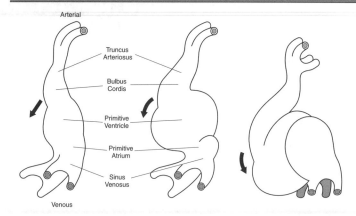

The primitive heart tube is formed from lateral plate mesoderm. The primitive heart tube undergoes dextral looping (bends to the right) and forms five dilatations. Four of the five dilatations become subdivided by a septum. Most of the common congenital cardiac anomalies result from defects in the formation of these septa.

## ADULT STRUCTURES DERIVED FROM THE DILATATIONS OF THE PRIMITIVE HEART

| Embryonic Dilatation | Adult Structure |
|---|---|
| Truncus arteriosus (neural crest) | Aorta<br>Pulmonary trunk |
| Bulbus cordis | Smooth part of right ventricle (**conus arteriosus**)<br>Smooth part of left ventricle (**aortic vestibule**) |
| Primitive ventricle | Trabeculated part of right ventricle<br>Trabeculated part of left ventricle |
| Primitive atrium | Trabeculated part of right atrium<br>Trabeculated part of left atrium |
| Sinus venosus (the only dilatation that does not become subdivided by a septum) | Right—smooth part of right atrium (**sinus venarum**)<br>Left—coronary sinus<br>Oblique vein of left atrium |

## ATRIAL SEPTUM

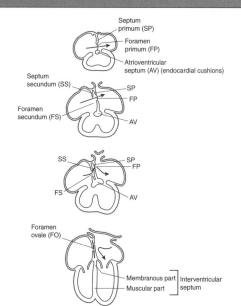

**Atrial septal defects** are called **ASDs**.

**Secundum-type ASDs** are caused by excessive resorption of the SP or reduced size of the SS or both. This results in an opening between the right and left atria. If the ASD is small, clinical symptoms may be delayed as late as age 30. This is the most clinically significant ASD.

The **foramen ovale** (FO) is the fetal communication between the right and left atria. It remains patent in up to 25% of normal individuals throughout life, although paradoxical emboli may pass through a large patent FO. **Premature closure of the FO** is the closure of the FO during prenatal life. This results in hypertrophy of the right side of the heart and underdevelopment of the left side.

## VENTRICULAR SEPTUM

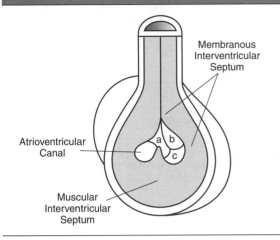

A **membranous ventricular septal defect (VSD)** is caused by the failure of the membranous interventricular septum to develop, and it results in **left-to-right shunting** of blood through the interventricular foramen. Patients with left-to-right shunting complain of **excessive fatigue upon exertion**. Left-to-right shunting of blood is not cyanotic but causes increased blood flow and pressure to the lungs (pulmonary hypertension). Pulmonary hypertension causes marked proliferation of the tunica intima and media of pulmonary muscular arteries and arterioles. Ultimately, the pulmonary resistance becomes higher than systemic resistance and causes **right-to-left shunting** of blood and "late" **cyanosis**. At this stage, the condition is called **Eisenmenger complex**. VSD is the most common congenital cardiac anomaly.

*Figure legend:* a, right bulbar ridge; b, left bulbar ridge; c, AV cushions.

## AORTICOPULMONARY SEPTUM

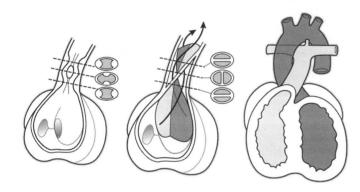

Neural crest cells migrate into the truncal and bulbar ridges of the truncus arteriosus, which grow in a spiral fashion and fuse to form the aorticopulmonary (AP) septum. The AP septum divides the truncus arteriosus into the **aorta** (dark gray) and **pulmonary trunk** (light gray).

### Transposition of the Great Vessels

Occurs when the AP septum fails to develop in a spiral fashion and results in the aorta opening into the right ventricle and the pulmonary trunk opening into the left ventricle. This causes **right-to-left** shunting of blood with resultant **cyanosis**. Infants born alive with this defect must have other defects (like a PDA or VSD) that allow mixing of oxygenated and deoxygenated blood.

### Tetralogy of Fallot

Occurs when the AP septum fails to align properly and results in (1) pulmonary stenosis, (2) overriding aorta, (3) interventricular septal defect, and (4) right ventricular hypertrophy. This causes **right-to-left** shunting of blood with resultant "early" **cyanosis**, which is usually present at birth. Tetralogy of Fallot is the most common congenital cyanotic cardiac anomaly.

### Persistent Truncus Arteriosus

Occurs when there is only partial development of the AP septum. This results in a condition in which only one large vessel leaves the heart and receives blood from both the right and left ventricles. This causes **right-to-left** shunting of blood with resultant **cyanosis**. This defect is always accompanied by membranous ventricular septal defect.

*Definition of abbreviation:* PDA, patent ductus arteriosus.

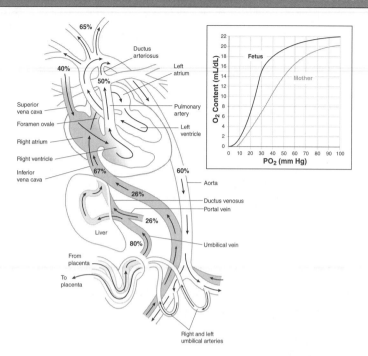

## Clinical Correlation

Normally, the ductus arteriosus closes within a few hours after birth, via smooth muscle contraction, to form the ligamentum arteriosum. **Patent ductus arteriosus (PDA)** occurs when the ductus arteriosus (connection between the pulmonary trunk and aorta) fails to close after birth.

Prostaglandin E and intrauterine or neonatal asphyxia **sustain the patency** of the ductus arteriosus.

Prostaglandin inhibitors (e.g., indomethacin), acetylcholine, histamine, and catecholamines **promote closure** of the ductus arteriosus.

PDA is common in premature infants and cases of maternal rubella infection. It causes a left-to-right shunting of blood. (Note: During fetal development, the ductus arteriosus is a right-to-left shunt).

In the fetal circulation pathway, the ductus venosus allows fetal blood to bypass the liver, and the foramen ovale and the ductus arteriosus allow fetal blood to bypass the lungs. Note the sites where the oxygen saturation level of fetal blood is the highest (umbilical vein) and the lowest (ductus arteriosus).

# CARDIOVASCULAR ANATOMY

## STRUCTURES OF THE MEDIASTINUM

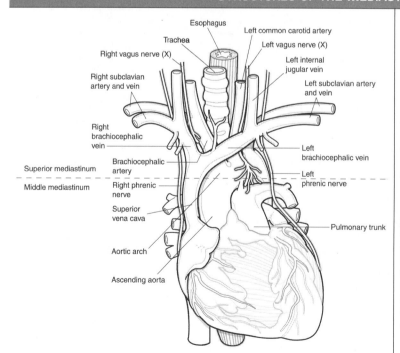

The thoracic cavity is divided into the **superior mediastinum** above the plane of the sternal angle and the **inferior mediastinum** (anterior, middle, and posterior mediastina) below that sternal plane. The superior mediastinum contains the thymic remnants, superior vena cava and its brachiocephalic tributaries, aortic arch and its branches, trachea, esophagus, thoracic duct, and the vagus and phrenic nerves.

The **anterior mediastinum** is anterior to the heart and contains remnants of the thymus. The **middle mediastinum** contains the heart and great vessels, and the **posterior mediastinum** contains the thoracic aorta, esophagus, thoracic duct, azygos veins, and the vagus nerves. The inferior vena cava passes through the diaphragm at the caval hiatus at the level of the eighth thoracic vertebra; the esophagus through the esophageal hiatus at the tenth thoracic vertebra; and the aorta courses through the aortic hiatus at the level of the twelfth thoracic vertebra.

ORGAN SYSTEMS

CARDIOVASCULAR

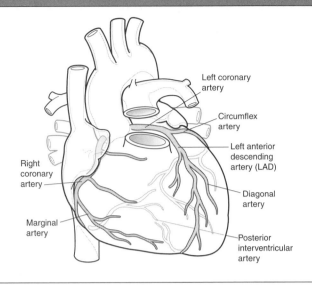

Arterial supply to the heart muscle is provided by the **right and left coronary arteries**, which are branches of the ascending aorta. The **right coronary artery** supplies the right atrium, the right ventricle, the sinoatrial and atrioventricular nodes, and parts of the left atrium and left ventricle. The distal branch of the right coronary artery (in 70% of subjects) is the **posterior interventricular artery** that supplies, in part, the posterior aspect of the interventricular septum. The **left coronary artery** supplies most of the left ventricle, the left atrium, and the anterior part of the interventricular septum. The two main branches of the left coronary artery are the anterior interventricular artery (LAD) and the circumflex artery.

In a myocardial infarction, the LAD is obstructed in 50% of cases, the right coronary in 30%, and the circumflex artery in 20% of cases.

## CHAMBERS AND VALVES OF THE HEART

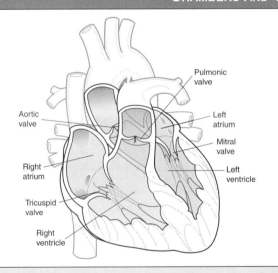

### Right Atrium

The right atrium receives venous blood from the entire body (except for blood from the pulmonary veins).

The **auricle** is derived from the fetal atrium; it has rough myocardium known as pectinate muscles.

The **sinus venarum** is the smooth-walled portion of the atrium, which receives blood from the superior and inferior venae cavae.

The **crista terminalis** is the vertical ridge that separates the smooth from the rough portion of the right atrium; it extends longitudinally from the superior vena cava to the inferior vena cava. The SA node is in the upper part of the crista terminalis.

The right AV **(tricuspid valve)** communicates with the right ventricle.

### Right Ventricle

The right ventricle receives blood from the right atrium via the tricuspid valve; outflow is to the pulmonary trunk via the pulmonary semilunar valve.

The **trabeculae carneae** are the ridges of myocardium in the ventricular wall.

The **papillary muscles** project into the cavity of the ventricle and attach to cusps of the AV valve by the strands of the chordae tendineae. Papillary muscles contract during ventricular contraction to keep the cusps of the AV valves closed.

The **chordae tendineae** control closure of the valve during contraction of the ventricle.

The **infundibulum** is the smooth area of the right ventricle leading to the pulmonary valve.

### Left Atrium

The left atrium receives oxygenated blood from the lungs via the pulmonary veins. There are four openings: the upper right and left and the lower right and left pulmonary veins.

The left AV orifice is guarded by the **mitral (bicuspid) valve**; it allows oxygenated blood to pass from the left atrium to the left ventricle.

*(Continued)*

### Left Ventricle

Blood enters from the left atrium through the mitral valve and is pumped out to the aorta through the aortic valve.

**Trabeculae carneae**, the ridges of myocardium in the ventricular wall, are normally three times thicker than those of the right ventricle.

**Papillary muscles** (usually two large ones) are attached by the chordae tendineae to the cusps of the bicuspid valve.

The **aortic vestibule** leads to the aortic semilunar valve and ascending aorta; the right and left coronary arteries originate from the right and left aortic sinuses at the root of the ascending aorta.

### Clinical Correlation

### Murmurs

Murmurs in valvular heart disease result when there is valvular insufficiency or a stenotic valve. For most of **ventricular systole**, the mitral valve should be closed and the aortic valve should be open, so that "common systolic valvular defects" include mitral insufficiency and aortic stenosis. For most of **ventricular diastole**, the mitral valve should be open and the aortic valve should be closed, so that "common diastolic valvular defects" include mitral stenosis and aortic insufficiency.

## BORDERS OF THE HEART

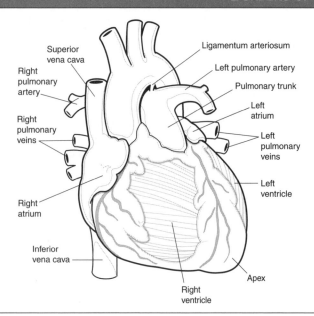

The **external** surface of the heart consists of several borders:

- the right border is formed by the right atrium
- the left border is formed by the left ventricle
- the base formed by the two atria
- the apex at the tip of the left ventricle

The **anterior** surface is formed by the right ventricle.

The **posterior** surface is formed mainly by the left atrium.

A **diaphragmatic** surface is formed primarily by the left ventricle.

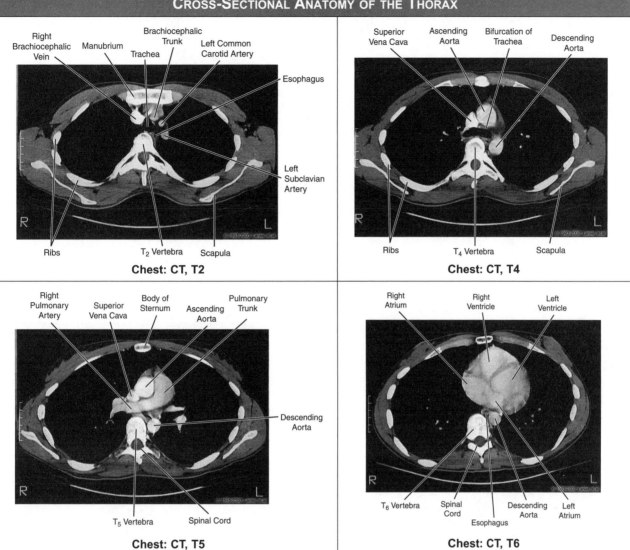

**Chest: CT, T2**

**Chest: CT, T4**

**Chest: CT, T5**

**Chest: CT, T6**

Images copyright 2005 DxR Development Group Inc. All rights reserved.

# CONDUCTING SYSTEM OF THE HEART

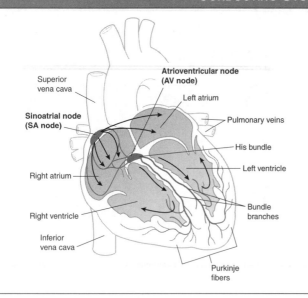

The **sinoatrial node** initiates the impulse for cardiac contraction. The **atrioventricular node** receives the impulse from the sinoatrial node and transmits that impulse to the ventricles through the **bundle of His**. The bundle divides into the **right and left bundle branches** and **Purkinje fibers** to the two ventricles.

**Sympathetic** innervation from the T1 to T5 spinal cord segments increases the heart rate, while the **parasympathetics** by way of the vagus nerves slow the heart rate.

# ASSOCIATIONS OF COMMON TRAUMATIC INJURIES WITH VESSEL AND NERVE DAMAGE

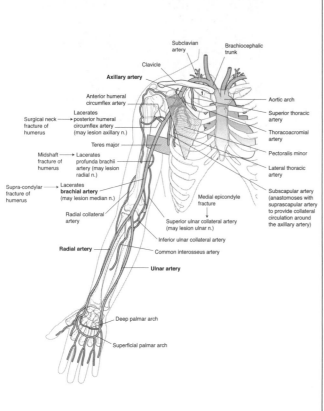

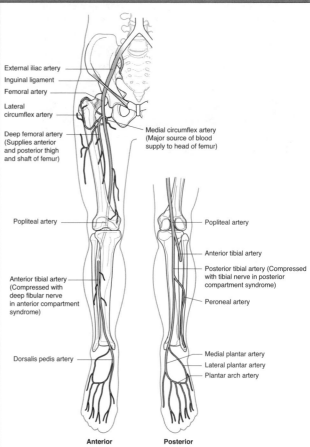

# CARDIOVASCULAR PHYSIOLOGY

## COMPARISON OF CARDIAC ACTION POTENTIALS

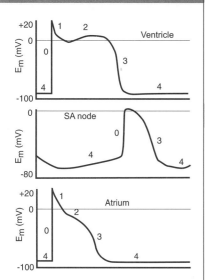

## IMPORTANT IMPLICATIONS OF ION CURRENTS

**Force development**
$Ca^{2+}$ current of plateau (phase 2) has major influence

**Timing/heart rate**
$i_f$ is increased by sympathetics → increased heart rate; parasympathetics decrease it

**Premature beats**
Action potential amplitude and shape not all-or-none; early beats abnormal with low force

**Susceptible period**
Arrhythmia risk high during relative refractory period

## CARDIAC ACTION POTENTIALS—IONIC MECHANISMS

### Unique Cardiac Ion Channels

| | |
|---|---|
| **iK** | Delayed rectifier; slow to open/close; depolarization opens |
| **iK$_1$** | Inward rectifier; open at rest; depolarization closes it |
| **L-type** | $Ca^{2+}$, slow channel, long acting; depolarization opens |
| **i$_f$** | $Na^+$; "funny channel"; repolarization opens it; causes the pacemaker spontaneous depolarization |

### Ionic Basis of Ventricular AP

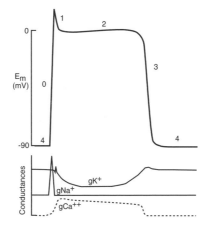

Conductances show changes only and do not reflect absolute values of different ions.

### Ionic Basis of SA Node AP

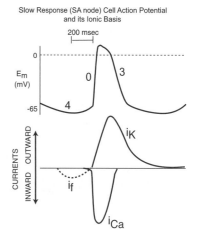

### Ventricles and Atria

**Phase 4**—resting potential
↑ $gK^+$ occurs via iK$_1$ channels
iK channels are closing or closed

**Phase 0**—upstroke
↑ $gNa^+$ via typical fast $Na^+$ channels
↓ $gK^+$ as iK$_1$ channels close

**Phase 1**—rapid partial repolarization
↓ $gNa^+$ as fast channels close
↑ $gK^+$ transiently via iK$_{to}$

**Phase 2**—plateau
↑ $gCa^{2+}$: slow (L-type) channels
at end of phase 2, ↑ $gK^+$ via iK channels

**Phase 3**—repolarization
↓ $gCa^{2+}$ as L-type channels close
↑ $gK^+$ via iK; then iK$_1$ opens

### SA Node and AV Node

**Phase 4**—pacemaker
↑ $gNa^+$ via i$_f$ "funny channel"
High $gK^+$ but ↓ as iK channels close

**Phase 0**—upstroke
↑ $gCa^{2+}$ via T-type (fast, transient) channels, then L-type (slow) open

No **phase 1** because no fast sodium channels

**Phase 2** usually absent

**Phase 3**—repolarization
↓ $gCa^{2+}$ as slow channels close
↑ $gK^+$ via iK channels

ORGAN SYSTEMS

CARDIOVASCULAR

## REFRACTORY PERIODS

Summation is difficult to achieve in cardiac muscle and tetany does not occur. In fact, the abnormal shape of action potentials initiated during the relative refractory period reduces calcium influx and thus contractile force, as shown.

| Muscle Twitch Versus Refractory Periods | Effect of AP Initiation During the Relative Refractory Period |
|---|---|

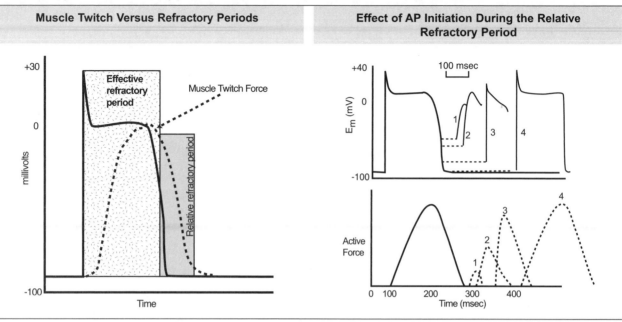

## BASIC PRINCIPLES OF THE ELECTROCARDIOGRAM

A moving wave of depolarization in the heart produces a positive deflection as it moves toward the positive terminals of the ECG electrodes. A depolarizing wave moving away from the positive (toward the negative) terminals produces a negative deflection. A wave of depolarization moving at right angles to the axis of the electrode terminals produces no deflection. Upon repolarization, the reverse occurs.

## SEQUENCE OF MYOCARDIAL EXCITATION AND CONDUCTION

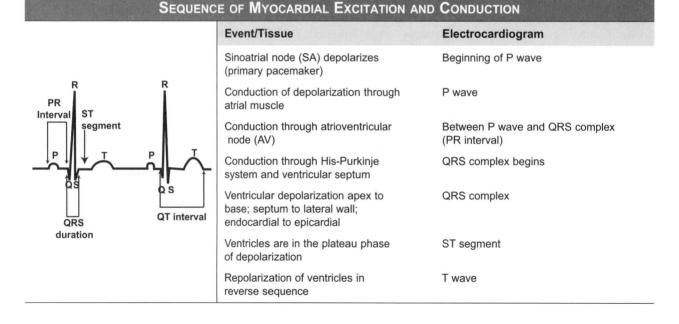

| Event/Tissue | Electrocardiogram |
|---|---|
| Sinoatrial node (SA) depolarizes (primary pacemaker) | Beginning of P wave |
| Conduction of depolarization through atrial muscle | P wave |
| Conduction through atrioventricular node (AV) | Between P wave and QRS complex (PR interval) |
| Conduction through His-Purkinje system and ventricular septum | QRS complex begins |
| Ventricular depolarization apex to base; septum to lateral wall; endocardial to epicardial | QRS complex |
| Ventricles are in the plateau phase of depolarization | ST segment |
| Repolarization of ventricles in reverse sequence | T wave |

## Important ECG Values

| | | |
|---|---|---|
| PR interval | 0.12–0.20 sec | Length measures AV conduction time |
| QRS duration | <0.12 sec | Measures ventricular conduction time |
| QT interval | 0.35–0.45 sec | Total time of ventricular depolarization and repolarization<br>Varies with heart rate, age |
| Heart rate, normal resting | 60–100 beats/min | <60/min = bradycardia;  >100/min = tachycardia |

## PRINCIPLES OF THE ELECTROCARDIOGRAM (EKG OR ECG)

| Moving Electrical Charge | | Creates Electrical Field Movement That Causes Ion Currents in Skin |
|---|---|---|
| Standard limb leads<br>(frontal plane) | I | ⊖ right arm; ⊕ left arm; positive lead at 0° |
| | II | ⊖ right arm; ⊕ left leg; positive lead at +60° |
| | III | ⊖ left arm; ⊕ left leg; positive lead at +120° |
| Augmented limb leads<br>(frontal plane) | aVR; aVL, aVF | aVR positive lead at –150°; aVL positive lead at –30°;<br>aVF positive lead at +90° |
| Precordial | $V_1$–$V_6$ (chest) | Horizontal plane; positive leads front; negative leads back of chest |
| Chart speed | 25 mm/sec | Each horizontal mm = 0.04 sec (40 msec) |
| Voltage | 1 mV/10 mm | Measure ± voltages of QRS, add to get net voltage of each lead |
| Mean electrical axis | Vector sum of two leads | Measure of overall wave of ventricular depolarization: normal axis, left or right axis deviation |

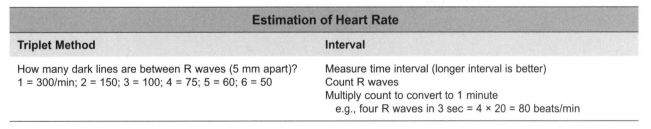

Begin    1 sec    2 sec    3 sec

300  150  100  75  60  50

Lead I

Four intervals = 75 beats/min
OR
Four beats in 3 sec = 4 X 20 = 80 beats/min

## Estimation of Heart Rate

| Triplet Method | Interval |
|---|---|
| How many dark lines are between R waves (5 mm apart)?<br>1 = 300/min; 2 = 150; 3 = 100; 4 = 75; 5 = 60; 6 = 50 | Measure time interval (longer interval is better)<br>Count R waves<br>Multiply count to convert to 1 minute<br>  e.g., four R waves in 3 sec = 4 × 20 = 80 beats/min |

## IMPORTANT RHYTHMS TO RECOGNIZE

| Rhythm | Characteristics |
|---|---|
| Sinus rhythm<br>    Normal      rate = 60–100<br>    Bradycardia  rate <60<br>    Tachycardia  rate >100 | Each beat originates in the SA node; therefore, the P wave precedes each QRS complex; PR interval is normal |
| AV conduction block | Abnormal conduction through AV node |
|     First degree | PR interval (> 0.20 sec); 1:1 correspondence; P wave:R wave |
|     Second degree Mobitz I (Wenckebach) | Progressively increased PR interval; then dropped (missing) QRS and then repeat of sequence |
|     Second degree Mobitz II | Regular but prolonged PR interval; unexpected dropped QRS; may be a regular pattern, such as 2:1 = 2 P waves:1 QRS complex or 3:1, etc. |
|     Third degree (complete) | No correlation of P waves and QRS complexes; usually high atrial rate and lower ventricular rate |
| Premature ventricular contraction (PVC) | Large, wide QRS complex originates in ectopic focus of irritability in ventricle; may indicate hypoxia |
| Ventricular tachycardia | Repeated large, wide QRS complexes like PVCs; Rate 150–250/min; acts like prolonged sequence of PVCs |
| Ventricular fibrillation | Total loss of rhythmic contraction; totally erratic shape |

## EVOLUTION OF AN INFARCTION: SIGNS ON THE EKG

| | | |
|---|---|---|
| Features to observe | QRS complex | Presence of prominent Q waves in leads where normally absent: infarct damage |
| | ST segment | Elevation or depression: acute injury |
| | T wave | Inversion; e.g., downward in lead where usually positive: acute ischemia |
| Acute myocardial infarction (MI) | Minutes to a few days | ST segment elevation or depression<br>Inverted T waves<br>Prominent Q waves |
| Resolving infarction (healing) | Weeks to months | Inverted T waves<br>Prominent Q waves |
| Stable (old) MI | Months to years | Prominent Q waves as result of MI persist for the rest of life |

*Caution:* Not all infarctions produce Q waves. Inverted T waves and/or ST abnormalities should always be investigated, even in absence of significant Q waves.

# MEAN ELECTRICAL AXIS (MEA)

| Definition | • Overall direction and force (vector) of the events of ventricular depolarization: obtained by vector sum of net voltage of two leads or by quadrant method using leads I and aVF<br>• MEA tends to shift toward large mass and away from an MI |
|---|---|
| Normal axis | • Expected in the absence of cardiac disease<br>• R wave: lead I, +; lead II, +; lead III, + |
| Left axis deviation | • May indicate left heart enlargement, as in hypertrophy or left dilated failure<br>• Abnormally prolonged (slow) left ventricular conduction<br>• Right heart MI, expiration, obesity, lying down<br>• R wave: lead I, +; lead II, +; lead III, − |
| Right axis deviation | • Right ventricular hypertrophy or dilation<br>• Prolonged right conduction<br>• Left heart MI, inspiration, tall lanky people, standing up<br>• R wave: lead I, −; lead II, +; lead III, + |
| Extreme right axis deviation | Difficult interpretation; one example: depolarization proceeding from abnormal focus in LV apex |

## Einthoven's Triangle: Leads I, II, and III*

## Vector Cardiogram

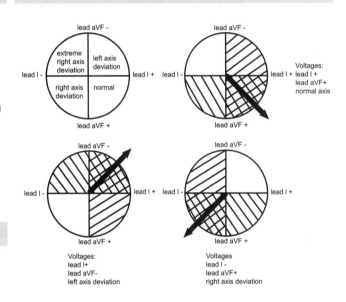

## Essentials of the EKG

Heart rate

Rhythm

Axis deviation

Hypertrophy

Infarction

*The figure adds aVF because the quadrant method of determining axis uses leads I and aVF.

## Cardiac Mechanical Performance

| Factor | Definition | Effects |
|--------|-----------|---------|
| Preload | Cardiac muscle cell length (sarcomere length) **before contraction begins** | ↑ preload causes ↑ active force development up to a limit |
| Afterload | Load on the heart during ejection of blood from the ventricle | ↑ afterload ↓ the volume of blood ejected during a beat |
| Contractility | Capacity of the heart to produce active force at a specified preload | High contractility ↑ ability to work <br> Low contractility ↓ ability to work |
| Rate | Heart rate (HR): number of cardiac cycles per minute | ↑ output of blood per minute, but ↓ output per beat; very high rate (>≈150/min) ↓ output |

## Cardiac Performance: Definitions

| | |
|--|--|
| **Stroke volume (SV)** | Blood ejected from ventricle per beat = EDV – ESV |
| **End diastolic volume (EDV)** | Volume of blood in ventricle at end of diastole; the preload |
| **End systolic volume (ESV)** | Volume of blood remaining in ventricle at end of systole |
| **Cardiac output (CO)** | Volume of blood per minute pumped by the heart; CO = SV × HR |
| **Ejection fraction (EF)** | Measure of contractility: EF = SV/EDV |
| **Left ventricular dP/dT (mm Hg/sec)** | Measure of contractility: maximum rate of change of pressure during isovolumic contraction |

## Cardiac and Vascular Function Curves

| | |
|--|--|
| **Cardiac function curve (CFC)** | • CFC generated by controlling preload and measuring cardiac output, stroke volume or other measure of systolic performance <br> • ↑ preload improves actin-myosin interdigitation and thus ↑ SV, CO, etc. <br> • CFC shifts **up** with ↑ **contractility; down** with ↓ **contractility**; so a new curve is produced when contractility changes <br> • Moving to a **different point on the same CFC** is a change only of **preload**: moving to a **different CFC** is change of **contractility** |
| **Vascular function curve (VFC)** | • VFC relates venous return to right atrial pressure <br> • ↑ **blood volume shifts VFC up, ↓ volume shifts VFC down** |
| **Equilibrium point** | Cardiac output is determined by both CFC and VFC. Intersection of the CFC and VFC is the stable operating point; if contractility or blood volume changes, the system will operate at the intersection of the two new curves. |

### Stability of Typical CFC and VFC

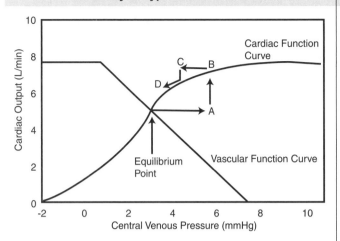

Diagram shows that cardiac output (CO, 5 L/min) changes only transiently when CFC and VFC are not changed. **Point A:** venous pressure is increased from 3 to 6 mm Hg because of sudden removal of blood from arterial system and injection into venous system. This causes **CO** to increase to **point B**. CO then returns to **equilibrium point** in steps (B → C, C → D) as blood is pumped from venous system back to arterial system.

### Changes in Blood Volume

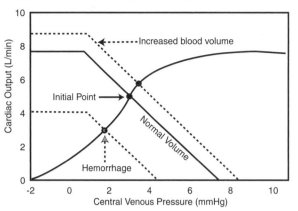

Increased blood volume (e.g., transfusion) shifts the VFC upward, which increases preload. Increased CO follows. Decreased blood volume (e.g., hemorrhage) shifts the VFC downward, which decreases preload. Decreased CO follows. Increases and decreases in preload produce increases and decreases in CO by the **Frank-Starling** mechanism.

### Sympathetic Stimulation of Heart

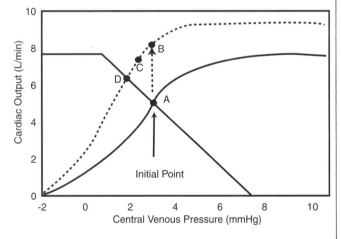

Increased contractility by cardiac sympathetic nerve stimulation shifts the CFC upward *(dashed line)*; however, this does not change the VFC. The initial large increase in CO *(point B)* returns to **point D** on the VFC as blood is transferred from the venous system to the arterial system.

### Changes in CO After Heart Failure

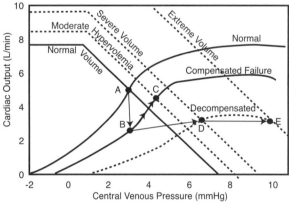

Reduced contractility shifts CO down **(point B)**, but preload immediately increases to intersect with the normal volume curve as shown. Within hours to days, blood volume increases, shifting VFC upward, and **point C** becomes the equilibrium point. With progressive failure, blood volume cannot increase enough to maintain CO at a normal level. **(point D)**. Blood volume continues to increase, which overstretches the heart **(point E)**.

ORGAN SYSTEMS

CARDIOVASCULAR

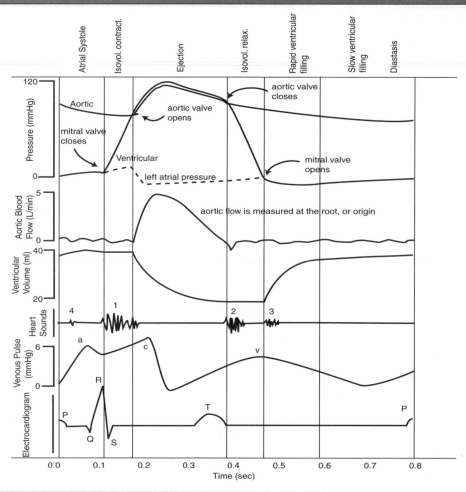

| Left ventricular pressure | **Systole:** begins at isovolumic contraction, ends at beginning of isovolumic relaxation: two phases are isovolumic contraction and ventricular ejection | **Diastole:** begins at beginning of isovolumic relaxation and ends at onset of isovolumic contraction: two phases are isovolumic relaxation and ventricular filling |
|---|---|---|
| Aortic pressure | Maximum is systolic pressure. During ejection, aortic pressure is slightly below ventricular pressure. | Minimum is diastolic pressure. Pressure falls during diastole as blood flows from aorta into capillaries and then veins. |
| Left atrial pressure | Systole; isolated from ventricular pressure because mitral valve is closed | Diastole, blood flows from atrium into ventricle because mitral valve is open. Note mitral closed during isovolumic relaxation. |
| Aortic flow (measured at root) | Systolic ejection begins when ventricular pressure exceeds aortic diastolic and aortic valve opens. | Ejection ends when rapidly falling ventricular pressure causes aortic valve to close. |
| Ventricular volume | Maximum at end of diastole; does not change during isovolumic contraction because mitral and aortic valves are closed. | Minimum at end of ejection phase; does not change during isovolumic relaxation (both valves closed). |
| Heart sounds | Systole: $S_1$ caused by sound of mitral closure | $S_2$ caused by sound of aortic valve closure |
| Venous pulse | Rises with atrial systole | Drops as atrium fills |
| EKG | QRS begins before isovolumic contraction | T wave begins during late ejection phase |

## CARDIAC PRESSURE–VOLUME LOOPS (PV LOOPS)

| Phase | Pressure | Volume |
|---|---|---|
| Filling | Slightly ↑ | Large ↑; point C = EDV |
| Isovolumic contraction | Rapid ↑; maximum dp/dt | No change, valves closed |
| Ejection | Continues to rise | ↓ as ejection proceeds |
| Isovolumic relaxation | Rapid ↓ | No change, valves closed |

### Applications

| | |
|---|---|
| **Area within loop = stroke work output** | Increase work by ↑ stroke volume (volume work) or by ↑ LVP (pressure work) |
| **Decreased blood volume (hemorrhage, dehydration, urination)** | Line C–D shift left (↓ preload); ↓ stroke volume ↓ stroke work |
| **Increase in contractility (sympathetics, or β-adrenergic drugs, digitalis)** | Line F–A shifts left (↓ ESV) a major effect; slight ↓ EDV; overall ↑ stroke volume, ↑ stroke work |
| **Decreased contractility, as in heart failure** | Loop shifts to right and systolic pressure is lower: ↑↑ ESV, ↑ EDP, ↓ SV, ↓ stroke work |
| **Volume expansion (normal heart)** | Line C–D shifts right (↑ EDV); ↑ SV; ↑ stroke work |

### Normal PV Curve

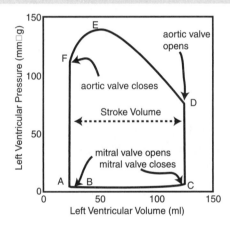

A–B: rapid filling
B–C: reduced or slower filling
C: end diastolic volume (EDV)
C–D: isovolumic contraction

D–F: ejection phase
F: end systolic volume (ESV)
F–A: isovolumic relaxation

- Area within loop = **stroke work**
- Increase work by ↑ stroke volume (volume work) or by ↑ LVP (pressure work)

### Blood Volume Changes

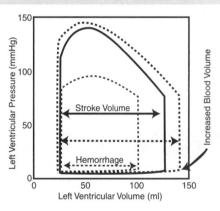

- **Decreased blood volume** (hemorrhage, dehydration): Line C–D shifts **left** (↓ preload); ↓ stroke volume, ↓ stroke work
- **Volume expansion** (normal heart): Line C–D shifts **right** (↑ EDV), ↑ SV, ↑ stroke work

*(Continued)*

| **Increased Afterload** | **Decreased Afterload** | **Progressive Heart Failure** |
|---|---|---|

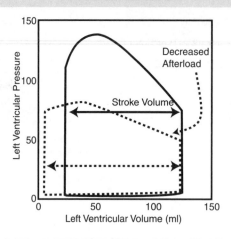

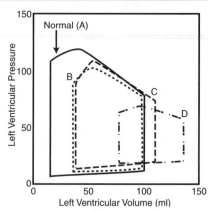

With increased afterload (e.g., ↑ aortic pressure), the velocity of shortening and the distance shortened are both decreased. Thus, ESV increases, causing SV to decrease.

Decreased afterload produces the opposite changes as increased afterload. Thus, ESV decreases and SV increases.

A: Normal

B: Acute loss of contractility without compensation

C: Compensated LV failure (SV partially restored because of moderate increase in preload)

D: Decompensated failure (SV remains low despite ↑↑↑ in preload)

Overall: Curves shift to the right and systolic pressures ↓.

Heart failure: ↑↑↑ ESV, ↑ EDV, ↓ SV, ↓ stroke work

## THE CARDIAC VALVES

| **Mitral** | Between LA and LV | Open during filling | Closed during ventricular systole and isovolumic relaxation |
|---|---|---|---|
| **Aortic** | Between LV and aorta | Open during ejection | Closed during diastole and isovolumic contraction |
| **Tricuspid** | Between RA and RV | Open during filling | Closed during ventricular systole and isovolumic relaxation |
| **Pulmonic** | Between RV and pulmonary artery | Open during ejection | Closed during diastole and isovolumic contraction |

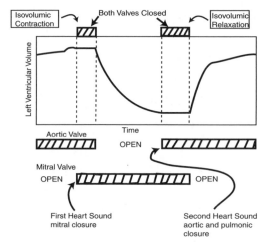

## Aortic Stenosis

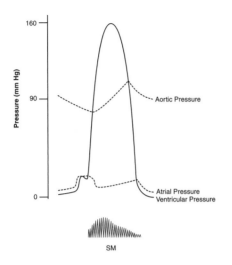

- Discrepancy of systolic LV and systolic aortic pressures
- Causes crescendo-decrescendo systolic murmur

## Aortic Regurgitation

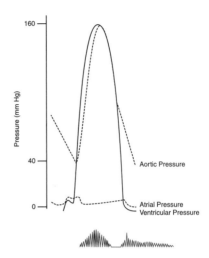

- Diastolic aortic decreases rapidly as blood flows back into ventricle; ventricular diastolic is elevated.
- Causes diastolic murmur

## Mitral Valve Stenosis

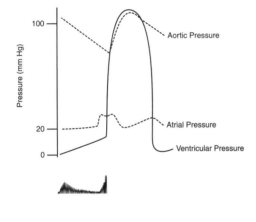

- Discrepancy of diastolic LVP and left atrial P during filling
- Causes diastolic murmur

## Mitral Regurgitation

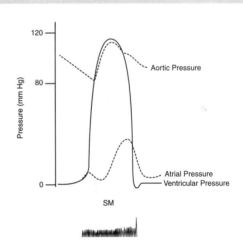

- Incompetent valve allows backflow into left atrium during ventricular systole
- Causes systolic murmur

*Definition of abbreviation:* SM, systolic murmur.

ORGAN SYSTEMS

CARDIOVASCULAR

## HEMODYNAMICS

| | |
|---|---|
| **Poiseuille's equation:**<br><br>$Q = (P_1 - P_2)/R$ | • Flow (Q); $P_1$ (input pressure); $P_2$ (output pressure); R (resistance); $(P_1 - P_2)$ = pressure gradient<br>• $\uparrow$ pressure gradient $\rightarrow$ $\uparrow$ flow<br>• $\uparrow$ resistance $\rightarrow$ $\downarrow$ flow |
| **Series circuits:**<br><br>$R_T = R_1 + R_2 + R_3 .....R_n$ | • $R_T$ = total resistance<br>• Flow is equal at all points in series circuit; pressure drops across each resistor<br>• **Adding more resistors in series increases $R_T$.** Pressure drop increases along circuit with constant flow, and flow decreases with constant input pressure $(P_1)$.<br>• Various types of blood vessels lie in series.<br><br><br>$P_i$ = input pressure   $P_o$ = output pressure |
| **Parallel circuits:**<br><br>$1/R_T = 1/R_1 + 1/R_2 + 1/R_3......1/R_n$ | • Flow divided between parallel resistors<br>• $R_T$ is always lower than the lowest resistor<br>• **Adding more resistors in parallel decreases $R_T$.**<br>• Produces low resistance circuit<br>• Organs lie in parallel<br><br><br>$Q_T = Q_1 + Q_2 + Q_3$<br>$\frac{1}{R_T} = \frac{1}{R_1} + \frac{1}{R_2} + \frac{1}{R_3}$ |
| **Hydraulic Resistance Equation:**<br><br>$R = (P_1 - P_2)/Q = 8\eta l/\pi r^4$ | • $\eta$ = viscosity; l = length; r = radius<br>• **Viscosity $\uparrow$ by $\uparrow$ hematocrit**<br>• **Viscosity $\downarrow$ in anemia**<br>• l is usually constant; r changes greatly for normal regulation and in disease.<br><br>• 2× radius = 1/16 R $\rightarrow$ 16 × flow<br>• ½ radius = 16 × R $\rightarrow$ 1/16 × flow<br>• **Control of radius is the dominant mechanism to control resistance.** |
| **Total peripheral resistance (TPR)** | • Resistance of peripheral circuit: aorta $\rightarrow$ right atrium<br>• **TPR $\uparrow$ by sympathetics, angiotensin II, and other vasoconstrictors**<br>• Highest TPRs in **arterioles**; also main site of blood flow regulation |
| **Total peripheral resistance equation**<br><br>**TPR = (MAP – RAP)/CO** | • Mean arterial pressure (MAP); right atrial pressure (RAP)<br>• Pressure gradient is between aorta and right atrium.<br>• TPR is calculated from MAP and cardiac output (CO). RAP is assumed to be 0 mm Hg, unless specified.<br>• TPR is also known as SVR (systemic vascular resistance) |
| **Compliance (C):**<br><br>$C = \Delta V / \Delta P$<br><br>**Pulse pressure (PP):**<br><br>**PP = SP – DP** | • $\Delta V$ = volume change; $\Delta P$ = pressure change<br>• High **compliance** means vessels easily distended by blood.<br>• **Elasticity** is inverse of compliance; vessels are stiff when elasticity is high<br><br>• SP = systolic pressure; DP = diastolic pressure<br><br>$\downarrow$ compliance (e.g., arteriosclerosis) $\rightarrow$ $\uparrow$ SP and $\downarrow$ DP, so PP $\uparrow$<br><br>• **Compliance:** systemic veins > pulmonary circuit > systemic arteries (volume of blood is in same order)<br><br><br><br>• **MAP = diastolic + 1/3 (pulse pressure)**<br>• MAP = 80 + 1/3(120 – 80) = 80 = 13 = 93 mm Hg |

*(Continued)*

| Cardiac output (Fick method) | $CO = \dot{V}O_2/(Ca - Cv)$ <br><br> $\dot{V}O_2$ = oxygen consumption, Ca = arterial oxygen content, Cv = venous oxygen content | Used to measure cardiac output; most accurate if Ca is pulmonary venous and Cv is pulmonary arterial |
|---|---|---|

## AREA-VELOCITY RELATIONSHIP

- **$V \propto$ 1/cross sectional area**
- **$V \propto 1/r^2$,**
- $V$ = velocity; $r$ = radius

- **Assuming total flow is equal in all vessel types, velocity increases as radius decreases.**

- **The aorta is a single large vessel, but its total area is small compared with numerous capillaries in parallel.**

- If low capillary velocity allows adequate time for diffusion, exchange is **perfusion limited**.

- If velocity is high, metabolic exchange may become **diffusion limited**.

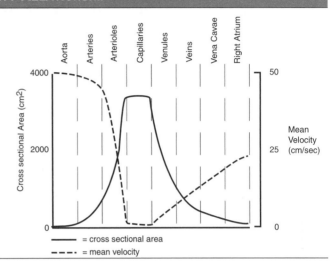

— = cross sectional area
--- = mean velocity

## PRESSURES OF THE CARDIOVASCULAR SYSTEM

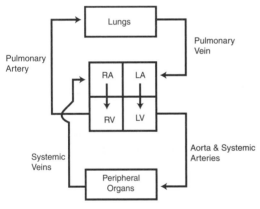

- The cardiac output and stroke volume of the left and right heart are nearly equal.

- The mean pressures are different because the systemic resistance is about 6× higher.

- The pulse pressure in the pulmonary circulation is lower because its compliance is higher.

| Pressures in the Pulmonary Circulation (mm Hg) | |
|---|---|
| Right ventricle | 25/0 |
| Pulmonary artery | 25/8 |
| Mean pulmonary artery | 14 |
| Capillary | 7–9 |
| Pulmonary vein | 5 |
| Left atrium | <5 |
| Pressure gradient | 15 – 5 = 10 |

| Pressures in the Systemic Circulation (mm Hg) | |
|---|---|
| Left ventricle | 120/0 |
| Aorta | 120/80 |
| MAP | 93 |
| Capillary: skeletal <br> Renal glomerular | <30 <br> 45–50 |
| Peripheral veins | <15 |
| Right atrium | 0 |
| Pressure gradient | 93 – 0 = 93 |

ORGAN SYSTEMS

CARDIOVASCULAR

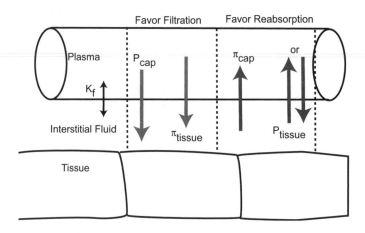

**Filtration = K_f (forces favor – forces opposed)**

$$\text{Filtration} = K_f [(P_{capillary} + \pi_{tissue}) - (P_{tissue} + \pi_{capillary})]$$

| | |
|---|---|
| **Ultrafiltration coefficient ($K_f$)** | • Related to surface area, capillary porosity; different in each tissue/organ<br>• Determines amount of ultrafiltration to given filtration pressure |
| **Capillary hydrostatic pressure ($P_{cap}$)** | • **Favors filtration;** $\uparrow P_{cap} \rightarrow \uparrow$ filtration<br>• Controlled by input pressure, arteriolar diameter, venous pressure |
| **Tissue (interstitial) oncotic pressure ($\pi_{tissue}$)** | • **Favors filtration;** $\uparrow \pi_{tissue} \rightarrow \uparrow$ filtration<br>• Directly related to [protein] in interstitial fluid<br>• **Example:** $\uparrow$ permeability (e.g., sepsis) $\rightarrow \uparrow \pi_{tissue} \rightarrow \uparrow$ filtration |
| **Capillary (plasma) oncotic pressure ($\pi_{cap}$)** | • **Opposes filtration;** $\uparrow \pi_{cap} \rightarrow \downarrow$ filtration<br>• Directly related to [protein] in plasma<br>• **Examples:**<br>  – Liver failure $\downarrow \pi_{cap} \rightarrow$ edema<br>  – Dehydration $\uparrow \pi_{cap} \rightarrow$ reabsorption |
| **Tissue (interstitial) hydrostatic pressure ($P_{tissue}$)** | • Increases filtration when negative (is normally negative in many but not all tissues)<br>• Opposes filtration when positive; edema causes positive pressure in interstitium, even when pressure is normally negative. |

ORGAN SYSTEMS

CARDIOVASCULAR

## FACTORS THAT ALTER CAPILLARY FLOW AND PRESSURE

| | Resistance | Capillary Flow | Capillary Pressure | Example |
|---|---|---|---|---|
| **Arteriole dilation** | ↓ | ↑ | ↑ | β-adrenergic agonist, α-adrenergic blocker, decreased sympathetic nervous system activity, metabolic dilation, ACE inhibitors |
| **Arteriole constriction** | ↑ | ↓ | ↓ | α-adrenergic agonist, β-adrenergic blocker, increased sympathetic nervous system activity, angiotensin II |
| **Venous dilation** | ↓ | ↑ | ↓ | Increased metabolism of tissue |
| **Venous constriction** | ↑ | ↓ | ↑ | Physical compression, increased sympathetic activity |
| **Increased arterial pressure** | N | ↑ | ↑ | Increased cardiac output, volume expansion |
| **Decreased arterial pressure** | N | ↓ | ↓ | Decreased cardiac output, hemorrhage, dehydration |
| **Increased venous pressure** | N | ↓ | ↑ | Congestive heart failure, physical compression |
| **Decreased venous pressure** | N | ↑ | ↓ | Hemorrhage, dehydration |

## WALL TENSION: LAW OF LAPLACE

| $T = P \times r$ | • Tension (T) in wall<br>• **↑ pressure and ↑ radius → ↑ tension** |
|---|---|
| **Applications** | **Arterial aneurysm:**<br>• Weak wall balloons<br>• Vessel radius ↑, causing ↑ wall tension.<br>• ↑ tension causes ↑ radius (vicious cycle), increasing risk of rupture<br><br>**Dilated heart failure:**<br>• ↑ ventricular volume → ↑ ventricular radius, which in turn causes ↑ wall tension.<br>• Thus, dilated ventricle must work harder than normal heart |

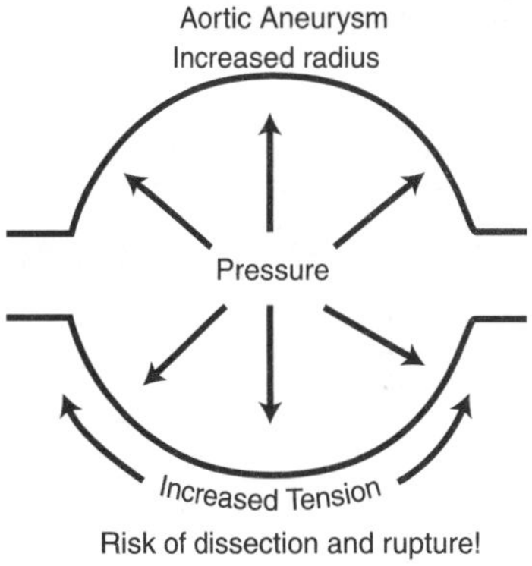

Aortic Aneurysm
Increased radius

Pressure

Increased Tension

Risk of dissection and rupture!

## AUTONOMIC CONTROL OF HEART AND CIRCULATION

| | Sympathetic | Parasympathetic |
|---|---|---|
| **Heart** | | |
| **Transmitter-receptor** | Norepinephrine: $\beta_1$-adrenergic | Acetylcholine: muscarinic |
| **Heart rate** | ↑ rate ($i_f$ and $Ca^{2+}$ currents): $\oplus$ chronotropic | ↓ rate (↑ gK, ↓ $i_f$ ): $\ominus$ chronotropic |
| **Contractility** | ↑ force (dp/dt, EF): $\oplus$ inotropic<br>↑ $gCa^{2+}$, ↑ cAMP, ↑ $Ca^{2+}$ release from SR,<br>↓ duration: fast, strong, short duration | Modest effects: $\ominus$ inotropic<br>↓cAMP; ↓$gCa^{2+}$ mainly at very high levels of activity only |
| **Conduction** | ↑ atrial and ventricular conduction<br>↑ conduction AV node<br>↓ PR interval of EKG | ↓ atrial and ventricular conduction<br>↓ conduction AV node<br>↑ PR interval of EKG |
| **Arteries/arterioles** | Norepinephrine: $\alpha_1$ (mainly) constriction<br><br>Epinephrine (adrenal): $\beta_2$ dilation<br>High levels: $\alpha_1$ constriction | No direct innervation of vascular smooth muscle |
| **Veins** | Norepinephrine: $\alpha_1$ (mainly) constriction but not usually much ↑ resistance, rather, ↓ capacitance shifts blood toward heart | No direct innervation |

## CONTROL OF ORGAN BLOOD FLOW

| Organ/Tissue | Neural | Metabolic/Other |
|---|---|---|
| **Skeletal muscle** | **Resting:** $\alpha$-adrenergic constriction<br>**Exercising:** $\beta$-adrenergic dilation (epinephrine, adrenal medulla) | • **Metabolic vasodilation dominates in exercise**<br>• Compression during static exercise blocks flow |
| **Skin** | • Thermoregulatory center<br>• $\alpha$-adrenergic constriction only | • Heat dilates, cold constricts, a direct effect |
| **Heart** | • $\alpha$-adrenergic constriction<br>• $\beta$-adrenergic dilation<br>• Overridden by metabolism | • **Metabolic dilation is dominant**<br>• ↑ Cardiac work → ↑ $O_2$ consumption →↑ coronary flow<br>• Compression during systole, so most coronary flow is during diastole |
| **Brain** | Not generally under neural control: autoregulation | • **Metabolism dominates:** ↑ $CO_2$ → dilation |

## AUTOREGULATION

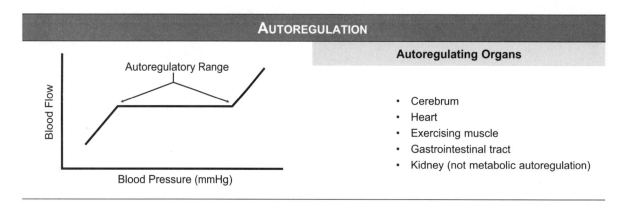

**Autoregulating Organs**

- Cerebrum
- Heart
- Exercising muscle
- Gastrointestinal tract
- Kidney (not metabolic autoregulation)

## BASICS OF INTEGRATED CONTROL OF ARTERIAL PRESSURE AND CARDIAC OUTPUT

| | Control | Major Actions |
|---|---|---|
| **Baroreceptors:** Carotid sinus (primary) Aortic arch (secondary) | ↑ pressure →↑ activity ↓ pressure →↓ activity | ↑ activity → ↑ PNS and ↓ SNS ↓ activity → ↓ PNS and ↑ SNS |
| Sympathetic (SNS) | ↑ pressure → ↓ SNS ↓ pressure → ↑ SNS | • Vasoconstriction (↑ α-adrenergic) → ↑ TPR • ↑ Contractility heart (↑ β-adrenergic) → ↓ ESV → ↑ SV • ↑ Heart rate (β-adrenergic) • ↑ Cardiac output (CO) |
| Parasympathetic (PNS) | ↑ pressure → ↑ PNS ↓ pressure → ↓ PNS | • ↓ heart rate (major); ↓ contractility (minor) • At rest, PNS dominant control of heart rate • ↓ cardiac output |
| Renal | ↑ MAP → ↓ renin, angiotensin II (AII) ↑ MAP →↑ urination →↓ volume →↓ preload | • AII vasoconstricts • **Renal control of blood volume and TPR dominant long-term control of blood pressure and CO** |

## SELECTED APPLICATIONS OF THE DIAGRAM

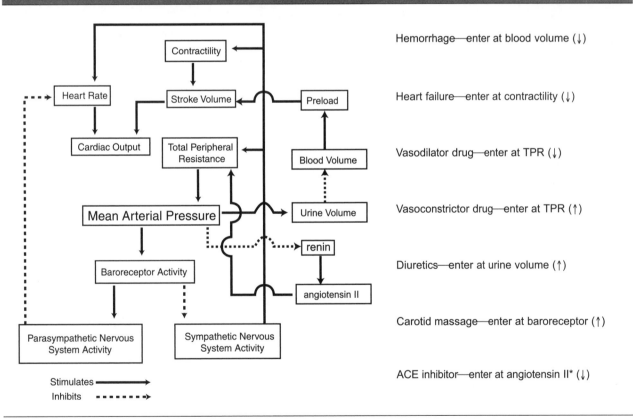

Hemorrhage—enter at blood volume (↓)

Heart failure—enter at contractility (↓)

Vasodilator drug—enter at TPR (↓)

Vasoconstrictor drug—enter at TPR (↑)

Diuretics—enter at urine volume (↑)

Carotid massage—enter at baroreceptor (↑)

ACE inhibitor—enter at angiotensin II* (↓)

Stimulates ———→
Inhibits ┄┄┄┄→

*Note:* also would increase urine flow through reduction of aldosterone (not shown in figure)

# CARDIOVASCULAR PATHOLOGY

## Congenital Abnormalities of the Heart

- Congenital abnormalities occur before the end of week 16 (completion of heart development).
- Clinical significance depends on degree of shunt.
- Up to 90% of congenital heart disease is of unknown etiology.
- **Maternal rubella:** exposure at fifth to tenth week can lead to PDA, ASDs, and VSDs.
- **Fetal alcohol syndrome:** cardiovascular defects, including VSD

### Acyanotic (Late Cyanosis) Congenital Heart Disease (Left-to-Right Shunts)

Initially a left-to-right shunt; causes chronic right heart failure and secondary pulmonary hypertension. Increased pressure causes **reversal of shunt flow** with late onset cyanosis: **Eisenmenger syndrome**

| | |
|---|---|
| Ventricular septal defect (VSD) | • Usually of membranous interventricular septum<br>• Often associated with other defects, including **trisomy 21** |
| Atrial septal defect (ASD) | **Ostium primum defect (5% of ASDs):**<br>• Defect in lower atrial septum above the atrioventricular valves<br>• Associated with anomaly of AV valves<br>• Requires antibiotic prophylaxis for invasive procedures<br><br>**Ostium secundum defects (90% of ASDs):**<br>• Defect is in center of the atrial septum at the foramen ovale<br>• Results from abnormalities of septum primum and/or septum secundum<br>• AV valves normal<br>• Antibiotic prophylaxis not needed |
| Complete endocardial cushion defect | Combination of ASD, VSD, and a common atrioventricular valve |
| Sinus venosus | • Defect in the upper part of the atrial septum<br>• May cause anomalous pulmonary venous return into superior vena cava or right atrium |
| Patent foramen ovale | • Remnant of the foramen ovale, usually not of clinical significance<br>• Risk of paradoxical emboli |
| Patent ductus arteriosus (PDA) | In the fetal circulation, the PDA shunts blood from the pulmonary artery into aorta. At birth, the pressure differential changes, and the flow is reversed (from aorta to pulmonary artery). This leads to pulmonary hypertension due to excess blood flowing through pulmonary artery.<br>**Pharmacology:**<br>• Indomethacin: closes PDA<br>• Prostaglandin E: keeps PDA open |

### Cyanotic Congenital Heart Disease (Right-to-Left Shunts)

- Right-to-left shunt bypasses the lungs and hence produces cyanosis as early as birth.
- Paradoxical embolism (DVT causes systemic infarct) may occur.

| | |
|---|---|
| Tetralogy of Fallot | • **Most common cyanotic congenital heart disease in older children and adults**<br>• Associated with trisomy 21<br>• Four lesions:<br>   *1)* VSD<br>   *2)* An overriding aorta that receives blood from both ventricles<br>   *3)* Right ventricular hypertrophy<br>   *4)* Pulmonic stenosis (right ventricular outflow obstruction) |

*(Continued)*

| Cyanotic Congenital Heart Disease (Right-To-Left Shunts; *Cont'd.*) | |
|---|---|
| Transposition of the great vessels | • Failure of the **truncoconal septum** to spiral<br>• The aorta arises from the right ventricle, and the pulmonary artery arises from the left ventricle, producing two closed loops. This is fatal if a shunt (e.g., PDA, VSD, ASD, patent foramen ovale) is not present to mix the venous and systemic blood. |
| Persistent truncus arteriosus | • Failure of the aorta and pulmonary arteries to separate<br>• Usually a membranous VSD<br>• Truncus arteriosus receives blood from both ventricles, so cyanosis results. |

*Definition of abbreviation:* DVT, deep venous thrombosis.

## OBSTRUCTIVE CONGENITAL HEART DISEASE

Does not usually cause cyanosis

| Coarctation of the aorta | **Preductal (infantile) type:**<br>• Narrowing of the aorta proximal to the opening of the ductus arteriosus<br>• Causes reversal of flow in intercostal arteries, leading to rib notching<br><br>**Postductal (adult) type:**<br>• Narrowing of the aorta distal to the opening of the ductus arteriosus<br>• **Most common type**; allows survival into adulthood<br>• **Disparity in pressure between the upper and lower extremities** |
|---|---|
| Pulmonic valve stenosis or atresia | • Unequal division of the truncus arteriosus so that the pulmonary trunk has no lumen or opening at the level of the pulmonary valve<br>• May cause cyanosis if severe |
| Aortic valve stenosis or atresia | **Complete atresia:** incompatible with life<br>**Bicuspid aortic valves:** asymptomatic, can lead to infective endocarditis, left ventricular overload, and sudden death<br>• Calcify fifth to sixth decade (tricuspid aortic valves usually calcify 10 years later)<br>• Most common cause of aortic stenosis (more than rheumatic fever) |

## Diseases Associated with Congenital Heart Defects

**Marfan syndrome:** 1/3 patients have aortic dilatation and incompetence, aortic dissection, and ASD

**Down syndrome:** 20% of patients may have congenital cardiovascular disease

**Turner syndrome:** Coarctation of the aorta

**22q11 syndromes (DiGeorge syndrome and velocardial facial syndrome):** Truncus arteriosus and tetralogy of Fallot

**Congenital rubella:** Septal defects, patent ductus arteriosus, pulmonary artery stenosis

**Maternal diabetes:** Transposition of great vessels

ORGAN SYSTEMS

CARDIOVASCULAR

# ISCHEMIC HEART DISEASE

- **Leading cause of death**
- Most angina pectoris caused by severe atherosclerotic narrowing of coronary arteries
- Result of decreased supply (anemia, carbon monoxide, pulmonary disease) and/or increased demand (exertion, hypertrophy)
- Sudden cardiac death the presenting symptom in 25% of patients with IHD

| | |
|---|---|
| **Angina pectoris** | • Paroxysmal substernal or precordial chest pain<br>• Transient **myocardial ischemia** without myocardial infarction |
| **Stable angina pectoris** | • Paroxysms are associated with a **fixed** amount of exertion, e.g., after walking three blocks<br>• Typical attacks last less than 10 minutes and are **relieved with rest** or sublingual nitroglycerin<br>• ECG may show **ST segment depression** (ischemia limited to subendocardium) |
| **Prinzmetal angina** | • Vasospasm causes decreased blood flow through atherosclerotic vessels<br>• This form of attack frequently occurs at rest with **ST-segment elevation** on ECG<br>• Treat with calcium channel blockers |
| **Unstable angina** | • Chest pain with progressively less exertion, then occurring at rest, **often precedes myocardial infarction**<br>• May be unresponsive to nitroglycerin |

# MYOCARDIAL INFARCTION

- Ischemic necrosis of myocardium, most commonly transmural, but can be subendocardial
- Highest incidence of fatal MI: 55 to 64 years old
- Risk factors: male sex, hypertension, hypercholesterolemia, cigarette smoking, family history, diabetes mellitus, oral contraceptive use, sedentary lifestyle, type A personality, family history of MI in men under 45, women under 55 years of age

| | |
|---|---|
| **Clinical features** | • Acute, severe, crushing chest pain, often radiating to the jaw or left arm; diaphoresis; little or no chest pain may be present in diabetic and elderly patients<br>• ECG: **ST elevation and T-wave inversion** with or without Q-waves<br>• **Elevated cardiac enzymes** |
| **Prognosis** | • Sudden cardiac death: secondary to a fatal arrhythmia, occurs in 25%<br>• Mortality after myocardial infarction: 35% in the first year, 45% in second year, and 55% in third year<br>• Complications: arrhythmias, CHF, cardiogenic shock, systemic emboli from mural thrombi, aneurysm<br>• Wall/papillary muscle rupture (3–7 days after infarct), postinfarction pericarditis (Dressler syndrome; 2–10 weeks postinfarction) |
| **Treatment and management** | • **Coronary artery bypass:** saphenous vein or internal mammary artery grafts restore circulation; grafts last approximately 10 years before restenosis typically occurs<br>• **Angioplasty** (balloon dilatation) also restores circulation, half re-stenose in 1 year |

ORGAN SYSTEMS

CARDIOVASCULAR

## Appearance of Infarcted Myocardium

| Time | Gross | Histologic |
|------|-------|-----------|
| 1 hour | No gross changes evident | Intracellular edema |
| 6–12 hours | | Wavy myocardial fibers, vacuolar degeneration, contraction band necrosis |
| 12–24 hours | Pale, cyanotic, edematous | |
| 24–48 hours | Well-demarcated, soft, pale | Neutrophilic infiltrate, increased cytoplasmic eosinophilia, and coagulation necrosis become evident |
| 3–10 days | Infarct becomes soft, yellow, surrounded by hyperemic rim | Monocytic infiltrate predominates at 72 hours |
| 2 weeks | Infarct area is surrounded by granulation tissue that is gradually replaced by scar tissue. | |

## Cardiac Enzymes

**Troponin I** peaks first (4 h): remains elevated

**CK-MB** peaks within 24 h: remains elevated

**LDH** peaks later (about 2 days): remains elevated

**AST** also rises and falls predictably in myocardial infarction, but may indicate liver damage instead

*Definition of abbreviations:* AST, aspartate aminotransferase; CK-MB, creatine kinase MB fraction; LDH, lactate dehydrogenase.

## Rheumatic Fever and Rheumatic Heart Disease

| Acute rheumatic fever | • Onset is typically 1–3 weeks after group A β-hemolytic streptococcal pharyngitis, otitis media<br>• Children: 5–15 years old<br>• Declining incidence secondary to penicillin use<br>• Antistreptococcal antibodies cross-react with host connective tissue<br>• Diagnosed using Jones criteria (two major or one major and two minor) | |
|---|---|---|
| **Jones Criteria** | **Major** | **Minor** |
| | • **Migratory polyarthritis**—large joints that become red, swollen, and painful<br>• **Erythema marginatum**—macular skin rash, often in "bathing suit" distribution<br>• **Sydenham chorea**—involuntary, choreiform movements of the extremities<br>• **Subcutaneous nodules**<br>• **Carditis**—may affect the endocardium, myocardium, or pericardium; myocarditis causes most deaths during the acute stage | • Previous rheumatic fever<br>• Fever<br>• Arthralgias<br>• Prolonged PR interval<br>• Elevated ESR<br>• Leukocytosis<br>• Elevated C-reactive protein |
| **Rheumatic heart disease** | • Repeated bouts of endocarditis and inflammatory insult lead to scarring and thickening of the valve leaflets with nodules along lines of closure<br>• **Mitral valve** most commonly (75–80%) affected; fibrosis and deformity lead to "fish mouth" or "buttonhole" stenosis. Next in frequency are the aortic and mitral valves together. Tricuspid and pulmonic valves are rarely affected.<br>• **Aschoff bodies** are pathognomonic lesions; focal collections of perivascular fibrinoid necrosis surrounded by inflammatory cells including large histiocytes (**Anitschkow cells**)<br>• Left atrial dilatation, mural thrombi, and right ventricular hypertrophy<br>• Predisposes to infective endocarditis | |

## CONGESTIVE HEART FAILURE (CHF)

| Types | Etiology | Comments |
|---|---|---|
| **Left-sided heart failure** | • Ischemic heart disease<br>• Aortic stenosis<br>• Aortic insufficiency<br>• Hypertension<br>• Cardiomyopathies | • Increased back pressure produces pulmonary congestion and edema<br>• Dyspnea, orthopnea, paroxysmal nocturnal dyspnea, and cough<br>• Renal hypoperfusion stimulates renin-angiotensin-aldosterone axis<br>• Retention of salt and water compounds the pulmonary edema |
| **Right-sided heart failure** | • Left-sided heart failure<br>• Cor pulmonale<br>• Pulmonary stenosis<br>• Pulmonary insufficiency | • Chronic passive congestion of the liver (**nutmeg liver**), peripheral edema, ascites, jugular venous distension<br>• Renal hypoperfusion with salt and water retention |
| **Cor pulmonale** | • Parenchymal disease (e.g., COPD, causing increased pulmonary vascular resistance)<br>• Vascular disease (e.g., vasculitis, shunts, multiple emboli) | • Cor pulmonale is right ventricular failure, resulting specifically from pulmonary hypertension<br>• May be acute (massive pulmonary embolus) or chronic. |

## SHOCK
### Decreased Effective Circulatory Volume

| | |
|---|---|
| **Causes** | • Decreased cardiac output (myocardial infarction, arrhythmia, tamponade)<br>• Reduction of blood volume (hemorrhage, adrenal insufficiency, fluid loss)<br>• Pooling in periphery: massive vasodilation caused by bacterial toxins and vasoactive substances |
| **Complications** | • Cellular hypoxia, lactic acidosis<br>• Encephalopathy<br>• Myocardial necrosis and infarcts<br>• Pulmonary edema, adult respiratory distress syndrome<br>• Acute tubular necrosis |
| **Stages** | **Compensated:** reflex tachycardia, peripheral vasoconstriction<br>**Decompensated:** ↓ blood pressure, ↑ tachycardia, metabolic acidosis, respiratory distress, and ↓ renal output<br>**Irreversible:** irreversible cellular damage, coma, and death |

## ENDOCARDITIS

### Classic Signs

**Janeway lesions**—erythematous, nontender lesions on palms and soles
**Roth spots**—retinal hemorrhages
**Osler nodes**—erythematous, tender lesions on fingers and toes
(Also see anemia, **splinter hemorrhages**)

| | |
|---|---|
| **Acute** | • Organism—high virulence; *Staphylococcus aureus* (50%) and streptococci (35%)<br>• Affects **previously normal valves**<br>• Often involves the **tricuspid valve in intravenous drug users**<br>• Vegetations may form myocardial abscesses, septic emboli, or destroy the valve, causing insufficiency.<br>• High fever with chills |
| **Subacute bacterial endocarditis** | • Organism—low virulence. ***Streptococcus viridans***, *Staphylococcus epidermidis*, gram-negative bacilli<br>• *Candida* is a rare cause (associated with indwelling vascular catheters)<br>• Affects **previously abnormal valves**<br>• More insidious onset, with positive blood cultures, fatigue, low-grade fever without chills, splinter hemorrhages |
| **Nonbacterial thrombotic (marantic) endocarditis** | • Associated with chronic illness<br>• Mitral valve most commonly affected<br>• Sterile, small vegetations, loosely adhering along lines of closure<br>• May embolize and provide a nidus for infective endocarditis |
| **Nonbacterial verrucous (Libman-Sacks) endocarditis** | • Mitral and tricuspid valvulitis in patients with systemic lupus erythematosus (SLE)<br>• Small, warty vegetations on **both sides** of their valve leaflets<br>• Does not embolize and rarely provides a nidus for infection |

## MYOCARDITIS

• Dilatation and hypertrophy of all four chambers, diffuse, patchy hemorrhage, peripheral edema
• Inflammatory lesions with characteristic cellular infiltrate:
    Neutrophilic—bacterial myocarditis
    Mononuclear—viral myocarditis
    Eosinophilic—Fiedler myocarditis

| | |
|---|---|
| **Noninfectious myocarditis** | Collagen vascular diseases, rheumatic fever, SLE, and drug allergies |
| **Viral myocarditis** | • **Most common form of myocarditis**<br>• **Coxsackie B** (positive-sense RNA viruses, picornavirus family); also, polio, rubella, and influenza<br>• Self-limited, but may be recurrent and lead to cardiomyopathy and death.<br>• 1/3 of AIDS patients show focal myocarditis on autopsy |
| **Bacterial myocarditis** | Diphtheria (toxin-mediated), meningococci |
| **Protozoal** | • ***Trypanosoma cruzi***: Chagas disease; myocardial pseudocysts can lead to CHF<br>• Toxoplasmosis also causes pseudocysts<br>• Myocardial involvement appears days to weeks after the primary infection<br>• May be asymptomatic versus acute onset of dyspnea, tachycardia, weakness, or severe CHF<br>• Most recover fully |

ORGAN SYSTEMS

CARDIOVASCULAR

| VALVULAR HEART DISEASE | |
|---|---|
| Mitral valve prolapse | • Mitral leaflets (usually posterior) project into left atrium during systole, leading to insufficiency<br>• 7% of the United States population, most commonly in **young women**<br>• Seen in most patients with **Marfan syndrome**<br>• Characteristic **midsystolic click** and high-pitched murmur<br>• Usually asymptomatic, but may have associated dyspnea, tachycardia, chest pain<br>• *Complications:* atrial thrombosis, calcification, infective endocarditis, systemic embolization |
| Mitral stenosis | • Stenosis may be combined with mitral valve prolapse<br>• Increased left atrial pressure and enlarged left atrium<br>• Early diastolic **opening snap**<br>• *Complications:* pulmonary edema, left atrial enlargement, chronic atrial fibrillation, atrial thrombosis and systemic emboli |
| Aortic valve insufficiency | • **Acute** (infective endocarditis)<br>• Sudden left ventricular failure, increased left ventricular filling pressure, inadequate stroke volume<br>• **Chronic** (aortic root dilation):<br>  – Volume overload, eccentric hypertrophy<br>  – Wide pulse pressure (**bounding pulse**)<br>  – Etiologies include congenitally bicuspid aortic valve, rheumatic heart disease, or syphilis |
| Aortic valve stenosis | • Rheumatic heart disease, bicuspid aortic valve<br>• Thickening and fibrosis of valve cusps without fusion of valve commissures (fusion present in rheumatic heart disease)<br>• Asymptomatic until late, presents with angina, syncope, and CHF<br>• Systolic ejection click<br>• *Complications:* sudden death, secondary to an arrhythmia or CHF |

| CARDIOMYOPATHIES<br>Diseases Not Related to Ischemic Injury | |
|---|---|
| Dilated (congestive) cardiomyopathy | • Gradual dilatation of all four chambers, producing cardiomegaly, ↓ contractility, stasis, formation of mural thrombi.<br>• Death from progressive CHF, thromboembolism, or arrhythmia<br>• *Etiologies:* idiopathic, alcohol (reversible), doxorubicin (irreversible), thiamine deficiency, pregnancy, postviral |
| Hypertrophic cardiomyopathy (idiopathic hypertrophic subaortic stenosis) | • Marked **asymmetric hypertrophy** of the ventricular septum, **left ventricular outflow obstruction**<br>• Decreased cardiac output may cause dyspnea, angina, atrial fibrillation, syncope, sudden death<br>• Classic case: **young adult athletes** who die during strenuous activity<br>• *Etiologies:* genetic (50%, autosomal dominant pattern) |
| Restrictive (infiltrative) cardiomyopathy | • Diastolic dysfunction (impaired filling)<br>• Infiltration of extracellular material within myocardium<br>• *Etiologies:* elderly—cardiac amyloidosis (may induce arrhythmias); young (<25 years old)—sarcoidosis associated with systemic sarcoidosis<br>• Secondary cardiomyopathy: metabolic disorders, nutritional deficiencies |

ORGAN SYSTEMS

CARDIOVASCULAR

## PERICARDIAL DISEASE

- Usually secondary; local spread from adjacent mediastinal structures
- Primary pericarditis is usually due to systemic viral infection, uremia, and autoimmune diseases

| | |
|---|---|
| **Fibrinous pericarditis** | - Exudate of fibrin<br>- *Etiologies:* post myocardial infarction, trauma, rheumatic fever, radiation, SLE<br>- Loud pericardial friction rub with chest pain, fever |
| **Serous pericarditis** | - Small exudative effusion with few inflammatory cells<br>- *Etiologies:* nonbacterial, immunologic reaction (rheumatic fever, SLE), uremia, or viral<br>- Usually asymptomatic |
| **Suppurative pericarditis** | - Purulent exudate; leads to constrictive pericarditis and cardiac insufficiency<br>- *Etiologies:* bacterial, fungal, or parasitic infection<br>- May have systemic signs of infection and a soft friction rub |
| **Hemorrhagic pericarditis** | - Exudate of blood with suppurative or fibrinous component<br>- *Etiologies:* tuberculosis or a malignant neoplasm; organization<br>- May lead to constrictive pericarditis |
| **Caseous pericarditis** | - Caseous exudate with fibrocalcific constrictive pericarditis<br>- *Etiologies:* tuberculosis |

## PERICARDIAL EFFUSION

Pericardial effusion is leakage of fluid (transudate or exudate) into the limited pericardial space. It may result in cardiac tamponade. Generally, the rate of filling rather than the absolute volume determines the degree of tamponade.

| | |
|---|---|
| **Serous effusion** | - *Etiology:* hypoproteinemia or CHF<br>- Develops slowly, rarely causing cardiac compromise |
| **Serosanguineous effusion** | - *Etiology:* history of trauma (e.g., cardiopulmonary resuscitation), tumor, or TB<br>- Develops slowly, rarely causing cardiac compromise |
| **Hemopericardium** | - *Etiology:* penetrating trauma, ventricular rupture (after myocardial infarction), or aortic rupture<br>- Develops quickly; **can cause cardiac tamponade** and death |

## CARDIAC NEOPLASMS

| | |
|---|---|
| **Primary tumors** (rare, majority benign) | **Myxoma: most common primary cardiac tumor in adults**<br>- Most occur in the left atrium<br>- May be any size; sessile or pedunculated<br>- Complications include ball-valve obstructions of the mitral valve, embolization of tumor fragments<br><br>**Rhabdomyoma: most common primary cardiac tumor in children** (especially those with **tuberous sclerosis**) |
| **Metastases** | Lung and lymphoma, involving the pericardium predominantly |

| VASCULITIDES | | | | |
|---|---|---|---|---|
| **Disease** | **Involvement** | **Clinical** | **Comments** | **Treatment** |
| **Buerger disease (thromboangiitis obliterans)** | • Involves **small and medium-sized arteries** and veins in the **extremities**<br>• **Microabscesses** and segmental **thrombosis** lead to vascular insufficiency, ulceration, **gangrene** | Causes severe pain (claudication) and Raynaud phenomenon in affected extremity | • Neutrophilic vasculitis that tends to involve the extremities of young men (usually under 40) who smoke heavily<br>• Common in Israel, India, Japan, and South America | Smoking cessation |
| **Churg-Strauss syndrome (allergic granulomatosis and angiitis)** | Lung, spleen, kidney | Associated with bronchial **asthma**, **granulomas**, and **eosinophilia** | • Variant of polyarteritis nodosa<br>• **P-ANCA** ⊕ | Corticosteroids, occasionally immunosuppressants |
| **Henoch-Schönlein purpura** | • Affects small vessels, most commonly in the skin, joints, and gastrointestinal system | • Typically develops after a URI<br>• "Palpable purpura" skin rash on buttocks and legs<br>• Arthralgias<br>• GI symptoms: abdominal pain, intestinal hemorrhage, melena<br>• Nephritis in cases with IgA nephropathy | • Most common form of childhood systemic vasculitis (peak at age 5)<br>• IgA-mediated leukocytoclastic vasculitis with circulating IgA immune complexes<br>• Linked to HLA-B35 and human parvovirus | • Most patients treated with supportive therapy<br>• Usually self-limited<br>• Cyclophosphamide sometimes used in cases with severe IgA nephropathy |
| **Kawasaki disease (mucocutaneous lymph node syndrome)** | • Segmental necrotizing vasculitis involves large, medium-sized, and small arteries<br>• **Coronary arteries** commonly affected (70%) | • Fever<br>• Conjunctivitis<br>• Erythema and erosions of the oral mucosa<br>• Generalized maculopapular skin rash<br>• Lymphadenopathy<br>• Mortality rate is 1–2% due to rupture of a **coronary aneurysm** or coronary thrombosis | Commonly affects infants and **young children** (age <4) in **Japan**, Hawaii, and U.S. mainland | IV immunoglobulin (IVIG), aspirin, sometimes anticoagulants |
| **Microscopic polyangiitis** | • Involves small vessels in a pattern resembling Wegener granulomatosis, but without granulomas<br>• Resembles polyarteritis nodosa in some vessels<br>• Segmental fibrinoid necrosis of the media may be present<br>• Some vessels show infiltration with fragmented neutrophils = **leukocytoclastic angiitis** | • Fever, malaise, myalgia, weight loss<br>• Skin rash in 50%, including ulcerations and gangrene<br>• Can affect vessels in many organ systems<br>• Roughly ¾ of patients survive 5 years | • 80% are ANCA positive, with 60% P-ANCA positive and 40% C-ANCA positive<br>• Immune complexes are rare<br>• Etiology unclear | Prednisone and cyclophosphamide to induce remission or treat relapse; methotrexate or azathioprine to maintain remission |

*(Continued)*

| Disease | Involvement | Clinical | Comments | Treatment |
|---------|-------------|----------|----------|-----------|
| Polyarteritis nodosa | • Small and medium-sized arteries in skin, joints, peripheral nerves, kidney, heart, and GI tract<br>• Lesions will be at different stages (acute, healing, healed) | • Affects young adults (male > female)<br>• Low-grade fever, weight loss, malaise<br>• Hematuria, renal failure, hypertension<br>• Abdominal pain, diarrhea, GI bleeding<br>• Myalgia and arthralgia | • Hepatitis B antigen (HBsAg) ⊕ in 30% of cases<br>• P-ANCA (anti-myeloperoxidase) found in many cases, but not diagnostic | Corticosteroids and cyclophosphamide (often fatal without treatment) |
| Sturge Weber syndrome | • Congenital vascular disorder affecting capillary-type vessels<br>• Angiomas of the leptomeninges and skin<br>• Cutaneous angiomas (**port-wine stains**) involving the skin of the face in the distribution of ophthalmic and maxillary divisions of trigeminal nerve<br>• Leptomeningeal angiomatosis | • Seizures and other neurologic manifestations due to altered blood flow ("vascular steal") in brain adjacent to leptomeningeal angiomas<br>• Glaucoma, blindness<br>• Mental deficiency may be present<br>• May have hemiparesis contralateral to leptomeningeal angiomatosis | • Thought to be due to a failure of regression of embryonal vessels that normally occurs around the ninth week of gestation<br>• Microscopically, the port-wine stain, which is a type of nevus flammeus, shows dilated and ectatic capillaries | • Laser therapy can ameliorate the port-wine stain<br>• Medical treatment of secondary conditions such as seizures, glaucoma, and headaches<br>• Some patients require surgery for intractable seizures or other major neurologic problems |
| Takayasu arteritis (pulseless disease) | • Granulomatous vasculitis with massive intimal fibrosis that tends to involve **medium-sized to large arteries**, including the aortic arch and major branches<br>• Produces characteristic narrowing of arterial orifices | • Fever, night sweats, muscle and joint aches, loss of pulse in upper extremities<br>• May lead to visual loss and other neurologic abnormalities | Most common in **Asia, especially in young and middle-aged women** (ages 15–45) | Corticosteroids |
| Temporal arteritis (giant cell arteritis) | • Usually segmental granulomatous involvement of small and medium-sized arteries, esp. the **cranial arteries** (temporal, facial, and ophthalmic arteries)<br>• Multinucleated giant cells and **fragmentation of the internal elastic lamina** seen in affected segments. | • Headache, facial pain, tenderness over arteries, and visual disturbances (**can progress to blindness**)<br>• Fever, malaise, weight loss, muscle aches, anemia<br>• Patient usually middle-aged to elderly female<br>• Elevated ESR | • Most common form of vasculitis<br>• Associated with HLA-DR4<br>• **Polymyalgia rheumatica:** systemic flu-like symptoms; joint involvement also present | Corticosteroids (important to avoid blindness) |
| Wegener granulomatosis | • Necrotizing granulomatous vasculitis that affects small arteries and veins<br>• Classically involves **nose, sinuses, lungs, and kidneys** | • Middle-aged adults, males > females<br>• Bilateral pneumonitis with nodular and cavitary pulmonary infiltrates<br>• Chronic sinusitis<br>• Nasopharyngeal ulcerations<br>• Renal disease (focal necrotizing glomerulonephritis) | Associated with **C-ANCA** (autoantibody against **proteinase 3**) | Corticosteroids, immunosuppressants |

ORGAN SYSTEMS

CARDIOVASCULAR

# Additional Vascular Diseases

## Arteriolosclerosis

- Refers to small artery and arteriolar changes, leading to luminal narrowing that are most often seen in patients with diabetes, hypertension, and aging
- Hyaline and hyperplastic (onion-skinning) types

## Atherosclerosis

Characterized by lipid deposition and intimal thickening of large and medium-sized arteries. Abdominal aorta more likely involved than the thoracic aorta. Within the abdominal aorta, lesions tend to be more prominent around the ostia. After the abdominal aorta, others commonly affected are the coronary, popliteal, and internal carotid arteries.

*Key process:* intimal thickening and lipid accumulation produces atheromatous plaques

The earliest lesion is the **fatty streak**, which is seen almost universally in children and may represent reversible precursor. The progression of the disease is thought in part due to a response to injury from such agents as hypertension, hyperlipidemia, and tobacco smoke. This leads to inflammatory cell adherence, migration, and proliferation of smooth muscle cells from the media into the intima.

The **mature plaque** has a **fibrous cap**, a cellular zone composed of **smooth muscle cells**, **macrophages**, and lymphocytes and a **central core** composed of necrotic cells, **cholesterol clefts, and lipid-filled foam cells** (macrophages). **Complicated plaques** are seen in advanced disease. These plaques may rupture, form fissures or ulcerate, leading to myocardial infarcts, strokes, and mesenteric artery occlusion. Damage to the cell wall predisposes to aneurysm formation.

| Major Risk Factors | Minor Risk Factors |
|---|---|
| Hyperlipidemia, hypertension, smoking, diabetes | Male sex, obesity, sedentary lifestyle, stress, elevated homocysteine, oral contraceptive use, increasing age, familial/genetic factors |

## Mönckeberg Medial Calcific Sclerosis

**Asymptomatic** medial calcification of medium-sized arteries

## Raynaud Disease

An idiopathic small artery vasospasm that causes **blanching and cyanosis of the fingers and toes**; the term Raynaud phenomenon is used when similar changes are observed secondary to a systemic disease, such as scleroderma or systemic lupus erythematosus.

ORGAN SYSTEMS

CARDIOVASCULAR

# HYPERTENSION

**Most cases (90%) are idiopathic and termed essential hypertension.** The majority of the remainder is secondary to intrinsic renal disease; less commonly, narrowing of the renal artery. Infrequent secondary causes include primary aldosteronism, Cushing disease, and pheochromocytoma.

Renal causes of hypertension can usually be attributed to increased renin release. This converts angiotensinogen to angiotensin I, which is converted to angiotensin II in the lung. Angiotensin II causes arteriolar constriction and stimulates aldosterone secretion and therefore sodium retention, which leads to an increased intravascular volume.

| Classification of Blood Pressure for Adults* | | |
|---|---|---|
| **BP Classification** | **Systolic BP (mm Hg)** | **Diastolic BP (mmHg)** |
| Normal | < 120 | and < 80 |
| Prehypertension | 120-139 | or 80-89 |
| Stage 1 Hypertension | 140-159 | or 90-99 |
| Stage 2 Hypertension | ≥ 160 | or ≥ 100 |

*Guidelines from 7th Report of the Joint National Committee on Prevention, Detection, Evaluation, and Treatment of High Blood Pressure (JNC 7)

# ANEURYSM

- A congenital or acquired weakness of the vessel wall media, resulting in a localized dilation or outpouching
- *Complications:* thrombus formation, compression of adjacent structures, and rupture with risk of sudden death

| Type of Aneurysm | Associations | Anatomic Location | Comments |
|---|---|---|---|
| **Atherosclerotic** | Atherosclerosis, hypertension | Usually involve **abdominal aorta**, often below renal arteries | Half of aortic aneurysms >6 cm in diameter will rupture within 10 years |
| **Syphilitic** | Syphilitic obliterative endarteritis of vasa vasorum | **Ascending aorta** (aortic root) | May dilate the aortic valve ring, causing aortic insufficiency |
| **Marfan syndrome** | Lack of **fibrillin** leads to poor elastin function | Ascending aorta (aortic root) | May dilate the aortic valve ring, causing aortic insufficiency |
| **Dissecting aneurysm (aortic dissection)** | **Hypertension, cystic medial necrosis** (e.g., Marfan syndrome) | Blood enters intimal tear in aortic wall and spreads through media | Presents with severe tearing pain |
| **Berry aneurysm** | Congenital; some associated with **adult polycystic kidney disease** | Classic location: **Circle of Willis** | Rupture leads to **subarachnoid hemorrhage** |

# VENOUS DISEASE

| **Deep vein thrombosis** | Involves deep leg veins | Major complication: **pulmonary embolus** |
|---|---|---|
| **Varicose veins** | Dilated, tortuous veins caused by increased intraluminal pressure | • Superficial veins of legs<br>• Hemorrhoids<br>• **Esophageal varices** |

## VASCULAR TUMORS

| | |
|---|---|
| **Angiosarcoma** | • Malignant vascular tumor with a high mortality<br>• Occurs most commonly in skin, breast, liver, soft tissues |
| **Glomus tumor** | • Small, painful tumors most often found under fingernails |
| **Hemangioma** | • Common, benign tumors that may involve skin, mucous membranes, or internal organs |
| **Hemangioblastoma** | • Associated with **von Hippel-Lindau disease**<br>• Tends to involve the central nervous system and retina |
| **Kaposi sarcoma** | • Low-grade malignancy of endothelial cells<br>• Viral etiology: **human herpesvirus 8** (HHV8)<br>• Most often seen in AIDS patients in the U.S. |

## EDEMA AND SHOCK

| | |
|---|---|
| **Edema** | • Fluid is maintained with vessels via balance between hydrostatic pressure ("pushing fluid out") and oncotic pressure ("pulling fluid in").<br>• Most causes of edema can be related to either increased hydrostatic pressure or reduced plasma osmotic pressure. Other causes included lymphatic obstruction, sodium retention.<br>• Clinically, may see pitting edema in extremities (dependent) or massive generalized edema (anasarca). |

| Increased Hydrostatic Pressure | Reduced Plasma Osmotic Pressure |
|---|---|
| *Local:* deep vein thrombosis<br>*Generalized:* congestive heart failure | Cirrhosis, nephrotic syndrome, protein losing enteropathy |

| **Shock** | Three major variants: cardiogenic, septic, and hypovolemic | | | |
|---|---|---|---|---|
| **Type** | **Comments** | **Heart Rate** | **Systemic Vascular Resistance** | **Cardiac Output** |
| **Cardiogenic** | Intrinsic pump failure. As the heart fails, stroke volume decreases, with compensatory increases in heart rate and systemic vascular resistance. | ↑ | ↑ | ↓ |
| **Septic** | Endotoxin mediated. Massive peripheral vasodilation with a decrease in systemic vascular resistance. There is peripheral pooling of blood (decreased effective circulatory volume). The heart compensates with an increase in heart rate. | ↑ | ↓ | ↑ |
| **Hypovolemic** | Blood loss. The effective circulatory volume decreases through actual loss. The heart is able to attempt to compensate with an increase in heart rate. | ↑ | ↑ | Unchanged |

# The Respiratory System

## DEVELOPMENT OF THE RESPIRATORY SYSTEM

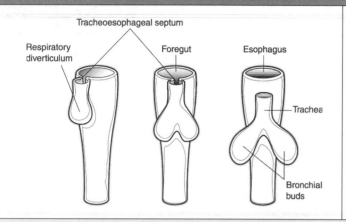

The **respiratory (laryngotracheal) diverticulum** forms in the ventral wall of the foregut. The lung bud forms at the distal end of the diverticulum and divides into two **bronchial buds**. These branch into the **main bronchi**, **lobar bronchi**, and **segmental bronchi**. The right bud divides into three main bronchi, and the left divides into two.

The **tracheoesophageal septum** divides the foregut into the esophagus and trachea.

### Clinical Correlate

A **tracheoesophageal fistula** is an abnormal communication between the trachea and esophagus caused by a malformation of the tracheoesophageal septum. 90% occur between the esophagus and **distal third of the trachea**. It is generally associated with **esophageal atresia** and **polyhydramnios**. Symptoms include gagging and cyanosis after feeding and the reflux of gastric contents into the lungs, causing pneumonitis.

## THE ALVEOLI AND BLOOD-GAS BARRIER

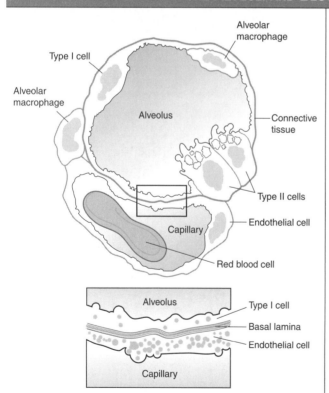

The **conducting zone** of the lungs does not participate in gas exchange and is **anatomic dead space**. It is composed of the trachea, bronchi, bronchioles, and terminal bronchioles. The trachea and bronchi contain pseudostratified ciliated columnar cells and goblet cells (secrete mucous). Bronchioles and terminal bronchioles contain ciliated epithelial cells and Clara cells (which secrete a surfactant-like substance, aid in detoxification, and are stem cells for the ciliated cells).

The **respiratory zone** carries out gas exchange and consists of respiratory bronchioles, alveolar ducts, and alveoli.

**Terminal bronchioles** divide into **respiratory bronchioles**, which contain alveoli and branch to form alveolar ducts. The ducts terminate in alveolar sacs and are lined by squamous alveolar epithelium.

**Alveoli** are thin-walled sacs responsible for gas exchange. They contain:

- **Type I epithelial cells**, which provide a thin surface for gas exchange.
- **Type II epithelial cells**, which produce **surfactant**.
- **Alveolar macrophages**, which are derived from monocytes and remove particles and other irritants via phagocytosis.

There are approximately 300 million alveoli in **each** lung.

ORGAN SYSTEMS

RESPIRATORY

# GROSS ANATOMY

## PHARYNX AND RELATED AREAS

The **pharynx** is a passageway shared by the digestive and respiratory systems. It has lateral, posterior, and medial walls throughout but is open anteriorly in its upper regions (**nasopharynx**, **oropharynx**), communicating with the nasal cavity and the oral cavity.

The **nasopharynx** is the region of the pharynx located directly posterior to the nasal cavity. It communicates with the nasal cavity through the **choanae** (i.e., posterior nasal apertures).

The **oropharynx** is the region of the pharynx located directly posterior to the oral cavity. It communicates with the oral cavity through a space called the **fauces**. The fauces are bounded by two folds, consisting of mucosa and muscle, known as the **anterior and posterior pillars**.

- The **anterior pillar of the fauces**, also known as the **palatoglossal fold**, contains the **palatoglossus muscle**.
- The **posterior pillar of the fauces**, also known as the **palatopharyngeal fold**, contains the **palatopharyngeus muscle**.
- The **tonsillar bed** is the space between the pillars that houses the **palatine tonsil**.

The **laryngopharynx** is the region of the pharynx that surrounds the larynx. It extends from the tip of the epiglottis to the cricoid cartilage. Its lateral extensions are known as the **piriform recesses**.

## THE LARYNX

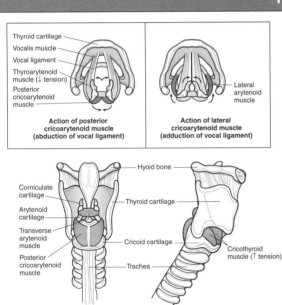

Action of posterior cricoarytenoid muscle (abduction of vocal ligament)

Action of lateral cricoarytenoid muscle (adduction of vocal ligament)

Posterior          Lateral

The larynx is the **voice box**. It also maintains a patent airway and acts as a sphincter during lifting and pushing.

**Skeleton of the larynx:**

- Three unpaired laryngeal cartilages (i.e., thyroid, cricoid, epiglottis) and three paired cartilages (i.e., arytenoid, cuneiform, corniculate)
- The fibroelastic membranes include the thyrohyoid membrane and the cricothyroid membrane (conus elasticus).The free, upper border of the latter is specialized to form the vocal ligament on either side.

## INTRINSIC MUSCLES OF THE LARYNX*

| Muscle | Function |
|--------|----------|
| Posterior cricoarytenoid | Abducts vocal fold |
| Lateral cricoarytenoid | Adducts vocal fold |
| Cricothyroid | Tenses vocal fold |
| Thyroarytenoid (including vocalis) | Relaxes vocal fold |
| Thyroepiglotticus | Opens laryngeal inlet |
| Aryepiglotticus | Closes laryngeal inlet |
| Oblique and transverse arytenoids | Close laryngeal inlet |

*Note that the cricothyroid is innervated by the external laryngeal nerve, a branch of the superior laryngeal branch of the vagus nerve. All other intrinsic laryngeal muscles are supplied by the recurrent laryngeal branch of the vagus nerve.

ORGAN SYSTEMS

RESPIRATORY

**Parietal pleura** lines the inner surface of the thoracic cavity; **visceral pleura** follows the contours of the lung itself. Inflammation of the central part of the diaphragmatic pleura may produce pain referred to the shoulder (phrenic nerve; C3, C4, and C5).

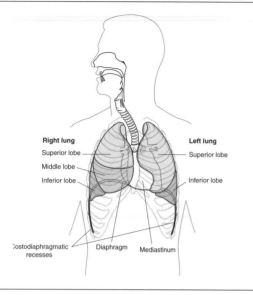

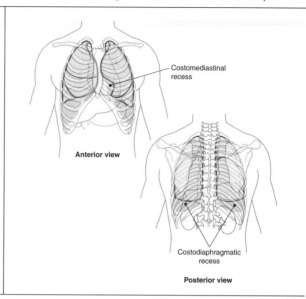

- The **costal line of reflection** is where the costal pleura becomes continuous with the diaphragmatic pleura from Rib 8 in the midclavicular line, to Rib 10 in the midaxillary line, and to Rib 12 lateral to the vertebral column.
- **Costodiaphragmatic recesses** are spaces below the inferior borders of the lungs where costal and diaphragmatic pleurae are in contact.
- The **costomediastinal recess** is a space where the left costal and mediastinal parietal pleurae meet, leaving a space due to the cardiac notch of the left lung. This space is occupied by the lingula of the left lung during inspiration.

## Structure of the Lungs

- The **right lung** is divided by the oblique and horizontal fissures into three lobes: superior, middle, and inferior.
- The **left lung** has only one fissure, the oblique, which divides the lung into upper and lower lobes. The **lingula** of the upper lobe corresponds to the middle lobe of the right lung.
- **Bronchopulmonary segments** of the lung are supplied by the segmental (tertiary) bronchus, artery, and vein. There are 10 on the right and eight on the left.

## Arterial Supply

- **Right and left pulmonary arteries** arise from the pulmonary trunk. The pulmonary arteries deliver deoxygenated blood to the lungs from the right side of the heart.
- **Bronchial arteries** supply the bronchi and nonrespiratory portions of the lung. They are usually branches of the thoracic aorta.

## Venous Drainage

- There are **four pulmonary veins**: superior right and left and inferior right and left.
- Pulmonary veins carry oxygenated blood to the left atrium of the heart.
- The **bronchial veins** drain to the azygos system. They share drainage from the bronchi with the pulmonary veins.

## Lymphatic Drainage

- Superficial drainage is to the bronchopulmonary nodes; from there, drainage is to the tracheobronchial nodes.
- Deep drainage is to the pulmonary nodes; from there, drainage is to the bronchopulmonary nodes.
- Bronchomediastinal lymph trunks drain to the right lymphatic and the thoracic ducts.

## Innervation of Lungs

- Anterior and posterior pulmonary plexuses are formed by vagal (parasympathetic) and sympathetic fibers.
- Parasympathetic stimulation has a bronchoconstrictive effect.
- Sympathetic stimulation has a bronchodilator effect.

## LUNG VOLUMES AND CAPACITIES

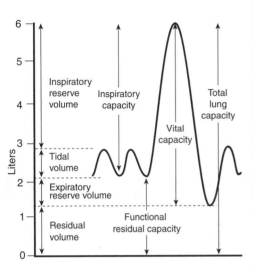

| | | |
|---|---|---|
| $V_T$ | Tidal volume | Air inspired and expired in normal breathing |
| TLC | Total lung capacity | Volume in lungs with maximal inspiration |
| FRC | Functional residual capacity | Volume in lungs at end of quiet, passive expiration; the equilibrium point of the system |
| RV | Residual volume | Volume at end of maximal forced expiration |
| VC | Vital capacity | Volume expired from maximal inspiration to maximal expiration |
| IRV | Inspiratory reserve volume | The volume inspired with a maximal inspiratory effort in excess of the tidal volume |
| ERV | Expiratory reserve volume | The volume expelled with an active expiratory effort after passive expiration |
| IC | Inspiratory capacity | The volume of air inspired with a maximal inspiratory effort after passive expiration |

*Note:* **FRC** and **RV** cannot be measured with a spirometer. Spirometry can only measure changes in volume.

## DEAD SPACE AND VENTILATION

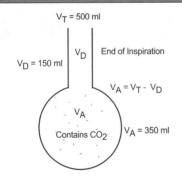

$V_T = 500$ ml

$V_D = 150$ ml

$V_D$ End of Inspiration

$V_A = V_T - V_D$

$V_A$

Contains $CO_2$

$V_A = 350$ ml

$V_D$ = dead space (no gas exchange)

**Anatomic $V_D$** = conducting airways

**Alveolar $V_D$** = alveoli with poor blood flow (ventilated but not perfused)

**Physiologic $V_D$** = anatomic + alveolar dead space

**Standard Symbols**

A = alveolar

a = arterial

V = volume

$\dot{V}$ = minute ventilation

P = pressure

$P_{ACO_2}$ = alveolar pressure of $CO_2$

$P_{aCO_2}$ = arterial pressure of $CO_2$

$P_{ECO_2}$ = $P_{CO_2}$ in expired air

| Abbreviation | Name | Definition | Normal Values |
|---|---|---|---|
| $V_D$ | Dead space | Volume that does not exchange gas with blood | 150 mL |
| $V_A$ | Alveolar volume | Portion of tidal volume that reaches alveoli during inspiration | 350 mL |
| $V_T$ | Tidal volume: $V_T = V_A + V_D$ | Amount of gas inhaled and exhaled during normal breathing – the sum of dead space volume and alveolar volume | 500 mL |
| n | Respiratory frequency | Breaths/minute | 15/min |
| $\dot{V}_E$ | Total ventilation: $V_{Tn} = V_{An} + V_{Dn}$ $\dot{V}_E = \dot{V}_A + \dot{V}_D$ | Total ventilation per minute $V_{Tn} = (350$ mL $\times 15$/min$) + (150$ mL $\times 15$/min$) = 7,500$ mL/min $\dot{V}_E = 5,250$ mL/min $+ 2,250$ mL/min $= 7,500$ mL/min | 7,500 mL/min |

*(Continued)*

ORGAN SYSTEMS

RESPIRATORY

| DEAD SPACE AND VENTILATION *(CONT'D.)* | | | |
|---|---|---|---|
| $\dot{V}_A$ | Alveolar ventilation $\dot{V}_A = (V_T - V_D) \times n$ | Amount of inspired air that reaches the alveoli each minute. It is the effective part of ventilation. | 5,250 mL/min |
| | $\dot{V}_A = \dfrac{\dot{V}_{CO_2}}{P_{CO_2}} \times K$ | The adequacy of alveolar ventilation can be determined from the concentration of expired carbon dioxide.<br>• $\dot{V}_{CO_2}$ = $CO_2$ production (generally assume is normal and constant)<br>• ↑ **alveolar ventilation** → ↓ $Pa_{CO_2}$<br>• ↓ **alveolar ventilation** → ↑ $Pa_{CO_2}$ | |

| Physiologic Dead Space | |
|---|---|
| $\dfrac{V_D}{V_T} = \dfrac{P_{a_{CO_2}} - P_{E_{CO_2}}}{P_{a_{CO_2}}}$ | All expired $CO_2$ comes from alveolar gas, not from dead space gas. Therefore, the fraction shows the dilution of $CO_2$ by the dead space. In the normal individual, anatomic dead space = physiologic dead space, and $V_D/V_T$ = 0.2–0.35. In lung disease, this number can increase. |

# MECHANICS OF BREATHING

## MUSCLES OF BREATHING

| Muscles of inspiration | • **Diaphragm—most important**<br>• Other muscles of inspiration are used primarily during exercise or in diseases that increase airway resistance (e.g., asthma):<br>  – **External intercostal muscles** (move ribs upward and outward)<br>  – **Accessory muscles** (elevate first two ribs and sternum) |
|---|---|
| Muscles of expiration | • Expiration is **passive** during quiet breathing.<br>• Muscles of expiration are used during exercise or increased airway resistance (e.g., asthma):<br>  – **Abdominal muscles** (help push diaphragm up during exercise or increased airway resistance)<br>  – **Internal intercostal muscles** (pull ribs downward and inward) |

## ELASTIC PROPERTIES OF THE LUNG

### Pressure-Volume Curve

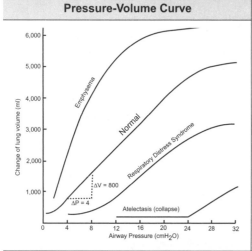

• **Compliance (ΔV/ΔP)** is used to estimate the distensibility of the lungs. It is inversely related to **elasticity** (tendency of a material to recoil when stretched).
• The steeper the slope, the higher the compliance. The flatter the slope, the lower the compliance (stiffer).
• Normal curve: Compliance = $\Delta V/\Delta P$ = 800 mL/4 cm $H_2O$ = 200 mL/cm $H_2O$
• Atelectasis requires an extreme effort to open collapsed alveoli.
• Compliance of lungs also ↑ with age.

| Clinical Correlation: Changes in Lung Compliance | | |
|---|---|---|
| ↑ **Compliance** | **Emphysema** | • Less elastic recoil of lungs, so FRC ↑<br>• Chest wall expands and becomes **barrel-shaped**<br>• Also, ↑ RV, ↑ TLC, ↓ FVC, ↑ $R_{aw}$ |
| ↓ **Compliance*** | **Fibrosis, respiratory distress syndrome** | • Tendency of lungs to collapse ↑, so FRC ↓<br>• Also, ↓↓ TLC, ↓ RV, ↓↓ FVC |

*Definition of abbreviation:* $R_{aw}$, airway resistance.
***Restrictive lung disease:** a condition that reduces the ability to inflate the lungs (e.g., ↓ compliance).

# ELASTIC PROPERTIES OF THE LUNG AND CHEST WALL

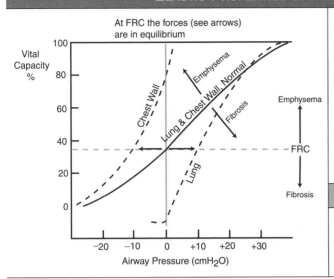

At FRC the forces (see arrows) are in equilibrium

Vital Capacity %

Airway Pressure (cmH₂O)

The figure to the left shows the pressure–volume relationships of the lung, the chest wall, and the lung and chest wall together.

- At FRC, the system is at equilibrium and the airway pressure = 0 cm $H_2O$. At FRC, the elastic recoil of the lungs tends to collapse the lungs. The tendency of the lungs to collapse is balanced exactly by the tendency of the chest wall to spring outward.
- The result of the opposing forces of the lungs and chest wall cause the intrapleural pressure (PIP) to be negative (a vacuum). The PIP is the pressure in the intrapleural space, which lies between the lungs and chest wall.

## Clinical Correlation

If sufficient air is introduced into the intrapleural space, the PIP becomes atmospheric (0 mm Hg), and the lungs and chest wall follow their normal tendencies: the lungs collapse and the chest wall expands. This is a **pneumothorax**.

# SURFACE TENSION

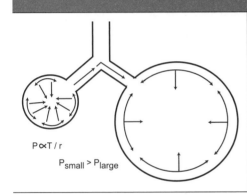

$P \propto T / r$

$P_{small} > P_{large}$

- The attractive forces between adjacent molecules of liquid are stronger than those between liquid and gas, creating a collapsing pressure.

- **Laplace's Law:** $P = \dfrac{2T}{r}$, where  P = collapsing pressure
  T = surface tension
  r = radius of alveoli
- Large alveoli ($\uparrow$r) have low collapsing pressures (easy to keep open).
- Small alveoli ($\downarrow$r) have high collapsing pressures (difficult to keep open).
- **Surfactant** reduces surface tension (T). With $\downarrow$ surfactant (e.g., premature infants), smaller alveoli tend to collapse (**atelectasis**).
- **Surfactant**, produced by **type II alveolar cells**, $\uparrow$ **compliance**.

# AIRWAY RESISTANCE

| Airflow | $Q = \dfrac{\Delta P}{R}$ | where  Q = airflow <br> $\Delta P$ = pressure gradient <br> R = airway resistance |
|---|---|---|
| Airway resistance | $R = \dfrac{8\eta l}{\pi r^4}$ | where  R = resistance <br> $\eta$ = viscosity of inspired gas <br> l = airway length <br> r = airway radius <br><br> **Medium-sized bronchi** are the major sites of airway resistance (not the smaller airways because there are so many of them). |
| Changes in airway resistance | | • **Bronchial smooth muscle:** <br> – Parasympathetic nervous system → bronchoconstriction via $M_3$ muscarinic receptors ($\uparrow$ resistance) <br> – Sympathetic nervous system → bronchodilation via $\beta_2$ receptors ($\downarrow$ resistance) <br> • **Lung volume:** <br> $\uparrow$ lung volume → $\downarrow$ resistance (greater radial traction on airways) <br> $\downarrow$ lung volume → $\uparrow$ resistance <br> • **Viscosity or density of inspired gas:** <br> $\uparrow$ density → $\uparrow$ resistance (deep sea diving) <br> $\downarrow$ density → $\downarrow$ resistance (breathing helium) |

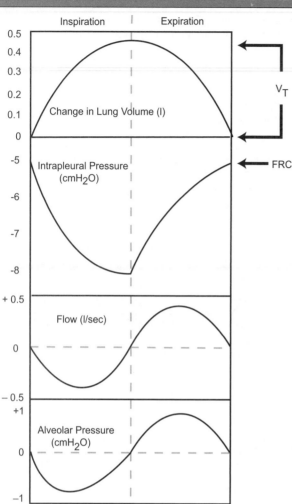

**At rest (FRC):** $P_A = P_{ATM} = 0$ mm Hg

## Inspiration

1. Inspiratory muscles contract.
2. Thoracic volume ↑.
3. $P_{IP}$ becomes more negative.
4. Lungs expand (also causes $P_{IP}$ to be more negative because of ↑ elastic recoil).
5. $P_A$ becomes negative.
6. Air flows in down pressure gradient ($P_{ATM} - P_A$).

## Expiration

1. Muscles relax.
2. Thoracic volume ↓.
3. $P_{IP}$ is less negative.
4. Lungs recoil inward (also causes $P_{IP}$ to be less negative).
5. $P_A$ becomes positive.
6. Air flows out down pressure gradient ($P_A - P_{ATM}$).

## Clinical Correlation

**Obstructive lung disease:** a condition that causes an abnormal increase in $R_{aw}$. **Chronic obstructive pulmonary disease (COPD)** such as emphysema → destruction of elastic tissue → ↑ lung compliance → collapse of airways on expiration (**dynamic compression**). This occurs in normal individuals during a forced expiration but can occur during normal expiration in COPD. COPD patients learn to expire slowly and with pursed lips.

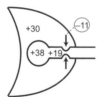

*Definition of abbreviations:* FRC, functional residual capacity; $P_A$, alveolar pressure; $P_{ATM}$, atmospheric pressure.

# PULMONARY DISEASE

| Normal 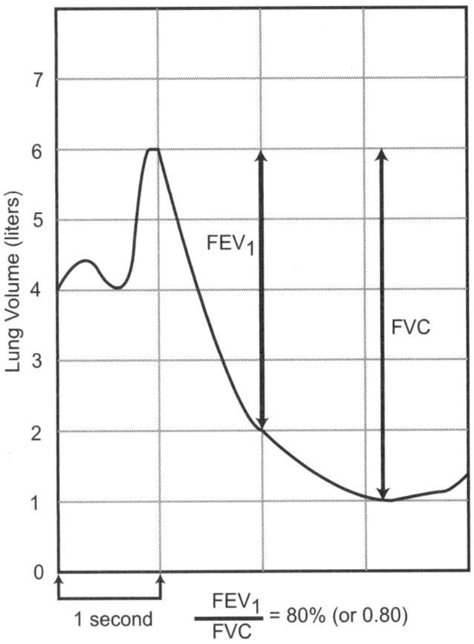 | Obstructive Disease 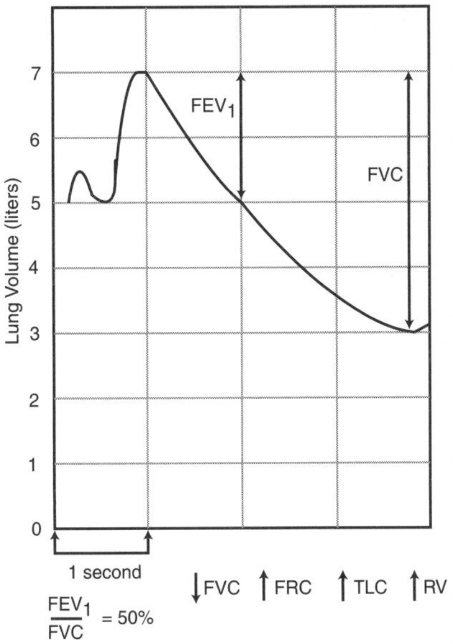 | Restrictive Disease 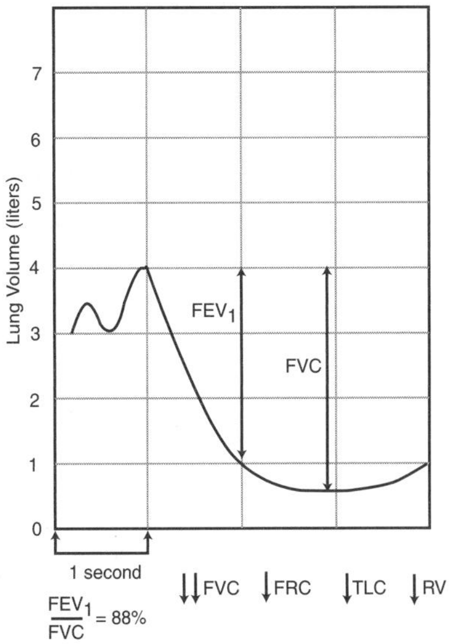 |
|---|---|---|

Normal:
FEV$_1$/FVC = 80% (or 0.80)
1 second

Obstructive:
↓FVC  ↑FRC  ↑TLC  ↑RV
FEV$_1$/FVC = 50%
1 second

Restrictive:
↓↓FVC  ↓FRC  ↓TLC  ↓RV
FEV$_1$/FVC = 88%
1 second

- **Forced vital capacity (FVC)** is the volume of air that can be expired with a maximal effort after a maximal inspiration.
- **Forced expiratory volume 1 (FEV$_1$)** is the volume of gas expired during the first second.

| | TLC | RV | FRC | FVC | FEV$_1$ | FEV$_1$/FVC | Most Diagnostic |
|---|---|---|---|---|---|---|---|
| **Obstructive pattern** | ↑ | ↑↑ | ↑↑ | NC or ↓ | ↓↓ | ↓↓ | ↓ FEV$_1$/FVC with ↑ TLC |
| **Restrictive pattern** | ↓↓ | ↓ | ↓ | ↓↓ | ↓ | NC or ↑ | ↓ FVC with ↓ TLC |

*Definition of abbreviation:* NC, no change.

## SUMMARY OF CLASSIC LUNG DISEASES

| Disease | Pattern | Characteristics |
|---|---|---|
| **Asthma** | Obstructive | R$_{aw}$ is ↑ and expiration is impaired. All measures of expiration are ↓ (FVC, FEV$_1$, FEV$_1$/FVC). Air is trapped →↑ FRC. |
| **COPD** | Obstructive | • Combination of **chronic bronchitis** and **emphysema**<br>• There is ↑ **compliance**, and expiration is impaired. Air is trapped →↑ FRC.<br>  – **"Blue bloaters"** (mainly bronchitis): impaired alveolar ventilation → severe hypoxemia with cyanosis and ↑ Paco$_2$. They are blue and edematous from right heart failure.<br>  – **"Pink puffers"** (mainly emphysema): alveolar ventilation is maintained, so they have normal Paco$_2$ and only mild hypoxemia. They have a reddish complexion and breathe with pursed lips at an ↑ respiratory rate. |
| **Fibrosis** | Restrictive | • There is ↓ **compliance**, and inspiration is impaired.<br>• **All lung volumes are decreased**, but because FEV$_1$ decreases less than FVC, FEV$_1$/FVC may be increased or normal. |

## Partial Pressures of $O_2$ and $CO_2$

**Dalton's Law of Partial Pressures:** Partial pressure $(p_{gas})$ = total pressure $(P_T)$ × fractional gas concentration $(F_{gas})$
**Alveolar gas equation:** $P_{AO_2} = P_{IO_2} - P_{CO_2}/R$
**Alveolar ventilation equation:** $\dot{V}_{CO_2}K/R$; $(K = P_B - P_{H_2O} = 760 - 47 = 713)$

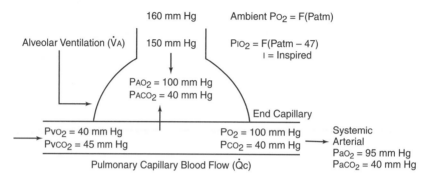

A = alveolar, a = systemic arterial

| | Equation | $O_2$ | $CO_2$ |
|---|---|---|---|
| **Dry inspired air** (any altitude) | $F_{gas}$ | 0.21 | 0 |
| **Dry air at sea level** | $P_{gas} = F_{gas} \times P_B$ | 0.21 (760) = 160 | 0 |
| **Inspired, humidified tracheal air** | $P_{gas} = F_{gas} \times (P_B - P_{H_2O})$ | 0.21 (760 − 47) = **150** | 0 |
| **Alveolar air (PA$_{gas}$)** | $O_2$: $P_{AO_2} = P_{IO_2} - P_{ACO_2}/R$ <br> $CO_2$: $\dot{V}_{CO_2}K/R$ | 150 − 40/0.8 = **100** | (280 mL/min × 713)/5,000 mL/min = **40** |
| **Systemic arterial blood (Pa$_{gas}$)** | — | 100 (completely equilibrates with alveolar $O_2$ if no lung disease) | 40 ($CO_2$ is from pulmonary capillaries and equilibrates with alveolar gas) |
| **Mixed venous blood (P$\bar{v}_{CO_2}$)** | — | 40 ($O_2$ has diffused from arterial blood into tissues) | 45 ($CO_2$ has diffused from tissues to venous blood) |

All pressures are expressed in mm Hg.

*Definition of abbreviations:* K, constant; $P_{ACO_2}$, partial pressure of alveolar carbon dioxide; $P_{AO_2}$, partial pressure of alveolar oxygen; $P_B$, barometric pressure; $P_{H_2O}$, water vapor pressure; $P_{IO_2}$, partial pressure of inspired oxygen; $\dot{V}_{CO_2}$, $CO_2$ production; R, respiratory exchange ratio.

| DIFFUSION | |
|---|---|
| **Fick's Law of Diffusion** | • $V_{gas} \propto D(P_1 - P_2) \times A/T$ <br><br> where $V_{gas}$ = diffusion of gas, D = diffusion coefficient of a specific gas, A = surface area, T = thickness. <br><br> • A and T are physical factors that change mainly in disease. <br> • D of $CO_2$ >>> $O_2$ |
| **Time course in pulmonary capillary** | 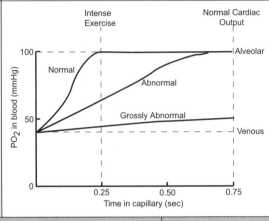 <br><br> • A red blood cell remains in capillary for 0.75 seconds (s) <br> • Equilibrium is reached in 0.25 s in normal lung at resting state. <br> • Exercise reduces equilibration time, but there is still enough reserve for full equilibration of oxygen in a healthy individual. |

| Perfusion-Limited Gases | Diffusion-Limited Gases |
|---|---|
| Gases that **equilibrate** between the alveolar gas and pulmonary capillaries are **perfusion-limited**. The amount of gas transferred is **not dependent** on the properties of the blood-gas barrier. <br><br> • $O_2$ (under normal conditions) <br> • $N_2O$ (nitrous oxide) <br> • $CO_2$ | Gases that **do not equilibrate** between the alveolar gas and the pulmonary capillaries are **diffusion-limited**. The amount of gas transferred **is dependent** on the properties of the blood-gas barrier. <br><br> • **$O_2$:** <br>  – Blood-gas barrier is thickened in **fibrosis**. <br>  – Surface area is ↓ in **emphysema**. <br>  – **Intense exercise** ↓ time for equilibration in pulmonary capillaries (can occur in normal lungs). <br>  – **Low $O_2$ gas mixture** (less partial pressure gradient, can occur in normal lungs) <br> • **CO:** Binds so avidly to Hb, Paco does not ↑ much. Used to measure the **pulmonary diffusing capacity**. |

ORGAN SYSTEMS

RESPIRATORY

## OXYGEN TRANSPORT AND THE HEMOGLOBIN–O$_2$ DISSOCIATION CURVE

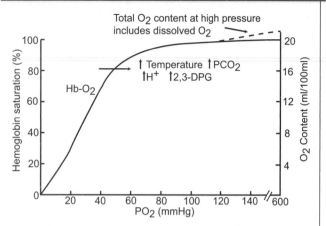

- Each hemoglobin (Hb) molecule has four subunits.
- Each subunit has a heme moiety with an iron in the ferrous state ($Fe^{2+}$), and two $\alpha$ and two $\beta$ polypeptide chains.
- **O$_2$ capacity:** maximal amount of O$_2$ that can bind to Hb
- **O$_2$ content\*:** Total O$_2$ in blood (bound + dissolved)

$$= (O_2 \text{ capacity} \times \% \text{ saturation}) + \text{dissolved } O_2$$

$$= (1.39 \times \text{Hb} \times \frac{\text{Sat}}{100}) + 0.003 \, P_{O2}$$

- **Content** reflects O$_2$ bound to Hb (the amount of O$_2$ that is dissolved is trivial compared to bound).
- **Partial pressure** reflects dissolved O$_2$.

| Key Pressures | Key Saturation % | Shift to Right ($\uparrow$ P$_{50}$) | Shift to Left ($\downarrow$ P$_{50}$) |
|---|---|---|---|
| Pao$_2$ = 100 mm Hg | Almost 100% saturated | • **Facilitates unloading**<br>• $\uparrow$ temperature, $\uparrow$ Pco$_2$, $\downarrow$ pH, $\uparrow$ 2,3-DPG | • **Facilitates loading**<br>• $\downarrow$ temperature, $\downarrow$ Pco$_2$, $\uparrow$ pH, $\downarrow$ 2,3-DPG |
| P$\bar{v}$o$_2$ = 40 mm Hg | 75% saturated | • Exercising muscle is hot, acidic, and hypercarbic | • CO poisoning |
| P$_{50}$ = 27 mm Hg | 50% saturated | | |

*Definition of abbreviations:* Hb, hemoglobin concentration; Sat, saturation; P$_{50}$, Po$_2$ at 50% saturation.
\*1.39 mL of O$_2$ binds 1 g of Hb (some texts use 1.34 or 1.36).

## ADDITIONAL CHANGES IN THE HEMOGLOBIN–O$_2$ DISSOCIATION CURVE

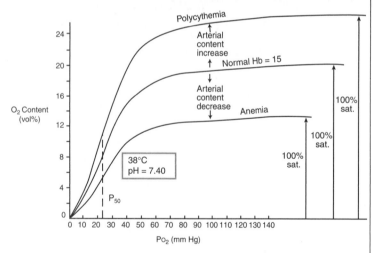

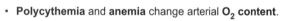

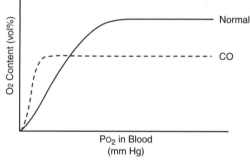

**CO poisoning** is dangerous for three reasons:

1. CO **left-shifts** the curve ($\downarrow$ P$_{50}$), causing $\downarrow$ O$_2$ unloading in tissues.
2. CO has 240 times greater affinity for Hb as O$_2$, thus $\downarrow$ **the O$_2$ content** of blood.
3. CO inhibits cytochrome oxidase

- **Polycythemia** and **anemia** change arterial **O$_2$ content**.
- Pao$_2$ and P$_{50}$ remain the same.

## $CO_2$ Transport

|  | Forms of $CO_2$ |
|---|---|
| | Percentages reflect contribution in arterial blood. <br><br> 1. $HCO_3^-$ = 90% <br><br> 2. Carbamino compounds (combination of $CO_2$ with proteins, especially Hb) = 5% <br><br> 3. Dissolved $CO_2$ = 5% |

## Pulmonary Blood Flow

| | |
|---|---|
| **Resistance (R)** | Very low |
| **Compliance** | Very high |
| **Pressures** | Very low compared with systemic circulation |
| **Effect of $P_{AO_2}$** | • **Alveolar hypoxia → vasoconstriction.** <br> • This is a local effect and the opposite of other organs, where hypoxia → vasodilation. <br> • This directs blood away from hypoxic alveoli to better ventilated areas <br> • This is also why fetal pulmonary vascular resistance is so high. Pulmonary resistance ↓ when the first breath oxygenates the alveoli, causing pulmonary blood flow to rise. |
| **Gravity** | Upright posture: greatest flow in base; lowest in apex |
| **Filter** | Removes small clots from circulation |
| **Vasoactive substances** | Converts angiotensin I → AII; inactivates bradykinin; removes prostaglandin $E_2$ and $F_{2\alpha}$ and leukotrienes |

$\dot{V}/\dot{Q}$: the ratio of alveolar ventilation ($\dot{V}$) to pulmonary blood flow ($\dot{Q}$).

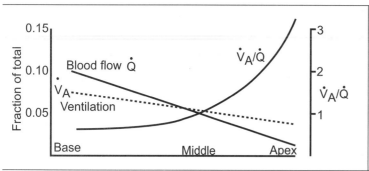

- **Blood flow** is lowest at the apex and highest at the base (gravity effect).
- **Ventilation** is lowest at the apex and highest at the base.
- The change in ventilation is not as great as blood flow, so the $\dot{V}/\dot{Q}$ **ratio** is highest at the apex and lowest at the base.

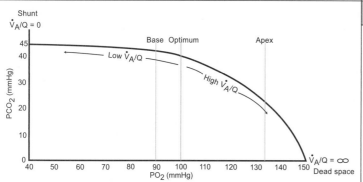

obstruction of ventilation | normal ventilation | obstruction of arterial vessel

## Changes in $\dot{V}/\dot{Q}$

A good way to remember the changes in partial pressures due to alterations in $\dot{V}/\dot{Q}$ is to think of the most extreme cases.

- If ventilation is 0 (airways blocked), $\dot{V}/\dot{Q} = 0$ (a **shunt**). No gas exchange occurs and the $P_{AO_2}$ and $P_{ACO_2}$ are the same as mixed venous blood.
- If perfusion is 0 (embolism), $\dot{V}/\dot{Q} = \infty$ (**dead space**). No gas exchange occurs and $P_{AO_2}$ and $P_{ACO_2}$ are the same as inspired air.

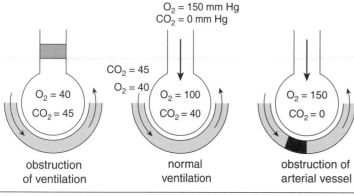

## Summary of Changes

|  | Apex | Base |
|---|---|---|
| $\dot{V}_A$ | ↓↓ | ↑ |
| $\dot{Q}$ | ↓↓↓ | ↑↑ |
| $\dot{V}_A/\dot{Q}$ | ↑↑ | ↓ |
| $P_{O_2}$ | ↑ | ↓ |
| $P_{CO_2}$ | ↓ | ↑ |

## DISORDERS THAT AFFECT ARTERIAL OXYGEN PRESSURE OR CONTENT

| | Notes | $Pa_{O_2}$ | $Pa_{CO_2}$ | $Ca_{O_2}$ | A-a* | Response to Supplemental $O_2$ ☃ |
|---|---|---|---|---|---|---|
| **Hypoventilation[1]** | Drugs (e.g., opiates, barbiturates), head trauma, chest wall dysfunction | ↓ | ↑ | ↓ | NC | ↑ $Pa_{O_2}$; ↑ $Ca_{O_2}$ |
| **↓ inspired $pO_2$** | ↑ altitude | ↓ | ↓[2] | ↓ | NC | ↑ $Pa_{O_2}$; ↑ $Ca_{O_2}$ |
| **Diffusion limitation[3]** | $PA_{O_2}$ and $Pa_{O_2}$ do not fully equilibrate | ↓ | NC[2] | ↓ | ↑ | ↑ $Pa_{O_2}$; ↑ $Ca_{O_2}$ |
| **Shunt[4]** | Venous blood mixes with arterial system, bypassing ventilated areas of lung | ↓ | NC[2] | ↓ | ↑ | Poor |
| **V̇/Q mismatch** | Ventilation and perfusion are mismatched in the lung | ↓ | NC[2] | ↓ | ↑ | ↑ $Pa_{O_2}$; ↑ $Ca_{O_2}$ |
| **CO poisoning** | Exhaust fumes | NC | NC | ↓ | NC | ↑ $Pa_{O_2}$; NC in $Ca_{O_2}$[5] |
| **↓ [Hb]** | Anemia | NC | NC | ↓ | NC | ↑ $Pa_{O_2}$; NC in $Ca_{O_2}$[6] |

*Definition of abbreviation:* NC, no change or minimal response.

*An increase in the A-a gradient indicates a problem with gas exchange.

☃ *Warning:* Supplemental $O_2$ in CNS depression and lung disease can shut off the hypoxic drive to ventilation and cause cessation of spontaneous breathing.

[1]Hypoventilation: ↓ $\dot{V}A$, so ↑ $Pa_{CO_2}$ → ↓ $PA_{O_2}$ → ↓ $Pa_{O_2}$ (As ↑ $CO_2$ diffuses into alveoli from blood, it displaces $O_2$.)

[2]Result of hypoxia-induced increase of ventilation

[3]Diffusion limitation causes disease (blood-gas barrier has less surface area or is thickened), ↓ transit time during intense exercise, exercise at high altitude

[4]Abnormal shunts (often congenital, e.g., Tetralogy of Fallot)

[5]Slow response of $Ca_{O_2}$ due to extremely high affinity of Hb for carbon monoxide

[6]Can only increase dissolved $O_2$ because Hb is saturated at normal $Pa_{O_2}$.

ORGAN SYSTEMS

RESPIRATORY

## Control of Ventilation

### Brainstem Respiratory Centers

| | | |
|---|---|---|
| **Medulla** | Rhythm generator | **Inspiratory center:** generates breathing rhythm<br>**Expiratory center:** not active during normal, passive expiration; involved in active expiration (e.g., exercise) |
| **Pons** | Regulates medulla | **Apneustic center:** stimulates prolonged inspiration<br>**Pneumotaxic center:** terminates inspiration |
| **Cortex** | Conscious and emotional response | Lesions above the pons eliminate voluntary control, but basic breathing pattern remains intact. |

### Chemoreceptors

| | Central (Medulla) Chemoreceptors (Respond to Changes in pH of CSF) | Peripheral Chemoreceptors (Carotid and Aortic Bodies) |
|---|---|---|
| **$O_2$** | No response | • ↓ $PaO_2$ (<60 mm Hg) → stimulates chemoreceptors → increased ventilation.<br>• *Note:* stimulated by changes in pressure, not $O_2$ content; thus, not stimulated by anemia. |
| **$CO_2$** | ↑ $Pco_2$ → stimulate chemoreceptors → ↑ **ventilation (via $H^+$)** | • ↑ $Paco_2$ → stimulation → ↑ ventilation.<br>• Central chemoreceptor response is most important during normal breathing. |
| **$H^+$** | ↑ $H^+$ → stimulation ↑ ventilation detects $H^+$ in CSF; 80–95% of response to hypercapnia | • ↑ $H^+$ → stimulation → ↑ ventilation.<br>• *Note:* Most of the response to metabolic acidosis is peripheral because fixed acids penetrate blood/brain barrier poorly. |

#### Clinical Correlation

Patients with severe lung disease can have chronic $CO_2$ retention, and the pH of their CSF can return to normal despite their hypercapnia. Having lost their $CO_2$ stimulus to ventilate, their hypoxic ventilatory drive becomes very important. If these patients are given enriched $O_2$ to breathe to correct their hypoxemia, their primary ventilatory drive will be removed, which can cause severe depression of ventilation.

*Note:* Other receptors such as pulmonary stretch receptors, irritant receptors, and joint and muscle receptors also have roles in the regulation of ventilation.

## Response to High Altitude

| Parameter | Response |
|---|---|
| $PAO_2$ | ↓ (because $P_B$ is ↓) |
| $PaO_2$ | ↓ (hypoxemia because $PAO_2$ is ↓) |
| Respiratory rate | ↑ (hypoxic stimulation of peripheral chemoreceptors) |
| $Paco_2$ and $PAco_2$ | ↓ (hyperventilation due to hypoxemia) |
| Arterial pH | ↑ (because of respiratory alkalosis); later becomes normal (renal compensation) |
| [Hb] | ↑ (polycythemia) |
| Hb % saturation | ↓ (because ↓ $Po_2$) |
| Pulmonary vascular resistance | ↑ (hypoxic vasoconstriction); this plus polycythemia lead to ↑ work and hypertrophy of right heart |
| [2,3-DPG] | ↑ |
| Hemoglobin-$O_2$ curve | Right-shift (because of ↑ 2,3-DPG) |
| Acute mountain sickness | Hypoxemia and alkalosis cause headache, fatigue, nausea, dizziness, palpitations, and insomnia. Treatment with acetazolamide can be therapeutic. |
| Chronic mountain sickness | Reduced exercise tolerance, fatigue, hypoxemia, polycythemia |

## EAR, NOSE, THROAT, AND UPPER RESPIRATORY SYSTEM INFECTIONS

| Type of Infection | Case Vignette/Key Clues | Common Causative Agents | Pathogenesis | Diagnosis | Treatment |
|---|---|---|---|---|---|
| **Sinusitis** | Sinus pain; low-grade fever | *Streptococcus pneumoniae* | Capsule, IgA protease | Gram ⊕ coccus, catalase ⊖ | Penicillin |
| | | *Haemophilus influenzae* | Capsule, IgA protease, endotoxin | Gram ⊖ rod, chocolate agar | Amoxicillin |
| | | *Moraxella catarrhalis* | β-lactamase producer | Gram ⊖ coccus | Ceftriaxone |
| **Oral cavitary disease** | Sore mouth with thick, white coating that can be scraped off easily to reveal painful red base | *Candida albicans* | Overgrowth of normal flora, immunocompromised, overuse of antibiotics | Gram ⊕ yeast, germ tube test | Nystatin, miconazole |
| **Sore throat** | Inflamed tonsils/pharynx, abscesses; cervical lymphadenopathy, fever, ± stomach upset; ± sandpaper rash | *Streptococcus pyogenes* | Exotoxins A–C (superantigens) | Rapid antigen test; gram ⊕, catalase ⊖ coccus; β-hemolytic, bacitracin sensitive | Penicillin |
| | White papules with red base on posterior palate and pharynx, fever | Coxsackie A | Unknown | Virus culture or PCR | None |
| | Throat looks like *Streptococcus* with severe fatigue, lymphadenopathy, fever, ± rash | Epstein-Barr virus | Infects B lymphocytes by attachment to CD21, causes ↑ CTLs | Heterophile ⊕ (Monospot test); mononucleosis; 70% lymphocytosis (Downey type II cells = CTLs) | Supportive |
| | Low-grade fever with a 1–2 day gradual onset of membranous nasopharyngitis and/or obstructive laryngotracheitis; bull neck from lymphadenopathy; elevated BUN; abnormal ECG; little change in WBC; unvaccinated, dislodged membrane bleeds profusely | *Corynebacterium diphtheriae* | Diphtheria toxin inactivates eEF-2 in heart, nerves, epithelium; pseudomembrane → airway obstruction when dislodged | Gram ⊕ nonmotile rod, Loeffler medium, ELEK test | Penicillin, antitoxin |
| **Common cold** | Rhinitis, sneezing, coughing; seasonal peaks | Rhinoviruses (summer–fall) Coronaviruses (winter–spring) | Virus attaches to ICAM-1 on respiratory epithelium | Clinical | Supportive |
| **Acute otitis media** | Red, bulging tympanic membrane, fever 102–103°F; pain goes away if drum ruptures or if ear tubes are patent | *Streptococcus pneumoniae* | Capsule, IgA protease | Gram ⊕ coccus, catalase ⊖ | Penicillin |
| | | *H. influenzae* (nontypeable) | Capsule, IgA protease, endotoxin | Gram ⊖ rod, chocolate agar | Amoxicillin |
| | | *Moraxella catarrhalis* | β-lactamase producer | Gram ⊖ diplococcus | Ceftriaxone |

*(Continued)*

ORGAN SYSTEMS

RESPIRATORY

## EAR, NOSE, THROAT, AND UPPER RESPIRATORY SYSTEM INFECTIONS (CONT'D.)

| Type of Infection | Case Vignette/Key Clues | Common Causative Agents | Pathogenesis | Diagnosis | Treatment |
|---|---|---|---|---|---|
| **Otitis externa** | Ear pain | *Staphylococcus aureus* | Normal flora enter abrasions | Gram ⊕, catalase ⊕, coagulase ⊕ | β-lactamase-resistant penicillin |
| | | *Candida albicans* | Normal flora enter abrasions | Gram ⊕ yeast, germ tube test | Nystatin, miconazole |
| | | *Proteus* | From water source | Gram ⊖ rod, urease ⊕, oxidase ⊖, swarming motility | Susceptibility testing* |
| | | *Pseudomonas aeruginosa* | From water source | Gram ⊖ rod, oxidase ⊕, blue-green pigments | Susceptibility testing* |
| **Malignant otitis externa** | Severe ear pain in diabetic; life-threatening | *Pseudomonas aeruginosa* | Capsule | Gram ⊖ rod, oxidase ⊕, blue-green pigments, fruity odor | Susceptibility testing* |

*Definition of abbreviations:* CTLs, cytotoxic T lymphocytes.

*Because there is so much drug resistance in these genera, susceptibility testing is necessary.

## MIDDLE RESPIRATORY TRACT INFECTIONS

| Disease | Case Vignette/ Key Clues | Common Causative Agents | Pathogenesis | Diagnosis | Treatment |
|---|---|---|---|---|---|
| Epiglottitis | Inflamed epiglottis; patient often 2–3 years old and **unvaccinated** | *Haemophilus influenzae* | Capsule (polyribitol phosphate) inhibits phagocytosis; IgA protease | Gram ⊖ rod, chocolate agar (requires hemin and NAD) | Ceftriaxone |
| Croup | **Infant** with fever, sharp barking cough, inspiratory stridor, hoarse phonation | Parainfluenza virus (croup) | Viral cytolysis; multinucleated giant cells formed | Detect virus in respiratory washings | Ribavirin |
| Laryngotracheitis, laryngotracheobronchitis | Hoarseness, burning retrosternal pain | Parainfluenza virus | Viral cytolysis; multinucleated giant cells formed | Detect virus in respiratory washings | Ribavirin |
| Bronchitis, bronchiolitis | Wheezy; **infant** or child ≤5 years old | RSV | Fusion protein creates syncytia | Direct immunofluorescence for viral Ags | Ribavirin |
| | >5 years old | *Mycoplasma pneumoniae*, viruses | Release of $O_2$ radicals causes necrosis of epithelium | Slow growth on Eaton medium, cold agglutinins | Symptomatic |

*Definition of abbreviations:* Ag, antigens; NAD, nicotinamide adenine dinucleotide; RSV, respiratory syncytial virus.

**Lobar pneumonia and bronchopneumonia**—acute inflammation and consolidation (solidification) of the lung due to an extracellular bacterial agent. Lobar affects entire lobe (opacification = consolidation on x-ray); bronchopneumonia (patchy consolidation around bronchioles on x-ray). Associated with high fever and productive cough.

**Interstitial (atypical) pneumonia** causes interstitial pneumonitis without consolidation and can be due to viral agents (influenza virus; parainfluenza; RSV, especially in young children; adenovirus; CMV, especially in immunocompromised; varicella), *Mycoplasma pneumoniae, and Pneumocytis jiroveci.*

**Clinical:**
- Fever and chills
- Cough (may be productive)
- Tachypnea
- Pleuritic chest pain
- Decreased breath sounds, rales, and dullness to percussion
- Elevated WBC count with a left shift

| Type of Infection | Case Vignette/ Key Clues | Most Common Causative Agents | Pathogenesis | Diagnosis | Treatment |
|---|---|---|---|---|---|
| **Pneumonia— typical** | Adults (including alcoholics), **rust-colored sputum** Lobar pneumonia or less commonly, bronchopneumonia | *Streptococcus pneumoniae, Haemophilus influenzae* (much less common) | Capsule antiphagocytic IgA protease | Gram ⊕ diplococcus, α hemolytic, catalase ⊖ lysed by bile, inhibited by Optochin | Third-generation cephalosporin, azithromycin |
| | Neutropenic patients, burn patients, CGD, CF | *Pseudomonas aeruginosa* | Opportunist | Gram ⊖ rod, oxidase ⊕, blue-green pigments | Sensitivity testing required |
| | Foul-smelling sputum, aspiration possible | Anaerobes, mixed infection *(Bacteroides, Fusobacterium, Peptococcus)* | Aspiration of vomitus → enzyme damage → anaerobic foci | Culture of sputum | Empiric antibiotic therapy (amoxicillin/ clavulanate, gentamicin) |
| | Alcoholic with aspiration, facultative anaerobic, gram ⊖ bacterium with huge capsule, **currant jelly sputum** | *Klebsiella pneumoniae* | Capsule protects against phagocytosis | Gram ⊖ rod, lactose fermenting, oxidase ⊖ | Susceptibility testing necessary |
| **Pneumonia— atypical** | Poorly nourished, unvaccinated baby/ child; giant cell pneumonia with hemorrhagic rash, Koplik spots | Measles: malnourishment ↑ risk of pneumonia and blindness | Cytolysis in lymph nodes, skin, mucosa Syncytia → giant cell pneumonia | Serology | Supportive |
| | Pneumonia teens/ young adults; bad hacking, dry cough "walking pneumonia" | *Mycoplasma pneumoniae* (most common cause of pneumonia in school-age children) | Adhesin causes adhesion to mucus; oxygen radicals cause necrosis of epithelium | Serology, cold agglutinins | Tetracycline, erythromycin |

*(Continued)*

ORGAN SYSTEMS

RESPIRATORY

| | PNEUMONIA (CONT'D.) | | | | |
|---|---|---|---|---|---|
| **Type of Infection** | **Case Vignette/ Key Clues** | **Most Common Causative Agents** | **Pathogenesis** | **Diagnosis** | **Treatment** |
| **Pneumonia— atypical (cont'd.)** | Air-conditioning exposure, common showers, especially >50 years, heavy smoker, drinker | *Legionella* spp. | Intracellular in macrophages | Direct fluorescent antibody | Erythromycin |
| | Bird exposure ± hepatitis | *Chlamydophilia psittaci* | Obligate intracellular | Direct fluorescent antibody, intracytoplasmic inclusions | Tetracycline, erythromycin |
| | AIDS patients with staccato cough; "ground glass" x-ray; biopsy: honeycomb exudate with silver staining cysts; premature infants | *Pneumocystis jiroveci (carinii)* | Attaches to type I pneumocytes, causes excess replication of type II pneumocytes | Silver-staining cysts in alveolar lavage | Trimethoprim sulfamethoxazole, pentamidine |
| | Primary influenza pneumonia Secondary (bacterial) | Influenza virus | Cytolysis in respiratory tract; cytokines contribute; secondary infections common | Virus culture | Amantadine, rimantadine |
| Acute pneumonia or chronic cough with weight loss, night sweats | Over 55 years, HIV ⊕, or immigrant from developing country | *Mycobacterium tuberculosis* | Facultative intracellular parasite → cell-mediated immunity and DTH | Auramine-rhodamine stain of sputum acid-fast bacilli | Multidrug therapy |
| | Dusty environment with bird or bat fecal contamination (Missouri chicken farmers, Ohio river) | *Histoplasma capsulatum* | Facultative intracellular | Intracellular yeast cells in sputum | Amphotericin B |
| | Desert sand S.W. United States | *Coccidioides immitis* | Acute, chronic lung infection, dissemination | Endospores in spherules in tissues | Amphotericin B |
| | Rotting, contaminated wood, same endemic focus as *Histoplasma* and east coast states | *Blastomyces dermatitidis* | Acute, chronic lung infection, dissemination | Broad-based budding yeast cells in sputum or skin | Ketoconazole |
| Sudden acute respiratory syndromes | Travel to Far East, Toronto, winter, early spring | SARS agent | Replication in cells of upper respiratory tree | Serology, virus, isolation | None |
| | "Four Corners" region (CO, UT, NM, AZ), spring, inhalation rodent urine | Hantavirus (Sin Nombre) | Virus disseminates to CNS, liver, kidneys, endothelium | Serology, virus, isolation | Ribavirin |

*Definition of abbreviations:* CGD, chronic granulomatous disease; CMV, cytomegalovirus; CF, cystic fibrosis; DTH, delayed-type hypersensitivity; RSV, respiratory syncytial virus.

## GRANULOMATOUS DISEASES

### Tuberculosis

Causes **caseating granulomas** containing acid-fast mycobacteria; transmission is by inhalation of aerosolized bacilli; increasing incidence in the U.S., secondary to AIDS

- Primary tuberculosis (initial exposure) can produce a **Ghon complex**, characterized by a subpleural caseous granuloma above or below the lobar fissure, accompanied by hilar lymph node granulomas.
- Secondary tuberculosis (reactivation or reinfection) tends to involve the **lung apex**.
- Progressive pulmonary tuberculosis can take the forms of cavitary tuberculosis, miliary pulmonary tuberculosis, and tuberculous bronchopneumonia. Miliary tuberculosis can also spread to involve other body sites.

**Clinical:** fevers and night sweats, weight loss, cough, hemoptysis, positive skin test (PPD)

### Sarcoidosis

**Sarcoidosis** is a granulomatous disease of unknown etiology; affects females > males, ages 20–60; most common in African American women. **Noncaseating granulomas** occur in any organ of the body; hilar and mediastinal adenopathy are typical.

**Clinical:** Cough, shortness of breath, fatigue, malaise, skin lesions, eye irritation or pain, fever/night sweats

**Labs:** ↑ serum **angiotensin-converting enzyme** (ACE)
**Schaumann bodies:** laminated calcifications
**Asteroid bodies:** stellate giant-cell cytoplasmic inclusions

## OBSTRUCTIVE LUNG DISEASE

Increased resistance to airflow secondary to obstruction of airways

**Chronic obstructive pulmonary disease (COPD)** includes chronic bronchitis, emphysema, asthma, and bronchiectasis.

| Disease | Characteristics | Clinical Findings |
|---------|-----------------|-------------------|
| **Chronic bronchitis** | • Persistent cough and copious **sputum production for at least 3 months** each year in 2 consecutive years<br>• Highly **associated with smoking** (90%) | • Cough, sputum production, dyspnea, frequent infections<br>• Hypoxia, cyanosis, weight gain |
| **Emphysema** | • Associated with destruction of alveolar septa, resulting in enlarged air spaces and a loss of elastic recoil, and producing overinflated, enlarged lungs<br>• Thought to be due to protease/antiprotease imbalance<br>*Gross:*<br>• **Overinflated, enlarged lungs**<br>• Enlarged, grossly visible air spaces<br>• Formation of apical blebs and bullae (centriacinar type) | • Progressive dyspnea<br>• Pursing of lips and **use of accessory muscles** to breathe<br>• **Barrel chest**<br>• Weight loss |
| **Centriacinar (centrilobular) emphysema** | • **Proximal respiratory bronchioles** involved<br>• Most common type (95%)<br>• **Associated with smoking**<br>• Worst in apical segments of upper lobes | |
| **Panacinar (panlobular) emphysema** | • **Entire acinus involved**; distal alveoli spared<br>• Less common<br>• **Alpha-1-antitrypsin deficiency**<br>• *Distribution:* entire lung; worse in bases of lower lobes | |
| **Asthma** | • Due to hyperreactive airways, resulting in episodic **bronchospasm**, producing **wheezing**, severe **dyspnea**, and coughing.<br>• Inflammation, edema, hypertrophy of mucous glands with **goblet cell hyperplasia** and **mucus plugs** are characteristic findings.<br>• Hypertrophy of bronchial wall smooth muscle, thickened basement membranes | |

*(Continued)*

## OBSTRUCTIVE LUNG DISEASE (CONT'D.)

| | |
|---|---|
| Extrinsic asthma | • **Type I hypersensitivit**y reaction<br>• **Allergic (atopic)**—most common type<br>• Childhood and young adults; ⊕ **family history**<br>• Allergens: pollen, dust, food, molds, animal dander, etc.<br>• Occupational exposure: fumes, gases, and chemicals |
| Intrinsic asthma | • Unknown mechanism<br>• **Respiratory infections** (usually viral)<br>• **Stress**<br>• **Exercise**<br>• **Cold** temperatures<br>• Drug induced (**aspirin**) |
| Bronchiectasis | • An abnormal permanent airway dilatation due to **chronic necrotizing infection**<br>• Most patients have underlying lung disease, such as bronchial obstruction, necrotizing pneumonias, **cystic fibrosis**, or **Kartagener syndrome**. |

## DRUGS FOR ASTHMA

| Class | Agents | Mechanism | Comments |
|---|---|---|---|
| **Bronchodilators** | | | |
| $\beta_2$ agonists | Albuterol<br>Terbutaline<br>Metaproterenol<br>Salmeterol<br>Formoterol | Stimulate $\beta_2$ receptors → ↑ cAMP → smooth muscle relaxation | • Generally have the advantage of **minimal cardiac side effects**<br>• Most often used as **inhalants**<br>• Salmeterol and formoterol are **long-acting** agents, so are useful for prophylaxis<br>• Cause skeletal muscle **tremors**; some **CV** side effects (tachycardia, arrhythmias) can still occur |
| Non-selective β agonists | Epinephrine ($\alpha_1,\alpha_2,\beta_1,\beta_2$)<br>Isoproterenol ($\beta_1, \beta_2$) | Stimulate $\beta_2$ receptors → ↑ cAMP → smooth muscle relaxation | • Not used as much as the $\beta_2$ agonists<br>• Epinephrine is used for **acute** asthma attacks and for **anaphylaxis** |
| Muscarinic antagonists | Ipratropium<br>Tiotropium | Block muscarinic receptors, inhibiting vagally induced bronchoconstriction | • Used as an inhalant; there are minimal systemic side effects<br>• Used in asthma and COPD<br>• $\beta_2$ agonists are generally preferred for acute bronchospasm<br>• These are useful in **COPD** because it decreases bronchial secretions and has fewer CV side effects<br>• Tiotropium is longer-acting |
| Methylxanthines | Theophylline | Inhibit PDE; block adenosine receptors | • Available orally<br>• Major use is for asthma (although $\beta_2$ agonists are first-line) |
| **Leukotriene Antagonists** | | | |
| Leukotriene antagonists | Zafirlukast<br>Montelukast | Block $LTD_4$ (and $LTE_4$) leukotriene receptors | • Orally active; not used for acute asthma episodes<br>• Prevents exercise-, antigen-, and aspirin-induced asthma |
| 5-lipoxygenase inhibitors | Zileuton | Block leukotriene synthesis | |
| **Anti-inflammatory Agents** | | | |
| Corticosteroids | Beclomethasone<br>Prednisone, prednisolone<br>Others | Inhibit phospholipase $A_2$ → ↓ arachidonic acid synthesis | • ↓ inflammation and edema<br>• Used orally and inhaled<br>• IV use in status asthmaticus |
| Release inhibitors | Cromolyn<br>Nedocromil | Inhibit mast cell degranulation | • Can prevent allergy-induced bronchoconstriction<br>• Available as nasal spray, oral, eye drops |

## RESTRICTIVE LUNG DISEASE
### (Decreased Lung Volumes and Capacities)

### Examples

**Chest wall disorders:** obesity, kyphoscoliosis, polio, etc.

**Intrinsic lung disease:**

Adult respiratory distress syndrome (ARDS)

Neonatal respiratory distress syndrome (NRDS)

Pneumoconioses (silicosis, asbestosis, "black lung" disease from coal dust)

Sarcoidosis

Idiopathic pulmonary fibrosis (Hamman-Rich syndrome)

Goodpasture syndrome

Wegener granulomatosis

Eosinophilic granuloma

Collagen-vascular diseases

Hypersensitivity pneumonitis

Drug exposure

## RESPIRATORY DISTRESS SYNDROMES

### Adult Respiratory Distress Syndrome (ARDS)

- Diffuse damage to the alveolar epithelium and capillaries, resulting in progressive respiratory failure unresponsive to oxygen therapy
- **Causes:** shock, sepsis, trauma, gastric aspiration, radiation, oxygen toxicity, drugs, pulmonary infections, and many others
- **Clinical presentation:** dyspnea, tachypnea, hypoxemia, cyanosis, and use of accessory respiratory muscles
  - X-ray: **bilateral lung opacity** ("white out")
  - Gross: heavy, **stiff, noncompliant lungs**
  - Micro:

    Interstitial and intra-alveolar edema

    Interstitial inflammation

    Loss of type I pneumocytes

    **Hyaline membrane formation**
  - Overall mortality 50%

### Neonatal Respiratory Distress Syndrome (NRDS)

Also known as **hyaline membrane disease of newborns**. Causes respiratory distress within hours of birth and is seen in infants with **deficiency of surfactant** secondary to prematurity (gestational age of <28 weeks has a 60% incidence), maternal diabetes, multiple births, or C-section delivery

- Clinical presentation: often normal at birth, but within a few hours develop increasing respiratory effort, tachypnea, nasal flaring, use of accessory muscle of respiration, an expiratory grunt, cyanosis
- X-ray: **"ground-glass"** reticulogranular densities
- Labs: lecithin: sphingomyelin ratio <2
- Micro: atelectasis and **hyaline membrane formation**
- Treatment: surfactant replacement and oxygen
- Complications of oxygen treatment in newborns:
  - **Bronchopulmonary dysplasia**
  - **Retrolental fibroplasia** (retinopathy of prematurity)
- **Prevention:** delay labor and corticosteroids to mature the lung

ORGAN SYSTEMS

RESPIRATORY

**Bronchogenic carcinoma** is the leading cause of cancer deaths among both men and women.

## Major Risk Factors

- **Cigarette smoking**
- Occupational exposures (asbestosis, uranium mining, radiation)
- Air pollution

## Histologic Types

Adenocarcinoma, bronchioloalveolar carcinoma, squamous cell carcinoma, small cell carcinoma, and large cell carcinoma

- Oncogenes
    - **L-*myc*:** small cell carcinomas
    - **K-*ras*:** adenocarcinomas
- Tumor suppressor genes
    - **p53** and the retinoblastoma gene

## Complications

- **Spread to hilar, bronchial, tracheal, or mediastinal nodes** in 50% of cases
- **Superior vena cava syndrome** (obstruction of SVC by tumor)
- Esophageal obstruction
- **Recurrent laryngeal nerve** involvement (hoarseness)
- **Phrenic nerve** damage, causing diaphragmatic paralysis
- Extrathoracic metastasis to adrenal, liver, brain, and bone
- **Pancoast tumor:** compression of cervical sympathetic plexus, leading to ipsilateral **Horner syndrome** (miosis, ptosis, anhidrosis)

| Type of Cancer/ (Percentage of Total) | Association with Smoking; Sex Preference | Location | Pathology |
|---|---|---|---|
| **Adenocarcinoma/35%** **Bronchioloalveolar carcinoma** (5%)—subset of adenocarcinoma | **Less strongly related;** female > male; most common lung cancer in nonsmokers | **Peripheral**, may occur in scars; can have associated pleural involvement | Forms glands and may produce mucin |
| **Squamous cell/30%** | **Strongly related;** male > female | **Central** | • Invasive nests of squamous cells, intercellular bridges (desmosomes); keratin production ("**squamous pearls**")<br>• Hyperparathyroidism secondary to increased secretion of parathyroid related peptide |
| **Small cell (oat cell) carcinoma/20%** | **Strongly related;** male > female | **Central** | • Very aggressive; micro: small round cells<br>• Frequently associated with paraneoplastic syndromes, including production of ACTH (Cushing syndrome), ADH, and parathyroid related peptide |
| **Large cell/10%** | — | — | Large anaplastic cells without evidence of differentiation |
| **Carcinoid/<5%** | — | Bronchial | May produce carcinoid syndrome |

## DISEASES OF THE PLEURA

| Pleural effusion | • Accumulation of **fluid in the pleural cavity**; may be a transudate or exudate |
|---|---|
| | • Chylous fluid in pleural space secondary to obstruction of thoracic duct (usually by tumor) = chylothorax |
| **Pneumothorax** | • **Air in the pleural cavity**, often due to penetrating chest wall injuries |
| | • *Spontaneous pneumothorax:* young adults with rupture of emphysematous blebs |
| | • *Tension pneumothorax:* life-threatening shift of thoracic organs across midline |
| | • Clinical: ↓ breath sounds, hyperresonance, tracheal shift to opposite side |
| **Mesothelioma** | • Highly malignant tumor of pleura (and peritoneum) |
| | • Pleural mesothelioma is associated with **asbestos exposure** in 90% of cases (**bronchogenic carcinoma** also strongly associated with asbestos exposure) |

## PULMONARY VASCULAR DISORDERS

| Pulmonary edema | Fluid accumulation within the lungs that can be due to many causes, including left-sided heart failure, mitral valve stenosis, fluid overload, nephrotic syndrome, liver disease, infections, drugs, shock, and radiation |
|---|---|
| **Pulmonary emboli** | Mostly arise from **deep vein thrombosis** in the leg (also arise from pelvic veins) and may be asymptomatic, cause pulmonary infarction, or cause sudden death; severity related to size of embolus and other comorbid conditions |
| **Pulmonary hypertension** | Pulmonary hypertension is increased artery pressure, usually due to increased vascular resistance or blood flow; can be idiopathic or related to underlying COPD, interstitial disease, pulmonary emboli, mitral stenosis, left heart failure, and congenital heart disease with left-to-right shunt |

ORGAN SYSTEMS

RESPIRATORY

# The Renal and Urinary System

## DEVELOPMENT OF THE KIDNEY AND URETER (MESODERM)

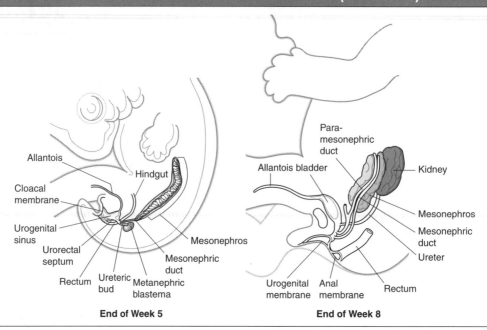

**End of Week 5**  **End of Week 8**

The **ureteric bud** penetrates the **metanephric mass**, which condenses around the diverticulum to form the metanephrogenic blastema. The **bud** dilates to form the **renal pelvis**, which subsequently splits into the cranial and caudal **major calyces**, which form the **minor calyces**. One to 3 million collecting tubules develop from the minor calyces, forming the renal pyramids.

Penetration of collecting tubules into the metanephric mass induces cells of the tissue cap to form nephrons, or excretory units.

- The **proximal nephron forms Bowman capsule**, whereas the **distal nephron connects to a collecting tubule**.
- Lengthening of the excretory tubule gives rise to the **proximal convoluted tubule**, the **loop of Henle**, and the **distal convoluted tubule**.

The kidneys develop in the pelvis but appear to ascend into the abdomen as a result of fetal growth of the lumbar and sacral regions. With their ascent, the ureters elongate, and the kidneys become vascularized by lateral splanchnic arteries, which arise from the abdominal aorta.

## DEVELOPMENT OF THE BLADDER AND URETHRA (ENDODERM)

### Bladder

- The **urorectal septum** divides the cloaca into the **anorectal canal** and the **urogenital sinus** by Week 7. The upper and largest part of the urogenital sinus becomes the **urinary bladder**, which is initially continuous with the **allantois**. As the lumen of the allantois becomes obliterated, a fibrous cord, the **urachus**, connects the apex of the bladder to the umbilicus. In the adult, this structure becomes the **median umbilical ligament**.

- The **mucosa** of the trigone of the bladder is initially formed from mesodermal tissue, which is replaced by **endodermal epithelium**. The smooth muscle of the bladder is derived from splanchnic mesoderm.

### Urethra

- The **male urethra** is anatomically divided into three portions: **prostatic**, **membranous**, and **spongy** (penile). The **prostatic urethra, membranous urethra, and proximal penile urethra** develop from the narrow portion of the **urogenital sinus** below the urinary bladder. The **distal spongy urethra** is derived from the **ectodermal cells** of the glans penis.

- The **female urethra** is derived entirely from the **urogenital sinus** (endoderm).

## CONGENITAL ABNORMALITIES

| | |
|---|---|
| **Renal agenesis** | Failure of one or both kidneys to develop because of early degeneration of the ureteric bud. Unilateral genesis is fairly common; bilateral agenesis is fatal (associated with oligohydramnios, and the fetus may have **Potter sequence**: clubbed feet, pulmonary hypoplasia, and craniofacial anomalies). |
| **Pelvic and horseshoe kidney** | Pelvic kidney is caused by a failure of one kidney to ascend. **Horseshoe kidney** (usually **normal renal function**, predisposition to calculi) is a fusion of both kidneys at their ends and failure of the fused kidney to ascend. |
| **Double ureter** | Caused by the early splitting of the ureteric bud or the development of two separate buds. |
| **Patent urachus** | **Failure of the allantois to be obliterated**. It causes urachal fistulas or sinuses. In male children with congenital valvular obstruction of the prostatic urethra or in older men with enlarged prostates, a patent urachus **may cause drainage of urine through the umbilicus**. |

## GROSS ANATOMY OF THE KIDNEY

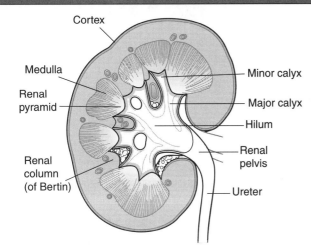

The kidney is divided into three major regions:

### Hilum

Located medially and is the point of entrance and exit for the renal artery and vein, and ureter

### Cortex

Forms the outer zone of the kidney, as well as several renal columns, which penetrate the entire depth of the kidney

### Medulla

Appears as a series of medullary pyramids. The apex of each pyramid directs the urinary stream into a minor calyx, which then travels to the major calyx, through the renal pelvis, and into the ureter

### Relation of the Kidneys to the Posterior Abdominal Wall

### Clinical Correlation

**Blockage by Renal Calculi**

The most common sites of ureteral constriction susceptible to blockage by renal calculi are:

- where the renal pelvis joins the ureter
- where the ureter crosses the pelvic inlet
- where the ureter enters the wall of the urinary bladder

# RENAL PHYSIOLOGY

## BASIC FUNCTIONS OF THE KIDNEYS

| | |
|---|---|
| **Fluid balance** | Maintain normal extracellular (ECF) and intracellular (ICF) fluid volumes |
| **Electrolytes** | Balance excretion with intake to maintain normal plasma concentrations |
| **Wastes** | Excrete metabolic wastes (nitrogenous products, acids, toxins, etc.) |
| **Fuels** | Reabsorb metabolic fuels (glucose, lactate, amino acids, etc.) |
| **Blood pressure** | Regulate ECF volume for the long-term control of blood pressure |
| **Acid–base** | Regulate absorption and excretion of $H^+$ and $HCO_3^-$ to control acid–base balance |

## FLUID BALANCE: ESTIMATION OF FLUID VOLUMES

### Basic Concepts

**Body fluid compartments:** TBW = ICF + ECF      ECF = plasma + ISF      TBW = ICF + (plasma + ISF)

---

**Estimating body fluid volumes:**
(must assume normal hydration)

TBW in Liters = 0.6 × weight in kg
ICF = 0.4 × weight
ECF = 0.2 × weight

---

**Measuring body fluid volumes** (indicator dilution principle):

$V = Q/C$, where V = body fluid volume, Q = quantity of indicator administered, C = concentration of indicator after dilution in body fluid compartment

**Indicators:** must disperse evenly in compartment, must disperse only in compartment of interest, and cannot be metabolized or excreted (no indicator is perfect)

TBW indicators: $D_2O$, $^3H_2O$, antipyrine ($C_{11}H_{12}N_2O$)
ECF indicators: $^{22}Na$, inulin, mannitol
PV indicators: $^{125}I$-albumin, Evans blue dye, $^{51}Cr$-red blood cells

---

**Osmolarity vs. molarity:**    Ionic substances dissociate, covalently bonded substances do not, therefore:
- 100 mM glucose = 100 mOsm/L
- 100 mM NaCl = 200 mOsm/L

---

**Osmolarity of ECF always = osmolarity of ICF:**    Estimate by 2× plasma $[Na^+]$

---

**All water and solutes pass through ECF:**    Evaluate changes in ECF first, then ICF

---

**ICF volume is controlled by ECF osmolarity:**
- ECF volume does not control ICF volume
- Water enters/leaves ICF to keep osmolarity of ICF = ECF

*Definition of abbreviations:* ECF, extracellular fluid; ICF, intracellular fluid; ISF, interstitial fluid; PV, plasma volume; TBW, total body water.

## NORMAL VALUES
### (Body weight = 100 kg, 300 mOsm/L)

| | ECF | ICF | TBW |
|---|---|---|---|
| **Volume (liters)** | 20 | 40 | 60 |
| **Osmolarity (mOsm/L)** | 300 | 300 | 300 |
| **Solute mass in compartment (mOsm)** | 6,000 | 12,000 | 18,000 |

# FLUID AND ELECTROLYTE ABNORMALITIES

## Diarrhea

- Weight loss = 4 kg (assume all weight loss is fluid loss)
- Solutes lost from ECF
- Isoosmotic loss: osmolarity remains at 300 mOsm/L; calculate TBW, ECF, ICF

|  | ECF | ICF | TBW |
|---|---|---|---|
| Volume (liters) | V = 4,800/300 = 16 | ICF = TBW − ECF<br>56 − 16 = 40 | 60 − 4 = 56 |
| Osmolarity (mOsm/L) | 300 | 300 | 300 |
| Solute mass in compartment (mOsm) | 6,000 − (300 × 4) = 4,800 | 12,000 | 56 × 300 = 16,800 |

*Conclusion: Isoosmotic volume gain or loss only changes ECF volume; ICF volume is unchanged.*

## Sweating

- Weight loss = 8 kg (assume all weight loss is fluid loss)
- Solutes lost from ECF
- Loss of hypoosmotic fluid, osmolarity = 330 mOsm/L; calculate TBW, ECF, ICF

|  | ECF | ICF | TBW |
|---|---|---|---|
| Volume (liters) | V = 5,160/330 = 15.6 | ICF = TBW − ECF<br>52 − 15.6 = 36.4 | 60 − 8 = 52 |
| Osmolarity (mOsm/L) | 330 | 330 | 330 |
| Solute mass in compartment (mOsm) | 6,000 − 840 = 5,160 | 12,000 | 52 × 330 = 17,160<br>= loss of 840 from ECF |

*Conclusion: ECF loss of water and solutes, but ↑ osmolarity → ↓ ICF volume due to water shift.*

## Drink 3 L Pure Water

- Weight gain = 3 kg
- No solutes lost or gained
- Gain of hypoosmotic fluid; calculate new osmolarity, TBW, ECF, ICF

|  | ECF | ICF | TBW |
|---|---|---|---|
| Volume (liters) | V = 6,000/285.7 = 21 | V = 12,000/285.7 = 42 | 60 + 3 = 63 |
| Osmolarity (mOsm/L) | 285.7 | 285.7 | 18,000/63 = 285.7 |
| Solute mass in compartment (mOsm) | 21 × 285.7 = 6,000 | 42 × 285.7 = 12,000 | 63 × 285.7 = 18,000 |

*Conclusion: Addition of pure water ↓ osmolarity, causing proportionate increases in ICF and ECF volumes.*

## PROCESSES IN THE FORMATION OF URINE

| | |
|---|---|
| **Filtration** | • Glomerular capillaries—same forces as described in cardiovascular section<br>• Glomerular filtration rate **(GFR)** |
| **Secretion (S)** | Active transport of solutes from plasma (via interstitial fluid) into tubular fluid |
| **Reabsorption (R)** | Passive or active movement of solutes and water from tubular fluid back into capillaries |
| **Excretion of X ($E_x$)** | • Result of the balance of filtration, secretion, and reabsorption<br>• $E_x = \dot{V} \times [X]_{urine}$; $\dot{V}$ = urine flow; $[X]_{urine}$ = urinary concentration of X |
| **Filtered load (F)** | • $F = GFR \times [solute]_{plasma}$<br>• Solute fraction bound to plasma protein does not filter |
| **Mass balance** | $E = F + S - R$ |

## EXAMPLES USING MASS BALANCE TO EVALUATE RENAL PROCESSING OF A SOLUTE

| Data | Calculations | Conclusions |
|---|---|---|
| • GFR = 100 mL/min<br>• $[Subst.]_{plasma}$ = 1 μg/mL<br>• $\dot{V}$ = 2 mL/min<br>• $[Subst.]_{urine}$ = 75 μg/mL | F = 100 × 1 = 100 μg/min<br>E = 2 × 75 = 150 μg/min | Subst. must be secreted because the amount excreted is > the amount filtered. S ≈ 50 μg/min* |
| • GFR = 100 mL/min<br>• $[Subst.]_{plasma}$ = 3 μg/mL<br>• $\dot{V}$ = 1 mL/min<br>• $[Subst.]_{urine}$ = 100 μg/mL | F = 100 × 3 = 300 μg/min<br>E = 1 × 100 = 100 μg/min | Subst. must be reabsorbed because the amount filtered is > the amount excreted. R ≈ 200 μg/min† |
| • GFR = 100 mL/min<br>• $[Subst.]_{plasma}$ = 2 μg/mL<br>• $\dot{V}$ = 4 mL/min<br>• $[Subst.]_{urine}$ = 50 μg/mL | F = 100 × 2 = 200 μg/min<br>E = 4 × 50 = 200 μg/min | Subst. is neither secreted nor reabsorbed because the amount excreted = the amount filtered.¶ |

*Definition of abbreviation:* Subst., substance.

*Assumes no reabsorption

†Assumes no secretion

¶Still possible that S = R, but this is unlikely.

| CLEARANCE AND ITS APPLICATIONS | |
|---|---|
| **Definition** | Volume of plasma from which a substance is removed (cleared) per unit time |
| **Concept** | Relates the excretion of a substance to its concentration in plasma |
| **Calculation** | $C_s = (U_s \times \dot{V})/P_s$          where, $C_s$ = clearance of substance, $U_s$ = urine concentration of substance, $\dot{V}$ = urine flow, $P_s$ = plasma concentration of substance |
| **Application: GFR** | • **Inulin clearance** can be used to calculate **GFR**.<br>• Rationale: inulin is filtered, but is neither secreted nor reabsorbed. Therefore,<br><br>$$\text{Clearance of inulin} = (U_{[inulin]} \times \dot{V})/P_{[inulin]} = \text{GFR}$$<br><br>• **Creatinine clearance** is the best clinical measure of GFR because it is produced continually by the body and is freely filtered but not reabsorbed. Creatinine is partially secreted, but its clearance is still a reasonable clinical estimate of GFR. |
| **Application:**<br><br>**Renal plasma flow (RPF)**<br><br>**Renal blood flow (RBF)** | **Para-aminohippuric acid (PAH)** is filtered and secreted; at low doses it is almost completely cleared from blood flowing through the kidneys during a single pass. Therefore, PAH clearance = RPF. However, PAH clearance is a measure of *plasma* flow rather than *blood* flow. Renal blood flow (RBF) can be calculated as follows:<br><br>**RBF = RPF / (1 − hematocrit)**, using hematocrit as decimal proportion, e.g., 0.40 |
| **Application:**<br><br>**Free water clearance ($C_{H_2O}$)** | • $C_{H_2O}$ is not a true clearance. It is the volume of water that would have to be added to or removed from urine to make the urine isoosmotic to plasma.<br><br>• $C_{H_2O}$ is the difference between water excretion (urine flow) and osmolar clearance. Thus:<br><br>$$C_{H_2O} = \dot{V} - C_{osm} = \dot{V} - (U_{osm} \times \dot{V})/P_{osm}$$<br><br>• **Positive $C_{H_2O}$:** Urine is hypotonic, ADH is low, "free water" has been removed from body, and plasma osmolarity is being increased.<br>• **Negative $C_{H_2O}$:** Urine is hypertonic, ADH is high, water is being conserved, and plasma osmolarity is being decreased. |

*Definition of abbreviation:* ADH, antidiuretic hormone.

ORGAN SYSTEMS

RENAL/URINARY

## STRUCTURE OF THE NEPHRON
### (Approximately 1 million nephrons/kidney)

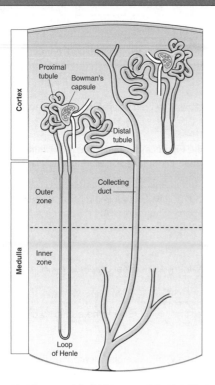

### Sequence of Fluid Flow in a Nephron

| Structure | Basic Function |
|---|---|
| Bowman capsule | Formation of filtrate |
| Proximal tubule (PT) | Reabsorption of $H_2O$, solutes; some secretion |
| Descending thin loop of Henle (DTL) | Reabsorption of $H_2O$, no solute transport |
| Ascending thin loop of Henle (ATL) | Reabsorption of solutes, not water |
| Thick ascending loop of Henle (TAL) | Reabsorption of solutes, not water |
| Early distal tubule (EDT) | Reabsorption of solutes; special sensory region |
| Late distal tubule (LDT); cortical collecting duct (CCD) | Reabsorption of solutes and water; regulation of acid–base status |
| Medullary collecting duct (MCD) | Reabsorption of $H_2O$; final control of urine volume and osmolarity |

## ASSOCIATION OF BLOOD VESSELS WITH THE NEPHRON

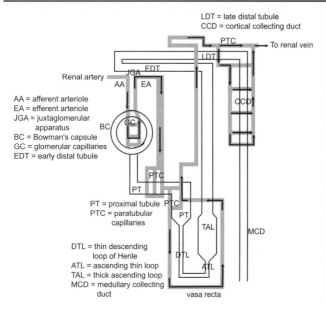

AA = afferent arteriole
EA = efferent arteriole
JGA = juxtaglomerular apparatus
BC = Bowman's capsule
GC = glomerular capillaries
EDT = early distal tubule

PT = proximal tubule
PTC = paratubular capillaries

DTL = thin descending loop of Henle
ATL = ascending thin loop
TAL = thick ascending loop
MCD = medullary collecting duct

LDT = late distal tubule
CCD = cortical collecting duct

Each tubular segment has a blood supply that allows exchange of water and/or solute.

### Sequence of Blood Flow in Nephrons

| Blood Vessel | Tubular Segment |
|---|---|
| Afferent arteriole | No exchange |
| Glomerular capillaries | Bowman capsule |
| Efferent arteriole | No exchange |
| Peritubular capillaries | Sequence: proximal tubule → loop of Henle → distal tubule → collecting duct |
| Vasa recta: specialized portion of peritubular capillaries that perfuse medulla<br>1–2% of blood flow | Loop of Henle, collecting duct |

# THE JUXTAGLOMERULAR APPARATUS (JGA)

The **juxtaglomerular apparatus** includes the site of **filtration** (Bowman capsule [BC] and glomerular capillaries), as well as the arterioles and macula densa tubule cells found at the end of the thick ascending limb. Macula densa cells sense tubular fluid NaCl and contribute to **autoregulation** and regulation of **renin secretion**.

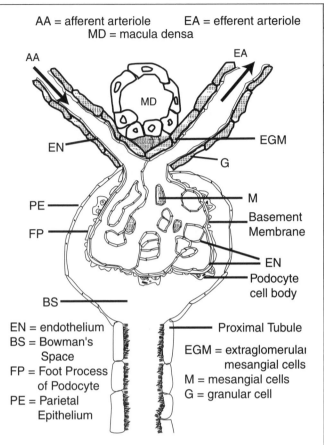

AA = afferent arteriole    EA = efferent arteriole
MD = macula densa

EN = endothelium
BS = Bowman's Space
FP = Foot Process of Podocyte
PE = Parietal Epithelium

EGM = extraglomerular mesangial cells
M = mesangial cells
G = granular cell

| Filtration | |
|---|---|
| **Bowman capsule** | A pouch wrapped around capillaries |
| **Podocytes** | Specialized cells of BC, which help prevent protein filtration |
| **Glomerular capillaries (GC)** | Fenestrated, which allows rapid filtration of water and small solutes, but prevents protein filtration |

$$\text{Filtration} = \text{GFR} = K_f[(P_{GC} - P_{BC}) - (\pi_{GC} - \pi_{BC})]$$
(same forces as discussed in CV)

| | |
|---|---|
| $K_f$ | Filtration coefficient is high for $H_2O$, electrolytes, small solutes |
| $P_{GC}$ | Remains high along GC due to very low GC resistance, favoring filtration |
| $P_{BC}$ | Remains low unless urinary tract obstruction is present |
| $\pi_{GC}$ | Rises along GC due to high filtration, until filtration ceases in distal capillary; reduced with low plasma protein |
| $\pi_{BC}$ | ≈ zero normally, proteinuria increases it |

| Filtration Fraction = GFR/RPF |
|---|
| Ranges from 15–30%, usually ≈20%<br>• Nonrenal capillary filtration fraction ≈1–2%<br>• Nonrenal $P_{cap}$ falls along capillary due to capillary resistance, so filtration only occurs at proximal end and reabsorption occurs distally. |

# AUTOREGULATION OF GFR AND RBF

An isolated change in renal perfusion pressure between 75 and 175 mm Hg will not change RBF or GFR significantly because **autoregulation** maintains RBF at a constant level by adjusting afferent and efferent arteriolar resistances. Autoregulation occurs via a **myogenic response** and **tubuloglomerular feedback**.

| Mechanisms of Autoregulation | |
|---|---|
| **Myogenic** | ↑ arterial pressure stretches vessel wall, which ↑ calcium movement into smooth muscle cells, causing them to contract. |
| **Tubuloglomerular feedback (TGF)** | ↓ arterial pressure causes GFR to ↓, which in turn ↓ delivery of NaCl to macula densa. This results in an ↑ in efferent arteriolar resistance and a ↓ in afferent arteriolar resistance, both of which ↑ GFR to a normal level. The ↑ in efferent arteriolar resistance occurs in response to ↑ levels of angiotensin II. |

| **Autoregulatory range** | Between approximately 75–175 mm Hg mean arterial pressure (MAP) |
|---|---|
| **Renal shutdown** | Lower than 50 mm Hg MAP; both GFR and RBF are very low; kidney shuts down |

# REGULATION OF FILTRATION (GFR AND RBF)

| Vessel | Constriction | | | Dilation | | |
|---|---|---|---|---|---|---|
| | $P_{cap}$ | GFR | RBF | $P_{cap}$ | GFR | RBF |
| **Afferent arteriole** | ↓ | ↓ | ↓ | ↑ | ↑ | ↑ |
| **Efferent arteriole** | ↑ | ↑ | ↓ | ↓ | ↓ | ↑ |

# TUBULAR FUNCTION: REABSORPTION AND SECRETION

| Active Facilitated Transporters Display Maximum Transport ($T_{max}$) Rates | |
|---|---|
| **Transport maximum** | $T_{max}$ = mass of solute per time transported *when carriers saturated* |
| **Limited carrier population** | Transport mediated by these carriers is saturable under pathophysiologic conditions, e.g., glucose transporters |
| **Reabsorption < $T_{max}$** | None of solute in urine until filtered load > $T_{max}$ |
| **Secretion < $T_{max}$** | All of solute delivered in plasma appears in urine until delivery > $T_{max}$ |
| **Interpretation** | Reduced $T_{max}$ for glucose indicates reduced number of functioning nephrons |

## Estimation of $T_{max}$ by Graphical Interpretation

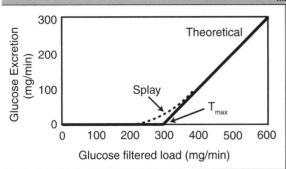

The *solid line* represents the theoretical relationship between glucose filtered load (FL) and glucose excretion (E). Actually, some glucose appears in the urine below the $T_{max}$ due to competition for binding sites. When the filtered load > $T_{max}$, $E = FL - T_{max}$.

Select a point on linear portion:

Reabsorption = excretion − filtered load

$T_{max}$ = 300 mg/min reabsorption

$FL_{glucose}$ = 500 mg/min; $E_{glucose}$ = 200 mg/min

$R_{glucose}$ = 200 mg/min − 500 mg/min = −300 mg/min

Therefore, $R_{glucose} = T_{max}$, and carriers are saturated

## Proximal Tubule

| First Half of the Proximal Tubule | Second Half of the Proximal Tubule |
|---|---|

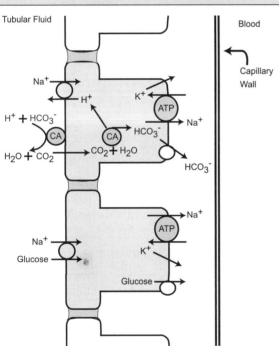

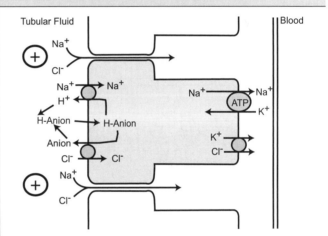

The processes in the left figure continue on in the second half of the proximal tubule and others are added:

3) Secondary active NaCl reabsorption is mediated by the parallel operation of the $Na^+/H^+$ antiport and $Cl^-$/anion antiport (e.g., $OH^-$, formate, oxalate, sulfate). $H^+$ plus anion associate into the neutral acid in the tubular fluid and diffuse passively into the cell, where they dissociate again to move through the antiports.
4) Water follows non-$Cl^-$ solute reabsorption in the first half of the PT and increases tubular fluid [$Cl^-$]. Passive $Cl^-$ diffusion pulls $Na^+$ electrically after it, but creates a small negative electrical potential in the tubular lumen.

1) $NaHCO_3^-$ reabsorption is depicted at the *top of the diagram*.
2) The $Na^+$-glucose symporter is depicted in the *bottom cell*; other symporters reabsorb amino acids, lactate, and phosphate.

*(Continued)*

| Proximal Tubule *(Cont'd.)* | | |
|---|---|---|
| **Substance** | **Action** | **Mechanism** |
| Water | 67% reabsorbed | • Simple diffusion; filtration forces favor reabsorption<br>• Solute reabsorption creates osmotic gradient, water follows it; paracellular and transcellular<br>• Cell membranes permeable to water |
| $Na^+$ | 67% reabsorbed | • $Na^+/K^+$-ATPase in the basolateral membrane creates an electrochemical gradient; secondary active transport, luminal (apical) surface; co- and countertransport<br>• Simple diffusion, paracellular |
| Glucose, lactate, amino acids, phosphate | $\approx$100% reabsorbed | • Secondary active transport at the luminal (apical) surface; cotransport with $Na^+$; $Na^+$ electrochemical gradient provides the power<br>• Transport maximum processes (*see* below) |
| $H^+$ | Secreted | Primary ATPase and secondary active antiport with $Na^+$ |
| $HCO_3^-$ | $\approx$100% reabsorbed | Reabsorbed as $CO_2$ at the apical surface; facilitated diffusion and exchange with $Cl^-$ on basolateral surface; carbonic anhydrase located at the apical surface and intracellularly |
| $Cl^-$ | $\approx$67% reabsorbed | • Transcellular: at the apical surface, exchange with anions; at the basolateral surface, facilitated diffusion and symport with $K^+$<br>• Paracellular, simple diffusion |
| $Ca^{2+}$ | $\approx$70% reabsorbed | 80% of proximal tubule reabsorption paracellular; 20% transcellular |
| Organic cations, anions | Mainly secreted | Various mechanisms |

| Loop of Henle: Overview | | | |
|---|---|---|---|
| | **Descending Thin Limb (DTL)** | **Ascending Thin Limb (ATL)** | **Thick Ascending Limb (TAL)** |
| **$H_2O$** | Reabsorbs 15% of GFR | Impermeable | Impermeable |
| **Solutes** | Diffuse into tubule | Slight active reabsorption | Reabsorbs 25% FL of NaCl, $K^+$; 20% FL of $Ca^{2+}$; 50–60% FL of $Mg^{2+}$ |
| **Tubular fluid volume** | Decreases | No change | No change |
| **Tubular fluid osmolarity** | Increases; DTL is called the "concentrating segment" | Decreases | Decreases below normal plasma; TAL is called the "diluting segment" |

*Definition of abbreviation:* FL, filtered load.

## Thick Ascending Loop of Henle

| | Mechanisms of Solute Transport, Thick Ascending Loop of Henle | |
|---|---|---|
| $Na^+$ | **Reabsorption:** <br>• Symport with $Cl^-$ and $K^+$ <br>• Antiport with $H^+$ <br>• Paracellular due to electrical force | |
| $K^+$ | **Reabsorption:** <br>• Paracellular reabsorption (electrical force) <br>• Symport with $Na^+$ and $Cl^-$ | |
| $Ca^{2+}$ | **Reabsorption:** <br>• Paracellular (electrical force) <br>• Transcellular, apical surface, simple diffusion <br>• Basolateral $Ca^{2+}$-ATPase, $Na^+$-$Ca^{2+}$ exchange <br>• $2H^+/Ca^{2+}$ ATPase antiport; parathyroid hormone stimulates | |
| $Mg^{2+}$ | **Reabsorption:** <br>• Paracellular (electrical force) <br>• Transcellular, active transport | |
| $H^+$ | **Secretion:** <br>• $Na^+/H^+$ exchange, $NH_4^+$ | |

**"Diluting segment":** reabsorption of solutes without reabsorption of water produces hyperosmotic interstitium of medulla; needed for descending loop water reabsorption and collecting duct ability to regulate water reabsorption

## Distal Tubule and Collecting Duct Overview

| | Tubular Fluid Volume | Tubular Fluid Osmolarity | Tubular Fluid Solutes |
|---|---|---|---|
| Delivered from TAL | ≈15% of GFR | Hypotonic at ≈1/2 $P_{OSM}$ | • ≈10% FL of NaCl, $K^+$, and $Ca^{2+}$ <br>• ≈5% FL of $HCO_3^-$ |
| **Early distal convoluted tubule (EDT)** | No $H_2O$ reabsorbed | Hypotonic at ≈1/3 $P_{OSM}$ | • Reabsorb ≈5% FL of NaCl via **apical $Na^+$-$Cl^-$ symporter** (NCC) in secondary active transport inhibited by **thiazide** diuretics <br>• Reabsorb ≈10% FL of $Ca^{2+}$ via secondary active transport stimulated by **parathyroid hormone (PTH)** and indirectly by **thiazide** diuretics |
| **Late distal tubule (LTD) and cortical collecting duct (CCD)** | $H_2O$ reabsorption regulated by **antidiuretic hormone (ADH)** | Varies primarily with $H_2O$ reabsorption | • Reabsorb ≈4% of FL of NaCl via active transport regulated by **aldosterone** <br>• Reabsorb ≈5% FL of $HCO_3^-$ via active transport regulated by **aldosterone** <br>• Secretion of $K^+$ determines total excretion; active secretion regulated by **aldosterone** |
| **Medullary collecting duct (MCD)** | $H_2O$ reabsorption regulated by **ADH** | Varies primarily with $H_2O$ reabsorption | Reabsorb ≈60% of FL of urea passively via transporter regulated by **ADH**; urea reabsorption is needed for medullary osmolarity |

*Definition of abbreviation:* FL, filtered load.
*Some refer to the LDT as the connecting tubule.

| Overview | | | | |
|---|---|---|---|---|
| **Steady-State Balance** (maintained by renal regulation of excretion) | | **Fractional E = (Excreted)/(Filtered)** | | **Major Regulators of Renal Excretion** |
| | | **Range** | **Typical** | |
| Water | Volume liquid drunk/day = $E_{H_2O}$ | 0.5–14% | ≈1% | **Antidiuretic hormone (ADH)** acting on LDT and **collecting duct** |
| Solute | Osmols generated as water soluble wastes = $E_{osmols}$ | | ≈1.5% | Major osmoles excreted are salts, acids, and nitrogenous wastes; excrete ≈600–900 mOsm/day |
| NaCl | Amount NaCl eaten/day = $E_{NaCl}$ | 0.1–5% | ≈0.5–1% | • **Aldosterone** acting on LDT and **CCD**; renal **SNS** tone acting on **PT**<br>• **Angiotensin II** on multiple segments<br>• Atrial natriuretic peptide, etc. |
| $K^+$ | Amount $K^+$ eaten/day ≈ $E_K^+$ | 1–80% | ≈15% | • **Aldosterone** acting on LDT and **CCD**; other factors described later |
| $Ca^{2+}$ | Amount $Ca^{2+}$ absorbed from GI/day = $E_{Ca}^{2+}$ | 0.1–3% | ≈1% | **Parathyroid hormone** (PTH) acting on **DCT** |
| $HCO_3^-$ | • *New* $HCO_3^-$ added to blood/day = net acid excretion (NAE) = $(E_{ammonium})$ + $(E_{H_2PO_4^-})$ − $(E_{bicarbonate})$<br>• NAE determines $[HCO_3^-]_{plasma}$ | $HCO_3^-$<br><br>$H_2PO_4^-$ | ≈0%<br><br>≈20% | **Aldosterone** acting on LDT and **CCD**; plasma pH and other factors described later |
| Urea | Amount generated/day = $E_{urea}$ | 20% – 80% | ≈40% | Synthesis depends on protein metabolism; regulated by **ADH** acting on medullary **collecting duct** |

*Definition of abbreviations:* CCD, cortical collecting duct.

ORGAN SYSTEMS

RENAL/URINARY

# Regulation of Urine Osmolarity and Urine Flow—Antidiuretic Hormone (ADH)

## Collecting Duct

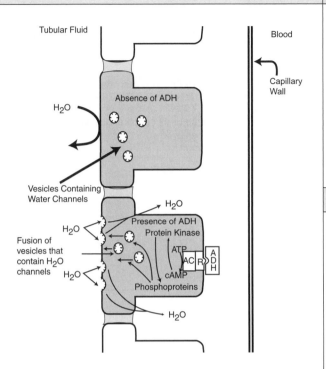

The ADH-receptor complex on the basolateral membrane activates adenylate cyclase. cAMP activates a kinase that phosphorylates proteins involved in movement of vesicles and fusion with the membrane. The resulting channels allow diffusion of water across the apical membrane.

## Effect of Plasma ADH on Urine Osmolarity, Urine Flow, and Total Solute Excretion

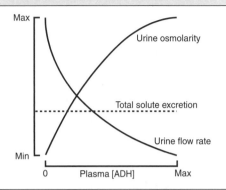

## Urine Osmolarity Versus Urine Flow

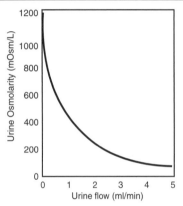

In the normal system, urine flow and osmolarity have an inverse relationship.

## Loop of Henle and the Countercurrent Mechanism Antidiuresis (Presence of ADH)

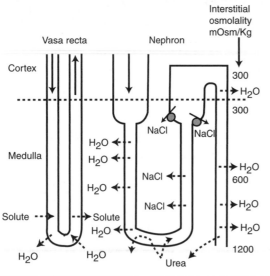

In the presence of ADH, the collecting duct is permeable to water. Because of the high osmolarity of the medulla, water is reabsorbed, so the urine volume is small and the urine concentration is the same as the medulla (hyperosmotic).

| | |
|---|---|
| **Vasa recta** | • Only 1–2% of renal blood flow<br>• Reabsorbed solutes "trapped" in medulla |
| **Balance of solutes and water** | • In total loop, more solute than $H_2O$ reabsorbed<br>• Produces hyperosmotic interstitium of medulla |
| **Descending thin loop** | • Fluid enters isoosmotic with normal plasma<br>• $H_2O$ reabsorption → ↓volume with ↑ osmolarity |
| **Ascending loop** | • Solute reabsorption only, not $H_2O$ → hypoosmotic tubular fluid<br>• Accumulation of solutes in interstitium of medulla |
| **Collecting duct** | • With ADH, collecting duct permeable to $H_2O$ and urea<br>• As duct passes through hyperosmotic interstitium, reabsorption of $H_2O$ → small volume of concentrated urine<br>• Negative $CH_2O$; dilutes plasma |

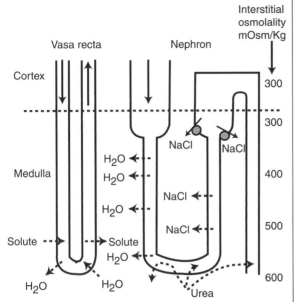

In the absence of ADH, the collecting duct is impermeable to water, so urine flow is high and the urine is dilute. Note that medullary osmolality is also lower than when ADH is present.

| | |
|---|---|
| **Vasa recta** | • ↑ blood flow with lower-than-normal osmolarity<br>• Washes out solutes, medullary osmolarity reduced |
| **Balance of solutes and water** | Medullary osmolarity still higher than normal plasma, but not as high as during antidiuresis |
| **Descending thin loop** | Less $H_2O$ is reabsorbed because the medulla is not as concentrated as during antidiuresis |
| **Ascending loop** | Solute reabsorption continues, but a significant portion of solutes that are reabsorbed are washed into the vasa recta |
| **Collecting duct** | • Without ADH, the collecting duct is impermeable to $H_2O$ and urea<br>• No $H_2O$ reabsorption because tubular fluid passes through medulla<br>• ↑ urine flow, ↓ urine osmolarity<br>• Positive $CH_2O$; acts to concentrate plasma |

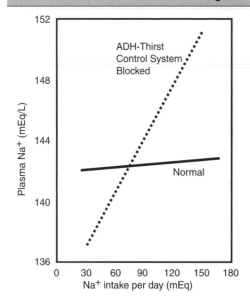

ADH secretion is increased by elevated plasma sodium or osmolarity and decreased by high blood volume or high pressure. This acts as a negative feedback system to control plasma osmolarity. (See **Antidiuretic Hormone and Control of Osmolarity and Volume** in the Endocrine section.)

| Calculation of Plasma Osmolality (mOsm/kg solution) |
|---|
| Plasma osmolality = 2 (plasma [Na$^+$]) + [glucose mg/dL]/18 + [urea mg/dL]/2.8 |
| Example: sodium = 145 mEq/L, glucose = 180 mg/dL, urea = 28 mg/dL |
| Plasma osmolality = 290 + 10 + 10 = 310 mOsm/kg |
| However: plasma Na$^+$ dominates control of ADH because of its osmotic effect; urea and glucose usually irrelevant. |
| *Note:* glucose may be important part of **urine** osmolality (especially in diabetes); when present, it causes osmotic diuresis. |

Normal function of the control system for ADH secretion and water consumption prevents large changes of plasma sodium concentration. Loss of this system causes plasma sodium concentration to increase in proportion to sodium intake.

| Control Signals for Na$^+$ and H$_2$O Excretion | | |
|---|---|---|
| **System** | **Action** | **Segment/Site** |
| Renal sympathetic nerves | ↓ GFR | Afferent arteriole constriction |
| | ↑ NaCl reabsorption | Proximal, TAL, DT, CD → ↑ H$_2$O reabsorption (except TAL, due to impermeability of water) |
| Renin–angiotensin II–aldosterone | Angio II → ↑ NaCl reabsorption | Proximal → ↑ H$_2$O reabsorption |
| | Aldosterone →↑ NaCl reabsorption | TAL, DT, CD →↑ H$_2$O reabsorption (except TAL, due to impermeability of water) |
| Atrial natriuretic peptide (ANP) | ↑ GFR | Glomerulus |
| | ↓ renin, angio II, aldosterone | JGA and adrenal cortex |
| | ↓ NaCl and H$_2$O reabsorption | CD (urodilatin* assists) |
| | ↓ ADH secretion and actions | Posterior pituitary and CD |
| ADH | ↑ permeability to H$_2$O | CD → ↑ H$_2$O reabsorption → ↓ urine flow and ↑ urine osmolarity |

*Urodilatin is a peptide produced by DT and CD when blood pressure/volume increase. Very potent inhibition of NaCl and water reabsorption, but only local action; it does not circulate.

## Disorders of Solute and Water Regulation

| Disorder | ECF Volume | $[Na^+]_{plasma}$ | Blood Pressure | Urine Volume and Osmolarity | Arterial pH | $[K^+]_{plasma}$ |
|---|---|---|---|---|---|---|
| Diabetes insipidus* | ↓ | ↑ | – or ↓ | ↑ volume<br>↓ osmolarity | ↑ | ↓<br>(↑ aldosterone and alkalosis) |
| SIADH | ↑ | ↓ | ↑ or – | ↓ volume<br>↑ osmolarity | ↓ | ↑<br>(but negative balance) |
| Aldosterone deficiency (primary) | ↓ | ↓ | ↓ | ↑ volume<br>↑ osmolarity | ↓ | ↑<br>positive balance |
| Aldosterone excess (primary) | ↑ | ↑ | ↑ | ↓ volume<br>↓ osmolarity | ↑ | ↓<br>negative balance |
| Polydipsia | ↑ | ↓ | – | ↑ volume<br>↓ osmolarity | ↓ | ↑<br>balance variable |
| Water deprivation (dehydration) | ↓ | ↑ | ↓ | ↓ volume<br>↑ osmolarity | ↑ | ↑, ↓, –<br>depends on multiple factors |

*Definition of abbreviation:* SIADH, syndrome of inappropriate (excessive) ADH secretion.

*ADH deficiency is called primary, central, or neurogenic; ↓ renal response to ADH is nephrogenic. Distinguish by response to administration of ADH; ↑ urine osmolarity in response to ADH injection indicates primary.

## Osmotic Diuresis

| Cause | Effect |
|---|---|
| Excessive solute in tubular fluid | Decrease reabsorption of $H_2O$ |
| Diabetic ketoacidosis | • Glucose and ketones in urine → polyuria, $K^+$ wasting<br>• $Na^+$ loss → hyponatremia |
| Starvation and alcoholic ketoacidosis | Ketonuria → polyuria, $K^+$ wasting, hyponatremia |
| Osmotic diuretics (mannitol, carbonic anhydrase inhibitors) | Inhibit proximal tubule $H_2O$ reabsorption → diuresis, $K^+$ wasting (due to ↑ flow) |
| Loop diuretics (furosemide) and distal tubule diuretics (thiazides) | Inhibit NaCl reabsorption →↑ tubular solutes → diuresis and $K^+$ wasting |

## Causes of Increased Potassium Excretion

| Tubular Flow and K⁺ Secretion | Factor | Mechanism |
|---|---|---|
| 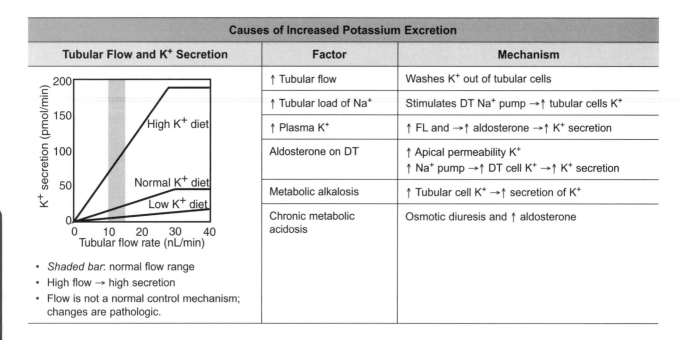 | ↑ Tubular flow | Washes K⁺ out of tubular cells |
| | ↑ Tubular load of Na⁺ | Stimulates DT Na⁺ pump →↑ tubular cells K⁺ |
| | ↑ Plasma K⁺ | ↑ FL and →↑ aldosterone →↑ K⁺ secretion |
| | Aldosterone on DT | ↑ Apical permeability K⁺<br>↑ Na⁺ pump →↑ DT cell K⁺ →↑ K⁺ secretion |
| | Metabolic alkalosis | ↑ Tubular cell K⁺ →↑ secretion of K⁺ |
| | Chronic metabolic acidosis | Osmotic diuresis and ↑ aldosterone |

- *Shaded bar*: normal flow range
- High flow → high secretion
- Flow is not a normal control mechanism; changes are pathologic.

## Effects of Volume Expansion and Contraction on K⁺ Secretion

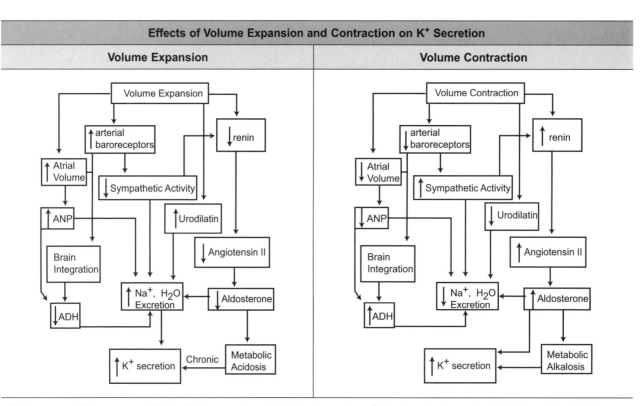

Volume expansion causes acidosis due to responses that ↓ reabsorption of bicarbonate in proximal tubule and ↓ aldosterone. Volume contraction causes alkalosis due to ↑ proximal tubular reabsorption of bicarbonate and ↑ aldosterone. Both can cause K⁺ wasting because metabolic alkalosis and chronic metabolic acidosis both ↑ K⁺ secretion in distal tubule and collecting duct.

ORGAN SYSTEMS

RENAL/URINARY

## Effects of Metabolic Alkalosis and Acidosis on K⁺ Excretion

| Metabolic Alkalosis | Metabolic Acidosis |
|---|---|

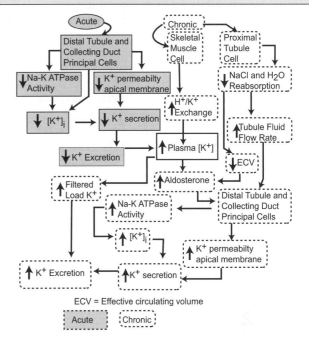

Both acute and chronic metabolic alkalosis cause hypokalemia with a negative potassium balance.

ECV = Effective circulating volume

Acute (<24 hours) and chronic metabolic acidosis **both** increase extracellular [K⁺]. However, acute decreases K⁺ excretion, but chronic increases K⁺ excretion.*

*Elevated aldosterone is the key to the reversal of the effect of acidosis on K⁺ excretion. Also, increased cellular H⁺ causes efflux of K⁺ from cells; low cellular H⁺ causes influx. Acidosis impairs metabolism; thus, ↓ solute reabsorption causes osmotic diuresis.

## RENAL MECHANISMS FOR ACID/BASE REGULATION

### Fundamental Principles

| | |
|---|---|
| **Tubular cell pH** | • If a cell is acidotic, it will secrete acid. <br> • If a cell is alkalotic, it will ↓ reabsorption of bicarbonate or secrete it. |
| **Fluid volume** | If ECV is decreased, ↑ $Na^+$ reabsorption will be accompanied by ↑ bicarbonate reabsorption. |
| **Overall role of kidneys** | This is the only significant mechanism for excretion of nonvolatile, metabolic acids. |
| **Response time** | Requires 24–72 hours for maximal compensatory response |
| **Net acid excretion (NAE)** | There is no net excretion of newly formed acid unless all bicarbonate is reabsorbed. <br> $NAE = \dot{V} \times [NH_4^+] + \dot{V} \times [H_2PO_4^-] - \dot{V} \times [HCO_3^-]$ |
| **Free H⁺ excretion** | Trivial amount even at most acidic urine pH $\cong$ 4.4 |
| **NH₄⁺ excretion** | Largest quantity of excreted acid; metabolized from glutamine; "nontitratable acid" |
| **H₂PO₄⁻ excretion** | Second largest quantity; "titratable acid" |
| **NH₄⁺ secretion** | $NH_4^+$ secreted in the proximal tubule is reabsorbed in TAL and added to interstitium; it is then taken up by DT and CD cells and secreted. |

## Tubular Handling of Bicarbonate

### Proximal Tubule Reabsorption of Bicarbonate Ion

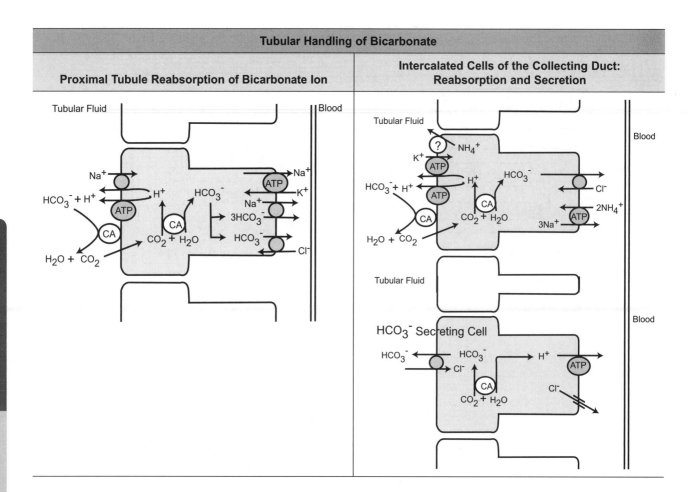

### Intercalated Cells of the Collecting Duct: Reabsorption and Secretion

$HCO_3^-$ Secreting Cell

## Tubular Handling of Ammonia

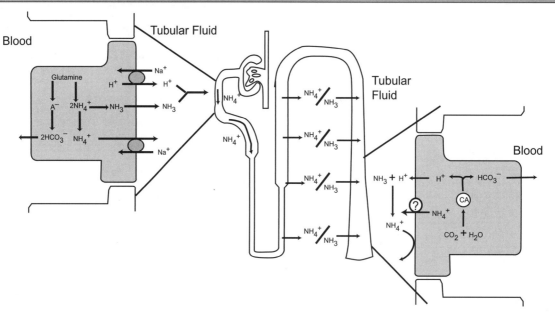

$NH_4^+$ can substitute for $K^+$ in the sodium pump. Apical secretion may be by substitution for $H^+$ in the $H^+$-$K^+$ exchanger or the $H^+$-ATPase. Production of $NH_4^+$ adds $HCO_3^-$ to blood.

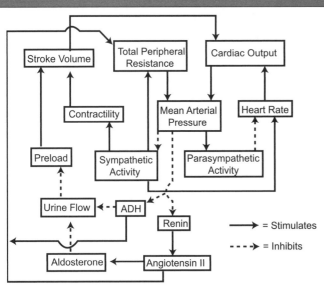

### Notes on Use of Feedback Diagram

- Many intermediate steps omitted.
- ADH (vasopressin) also vasoconstricts.
- Diagram merges elements of cardiovascular and endocrine physiology.
- For applications, make the most direct connection; e.g., hemorrhage: begin at reduced preload →↓ stroke volume, and so on. For an understanding of ACE inhibition, begin at ↓ angiotensin II.

$\longrightarrow$ = Stimulates

$\dashrightarrow$ = Inhibits

## ACID/BASE AND ITS REGULATION

### Fundamental Principles

| | |
|---|---|
| **Carbonic anhydrase reaction** | Produces strong acid and weak base → acidic solution |
| **Respiratory contribution** | Determined by arterial $P_{CO_2}$: ↑ $P_{CO_2}$ → acidosis; ↓ $P_{CO_2}$ → alkalosis |
| **Metabolic contribution** | Determined by arterial $HCO_3^-$: ↑ $HCO_3^-$ → alkalosis ; ↓ $HCO_3^-$ → acidosis |
| **Simple disorder** | One disorder with or without compensation |
| **Mixed or combined disorder** | Two simultaneous disorders |
| **Compensation** | • A response that tends to correct pH: compensation is never perfect.<br>• Fully compensated means that the mechanism has come as close as possible to restoring normal pH. |
| **Normal arterial blood gas** | pH = 7.40; $P_{CO_2}$ = 40 mm Hg; $P_{O_2}$ = 83 – 100 mm Hg; $HCO_3^-$ = 24 mEq/L |
| **Henderson-Hasselbalch Eq.** | Several forms; they show relationship between pH, $P_{CO_2}$, and $HCO_3^-$. |

| The Carbonic Anhydrase Reaction | Henderson-Hasselbalch Equation |
|---|---|
| $$CO_2 + H_2O \overset{CA}{\rightleftharpoons} H_2CO_3 \rightleftharpoons H^+ + HCO_3^-$$ <br><br> CA, carbonic anhydrase | $$pH = 6.1 \log \frac{[HCO_3^-]}{0.03\, P_{CO_2}}$$ <br> • ↑ $P_{CO_2}$ → ↓ pH <br> • ↑ $HCO_3^-$ → ↑ pH |

### Examples of Calculations

| | |
|---|---|
| $P_{CO_2}$ = 60 mm Hg; $HCO_3^-$ = 18 mEq/L | pH = 6.1 + log (18/1.8) = 6.1 + log 10 = 6.1 + 1 = 7.1 |
| $P_{CO_2}$ = 40 mm Hg; $HCO_3^-$ = 24 mEq/L | pH = 6.1 + log (24/1.2) = 6.1 + log 20 = 6.1 + 1.3 = 7.4 |
| $P_{CO_2}$ = 20 mm Hg; $HCO_3^-$ = 24 mEq/L | pH = 6.1 + log (24/0.6) = 6.1 + log 40 = 6.10 + 1.60 = 7.70 |
| $P_{CO_2}$ = 60 mm Hg; $HCO_3^-$ = 36 mEq/L | pH = 6.1 + log (36/1.8) = 6.1 + log 20 = 6.1 + 1.3 = 7.4 |

*Note:* pH is normal, but this is not normal acid/base status; both $P_{CO_2}$ and $HCO_3^-$ are abnormal.

## Fundamental Mechanisms to Control pH

| Buffers | Fast, seconds: ECF bicarbonate (largest), phosphate, and proteins |
|---|---|
| Respiratory | Ventilation response fast, within a few minutes: change $P_{CO_2}$ by changing ventilation.<br>• $\uparrow$ ventilation $\rightarrow \downarrow P_{CO_2} \rightarrow$ alkalosis<br>• $\downarrow$ ventilation $\rightarrow \uparrow P_{CO_2} \rightarrow$ acidosis |
| Renal | • Slow; 24–72 hours; powerful: major mechanism to excrete nonvolatile acids.<br>• Change in renal acid excretion and $HCO_3^-$ production is called a metabolic response. |
| Primary disorders | • Primary disorder ventilation = respiratory acid/base disorder<br>• Primary disorder excess production of acid, $\downarrow$ renal excretion of acid, or loss of bicarbonate in urine or feces = metabolic disorder |

## The Davenport Diagram

- Above the base buffer line, there is excess metabolic base (a positive base excess).
- Below it, there is excess metabolic acid (negative base excess).
- Read pH perpendicular to the x-axis; $HCO_3^-$ perpendicular to the y-axis, but $P_{CO_2}$ along the curves.

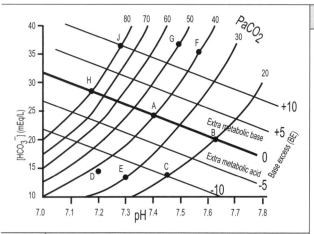

### Patient Examples

Predicted bicarbonate concentration with changes of $PCO_2$

| $PCO_2$ (mm Hg) | 80 | 60 | 40 | 20 |
|---|---|---|---|---|
| $HCO_3^-$ (mEq/L) | 29 | 27 | 24 | 21 |

Draw a vertical line through the $PCO_2$ to get the predicted $HCO_3^-$

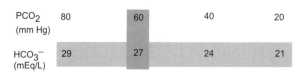

A patient has $PCO_2$ = 60 mm Hg and $[HCO_3^-]$ = 28 mEq/L
Has metabolism changed?
No: the bicarbonate is almost exactly as expected from the $PCO_2$

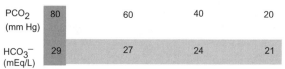

A patient has $PCO_2$ = 80 mm Hg and $[HCO_3^-]$ = 35 mEq/L

What is the predicted bicarbonate?   29 mEq/L
Is there more or less bicarbonate than predicted?   More
Has metabolism changed?     Yes, there is excess bicarbonate.
What is the metabolic contribution?  Alkalosis

| Point | Interpretation |
|---|---|
| A | Normal acid/base status |
| B | Uncompensated respiratory alkalosis |
| C | Respiratory alkalosis with compensatory metabolic acidosis |
| D | Uncompensated metabolic acidosis |
| E | Metabolic acidosis with compensatory respiratory alkalosis |
| F | Uncompensated metabolic alkalosis |
| G | Metabolic alkalosis with compensatory respiratory acidosis |
| H | Uncompensated respiratory acidosis |
| J | Respiratory acidosis with compensatory metabolic alkalosis |

| Simple Acid–Base Disorders | | | |
|---|---|---|---|
| Type of Disorder | pH | Paco$_2$ | HCO$_3^-$ |
| Metabolic acidosis | ↓ | ↓* | ↓ |
| Metabolic alkalosis | ↑ | ↑* | ↑ |
| Respiratory acidosis | ↓ | ↑ | ↑* |
| Respiratory alkalosis | ↑ | ↓ | ↓* |

*Change due to compensation

## A Step-by-Step Approach to Diagnosis of Simple Disorders

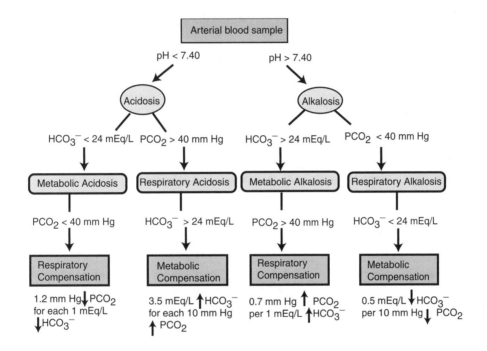

1. What is the pH? Acidotic or alkalotic?
2. What is the respiratory contribution? Acidosis, alkalosis, or no change?
3. What is the metabolic contribution? Acidosis, alkalosis, or no change?
4. What causes the acid–base disorder? *Ans:* the factor (respiratory or metabolic) that would produce the abnormal pH.
5. Is there compensation? Did the other factor change in the direction that would help offset the disorder?

| Use of the Plasma Anion Gap (PAG) | |
|---|---|
| Use | To determine whether the cause of a metabolic acidosis is due to ↑ concentration of nonvolatile acid |
| Discriminates | Whether the primary disorder is loss of bicarbonate in urine or feces |
| Principle | Cations = anions in plasma, if all were measured; commonly measure $Na^+$, $Cl^-$, and $HCO_3^-$; metabolic acids are not measured. So there is a gap between cations and anions as measured. |
| Calculation | PAG = $[Na^+]$ – ($[Cl^-]$ + $[HCO_3^-]$); normal = $12 \pm 2$ |
| Interpretation ↑ PAG | Excess molecules of acid, e.g., diabetic ketoacidosis, aspirin, lactic acidosis, etc. |
| Non-anion gap acidosis (normal PAG) | Acidosis due to loss of bicarbonate in urine or diarrhea results in hyperchloremic acidosis; kidneys reabsorb excess $Cl^-$ in replacement for bicarbonate |

| Urinary Anion Gap (UAG) | |
|---|---|
| Principle | Hard to measure $NH_4^+$ in urine, but it is the major form of acid excreted <br> Cations = anions in urine, if all are measured |
| Ions measured | $Na^+$, $K^+$, $Cl^-$: anions > cations because did not measure $NH_4^+$ |
| UAG calculation | UAG = $[Na^+]$ + $[K^+]$ – $[Cl^-]$ |
| Interpretation of negative | Kidneys are excreting acid |
| Interpretation of positive | Kidneys are excreting base |
| In acidosis | UAG should be negative if kidneys are compensating appropriately |
| In alkalosis | UAG should be positive if kidneys are compensating appropriately |

**Sample case:**

*Arterial:* pH = 7.15, $Paco_2$ = 30 mm Hg, $[HCO_3^-]$ = 10 mEq/L, $Cl^-$ = 100 mEq/L, $Na^+$ = 145 mEq/L

*Urine:* $Na^+$ = 100 mEq/L, $K^+$ = 90 mEq/L, $Cl^-$ = 140 mEq/L

**Diagnosis:** metabolic acidosis with respiratory compensation; PAG = 35; therefore, grossly excessive acid in the body. UAG is positive, so kidneys are not excreting acid. Primary cause is likely to be retention of acid by kidneys.

# RENAL PATHOLOGY

## CYSTIC DISEASE OF THE KIDNEY

| | |
|---|---|
| **Childhood polycystic disease** | • Rare **autosomal recessive** disease, presenting in infancy with renal (and often hepatic) cysts and progressive renal failure<br>• *Gross:* bilaterally enlarged kidneys with smooth surfaces. *Cut section:* sponge-like appearance with multiple small cysts in the cortex and medulla |
| **Adult polycystic disease** | • **Autosomal dominant**, usually have normal renal function until middle age<br>• Present with renal insufficiency, hematuria, flank pain, and hypertension<br>• *Extrarenal manifestations:* liver cysts, **circle of Willis berry aneurysms**, mitral valve prolapse<br>• *Gross:* marked bilateral enlargement with large cysts bulging through the surface<br>• *Micro:* cysts involve <10% of nephrons |
| **Simple cysts** | Common, can be single or multiple; have little clinical significance |
| **Medullary sponge kidney** | • Multiple **cystic dilatations of collecting ducts in medulla**<br>• Most are asymptomatic |
| **Acquired cystic disease** | • Multiple cortical and medullary cysts may result from **prolonged renal dialysis**<br>• Unclear whether ↑ risk for development into renal cell carcinoma |

## GLOMERULAR DISEASES

| Type | Clinical Presentation | Mechanism | Light Microscopy | Electron Microscopy | Immuno-fluorescence |
|---|---|---|---|---|---|
| Poststreptococcal glomerulonephritis | Nephritis; **elevated ASLO**; low complement; children > adults<br><br>Usually recover completely; occasionally progress to RPGN | Immunologic (type III hypersensitivity) | Polymorpho-nuclear neutrophil leukocyte infiltration; proliferation | **Subepithelial humps** | **Granular pattern**; GBM and mesangium contain IgG and C3 |
| Lipoid nephrosis (minimal change) | **Nephrotic syndrome; children > adults**<br><br>Usually normal renal function; may respond to steroids | Unknown | Normal | No deposits; **loss of epithelial foot processes** | Negative |
| Membranous glomerulonephritis | **Nephrotic syndrome; adults > children**<br><br>May respond to steroids | Immunologic | Capillary wall thickening | **Subepithelial spikes**; loss of epithelial foot processes | Granular pattern of IgG and C3 |
| Membranoproliferative glomerulonephritis | Variable: mild proteinuria, mixed nephritic/nephrotic, or frank nephrotic syndrome<br><br>Poor response to steroids | *Type I:* immune complex and both classic and alternate complement pathways<br><br>*Type II:* immune complex and alternate complement pathway | Basement membrane thick and split; mesangial proliferation | *Type I:* **subendothelial deposits**<br><br>*Type II:* **dense deposit disease** | *Type I:* IgG and C3, C1q, and C4<br><br>*Type II:* C3 (IgG, C1q, and C4 usually absent)<br><br>"C3 nephritic factor" |
| Focal segmental glomerulosclerosis | Nephrotic syndrome<br><br>Poor prognosis; rarely responds to steroids | Immunologic; aggressive variant of lipoid nephrosis; **IV drug use; HIV nephropathy** | Focal and segmental sclerosis and hyalinization | Epithelial damage; loss of foot processes | IgM and C3 focal deposits |

*(Continued)*

## GLOMERULAR DISEASES (CONT'D.)

| Type | Clinical Presentation | Mechanism | Light Microscopy | Electron Microscopy | Immuno-fluorescence |
|------|----------------------|-----------|------------------|---------------------|---------------------|
| Goodpasture syndrome | RPGN + pulmonary hemorrhage<br><br>Often poor prognosis; may respond to steroids, plasmapherisis, cytotoxic agents | **Anti-GBM antibodies** (type II hyper-sensitivity) | **Crescents**; mesangial proliferation in early cases | GBM disruption; no deposits | **Linear IgG and C3** |
| Idiopathic RPGN | RPGN; may follow flu-like syndrome<br><br>Extremely poor prognosis | Immunologic | **Crescents** | Variable, ± deposits; all have GBM ruptures | Granular or linear |
| Focal proliferative glomerulonephritis | Primary focal glomerulonephritis or part of multisystem disease; may be subclinical or present with hematuria, proteinuria, nephrotic syndrome<br><br>Variable prognosis | Immunologic | Proliferation limited to certain segments of particular glomeruli | Variable; may show mesangial deposits | Variable; may show mesangial deposits |
| IgA nephropathy (Berger disease) | Variable: recurrent hematuria, mild proteinuria, nephrotic syndrome; children and young adults<br><br>Usually slowly progressive course | Unknown | Variable: normal or segmental/mesangial proliferation or crescentic | Mesangial deposits | **Mesangial IgA deposition** |
| Diabetic glomerulopathy | Microscopic proteinuria; or can eventually cause nephrotic syndrome<br><br>Prognosis variable, depends on diabetic control | Nonenzymatic glycosylation causes glomerular basement membrane thickening and mesangial matrix expansion | Capillary basement membrane thickening; diffuse and nodular glomerular sclerosis (Kimmelstiel-Wilson) | Thickened glomerular basement membrane and well-demarcated, roughly round nodules in the glomeruli | Not really helpful; may show non-specific immunoglobulin G deposition along the basement membrane |
| Chronic glomerulonephritis | Chronic renal failure; may follow a variety of acute glomerulopathies<br><br>Poor prognosis | Variable | **Hyalinized glomeruli** | Negative | Negative or granular |
| Amyloidosis | Nephrotic syndrome<br><br>Prognosis variable, depends in underlying condition | Amyloid deposition, often accompanying diseases e.g., multiple myeloma, chronic infections, tuberculosis, and rheumatoid arthritis | Eosinophilic amorphous deposits in glomeruli and interstitium that show apple-green birefringence when stained with Congo Red | Fibrillar depositions of amyloid material | Immuno-fluorescence is not usually helpful |
| Alport syndrome | Hematuria, proteinuria, which slowly progress to renal failure; **deafness**; ocular disorders<br><br>Renal failure common by age 50 | **X-linked** disorder of collagen | Segmental and focal glomerulo-sclerosis, tubular atrophy, interstitial fibrosis, chronic inflammation | **Thickening** (sometimes thinning) and **splitting the basement membrane** | **Immuno-fluorescence for individual chains of type IV collagen** can be diagnostic |

*Definition of abbreviations:* ASLO, antistreptolysin O; GBM, glomerular basement membrane; RPGN, rapidly progressive glomerulonephritis.

| TUBULAR DISEASES OF THE KIDNEY | |
|---|---|
| **Acute Tubular Necrosis (ATN)** | **Most common cause of acute renal failure**; associated with reversible injury to the tubular epithelium; excellent prognosis if patient survives disease responsible for the ATN |
| **Ischemic ATN** | • Most common cause of ATN<br>• ↓ blood flow caused by severe renal vasoconstriction, hypotension, or shock |
| **Nephrotoxic ATN** | Caused by heavy metals such as mercury, drugs, and myoglobin |
| **Four Phases of ATN** | |
| **Initial phase** | *36 hours*: after precipitating event occurs |
| **Oliguric phase** | *10 days:* ↓ urine output; uremia, fluid overload, and hyperkalemia may occur |
| **Diuretic phase** | *2–3 weeks:* gradual ↑ in urine volume (up to 3 L/day); hypokalemia, electrolyte imbalances, and infection may occur |
| **Recovery phase** | *3 weeks:* improved concentrating ability, restoration of tubular function; normalization of BUN and creatinine |

| TUBULOINTERSTITIAL DISEASES OF THE KIDNEY | |
|---|---|
| **Pyelonephritis** | • Infection of the renal pelvis, tubules, and interstitium<br>• **Ascending infection is the most common route** with organisms from the patient's fecal flora; hematogenous infection is much less common.<br>• Etiologic agents usually gram-negative bacilli (e.g., *E. coli, Proteus,* and *Klebsiella*). *E. coli* pili mediate adherence, motility aids movement against flow of urine. *Proteus* (urease, alkaline urine, struvite stones), *Klebsiella* (large capsule) |
| **Acute pyelonephritis** | • Risk factors: urinary obstruction, vesicoureteral reflux, pregnancy, instrumentation, diabetes mellitus<br>• Under 40 more common in women (shorter urethra); over 40, ↑ incidence in men due to benign prostatic hypertrophy<br>• **Symptoms:** fever, malaise, dysuria, frequency, urgency, and costovertebral angle (CVA) tenderness. **Fever, CVA tenderness,** and **WBC casts** distinguish pyelonephritis from cystitis.<br>• **Urine:** many WBCs and WBC casts<br>• **Gross:** scattered yellow microabscesses on the renal surface<br>• **Micro:** foci of interstitial suppurative necrosis and tubular necrosis<br>• Blunting of the calyces may be seen on intravenous pyelogram |
| **Chronic pyelonephritis** | • **Reflux nephropathy** most common cause<br>• Interstitial parenchymal scarring deforms the calyces and pelvis<br>• **Symptoms:** onset can be insidious or acute; present with renal failure and hypertension<br>• **Gross:** irregular scarring and deformed calyces with overlying corticomedullary scarring<br>• **Micro:** chronic inflammation with tubular atrophy<br>• Pyelogram diagnostic |
| **Acute allergic interstitial nephritis** | • **Hypersensitivity reaction** to infection or drugs (e.g., NSAIDs, penicillin)<br>• Leads to interstitial edema with a mononuclear infiltrate<br>• Presents 2 weeks after exposure with hematuria, pyuria, eosinophilia, and azotemia |
| **Analgesic nephritis** | Interstitial nephritis and renal papillary necrosis, induced by large doses of analgesics |
| **Gouty nephropathy** | • **Urate crystals** in tubules, inducing tophus formation and a chronic inflammatory reaction<br>• *Note:* Urate crystals appear as **birefringent, needle-shaped crystals** on light microscopy. |
| **Acute urate nephropathy** | • Precipitation of crystals in the collecting ducts, causing obstruction<br>• Seen in **lymphoma and leukemia**, especially after chemotherapy |
| **Multiple myeloma** | **Bence-Jones proteins** are directly toxic to tubular epithelium |
| **Diffuse cortical necrosis** | • Generalized infarction of both kidneys; preferentially involves the renal cortex<br>• Seen in settings of obstetric catastrophes (abruptio placentae) and shock<br>• Mechanism thought to be a combination of vasospasm and DIC |

## VASCULAR DISEASES OF THE KIDNEY

| | |
|---|---|
| **Ischemia** | • Caused by embolization of mural thrombi usually left side of heart or aorta<br>• **Gross:** sharply demarcated, wedge-shaped pale regions, which undergo necrosis with subsequent scarring<br>• **Symptoms:** infarcts may be asymptomatic or may cause pain, hematuria, and hypertension |
| **Renal vein thrombosis** | • Thrombosis of one or both renal veins may occur<br>• Associated with the nephrotic syndrome, particularly membranous glomerulonephritis<br>• Renal cell carcinoma may also provoke renal vein thrombosis as a result of direct invasion by tumor<br>• Presents with hematuria, flank pain, and renal failure<br>• **Gross:** kidney enlarged<br>• **Micro:** hemorrhagic infarction of renal tissue |

## UROLITHIASIS

• Affects 6% of the population; men > women
• Renal colic may occur if small stones pass into the ureter, where they may also cause hematuria and urinary obstruction and predispose to infection

| | |
|---|---|
| **Calcium stones** | • **75% of stones**; most patients have hypercalciuria without hypercalcemia<br>• Calcium stones are **radiopaque**; they are the only ones that can be seen on x-ray |
| **Magnesium-ammonium phosphate stones** | • 15% of stones; occur after infection by urease-producing bacteria, such as *Proteus*<br>• Urine becomes alkaline, resulting in precipitation of **magnesium-ammonium phosphate salts**; may form large stones (e.g., **staghorn calculi**) |
| **Uric acid stones** | Seen in **gout**, **leukemia**, and in patients with acidic urine |
| **Cystine stones** | • Very rare<br>• Associated with an autosomal recessive amino acid transport disorder, leading to **cystinuria**<br>• Most stones are unilateral and formed in calyx, pelvis, bladder |

## OBSTRUCTIVE UROPATHY AND HYDRONEPHROSIS

| | |
|---|---|
| **Hydronephrosis** | • Multiple etiologies, including stones, benign prostatic hypertrophy, pregnancy, neurogenic bladder, tumor, inflammation, and posterior urethral valves<br>• Persistence of glomerular filtration despite urinary obstruction, causing dilation of calyces and pelvis. High pressure in the collecting system causes atrophy and ischemia.<br>• **Gross:** dilatation of the pelvis and calyces with blunting of renal pyramids<br>• **Symptoms:**<br>  – *Unilateral:* may remain asymptomatic as the kidney atrophies<br>  – *Bilateral incomplete:* loses concentrating ability, causing urinary frequency, polyuria and nocturia<br>  – *Bilateral complete:* causes anuria, uremia, and death if untreated |

## TUMORS OF THE KIDNEY

### Benign

| | |
|---|---|
| **Cortical adenomas** | • Common finding at autopsy<br>• **Gross:** yellow, encapsulated cortical nodules<br>• **Micro:** may be identical to renal cell carcinoma, distinguished by size |
| **Angiomyolipomas** | • Hamartomas, composed of fat, smooth muscle, and blood vessels<br>• Particularly common in patients with tuberous sclerosis |

### Malignant

| | |
|---|---|
| **Renal cell carcinomas** | • 90% of all renal cancers in adults; seen in ages 50–70 with no sex predilection<br>• Moderate association with smoking and a familial predisposition<br>• Occurs in 2/3 of patients with von Hippel-Lindau disease<br>• **Symptoms:** "classic" triad of hematuria, palpable mass, and costovertebral pain (10% of cases); hematuria in middle-aged patient should raise concern<br>• **Gross:** most common in the upper pole; usually solitary, with areas of necrosis and hemorrhage; often invades the renal vein and extends into the vena cava and heart<br>• **Micro:** polygonal clear cells with abundant clear cytoplasm<br>• Paraneoplastic syndrome: polycythemia<br>• High incidence of metastasis on initial presentation<br>• 5-year survival depends on stage, especially poor (25–50%) if tumor extends into the renal vein |
| **Wilms tumor (nephroblastoma)** | • Common childhood malignancy with peak incidence at age 2<br>• **Symptoms:** abdominal mass and hypertension, nausea, hematuria, intestinal obstruction<br>• May be associated with other congenital anomalies<br>• **Gross:** very large, demarcated masses; most are unilateral, but may be bilateral if familial<br>• **Micro:** embryonic glomerular and tubular structures surrounded by mesenchymal spindle cells<br>• 90% survival rate when patients are treated with surgery, chemotherapy, radiotherapy |
| **Transitional cell carcinoma** | • Can involve the epithelium of the renal pelvis<br>• Histology similar to transitional cell carcinoma of the bladder, but is less common<br>• Can present with hematuria |

## ANOMALIES OF THE URETERS

| | |
|---|---|
| **Double ureters** | • Form when two same-sided ureters join at some point before the junction to the bladder or enter the bladder separately<br>• Associated with double renal pelvises or an abnormally large kidney |

### Ureteral Obstruction in Hydroureter and Hydronephrosis

| | |
|---|---|
| **Internal obstruction** | • **Renal calculi** are most common cause; usually impact at the ureteropelvic junction, entrance to the bladder, and where they cross iliac vessels<br>• Other causes: strictures, tumors |
| **External obstruction** | • Pelvic tumors may compress or invade the ureteral wall; sclerosing retroperitonitis, a fibrosis of retroperitoneal structures, can cause obstruction.<br>• Pregnancy does not cause obstruction, but does cause dilation (secondary to progesterone). |

ORGAN SYSTEMS

RENAL/URINARY

## PATHOLOGY OF THE BLADDER

| | |
|---|---|
| **Diverticula** | • **Pouch-like evaginations** of the bladder wall<br>• Occur in older men and women and may lead to urinary stasis and therefore infection |
| **Exstrophy of bladder** | • Caused by **absence of the anterior musculature** of the bladder and abdominal wall; developmental failure of downgrowth of mesoderm over the anterior bladder<br>• Site of severe chronic infections, with ↑ incidence of adenocarcinoma |
| **Patent urachus** | • Fistula that **connects the bladder with the umbilicus**; isolated persistence of the central urachus termed a urachal cyst<br>• Carcinomas may develop in these cysts |
| **Infectious cystitis** | • Cystitis causes frequency, urgency, dysuria, and suprapubic pain<br>• **Causative organisms:** *E. coli, Staphylococcus saprophyticus* (associated with intercourse), *Proteus, Klebsiella* (esp. in diabetics), *Pseudomonas (*capsule is antiphagocytic, exotoxin A inhibits EF-2, esp. in patients with structural abnormalities and antibiotic usage), *Enterococcus* (esp. in males with prostate problems)<br>• No WBC casts in urine (as compared with pyelonephritis)<br>• Systemic signs, such as fever and chills, are also uncommon with lower urinary tract infections; CVA tenderness usually absent |
| **Hemorrhagic cystitis** | Marked mucosal hemorrhage secondary to viruses, radiation, or chemotherapy (**cyclophosphamide**) |
| **Cystitis emphysematosa** | • Submucosal gas bubbles<br>• Occurs mostly in diabetics |
| **Bladder obstruction** | • **Men:** benign prostatic hyperplasia or carcinoma most common cause<br>• **Women:** cystocele of the bladder most common cause<br>• **Gross:** thickening, hypertrophy, and trabeculation of the smooth muscle bladder wall |
| **Carcinoma of the bladder** | • **Transitional cell carcinoma:** 90% of primary bladder neoplasms<br>• **Risk factors: Smoking,** occupational exposure **(e.g., naphthylamine),** infection with *Schistosoma haematobium* **(more commonly associated with squamous cell carcinoma)**<br>• 3% of all cancer deaths in the United States - peak incidence between 40 and 60 years of age.<br>• Usually presents with painless hematuria, may also cause dysuria, urgency, frequency, hydronephrosis, and pyelonephritis.<br>• Prognosis. High incidence of recurrence at multiple locations. |

# The Gastrointestinal System

# EMBRYOLOGY OF THE GASTROINTESTINAL SYSTEM

## DEVELOPMENT OF THE GASTROINTESTINAL TRACT

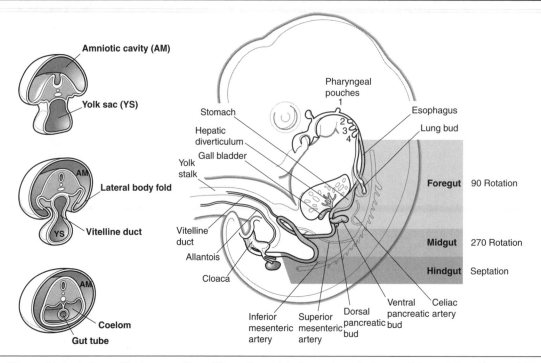

The **primitive gut tube** is formed by incorporation of the yolk sac into the embryo during cranial–caudal and lateral folding.

- The epithelial lining and glands of the mucosa are derived from **endoderm**. The epithelial lining of the gut tube proliferates rapidly and obliterates the lumen, followed by recanalization.
- The lamina propria, muscularis mucosa, submucosa, muscularis externa, and adventitia/serosa are derived from **mesoderm**.

The primitive gut tube is divided into the **foregut**, **midgut**, and **hindgut**, each supplied by a specific artery, each receiving a slightly different autonomic innervation, and each having slightly different relationships to a mesentery.

| ADULT STRUCTURES DERIVED FROM EACH OF THE THREE DIVISIONS OF THE PRIMITIVE GUT TUBE | | |
| --- | --- | --- |
| **Foregut** | **Midgut** | **Hindgut** |
| **Artery:** celiac | **Artery:** superior mesenteric | **Artery:** inferior mesenteric |
| **Parasympathetic innervation:** vagus nerves | **Parasympathetic innervation:** vagus nerves | **Parasympathetic innervation:** pelvic splanchnic nerves |
| **Sympathetic innervation:** greater splanchnic nerves, T5–T9* | **Sympathetic innervation:** lesser and lowest splanchnic nerves, T9–T12* | **Sympathetic innervation:** lumbar splanchnic nerves L1–L2* |
| **Foregut Derivatives** | **Midgut Derivatives** | **Hindgut Derivatives** |
| Esophagus<br>Stomach<br>Duodenum (first and second parts)<br>Liver<br>Pancreas<br>Biliary apparatus<br>Gall bladder<br>Pharyngeal pouches†<br>Lungs†<br>Thyroid†<br>Spleen‡ | Duodenum (second, third, and fourth parts)<br>Jejunum<br>Ileum<br>Cecum<br>Appendix<br>Ascending colon<br>Transverse colon (proximal two thirds) | Transverse colon (distal third)<br>Descending colon<br>Sigmoid colon<br>Rectum<br>Anal canal (above pectinate line) |

*Referred pain—stimulation of visceral pain fibers that innervate a gastrointestinal structure results in a dull, aching, poorly localized pain that is referred over the T5 through L1 dermatomes. The **sites of referred pain** generally correspond to the spinal cord segments that provide the sympathetic innervation to the affected gastrointestinal structure.

†Derivatives of endoderm, but not supplied by the celiac artery or innervated as above.

‡Spleen is not a foregut derivative, but is supplied by the celiac artery.

# GASTROINTESTINAL HISTOLOGY

## LAYERS OF THE DIGESTIVE TRACT

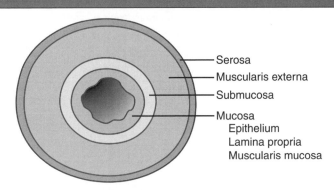

Serosa
Muscularis externa
Submucosa
Mucosa
  Epithelium
  Lamina propria
  Muscularis mucosa

*Submucosal plexus (Meissner plexus):* a collection of ganglia and interneurons of the enteric nervous system (ENS), predominantly responsible for regulating epithelial function and some circular smooth muscle function

*Myenteric plexus (Auerbach plexus):* a collection of ganglia and interneurons of the enteric nervous system (ENS), predominantly responsible for regulating longitudinal and some circular smooth muscle function

Note that the first third of esophageal muscle is skeletal, the middle third is mixed skeletal and smooth, and the final third is smooth muscle. Also, the stomach smooth muscle contains an oblique layer between the submucosa and circular layer of smooth muscle.

# HISTOLOGY OF SPECIFIC REGIONS

| Region | Major Characteristics | Mucosal Cell Types at Surface | Function of Surface Mucosal Cells |
|---|---|---|---|
| **Esophagus** | • Nonkeratinized stratified squamous epithelium<br>• Skeletal muscle in muscularis externa (upper 1/3)<br>• Smooth muscle (lower 1/3) | — | — |
| **Stomach** (body and fundus) | *Rugae:* shallow pits; deep glands | Mucous cells | Secrete mucus; form protective layer against acid; tight junctions between these cells probably contribute to the acid barrier of the epithelium. |
| | | Chief cells | Secrete pepsinogen and lipase precursor |
| | | Parietal cells | Secrete HCl and intrinsic factor |
| | | Enteroendocrine (EE) cells | Secrete a variety of peptide hormones |
| Pylorus | Deep pits; shallow branched glands | Mucous cells | Same as above |
| | | Parietal cells | Same as above |
| | | EE cells | High concentration of gastrin |
| **Small intestine** | Villi, plicae, and crypts | Columnar absorptive cells | Contain numerous microvilli that greatly increase the luminal surface area, facilitating absorption |
| Duodenum | Brunner glands, which discharge alkaline secretion | Goblet cells | Secrete acid glycoproteins that protect mucosal linings |
| | | Paneth cells | Contains granules that contain lysozyme. May play a role in regulating intestinal flora |
| | | EE cells | High concentration of cells that secrete cholecystokinin and secretin |
| Jejunum | Villi, well developed plica, crypts | Same cell types as found in the duodenal epithelium | Same as above |
| Ileum | Aggregations of lymph nodules called Peyer patches | M cells found over lymphatic nodules and Peyer patches | Endocytose and transport antigen from the lumen to lymphoid cells |
| **Large intestine** | Lacks villi, crypts | Mainly mucus-secreting and absorptive cells | Transports Na$^+$ (actively) and water (passively) out of lumen |

## ABDOMINAL VISCERA

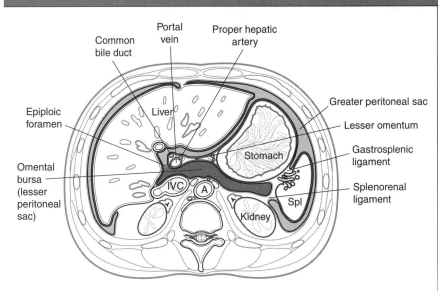

Viscera are classified as:

- **Peritoneal organs**—have a mesentery and are almost completely enclosed in peritoneum. These organs are mobile.

- **Retroperitoneal organs**—are partially covered with peritoneum and are immobile or fixed organs.

This figure is a cross-section of the abdomen that shows the greater and lesser peritoneal sacs and associated abdominal viscera.

| Major Peritoneal Organs (suspended by a mesentery) | Major Secondary Retroperitoneal Organs (lost a mesentery during development) | Major Primary Retroperitoneal Organs (never had a mesentery) |
|---|---|---|
| Stomach | Midgut duodenum | Kidneys |
| Liver and gallbladder | Head, neck, and body of pancreas | Adrenal glands |
| Spleen | Ascending colon | Ureter |
| Foregut duodenum | Descending colon | Aorta |
| Tail of pancreas | Upper rectum | Inferior vena cava |
| Jejunum | | Lower rectum |
| Ileum | | Anal canal |
| Appendix | | |
| Transverse colon | | |

ORGAN SYSTEMS

GASTROINTESTINAL

ORGAN SYSTEMS

GASTROINTESTINAL

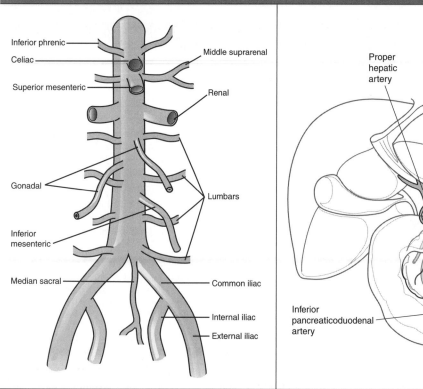

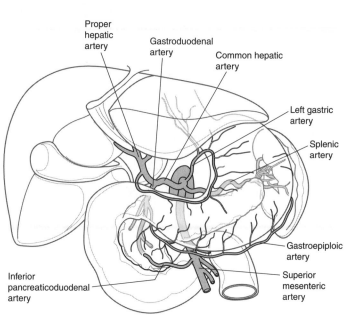

## Clinical Correlations

In an **occlusion of the celiac artery** at its origin from the abdominal aorta, collateral circulation may develop in the **head of the pancreas** by way of anastomoses between the **pancreaticoduodenal branches of both the superior mesenteric** and the gastroduodenal arteries.

Branches of the **celiac circulation** may be subject to **erosion** if an ulcer penetrates the posterior wall of the stomach or the posterior wall of the duodenum.

- The **splenic artery** may be subject to erosion by a penetrating ulcer of the **posterior wall** of the stomach.
- The **left gastric artery** may be subject to erosion by a penetrating ulcer of the **lesser curvature** of the stomach.
- The **gastroduodenal artery** may be subject to erosion by a penetrating ulcer of the **posterior wall** of the first part of the duodenum.

Patients with a penetrating ulcer may have **pain referred to the shoulder**, which occurs when air escapes through the ulcer and stimulates the peritoneum covering the inferior aspect of the diaphragm. The contents of a **penetrating ulcer** of the posterior wall of the stomach or the duodenum may enter the **omental bursa**.

**Hematemesis** may result from bleeding into the lumen of the esophagus, stomach, or duodenum proximal to the ligament of Treitz. Hematemesis is commonly caused by a duodenal ulcer, a gastric ulcer, or esophageal varices.

## Superior and Inferior Mesenteric Arteries

| Superior Mesenteric Artery Distribution | Inferior Mesenteric Artery Distribution |
| --- | --- |

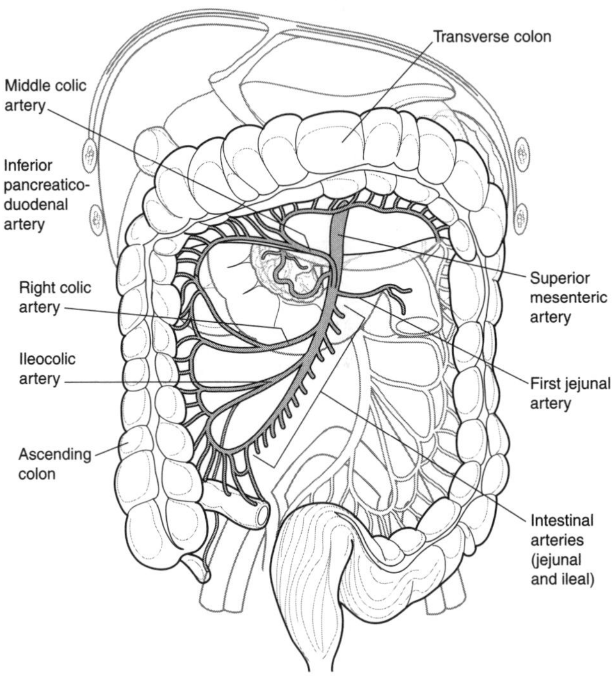
Transverse colon
Middle colic artery
Inferior pancreaticoduodenal artery
Right colic artery
Ileocolic artery
Ascending colon
Superior mesenteric artery
First jejunal artery
Intestinal arteries (jejunal and ileal)

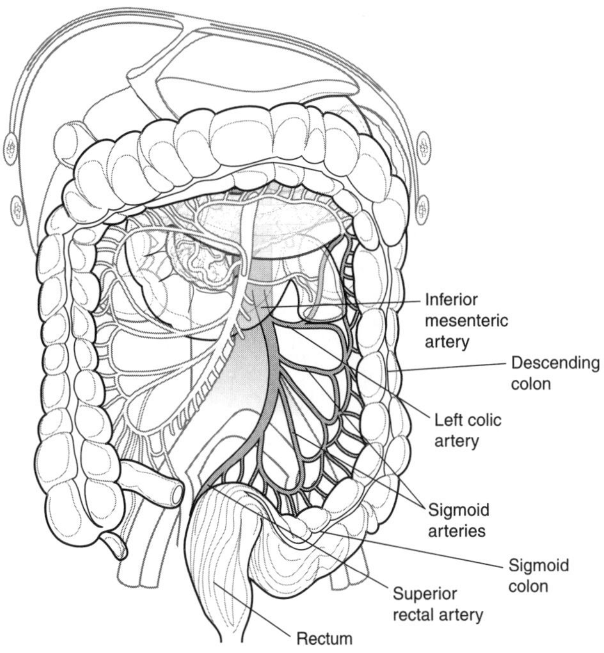
Inferior mesenteric artery
Descending colon
Left colic artery
Sigmoid arteries
Sigmoid colon
Superior rectal artery
Rectum

### Clinical Correlation

- Common sites of **ischemic bowel infarction** are in the transverse colon near the splenic flexure and in the rectum.
- **Infarction of the transverse colon** occurs between the distal parts of the middle colic branches of the superior mesenteric and left colic branches of the inferior mesenteric arteries.
- **Infarction of the rectum** occurs between the distal parts of the superior rectal branches of the inferior mesenteric artery and the middle rectal branches of the internal iliac artery.

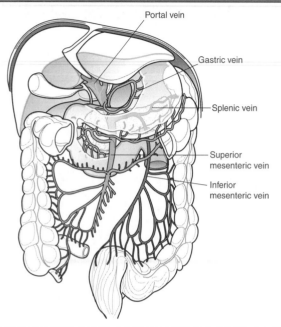

**Portal vein**

**Gastric vein**

**Splenic vein**

**Superior mesenteric vein**

**Inferior mesenteric vein**

### Clinical Correlation

Patients with cirrhosis of the liver may develop **portal hypertension**, in which venous blood from gastrointestinal structures, which normally enters the liver by way of the portal vein, is forced to flow in the retrograde direction in tributaries of the portal vein.

Retrograde flow forces portal venous blood into tributaries of the superior or inferior vena cava; **portacaval anastomoses** are established at these sites, permitting portal venous blood to bypass the liver.

| Sites of Anastomoses | Portal | Caval | Clinical Signs |
|---|---|---|---|
| 1. Umbilicus | Paraumbilical veins | Superficial veins of the anterior abdominal wall | Caput medusa |
| 2. Rectum | Superior rectal veins (inferior mesenteric vein) | Middle and inferior rectal veins (internal iliac vein) | Internal hemorrhoids |
| 3. Esophagus | Gastric veins | Veins of the lower esophagus, which drain into the azygos system | Esophageal varices |
| 4. Retroperitoneal organs | Tributaries of the superior and inferior mesenteric veins | Veins of the posterior abdominal wall | Not clinically relevant |

## INFERIOR VENA CAVA (IVC) AND TRIBUTARIES

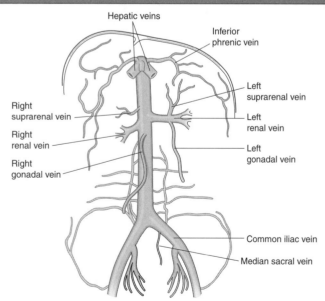

**Hepatic veins**

**Inferior phrenic vein**

**Left suprarenal vein**

**Left renal vein**

**Left gonadal vein**

**Right suprarenal vein**

**Right renal vein**

**Right gonadal vein**

**Common iliac vein**

**Median sacral vein**

The **inferior vena cava** is formed at about the level of the L5 vertebra by the union of the common iliac veins. It ascends just to the right of the midline.

On the right, the renal, adrenal, and gonadal veins drain directly into the inferior vena cava.

On the left, only the **left renal vein** drains directly into the inferior vena cava; the left gonadal and the left adrenal veins drain into the left renal vein. The left renal vein crosses the anterior aspect of the aorta just inferior to the origin of the superior mesenteric artery.

### Clinical Correlation

The **left renal vein may be compressed** by an **aneurysm of the superior mesenteric artery** as the vein crosses anterior to the aorta. Patients with compression of the left renal vein may have renal and adrenal hypertension on the left, and, in males, a varicocele on the left.

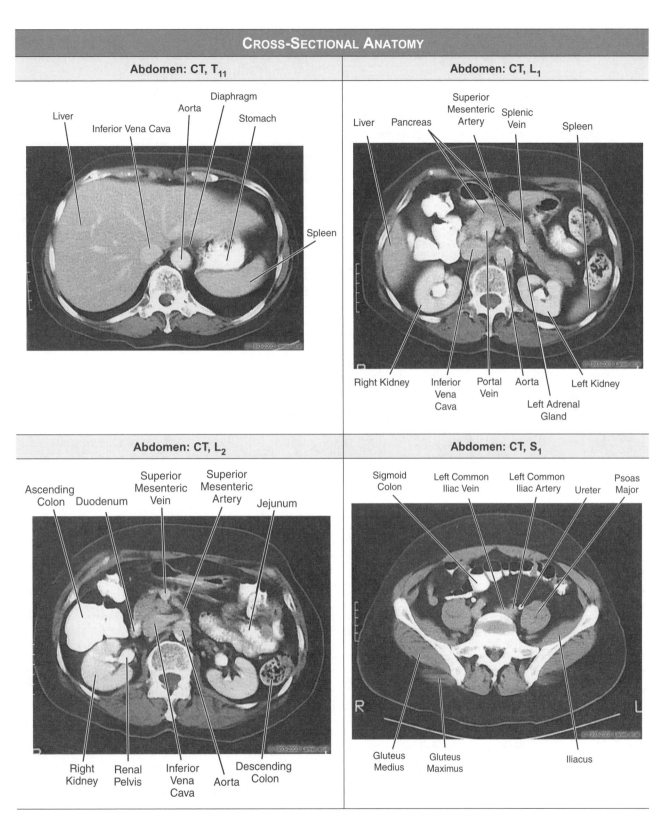

**Abdomen: CT, T₁₁**

Liver
Inferior Vena Cava
Aorta
Diaphragm
Stomach
Spleen

**Abdomen: CT, L₁**

Liver
Pancreas
Superior Mesenteric Artery
Splenic Vein
Spleen

Right Kidney
Inferior Vena Cava
Portal Vein
Aorta
Left Kidney
Left Adrenal Gland

**Abdomen: CT, L₂**

Ascending Colon
Duodenum
Superior Mesenteric Vein
Superior Mesenteric Artery
Jejunum

Right Kidney
Renal Pelvis
Inferior Vena Cava
Aorta
Descending Colon

**Abdomen: CT, S₁**

Sigmoid Colon
Left Common Iliac Vein
Left Common Iliac Artery
Ureter
Psoas Major

Gluteus Medius
Gluteus Maximus
Iliacus

ORGAN SYSTEMS

GASTROINTESTINAL

# GASTROINTESTINAL PHYSIOLOGY

## APPETITE

Appetite is primarily regulated by two regions of the hypothalamus: a feeding center and a satiety center. Normally, the feeding center is active, but is transiently inhibited by the satiety center.

### Hypothalamus

| | Location | Stimulation | Destruction |
|---|---|---|---|
| **Feeding center** | Lateral hypothalamic area | Feeding | Anorexia |
| **Satiety center** | Ventromedial nucleus of hypothalamus | Cessation of feeding | Hypothalamic obesity syndrome |

### Hormones That May Affect Appetite

| | |
|---|---|
| **Cholecystokinin (CCK)** | • Released from I-cells in the mucosa of the small intestine<br>• CCK-A receptors are in the periphery<br>• CCK-B receptors are in the brain—both reduce appetite when stimulated |
| **Calcitonin** | • Released mainly from the thyroid gland<br>• Has also been reported to decrease appetite by an unknown mechanism |

### Mechanical Distention

- Distention of the alimentary tract inhibits appetite, whereas the contractions of an empty stomach stimulate it.
- Some satiety is derived from mastication and swallowing alone.

### Miscellaneous

Other factors that help to determine appetite and body weight include body levels of fat and genetic factors.

## SALIVA

| | |
|---|---|
| **Salivary glands**<br>Submandibular<br>Parotid<br>Sublingual | • Produce approximately 1.5 L/day of saliva<br>• The presence of food in the mouth, the taste, smell, sight, or thought of food, or the stimulation of vagal afferents at the distal end of the esophagus increase the production of saliva. |
| **Functions** | • Initial triglyceride digestion (lingual lipase)<br>• Initial starch digestion ($\alpha$-amylase)<br>• Lubrication |
| **Composition** | **Ions:** $HCO_3^-$ 3× [plasma]; $K^+$ 7 × [plasma]; $Na^+$ 0.1 × [plasma]; $Cl^-$ 0.15 × [plasma]<br>**Enzymes:** $\alpha$-amylase, lingual lipase<br>**Hypotonic**<br>**pH:** 7–8<br>**Flow rate:** alters the composition<br>**Antibacterial:** lysozyme, lactoferrin, defensins, IgA |
| **Regulation** | **Parasympathetic** — ↑ synthesis and secretion of **watery** saliva via muscarinic receptor stimulation; (anticholinergics → dry mouth)<br>**Sympathetic** — ↑ synthesis and secretion of **viscous** saliva via β-adrenergic receptor stimulation |

ORGAN SYSTEMS

GASTROINTESTINAL

## SWALLOWING

Swallowing is a reflex action coordinated in the **swallowing center** in the medulla. Afferents are carried by the glossopharyngeal (CN IX) and vagus (CN X) nerves. Food is moved to the esophagus by the movement of tongue (hypoglossal nerve, CN XII) and the palatal and pharyngeal muscles (CNs IX and X).

1. **Initiation of swallowing** occurs voluntarily when the mouth is closed on a bolus of food and the tongue propels it from the oral cavity into the pharynx.
2. **Involuntary contraction** of the **pharynx** advances the bolus into the esophagus.
3. Automatic **closure of the glottis** during swallowing inhibits breathing and prevents aspiration.
4. Relaxation of the **upper esophageal sphincter (UES)** allows food to enter the esophagus.
5. **Peristaltic contraction of the esophagus** propels food toward the **lower esophageal sphincter (LES)**, the muscle at the gastroesophageal junction.
6. The LES is tonically contracted, relaxing on swallowing. **Relaxation of the LES** is mediated via the vagus nerve; **VIP** (vasoactive inhibitory peptide) is the major neurotransmitter causing LES relaxation.

### Clinical Correlation

| | |
|---|---|
| **Achalasia** | **Pathologic inability of the LES to relax** during swallowing. Food accumulates in the esophagus, sometimes causing **megaesophagus**. |
| **Gastric reflux** | **LES tone** is low, allowing acid reflux into the esophagus; can lead to gastroesophageal reflux disease (**GERD**). |

## THE STOMACH

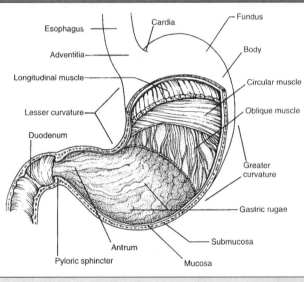

- The stomach has **three layers of smooth muscle**: longitudinal (outer, for peristalsis), circular (for mixing), and oblique (inner).

- The stomach is composed of the **fundus**, **body**, and **antrum**.

- **Receptive relaxation** mediated by VIP occurs in the fundus. As the stomach fills, a vagovagal-mediated receptive relaxation occurs, allowing storage.

- The bolus of swallowed food received by the stomach is further macerated and mixed with HCl, mucus, and pepsin. The food **(chyme)** is then discharged at a controlled rate into the duodenum. Only a small amount of chemical digestion actually occurs in the stomach.

### Gastric Motility

- A pacemaker within the greater curvature produces a **basal electric rhythm (BER)** of 3 to 5 waves/min.
- The **magnitude** of the gastric contractions are **increased by parasympathetic** and **decreased by sympathetic stimulation**.
- **Migrating motor complexes (MMC)** are propulsive contractions initiated during fasting that begin in the stomach and move undigested material from the stomach and small intestine into the colon. They repeat every 90 to 120 minutes and are mediated by **motilin**. This housekeeping function lowers the bacterial count in the gut.

### Gastric Emptying

- The **pylorus** is continuous with the circular muscle layer and acts as a "valve" to control gastric emptying.
- The contractions of the stomach (peristalsis) propel chyme through the pylorus at a regulated rate.
- Pyloric sphincter contraction at the time of antral contraction limits the movement of chyme into the duodenum and promotes mixing by forceful regurgitation of antral contents back into the fundus (**retropulsion**).
- **Gastric emptying is delayed by:**
  - **Fat/protein in the duodenum stimulating CCK release**, which increases gastric distensibility
  - **$H^+$ in the duodenum** via neural reflexes
  - Stomach contents that are hypertonic or hypotonic

*Definition of abbreviation:* VIP, vasoactive intestinal peptide.

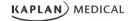

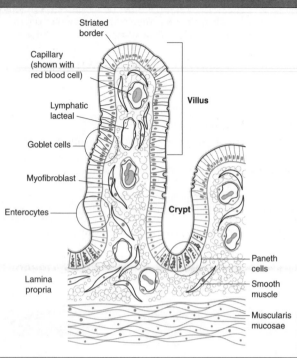

- The small intestine participates in the **digestion and absorption** of nutrients. It has specialized villi on the epithelial surface to aid in this function.

- The **duodenum** is the proximal pyloric end of the small intestine. Distal to the duodenum is the **jejunum**, and then the **ileum**.

- In the small intestine, the chyme from the stomach is **mixed** with mucosal cell secretions, exocrine pancreatic juice, and bile.

- **Mucus production** occurs in surface epithelial cells throughout the gastrointestinal tract, **Brunner glands** in the duodenum, and **goblet cells** in the mucosa throughout the intestine.

- **Mucus functions** include lubrication of the gastrointestinal tract, binding bacteria, and trapping immunoglobulins where they have access to pathogens.

- The **rate of mucus** secretion is increased by cholinergic stimulation, chemical irritation, and physical irritation.

### Clinical Correlate

Any compromise of the mucous protection can lead to significant damage and irritation of the gastrointestinal tract, leading to gastritis, duodenitis, or even peptic ulcer disease.

### Intestinal Motility

- **Small bowel slow waves** move caudally in the circular smooth muscle. The rate slows from approximately 12/min in the jejunum to approximately 9/min in the ileum.

- **Segmentation contractions** are ring-like contractions that **mix intestinal contents**. They occur at random "nodes" along the intestine. These relax, and then new nodes are formed at the former internodes. This action moves the chyme back and forth, increasing mucosal exposure to the chyme.

- **Peristalsis** is a reflex response initiated by stretching of the lumen of the gut. There is contraction of muscle at the oral end and relaxation of muscle at the caudal end, thus **propelling the contents caudally**. Although peristalsis is modulated by autonomic input, it can occur even in isolated loops of small bowel with no extrinsic innervation.

  - The intrinsic control system senses stretch with calcitonin gene-related polypeptide neurons (CGRP).
  - The contractile wave is initiated by acetylcholine (ACh) and substance P.
  - The relaxation caudal to the stimulus is initiated by nitric oxide (NO) and VIP.

- **Parasympathetic stimulation ↑ contractions** and **sympathetic stimulation ↓ contractions.**

- The **gastroileal reflex** is caused by food in the stomach, which stimulates peristalsis in the ileum and relaxes the ileocecal valve. This delivers intestinal contents to the large intestine.

- Small intestinal **secretions** are generally **alkaline**, serving to neutralize the acidic nature of the chyme entering from the pylorus.

### Clinical Correlation

Peristalsis is activated by the **parasympathetic system**. For those suffering from decreased intestinal motility manifesting as constipation (paralytic ileus, diabetic gastroparesis), dopaminergic and cholinergic agents are often used (e.g., metoclopramide).

# LARGE INTESTINE (COLON)

## General Features

- The colon is larger in diameter and shorter in length than is the small intestine. Fecal material moves from the **cecum**, through the colon (**ascending**, **transverse**, **descending**, and **sigmoid colons**), rectum, and anal canal.
- Three longitudinal bands of muscle, the **teniae coli**, constitute the outer layer. Because the colon is longer than these bands, pouching occurs, creating **haustra** between the teniae and giving the colon its characteristic "caterpillar" appearance.
- The mucosa has **no villi**, and mucus is secreted by short, inward-projecting colonic glands.
- Abundant lymphoid follicles are found in the cecum and appendix and more sparsely elsewhere.
- The major functions of the colon are **reabsorption of fluid and electrolytes** and **temporary storage of feces**.

## Colonic Motility

- **Peristaltic waves** briefly open the normally closed ileocecal valve, passing a small amount of chyme into the cecum. Peristalsis also advances the chyme in the colon. Slow waves, approximately 2/min, are initiated at the ileocecal valve and increase to approximately 6/min at the sigmoid colon.
- **Segmentation contractions** mix the contents of the colon back and forth.
- **Mass movement contractions** are found only in the colon. Constriction of long lengths of colon propels large amounts of chyme distally toward the anus. Mass movements propel feces into the rectum. Distention of the rectum with feces initiates the **defecation reflex**.

## Absorption

The mucosa of the colon has great absorptive capability. **$Na^+$ is actively transported with water following**, and **$K^+$ and $HCO_3^-$ are secreted into the colon**.

## Defecation

| | |
|---|---|
| **Feces** | Contains undigested plant fibers, bacteria, inorganic matter, and water. Nondietary material (e.g., sloughed-off mucosa) constitutes a large portion of the feces. In normal feces, 30% of the solids may be bacteria. Bacteria synthesize **vitamin K**, B-complex vitamins, and folic acid, split urea to $NH_3$, and produce small organic acids from unabsorbed fat and carbohydrate. |
| **Defecation** | Rectal distention with feces activates intrinsic and cord reflexes that cause relaxation of the internal anal sphincter (smooth muscle) and produce the urge to defecate. If the external anal sphincter (skeletal muscle innervated by the **pudendal nerve**) is then voluntarily relaxed, and intra-abdominal pressure is increased via the **Valsalva maneuver**, defecation occurs. If the external sphincter is held contracted, the urge to defecate temporarily diminishes. |
| **Gastrocolic reflex** | Distention of the stomach by food **increases the frequency of mass movements** and produces the urge to defecate. This reflex is mediated by **parasympathetic** nerves. |

# VOMITING

Vomiting occurs in three phases: **nausea**, **retching**, and **vomiting**.

- **Nausea**—hypersalivation, decreased gastric tone, increased duodenal and proximal jejunal tone → reflux of contents into stomach
- **Retching**—Gastric contents travel to the esophagus. Retching occurs if upper esophageal sphincter (UES) remains closed.
- **Vomiting**—If pressure increases enough to open the UES, vomiting occurs; vomiting can be triggered by oropharyngeal stimulation, gastric overdistention and gastroparesis, vestibular stimulation, or input from the **chemoreceptor trigger zone**, located in the **area postrema** in the floor of the fourth ventricle, which stimulates the medullary vomiting center.

| ANTIEMETICS | | |
|---|---|---|
| **Drug Class** | **Agents** | **Comments** |
| **5HT$_3$ antagonists** | **Ondansetron**<br>Granisetron, dolasetron | May act in chemoreceptor trigger zone and in peripheral sites |
| **DA antagonists** | **Phenothiazine**, metoclopramide* | Block D$_2$ receptors in chemoreceptor trigger zone |
| **Cannabinoids** | **Dronabinol** | Active ingredient in marijuana |

| EMETICS | |
|---|---|
| **Ipecac** | • Locally irritates the GI tract and stimulates the chemoreceptor trigger zone<br>• If emesis does not occur in 15-20 min, lavage must be used to remove ipecac |
| **Apomorphine** | • Dopamine-receptor agonist that stimulates the chemoreceptor trigger zone<br>• Vomiting should occur within 5 min |

*Also a prokinetic agent

## GASTROINTESTINAL HORMONES

Gastrointestinal hormones are released into the systemic circulation after physiologic stimulation (e.g., by food in gut), can exert their effects independent of the nervous system when administered exogenously, and have been chemically identified and synthesized. The five gastrointestinal hormones include **secretin, gastrin, cholecystokinin (CCK), gastric inhibitory peptide (GIP)**, and **motilin**.

| Hormone | Source | Stimulus | Actions |
|---|---|---|---|
| **Gastrin*, ‡** | **G cells** of gastric antrum | • **Small peptides, amino acids, Ca$^{2+}$ in lumen of stomach**<br>• Vagus (via **GRP**)<br>• **Stomach distension**<br>• **Inhibited by: H$^+$ in lumen of antrum** | • **↑ HCl secretion by parietal cells**<br>• **Trophic effects on GI mucosa**<br>• ↑ pepsinogen secretion by chief cells<br>• ↑ histamine secretion by ECL cells |
| **CCK*** | **I cells** of duodenum and jejunum | • **Fatty acids, monoglycerides**<br>• **Small peptides and amino acids** | • **Stimulates gallbladder contraction** and **relaxes sphincter of Oddi**<br>• **↑ pancreatic enzyme secretion**<br>• Augments secretin-induced stimulation of pancreatic HCO$_3^-$<br>• **Inhibits gastric emptying**<br>• Trophic effect on exocrine pancreas/gallbladder |
| **Secretin†** | **S cells** of duodenum | • **↓ pH** in duodenal lumen<br>• **Fatty acids** in duodenal lumen | • **↑ pancreatic HCO$_3^-$ secretion** (neutralizes H$^+$)<br>• Trophic effect on exocrine pancreas<br>• **↑ bile production**<br>• **↓ gastric H$^+$ secretion** |
| **GIP†** | K cells of duodenum and jejunum | **Glucose, fatty acids, amino acids** | • **↑ insulin release**<br>• **↓ gastric H$^+$ secretion** |
| **Motilin** | Enterochromaffin cells in duodenum and jejunum | Absence of food for >2 hours | Initiates MMC motility pattern in stomach and small intestine |

(Continued)

| Gastrointestinal Hormones *(Cont'd.)* | | | |
|---|---|---|---|
| **Paracrines/ Neurocrines** | **Source** | **Stimulus** | **Actions** |
| Somatostatin | D cells throughout GI tract | ↓ pH in lumen | • ↓ gallbladder contraction, pancreatic secretion<br>• ↓ gastric acid and pepsinogen secretion<br>• ↓ small intestinal fluid secretion<br>• ↓ ACh release from the myenteric plexus and decreases motility<br>• ↓ α-cell release of glucagon, and β-cell release of insulin in pancreatic islet cells |
| Histamine | Enterochromaffin cells | • Gastrin<br>• ACh | ↑ **gastric acid secretion** (directly, and potentiates gastrin and vagal stimulation) |
| VIP[†, ¶] | Neurons in GI tract | • Vagal stimulation<br>• Intestinal distention | • **Relaxation of intestinal smooth muscle, including sphincters**<br>• ↑ **Pancreatic HCO$_3^-$ secretion**<br>• **Stimulates intestinal secretion of electrolytes and H$_2$O** |
| GRP | Vagal nerve endings | Cephalic stimulation, gastric distension | **Stimulates gastrin release** from G cells |
| Pancreatic polypeptide | F cells of pancreas, small intestine | Protein, fat, glucose in lumen | ↓ pancreatic secretion |
| Enteroglucagon | L cells of intestine | — | • ↓ gastric, pancreatic secretions<br>• ↑ insulin release |

*Definition of abbreviations:* ECL, enterochromaffin-like cells; GIP, gastric inhibitory peptide; GRP, gastrin-releasing peptide.

*Member of gastrin-CCK family

[†]Member of secretin-glucagon family

**Clinical Correlates:**

[‡]**Zollinger-Ellison syndrome (gastrinoma)**—non-β islet-cell pancreatic tumor that produces gastrin, leading to ↑ in gastric acid secretion and development of peptic ulcer disease

[¶]**VIPoma**—tumor of non-α, non-β islet cells of the pancreas that secretes VIP, causing watery diarrhea

## GASTRIC SECRETIONS

| Secretion Product | Cell Type | Region of Stomach | Stimulus for Secretion | Inhibitors of Secretion | Action of Secretory Product |
|---|---|---|---|---|---|
| HCl | Parietal (oxyntic) cells | Body/fundus | • Gastrin<br>• ACh (from vagus)<br>• Histamine | • **Low pH** inhibits (by inhibiting gastrin)<br>• Prostaglandins<br>• Chyme in duodenum (via GIP and secretin) | • Kills pathogens<br>• Activates pepsinogen to pepsin |
| Intrinsic factor | | | | | Necessary for **vitamin B$_{12}$** absorption by the ileum; forms complex with vitamin B$_{12}$ |
| Pepsinogen (zymogen, precursor of **pepsin**) | Chief cells | Body/fundus | • ACh (from vagus)<br>• Gastrin<br>• HCl | H$^+$ (via somatostatin) | • Converted to pepsin by ↓ pH and pepsin (autocatalytic)<br>• **Digests up to 20% of proteins** |
| Gastrin | G cells | Antrum | • Small peptides/aa<br>• Vagus (via GRP)<br>• Stomach distention | H$^+$ (via somatostatin) | • **↑ HCl secretion (parietal cells)**<br>• ↑ pepsinogen secretion (chief cells)<br>• ↑ histamine secretion by ECL cells |
| Mucus | Mucous cells | Entire stomach | ACh (from vagus) | | Forms gel on mucosa to protect mucosa from HCl and pepsin; traps HCO$_3$$^-$ to help neutralize acid |

*Definition of abbreviations:* aa, amino acids; ECL, enterochromaffin-like cells.

## MECHANISM OF GASTRIC H$^+$ SECRETION

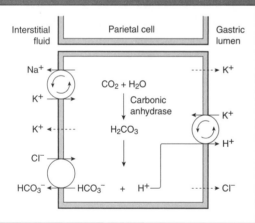

- In the parietal cell, CO$_2$ and H$_2$O are converted by carbonic anhydrase to H$^+$ and HCO$_3$$^-$.
- H$^+$ is secreted into the lumen of the stomach by H$^+$-K$^+$ pump (**H$^+$/K$^+$–ATPase**). Cl$^-$ is secreted with H$^+$.
- HCO$_3$$^-$ is absorbed into the bloodstream in exchange for Cl$^-$.
- After a meal, enough H$^+$ may be secreted to raise the pH of systemic blood and turn the urine alkaline (**"alkaline tide"**).

The three primary triggers of H$^+$ secretion are:

- **ACh** (from vagus), via the M$_3$ muscarinic receptor
- **Histamine**, via the H$_2$ histamine receptor
- **Gastrin**, via unidentified receptor

## Drugs for Peptic Ulcer Disease

| Drug Class | Agents | Comments |
|---|---|---|
| Antacids | Magnesium hydroxide, aluminum hydroxide, calcium carbonate | *Magnesium:* **laxative** effect<br>*Aluminum hydroxide:* **constipating** effect |
| H₂ antagonists | **Cimetidine**, ranitidine, famotidine, nizatidine | • Useful in PUD, GERD, Zollinger-Ellison syndrome, but not as effective as proton pump inhibitors<br>• **Cimetidine inhibits hepatic drug metabolizing enzymes** and has **antiandrogen effects** |
| Proton pump inhibitors | **Omeprazole**, lansoprazole, esomeprazole, pantoprazole, rabeprazole | • Irreversibly **inactivate $H^+/K^+$-ATPase**, thus blocking $H^+$ secretion.<br>• Work very well—useful in PUD, Zollinger-Ellison syndrome, and GERD |
| Mucosal protective agents | **Sucralfate** | Polymerizes in the stomach and forms protective coating over ulcer beds. |
| | Misoprostol | $PGE_1$ derivative used for peptic ulcers caused by NSAIDs |
| Antibiotics | Macrolides, metronidazole, tetracyclines (various combinations) | To treat *H. pylori* |

*Definition of abbreviations:* GERD, gastroesophageal reflux disorder; $PGE_1$, prostaglandin $E_1$; NSAIDs, nonsteroidal antiinflammatory drugs; PUD, peptic ulcer disease.

## Phases of Gastric Secretion

| | |
|---|---|
| Cephalic phase | The smell, sight, thought, or chewing of food can increase gastric secretion via parasympathetic (vagal) pathways. Responsible for approximately 30% of acid secreted. |
| Gastric phase | Food in the stomach ↑ secretion. The greatest effects occur with proteins and peptides, leading to **gastrin** release (alcohol and caffeine also exert a strong effect). Gastric distention initiates vagovagal reflexes. Accounts for approximately 60% of acid secreted. |
| Intestinal phase | Protein digestion products in the duodenum stimulate duodenal gastrin secretion. In addition, absorbed amino acids act to stimulate $H^+$ secretion by parietal cells. The intestinal phase accounts for less than 10% of the gastric secretory response to a meal. |

The exocrine secretions of the pancreas are produced by the **acinar cells**, which contain numerous enzyme-containing granules in their cytoplasm, and by the **ductal cells**, which secrete $HCO_3^-$. The secretions reach the duodenum via the **pancreatic duct**.

| | |
|---|---|
| **Bicarbonate ($HCO_3^-$)** | • $HCO_3^-$ in the duodenum **neutralizes HCl in chyme** entering from the stomach. This also deactivates pepsin. |
| | • When $H^+$ enters the duodenum, S cells secrete **secretin**, which acts on pancreatic ductal cells to increase $HCO_3^-$ production. |
| | • $HCO_3^-$ is produced by the action of **carbonic anhydrase** on $CO_2$ and $H_2O$ in the pancreatic ductal cells. $HCO_3^-$ is secreted into the lumen of the duct in exchange for $Cl^-$. |
| **Pancreatic enzymes** | • Approximately 15 enzymes are produced by the pancreas, which are responsible for **digesting proteins, carbohydrates, lipids, and nucleic acids**. |
| | • When small peptides, amino acids, and fatty acids enter the duodenum, **CCK** is released by I cells, stimulating pancreatic enzyme secretion. |
| | • **ACh** (via vagovagal reflexes) also stimulates enzyme secretion and potentiates the action of secretin. |
| | • **Protection of pancreatic acinar cells against self-digestion:**<br>  – **Proteolytic enzymes are secreted as inactive precursors**, which are activated in the gut lumen. For example, the duodenal brush border enzyme, **enterokinase**, converts trypsinogen to the active enzyme, trypsin. Trypsin then catalyzes the formation of more trypsin and activates chymotrypsinogen, procarboxypeptidase, and prophospholipases A and B. Ribonucleases, amylase, and lipase do not exist as proenzymes.<br>  – Produce **enzyme inhibitors** to inactivate trace amounts of active enzyme formed within. |

| Enzyme | Reaction Catalyzed |
|---|---|
| **Proteases:** | |
| Trypsin | Proteins → peptides |
| Chymotrypsin | Proteins → peptides |
| Carboxypeptidase | Peptides → amino acids |
| | |
| **Polysaccharidase:** | |
| Amylase | Starch and glycogen → maltose, maltotriose, and α-limit dextrins |
| | |
| **Lipases:** | |
| Phospholipases A and B | Phospholipids → phosphate, fatty acids, and glycerol |
| Esterases | Cholesterol esters → free cholesterol and fatty acids |
| Triacylglycerol lipases | Triglycerides → fatty acids and monoglycerides |
| | |
| **Nucleases:** | |
| Ribonuclease | RNA → ribonucleotides |
| Deoxyribonuclease | DNA → deoxyribonucleotides |

| Physiologic roles | • Excretion of **bilirubin**, **cholesterol**, drugs, and **toxins**<br>• Promotion of **intestinal lipid absorption**<br>• Delivery of **IgA** to small intestine |
|---|---|
| Components of bile | • Bile—composed of **bile salts, phospholipids, cholesterol, bilirubin (bile pigments), water, and electrolytes** |

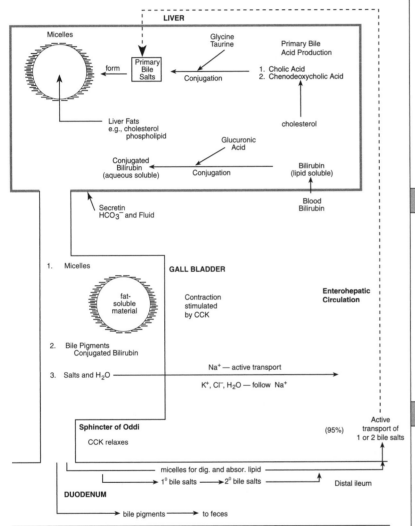

### Formation of Bile

• Bile, produced by hepatocytes, drains into **hepatic ducts** and is stored in the **gallbladder** for later release.

• **Primary bile acids** (cholic and chenodeoxycholic acids) are made from cholesterol in the liver. **Secondary bile acids** (deoxycholic and lithocholic) are products of bacterial metabolism of primary bile acids in the gut.

• All bile acids must be conjugated with **glycine** or **taurine** to form their **bile salt** before being secreted into bile.

• Above a **critical micellar concentration**, bile salts form **micelles**. Electrolytes and $H_2O$ are also added to the bile.

### Micelles

• Micelles are water soluble-spheres with a lipid-soluble interior.

• Micelles are vital in the digestion, transport, and absorption of lipid-soluble substances from the duodenum to the distal ileum, where bile salts are actively reabsorbed and recycled (**enterohepatic circulation**).

• A lack of reabsorbing mechanisms or distal ileal disease can lead to deficiency of bile salts. This can lead to malabsorption, gallstones, and **steatorrhea**.

### Gallbladder

• The gallbladder concentrates and stores bile for release during meals.

• During the interdigestive period, the **sphincter of Oddi** is closed and the gallbladder is relaxed, allowing it to fill with bile.

• Bile is **concentrated** in the gallbladder by water and electrolyte absorption.

• Small peptides and fatty acids in the duodenum cause **CCK** secretion, which causes **gallbladder contraction** and **relaxation of the sphincter of Oddi**. ACh also aids in this process.

*(Continued)*

ORGAN SYSTEMS

GASTROINTESTINAL

| Bilirubin | • Bilirubin is a product of **heme metabolism**.<br>• It is taken up by hepatocytes and **conjugated with glucuronic acid** prior to secretion into bile. This gives bile a golden yellow color. In the large intestine, bilirubin is deconjugated and metabolized by bacteria to form **urobilinogens** (colorless). Some of the urobilinogens are reabsorbed; most of the reabsorbed urobilinogens are secreted into bile, with the remainder excreted in the urine.<br>• Most urobilinogen remains in the gut and is further reduced to pigmented compounds (stercobilins and urobilins) and excreted in feces. **Stercobilins** give a brown color to feces.<br>• **Jaundice** (yellowing of the skin and whites of the eyes) is a result of **elevated bilirubin**. |
|---|---|
| **Regulation of bile secretion** | • **Secretin** stimulates the secretion of bile **high in $HCO_3^-$ content** from the biliary ductules, but does not alter bile salt output.<br>• Secretion of bile salts by hepatocytes is directly proportional to hepatic portal vein concentration of bile salts. |

## DIGESTION AND ABSORPTION

- Carbohydrates, lipids, and proteins are digested and absorbed in the small intestine.
- The brush border of the small intestine increases surface area, greatly facilitating absorption of nutrients.

| Carbohydrate digestion | Must be converted to **monosaccharides** in order to be absorbed |
|---|---|
| | **Mouth** |
| | • **Salivary amylase** normally hydrolyzes approximately 10 to 20% of ingested starch.<br>• It **hydrolyzes only** α-**(1:4)-glycosidic linkages** to maltose, maltotriose, and α-limit dextrins. |
| | **Intestine** |
| | • **Pancreatic amylase** is found in the highest concentration in the duodenal lumen, where it rapidly hydrolyzes starch to oligosaccharides, maltose, maltotriose, and α-limit dextrins.<br>• **Maltase, α-dextrinase, lactase, sucrase,** and **isomaltase** are found in the **brush border**, with the highest concentrations in the mid-jejunum and proximal ileum.<br>  – α-**dextrinase:** cleaves terminal α-1,4 bonds, producing free glucose<br>  – **Lactase:** converts lactose to glucose and galactose<br>  – **Sucrase:** converts sucrose to glucose and fructose<br>  – **Maltase:** converts maltose and maltotriose to 2 and 3 glucose units, respectively.<br>• The monosaccharide end products (**glucose, galactose,** and **fructose**) are readily absorbed from the small intestine, primarily in the jejunum. |
| | **Clinical Correlation** |
| | • **Lactase deficiency** causes an inability to digest lactose into glucose and galactose.<br>• *Consequence:* ↑ osmotic load, giving rise to **osmotic diarrhea** and **flatulence**.<br>• Very common in African Americans, Asians, and Mediterraneans, and to a lesser degree, in Europeans/Americans. |
| **Carbohydrate absorption** | **Luminal Membrane** |
| | • **Glucose and galactose** compete for transport across the brush border by a **$Na^+$-dependent coporter (SGLT-1)**. $Na^+$ moves down its gradient into the enterocyte and the sugars move up their concentration gradients into the enterocyte (secondarily active). A $Na^+$-$K^+$ ATPase in the basolateral membrane helps maintain the $Na^+$ gradient (by keeping intracellular $Na^+$ low).<br>• **Fructose:** facilitated diffusion (down its concentration gradient) via GLUT-5 transporter |
| | **Basolateral Membrane** |
| | **Glucose, galactose,** and **fructose** are transported across the basolateral membrane via facilitated diffusion (GLUT-2 transporter). |

*(Continued)*

| | DIGESTION AND ABSORPTION (CONT'D.) |
|---|---|
| **Lipid digestion** | **Stomach** |
| | • Fatty materials are **pulverized** to decrease particle size and increase surface area. |
| | • **CCK** slows gastric emptying to allow enough time for digestion and absorption in the small intestine. |
| | **Small Intestine** |
| | • **Bile acid micelles** emulsify fat. |
| | • **Pancreatic lipases** digest fat. |
| | • Fats are hydrolyzed by pancreatic lipases to **free fatty acids**, **monoacylglycerols**, and other lipids (e.g., **cholesterol**, and **fat-soluble vitamins A, D, E, K**), which collect in micelles. |
| **Lipid absorption** | • **Micelles** carry products of fat digestion in the aqueous fluid of the gut lumen to the brush border, where they can diffuse into the enterocyte. |
| | • Enterocytes **re-esterify the fatty acids** to form triacylglycerols, phospholipids, and cholesteryl esters, which are incorporated with **apoproteins** into **chylomicrons**. |
| | • Chylomicrons are **released by exocytosis** into the intercellular spaces, where they **enter the lacteals** of the lymphatic system. They then enter the venous circulation via the **thoracic duct**. |
| | • Glycerol diffuses into portal blood and is either oxidized for energy or stored as glycogen. |
| | • **Triacylglycerols** with **medium- and short-chain fatty acids** are hydrolyzed quickly and do not require micelle formation for absorption. They undergo little re-esterification and are absorbed directly into the portal venous system. |
| | **Clinical Correlation** |
| | **Abetalipoproteinemia** results from a deficiency of apoprotein B, causing an inability to transport chylomicrons out of intestinal cells. |
| **Protein digestion** | **Stomach** |
| | **Pepsin** begins protein digestion in the stomach. It functions best at pH 2 and is irreversibly deactivated above pH 5; therefore, it will be inactivated in the duodenum. Pepsin is not an essential enzyme. |
| | **Small Intestine** |
| | Protein digestion continues with **pancreatic proteases** (trypsin, chymotrypsin, elastase, carboxypeptidases A and B) activated by brush border peptidases. These are essential enzymes. |
| **Protein absorption** | **Luminal Membrane** |
| | • Protein products can be absorbed as **amino acids**, **dipeptides**, and **tripeptides**. |
| | • Amino acids are absorbed via $Na^+$**-dependent amino acid cotransport**. Many different transport systems have been identified, e.g., carriers for neutral, basic, acidic, and imino amino acids. |
| | • Dipeptides and tripeptides are absorbed via an $H^+$**-dependent cotransport** mechanism. |
| | **Basal Membrane** |
| | • Dipeptides and tripeptides are hydrolyzed to amino acids intracellularly. |
| | • Amino acids are transported to the blood by facilitated diffusion. |
| | **Clinical Correlation** |
| | **Hartnup disease** is a disorder in which neutral amino acids cannot be absorbed. |
| **Water and electrolyte absorption** | The absorption of water and electrolytes occurs mainly in the **small intestine**. Approximately 5–10 liters of fluid must be absorbed daily (intake and secretion), with 80–90% being absorbed in the small intestine at a maximal rate of 700 mL/h. |

*(Continued)*

| | DIGESTION AND ABSORPTION *(CONT'D.)* |
|---|---|
| **NaCl** | • In the **proximal intestine**, there is **Na$^+$-H$^+$ exchange, Na$^+$-glucose or Na$^+$-amino acid cotransport, Na$^+$-Cl$^-$ cotransport,** and **passive diffusion** through Na$^+$ channels.<br>• In the colon, passive diffusion through Na$^+$ channels is more important and is stimulated by **aldosterone**.<br>• **Cl$^-$** is absorbed via Na$^+$-Cl$^-$ cotransport, Cl$^-$-HCO$_3^-$ exchange, and passive diffusion. |
| **K$^+$** | • K$^+$ absorption occurs in the small intestine by passive diffusion.<br>• K$^+$ is secreted in the colon (stimulated by aldosterone). |
| **Ca$^{2+}$** | • Absorption in the small intestine is via a vitamin D-dependent carrier.<br>• Vitamin D deficiency → ↓ Ca$^{2+}$ absorption → **osteomalacia** (adults) and **rickets** (children). |
| **H$_2$O** | • Secondary to solute absorption<br>• Isoosmotic absorption in gallbladder and small intestine; permeability is lower in colon. |
| **Iron** | • Absorbed as **free Fe$^{2+}$** or as **heme** iron, primarily in the duodenum<br>• **Fe$^{2+}$** is bound to transferrin in the blood. |
| **Vitamins** | • **Fat-soluble (A, D, E, K)**—incorporated into micelles and absorbed<br>• **Water soluble**—usually via Na$^+$-dependent cotransporters<br>• **Vitamin B$_{12}$**—absorption occurs in ileum and is transported while bound to intrinsic factor; ↓ intrinsic factor (gastrectomy) → **pernicious anemia** |
| **H$_2$O, electrolyte secretion** | Secretion occurs in **crypts**. **Cl$^-$** is the main ion secreted, via cAMP-regulated channels in the luminal membrane. |
| | **Clinical Correlation** |
| | **Cholera toxin** stimulates adenylate cyclase → ↑ cAMP → open Cl$^-$ channels; Na$^+$ and H$_2$O follow → secretory diarrhea. |

# GASTROINTESTINAL PATHOLOGY

## LESIONS OF THE ORAL CAVITY

| | |
|---|---|
| **Leukoplakia** | • White plaques on oral mucosa, produced by hyperkeratosis of the epithelium<br>• 10% have epithelial dysplasia, a precancerous lesion<br>• *Predisposing factors:* smoking, smokeless tobacco, alcohol abuse, chronic friction, and irritants |
| **Erythroplakia** | • Flat, smooth, and red.<br>• Significant numbers of atypical epithelial cells<br>• High risk of malignant transformation |
| **Hairy leukoplakia** | • Wrinkled surface<br>• Patches on the side rather than the middle of tongue<br>• No malignant transformation |
| **Lichen planus** | White reticulate lesions on the buccal mucosa and tongue |
| **Tumors of the Oral Cavity** | |
| **Benign tumors** | Hemangiomas, hamartomas, fibromas, lipomas, adenomas, papillomas, neurofibromas, and nevi |
| **Malignant tumors** | • **Squamous carcinoma** most common. Peak incidence from ages 40–70 years.<br>• Associated with tobacco and alcohol use, particularly when used together<br>• **Lower lip** most common site, but may affect floor of mouth and tongue |

## ESOPHAGEAL PATHOLOGY

| | |
|---|---|
| **Achalasia** | • **Lack of relaxation of the LES** secondary to loss of myenteric plexus<br>• *Most common ages:* 30–50.<br>• *Symptoms:* dysphagia, regurgitation, aspiration, chest pain<br>• Can be idiopathic, secondary to Chagas disease (*Trypanosoma cruzi*), or malignancy |
| **Barrett esophagus** | • Gastric or intestinal **columnar epithelium** replaces normal squamous epithelium<br>• Occurs with chronic insult, usually reflux (**increases risk of adenocarcinoma** 30–40 times) |
| **Boerhaave syndrome** | • Violent retching causes potentially fatal esophageal rupture |
| **Diverticula** | • Sac-like protrusions of one or more layers of the pharyngeal or esophageal wall<br>• **Zenker diverticula:**<br>  – Occur at the junction of the pharynx and esophagus in elderly men<br>  – *Symptoms:* dysphagia and regurgitation of undigested food soon after ingestion<br>• **Traction diverticula:** true diverticula in mid-esophagus; usually asymptomatic |
| **Esophageal carcinoma** | • Most are **adenocarcinomas** occurring after 50 and have male:female ratio of 4:1<br>• Incidence higher in northern Iran, Central Asia<br>• Associated with smoking, alcohol, nitrosamines, achalasia, Barrett esophagus, and vitamin A deficiency<br>• Presents with dysphagia (first to solids)<br>• Liver and lung most common sites of metastasis; poor prognosis |
| **Esophageal strictures** | • Narrowing of the esophagus, often as a result of fibrosis after severe inflammation. Caused by reflux, Herpes virus, Cytomegalovirus, *Candida,* chemical burns (e.g., lye ingestion).<br>• Carcinoma should be ruled out |
| **Esophageal varices** | • Dilated tortuous vessels of the esophageal venous plexus resulting from **portal hypertension**<br>• Esophageal varices are prone to **bleeding**; may be life-threatening |

*(Continued)*

## ESOPHAGEAL PATHOLOGY (CONT'D.)

| | | |
|---|---|---|
| **Esophagitis** | • Most common cause is reflux; other causes include infections (Herpes virus, Cytomegalovirus, *Candida*) and eosinophilic esophagitis | |
| **Hernia** | **Sliding** | 90% of cases, gastroesophageal junction above diaphragm, associated with **reflux** |
| | **Paraesophageal** | Gastric cardia above diaphragm, gastroesophageal junction remains in the abdomen; herniated organ at risk for strangulation and infarction |
| **Mallory-Weiss tears** | Occur at gastroesophageal junction secondary to recurrent **forceful vomiting**, usually seen in **alcoholics** | |
| **Schatzki rings** | Mucosal rings at the squamocolumnar junction below the aortic arch | |
| **Tracheoesophageal fistula** | • Usually esophageal blind pouch with a fistula between the lower segment of the esophagus and trachea<br>• Associated with congenital heart disease and other gastrointestinal malformations | |
| **Webs** | • Mucosal folds in the upper esophagus above the aortic arch<br>• **Plummer-Vinson syndrome:** dysphagia, glossitis, iron-deficiency anemia, and esophageal webs | |

*Definition of abbreviation:* LES, lower esophageal sphincter.

## STOMACH

| | |
|---|---|
| **Acute gastritis (erosive)** | Can be caused by alcohol, aspirin, smoking, shock, steroids, and uremia<br>Patients experience heartburn, epigastric pain, nausea, vomiting, and hematemesis |
| **Chronic gastritis** | |
|   **Fundal (type A)** | Autoimmune; associated with **pernicious anemia**, achlorhydria, and intrinsic factor deficiency |
|   **Antral (type B)** | Caused by *Helicobacter pylori* and is most common form of chronic gastritis in U.S. |
| **Carcinoma** | • *Risk factors:* genetic predisposition, diet, hypochlorhydria, pernicious anemia, and nitrosamines<br>• Usually asymptomatic until late, then presents with anorexia, weight loss, anemia, epigastric pain. Virchow node (left supraclavicular lymph node) common site of metastasis<br>• *Pathology:* 50% arise in the antrum and pylorus<br>• *Linitis plastica:* infiltrating gastric carcinoma with a diffuse fibrous response<br>• *Histology:* signet ring cells characteristic of gastric carcinoma |
| **Hypertrophic gastropathy** | • **Menetrier disease:** markedly thickened rugae due to hyperplastic superficial mucus glands with atrophy of deeper glands<br>• **Hypertrophic-hypersecretory gastropathy:** hyperplasia of parietal and chief cells in gastric glands<br>• **Excessive gastrin secretion (e.g., gastrinoma, Zollinger-Ellison syndrome):** produces gastric gland hyperplasia. Risk of peptic ulcer disease. |
| **Peptic ulcers** | • *Common locations:* proximal duodenum, stomach, and esophagus<br>• *H. pylori* infection important etiologic factor. Modification of acid secretion coupled with antibiotic therapy that eradicates *H. pylori* is apparently curative in most patients.<br>• *Symptoms:* episodic epigastric pain; *complications:* hemorrhage, perforation<br>• Duodenal ulcers do not become malignant. Gastric ulcers only rarely<br>• *Stress ulcers:* burns → Curling ulcers; CNS trauma → Cushing ulcers |
| **Pyloric stenosis** | • Congenital hypertrophy of pyloric muscle<br>• *Classic case:* firstborn boy, presenting with **projectile vomiting** 3–4 weeks after birth; associated with a palpable **"olive" mass** in epigastric region<br>• *Treatment:* surgical |

| SMALL INTESTINE | |
|---|---|
| **Celiac sprue** | • Allergic reaction to the **gliadin** component of gluten; genetic predisposition<br>• Predisposes to neoplasm, especially lymphoma<br>• *Pathology:* atrophy of villi in the jejunum; affects only **proximal** small bowel |
| **Congenital anomalies** | • **Meckel diverticulum:** persistent omphalomesenteric vitelline duct. Located near ileocecal valve. May contain ectopic gastric, pancreatic, or endometrial tissue, which may produce ulceration<br>• **Vitelline fistula:** direct connection between the intestinal lumen and the outside of the body at the umbilicus due to persistence of the vitelline duct. Associated with drainage of meconium from the umbilicus<br>• Atresia: congenital absence of a region of bowel (e.g., **duodenal atresia**); polyhydramnios, obstruction, and bile-stained vomiting in neonate<br>• Stenosis: narrowing that may cause obstruction<br>• **Omphalocele:** when the midgut loop fails to return to the abdominal cavity, forming a light gray shiny sac at the base of the umbilical cord filled with loops of small intestine<br>• **Gastroschisis:** A failure of the lateral body folds to fuse causes extrusion of the intestines through a open defect in the abdominal wall that is usually to the right of the umbilicus; unlike omphalocele, the intestines are exposed to the open air rather than being covered with a membrane. |
| **Hernias** | • Cause 15% of small intestinal obstruction, most commonly at the inguinal and femoral canals<br>• **Inguinal hernias**<br>  – **Indirect inguinal hernia:** the intestinal loop goes through the internal (deep) inguinal ring, external (superficial) inguinal ring, and into the scrotum. Much more common in males; may present in infancy if there is a failure of the processus vaginalis to close.<br>  – **Direct inguinal hernia:** the intestinal loop protrudes through the inguinal (Hesselbach's) triangle to cause a bulge in the abdominal wall medial to the inferior epigastric artery. Hesselbach's triangle is defined by the inferior epigastric artery, the lateral border of the rectus abdominus, and the inguinal ligament. The typical patient is an older man, and the hernia is covered by the external spermatic fascia.<br>• **Femoral hernia:** the intestinal loop protrudes below the inguinal ligament through the femoral canal below and lateral to the pubic tubercle. More common in women. This type of hernia is particularly likely to produce a dangerous bowel incarceration.<br>• **Diaphragmatic hernia:** infants with defective development of pleuroperitoneal membrane may have intestines and other abdominal structures herniated into the thorax; potentially fatal because of impairment of lung expansion |
| **Ischemic bowel disease** | • Thrombosis or embolism of the **superior mesenteric artery** accounts for approximately 50% of cases; venous thrombosis for 25% of cases<br>• Internal hernias can strangulate entrapped loops of bowel<br>• Usually after age 60 and presents with abdominal pain, nausea, and vomiting |
| **Intussusception** | • Telescoping of one segment of bowel into another; lead point usually an intraluminal mass<br>• More common in infants and children; may be reduced with a diagnostic barium enema |
| **Lymphoma** | • Usually non-Hodgkin, large cell, diffuse type<br>• In immunosuppressed patients, the incidence of primary lymphomas of small intestine is increasing.<br>• **MALToma:** often follicular and follow a more benign course; associated with *H. pylori* infection; may regress after antibiotic therapy. |
| **Necrotizing enterocolitis** | • Life-threatening acute, necrotizing inflammation of the small and large intestines<br>• Usually in premature or low birth weight neonates<br>• Peak incidence when babies start oral foods at 2 to 4 days, but can occur any time in first three months of life<br>• If surgical treatment is required, it may cause short bowel syndrome |
| **Tropical sprue** | • Unknown etiology; high incidence in the tropics; especially Vietnam, Puerto Rico<br>• *Pathology:* similar to changes in celiac disease, but affects **entire** length of small bowel |
| **Volvulus** | • Twisting of the bowel about its mesenteric base; may cause obstruction and infarction<br>• May be associated with malrotation of the midgut<br>• Typical patient is elderly |
| **Whipple disease** | • Rare, periodic acid-Schiff (PAS)–positive **macrophages in the lamina propria** of intestines<br>• Caused by small bacilli (***Tropheryma whippelii***); more common in men (10:1) |

| APPENDIX | |
|---|---|
| **Appendicitis** | • The vermiform appendix may become inflamed as a result of either an obstruction by stool, which forms a **fecalith** (common in adults), or **hyperplasia** of its lymphatic tissue (common in children).<br>• An inflamed appendix may stimulate visceral pain fibers, which course back in the lesser splanchnic nerves and result in colicky pain referred over the umbilical region. |

| LARGE INTESTINE | |
|---|---|
| **Angiodysplasia** | • Dilated tortuous vessels of the right colon → lower gastrointestinal bleeding in elderly<br>• Highest incidence in the cecum |
| **Diverticular disease** | • Multiple outpouchings of colon present in 30–50% of adults; higher incidence with ↑ age<br>• Presents with pain and fever |
| **Hirschsprung disease** | • **Absence of ganglion cells** of Meissner and Auerbach plexus in distal colon<br>• Produces markedly distended colon, proximal to aganglionic portion<br>• **Failure to pass meconium**, with constipation, vomiting, and abdominal distention |
| **Imperforate anus** | Failure of perforation of the membrane that separates endodermal hindgut from ectodermal anal dimple |
| **Polyps** | |
| **Tubular adenomas** | • Pedunculated polyps; 75% of adenomatous polyps<br>• Sporadic or familial; average age of onset is 60; most occur in left colon<br>• Cancer occurs in approximately 4% of patients |
| **Villous adenomas** | • Largest, least common polyps; usually sessile<br>• **1/3 cancerous** |
| **Tubulovillous adenomas** | • Combined tubular and villous elements<br>• **Increased villous elements →↑ likelihood of malignant transformation** |
| **Polyposis Syndromes** | |
| **Peutz-Jeghers syndrome** | • **Autosomal dominant**; involves entire gastrointestinal tract; **melanin pigmentation** of the buccal mucosa<br>• Polyps—**hamartomas**; not premalignant |
| **Turcot syndrome** | Colonic polyps associated with brain tumors |
| **Familial multiple polyposis** | • **Autosomal dominant**; appearance of polyps during adolescence<br>• Start in rectosigmoid area and spread to cover entire colon<br>• **Virtually all patients develop cancers**; prophylactic total colectomy recommended |
| **Gardner syndrome** | • Colonic polyps associated with **desmoid tumors**<br>• **Risk of colon cancer nearly 100%** |
| **Malignant Tumors** | |
| **Adenocarcinoma** | • **98% of all colonic cancers;** third most common tumor in both women and men; peak incidence in 60s<br>• *Symptoms:* rectal bleeding, change in bowel habits, weakness, malaise, and weight loss<br>• Tumor spreads by direct extension and **metastasis to nodes, liver, lungs, bones**<br>• **Carcinoembryonic antigen (CEA) tumor marker** helps to monitor tumor recurrence after surgery<br>• 75% of tumors in rectum, sigmoid colon<br>• **Left-sided lesions:** annular constriction, infiltration of the wall, **obstruction**<br>• **Right-sided lesions:** often bulky, polypoid, protuberant masses; **rarely obstruct** because fecal stream is liquid on right side |
| **Squamous cell carcinoma** | • Occur in anal region, associated with **papilloma viruses**<br>• Incidence rising in homosexual men with AIDS |

ORGAN SYSTEMS

GASTROINTESTINAL

## INFLAMMATORY BOWEL DISEASE: CROHN DISEASE VERSUS ULCERATIVE COLITIS

|  | Crohn Disease | Ulcerative Colitis |
|---|---|---|
| Most common site | Terminal ileum | Rectum |
| Distribution | Mouth to anus | Rectum → colon; "backwash" ileitis |
| Spread | Discontinuous/"skip" | Continuous |
| Gross features | Focal ulceration with intervening normal mucosa, linear fissures, cobblestone appearance, thickened bowel wall, "creeping fat" | Extensive ulceration, pseudopolyps |
| Micro | Noncaseating granulomas | Crypt abscesses |
| Inflammation | Transmural | Limited to mucosa and submucosa |
| Complications | Strictures, "string sign" on barium studies, obstruction, abscesses, fistulas, sinus tracts | Toxic megacolon |
| Genetic association | Family history of any type of inflammatory bowel disease is associated with increased risk. | |
| Extraintestinal manifestations | Less common | Common (e.g., arthritis, spondylitis [HLA B27 positive], primary sclerosing cholangitis, erythema nodosum, pyoderma gangrenosum) |
| Cancer risk | Slight 1–3% | 5–25% |

## EXOCRINE PANCREAS

| | |
|---|---|
| **Acute hemorrhagic pancreatitis** | • Diffuse necrosis of the pancreas by release of activated enzymes<br>• Most often associated with **alcoholism** and **biliary tract disease**<br>• *Symptoms:* sudden onset of acute, continuous, and intense abdominal pain, often radiating to back; accompanied by nausea, vomiting, and fever → frequently results in shock<br>• *Lab values:* **high amylase**, **high lipase** (elevated after 3–4 days), leukocytosis<br>• *Gross:* gray areas of enzymatic destruction, white areas of fat necrosis, red areas of hemorrhage |
| **Chronic pancreatitis** | • Remitting and relapsing episodes of mild pancreatitis → progressive pancreatic damage<br>• X-rays reveal **calcifications** in pancreas<br>• Chronic pancreatitis may result in **pseudocyst formation**, **diabetes**, steatorrhea |
| **Pseudocysts** | • Possible sequelae of pancreatitis or trauma<br>• Up to 10 cm in diameter with a fibrous capsule; no epithelial lining or direct communication with ducts |
| **Carcinoma** | • *Risk factors:* smoking, high-fat diet, chemical exposure<br>• Commonly develop in **head of the pancreas**, may result in compression of bile duct and main pancreatic duct → obstructive jaundice<br>• **Asymptomatic until late** in course, then weight loss, abdominal pain (classically, epigastric pain radiating to back), jaundice, weakness, anorexia; **Trousseau syndrome (migratory thrombophlebitis)** often seen<br>• Very poor prognosis |
| **Cystic fibrosis** | • Autosomal recessive; *CFTR* (cystic fibrosis transmembrane conductance regulator protein) gene located on chromosome 7<br>• **Defective chloride channel**: secretion of very thick mucus and **high sodium and chloride levels in sweat**<br>• 15% present with **meconium ileus** (most present during first year with steatorrhea, **pulmonary infections**, and obstructive pulmonary disease)<br>• *Pseudomonas aeruginosa* is most common etiologic agent<br>• Mean survival age 20; mortality most often due to pulmonary infections |
| **Annular pancreas** | Occurs when the ventral and dorsal pancreatic buds form a ring around the duodenum → obstruction of the duodenum |

| CONGENITAL HEPATIC MALFORMATIONS | |
|---|---|
| **Extrahepatic biliary atresia** | • Incomplete recanalization → cholestasis, cirrhosis, portal hypertension<br>• **Within first weeks of life:** jaundice, dark urine, light stools, hepatosplenomegaly |
| **Intrahepatic biliary atresia** | • Diminished number of bile ducts; sometimes associated with α-**1-antitrypsin deficiency**<br>• **Presents in infancy** with cholestasis, pruritus, growth retardation, ↑ serum lipids<br>• Icterus visible when serum bilirubin exceeds 2 mg/dL (true in any case of jaundice) |
| **Conjugated hyperbilirubinemia** | • **Dubin-Johnson syndrome:** benign conjugated hyperbilirubinemia due to impaired transport; liver grossly **black**<br>• **Rotor syndrome:** asymptomatic, similar to Dubin-Johnson, but the liver **not pigmented** |
| **Unconjugated hyperbilirubinemia** | • Can be due to hemolysis, diffuse hepatocellular damage, enzymatic defect<br>• **Gilbert syndrome:** autosomal recessive disease; deficiency of glucuronyl transferase; benign<br>• **Crigler-Najjar syndrome:**<br>  – *Type 1:* autosomal recessive with **complete absence of glucuronyl transferase**, marked unconjugated hyperbilirubinemia, severe kernicterus, death<br>  – *Type 2:* autosomal dominant with **mild deficiency of glucuronyl transferase**; no kernicterus |
| **Cholestasis** | • Impaired excretion of conjugated bilirubin; can have chalky stool<br>• *Intrahepatic:* viral hepatitis, cirrhosis, drug toxicity<br>• *Extrahepatic:* gallstones, carcinoma of bile ducts, ampulla of Vater or head of pancreas |
| **Hepatic failure** | Causes jaundice, encephalopathy, renal failure, palmar erythema, spider angiomas, gynecomastia, testicular atrophy, prolonged prothrombin time, hypoalbuminemia |
| **Chronic passive congestion** | • Associated with **right heart failure**<br>• *Pathology:* congestion of central veins and centrilobular hepatic sinusoids (known as **"nutmeg liver"**) |

| | |
|---|---|
| **Alcoholic liver disease** | • Three major stages: 1) **fatty liver**, 2) **alcoholic hepatitis**, 3) **alcoholic cirrhosis**<br>• Alcoholic hepatitis usually associated with fatty change; occasionally seen with cirrhosis<br>• Results from prolonged alcoholic abuse<br>• *Note:* **Mallory bodies** may be seen, but may also be seen in Wilson disease, hepatocellular carcinoma, and primary biliary cirrhosis<br>• AST/ALT > 2.0 indicates alcoholic liver disease |
| **Alpha-1-antitrypsin deficiency** | • Autosomal recessive; characterized by deficiency of a protease inhibitor<br>• Results in **pulmonary emphysema** and **hepatic damage (cirrhosis)** |
| **Budd-Chiari syndrome** | • Congestive liver disease secondary to thrombosis of the inferior vena cava or hepatic veins<br>• Causes "nutmeg liver" (also seen in right heart failure) with centrilobular congestion and necrosis<br>• May develop rapidly or slowly; more likely to be fatal if it develops rapidly |
| **Cirrhosis** | • Third leading cause of death in the 25- to 65-year-old age group<br>• *Leading etiologies:* **alcoholism** and **hepatitis C** |
| **Hemochromatosis** | • **Primary** form **autosomal recessive** inheritance; **secondary** form usually **related to multiple blood transfusions**<br>• Deposits of iron in the liver, pancreas, heart, adrenal, skin **"bronze diabetes"**<br>• *Also seen:* cardiac arrhythmias, gonadal insufficiency, arthropathy<br>• High incidence of hepatocellular carcinoma |
| **Portal hypertension** | • **Intrahepatic:** most common cause and usually secondary to cirrhosis of the liver; *other causes:* schistosomiasis, sarcoid<br>• **Posthepatic:** right-sided heart failure, Budd-Chiari syndrome<br>• **Prehepatic:** portal vein obstruction<br>• *Clinical:* ascites, portosystemic shunts that form hemorrhoids, **esophageal varices**, periumbilical varices (**caput medusae**), **encephalopathy**, splenomegaly<br>• *Additionally,* impaired estrogen metabolism: **gynecomastia**, gonadal atrophy, amenorrhea in females, **spider angiomata**, palmar erythema |
| **Primary biliary cirrhosis** | • Autoimmune etiology; causes sclerosing cholangitis, cholangiolitis<br>• Associated with other autoimmune diseases; **primarily affects middle-aged women**<br>• Presents with fatigue and pruritus; elevated alkaline phosphatase<br>• **Antimitochondrial antibody** in over 90% of patients |
| **Secondary biliary cirrhosis** | • Longstanding large bile duct obstruction, stasis of bile, inflammation, secondary infection, and scarring<br>• Usually presents with jaundice |
| **Reye syndrome** | • Usually affects children between 6 months and 15 years of age<br>• Characterized by **fatty change in the liver, edematous encephalopathy**<br>• *Etiology:* unclear; **frequently preceded by a mild upper respiratory infection**, **varicella**, **influenza** A or B infection<br>• Also associated with **aspirin** administration at levels not ordinarily toxic |
| **Sclerosing cholangitis** | • Chronic fibrosing inflammatory disease of the extrahepatic and larger intrahepatic bile ducts<br>• Associated with inflammatory bowel disease; predisposition for cholangiocarcinoma |
| **Wilson disease (hepatolenticular degeneration)** | • **Autosomal recessive—inadequate excretion of copper**<br>• *Clinical:* rarely manifests before age 6, then presents with weakness, **jaundice**, fever, angiomas, and eventually **portal hypertension**; *CNS manifestations:* **tremor**, **rigidity**, disorders of affect and thought<br>• *Labs:* **low serum ceruloplasmin**; ↑ urinary copper excretion<br>• *Pathology:* macronodular cirrhosis, degenerative changes in the lenticular nuclei of brain, pathognomonic **Kayser-Fleischer rings**, a deposition of copper in Descemet membrane of the corneal limbus |

## HEPATIC TUMORS

| | |
|---|---|
| **Liver cell adenoma** (benign) | • ↑ incidence with **anabolic steroid** and **oral contraceptive use**<br>• Forms a mass, which may be mistaken for carcinoma, or may rupture (especially during pregnancy) |
| **Nodular hyperplasia** (benign) | • Appears as solitary nodule that often has a fibrous capsule and bile ductules<br>• Stellate fibrous core usually present<br>• Nodular regenerative hyperplasia—multiple nodules composed of normal hepatocytes with loss of normal architecture |
| **Cholangiocarcinomas** | • 10% of primary liver neoplasms; **associated with primary sclerosing cholangitis**<br>• In developing countries, also associated with **infection with *Clonorchis sinensis*** (liver fluke)<br>• *Clinical:* weight loss, jaundice, pruritus<br>• 50% metastasize to lungs, bones, adrenals, and brain, exhibiting both hematogenous and lymphatic spread |
| **Hepatoblastoma** | • Rare, malignant neoplasm of children<br>• Hepatomegaly, vomiting, diarrhea, weight loss, elevated serum levels of AFP |
| **Hepatocellular carcinoma** | • **90% of primary liver neoplasms; strongly associated with cirrhosis, HCV and HBV** infections<br>• *Clinical:* tender hepatomegaly, ascites, weight loss, fever, polycythemia, hypoglycemia<br>• **Alpha-fetoprotein is present in 50–90%** of patients' serum (AFP also found with other forms of liver disease, pregnancy, fetal neural tube defects, germ-cell carcinomas of the ovaries and testes)<br>• Death due to gastrointestinal bleed and liver failure; generally, metastases first occur in lungs |

## HEPATIC INFECTIONS

| | |
|---|---|
| **Acute viral hepatitis** | • Can be icteric or anicteric<br>• *Symptoms:* malaise, anorexia, fever, nausea, upper abdominal pain, hepatomegaly<br>• *Labs:* elevated transaminases |
| **Chronic hepatitis** | • 5–10% of HBV infections and **well over 50% of HCV**; *other etiologies:* drug toxicity, Wilson disease, alcohol, α-1-antitrypsin deficiency, autoimmune hepatitis<br>• *Histology:* chronic inflammation with hepatocyte destruction, cirrhosis, liver failure |
| **Fulminant hepatitis** | • **Massive hepatic necrosis** and progressive hepatic dysfunction; mortality of 25–90%<br>• *Etiologies:* HBV, HCV, delta virus (HDV) superinfection, HEV, chloroform, carbon tetrachloride, certain mushrooms, acetaminophen overdose<br>• *Pathology:* progressive shrinkage of liver as parenchyma is destroyed |
| **Liver abscesses** | Pyogenic:<br>• *E. coli, Klebsiella, Streptococcus, Staphylococcus*; ascending cholangitis most common cause<br>• Seeding of liver due to bacteremia another potential cause<br>Parasitic:<br>• *Entamoeba histolytica:* especially in men over age 40 following intestinal disease; thick, brown abscess fluid<br>• *Ascaris lumbricoides:* can cause blockage of bile ducts, eosinophilia, verminous abscesses |
| **Parasitic infections** | • **Schistosomiasis:** splenomegaly, portal hypertension, ascites<br>• **Amebiasis:** *Entamoeba histolytica*, bloody diarrhea, pain, fever, jaundice, hepatomegaly |

*Definition of abbreviations:* HBV, hepatitis B virus; HCV, hepatitis C virus.

| | CHARACTERISTICS OF VIRAL HEPATITIDES | | | | |
|---|---|---|---|---|---|
| | **Hepatitis A** | **Hepatitis B** | **Hepatitis C** | **Hepatitis D** | **Hepatitis E** |
| **Nucleic acid** | RNA (Picornavirus) | DNA (Hepadnavirus) | RNA (Flavivirus) | RNA | RNA (Hepevirus) |
| **Characteristics** | • 50% seropositivity in people >50<br>• *Clinical disease:* mild or asymptomatic; rare after childhood | • Worldwide carrier rate 300 million<br>• 300,000 new infections/year in U.S. | • 150,000 new cases/year in U.S.<br>• **Most important cause of transfusion-related hepatitis** | • Replication defective<br>• **Dependent on HBV coinfection** for multiplication | **Fulminant** hepatitis 0.3–3%; **20% in pregnant women** |
| **Transmission** | • **Fecal-oral**, raw shellfish (concentrate virus)<br>• Not shed in semen, saliva, urine<br>• Shed in stool 2 weeks before onset of jaundice and 1 week after | • **Parenteral**, close personal contact<br>• Transfusion<br>• Dialysis<br>• Needle-sticks<br>• IV drug use<br>• Male homosexual activity | • **Parenteral**, close personal contact<br>• **Route of transmission undetermined in 40–50%** of cases | **Parenteral**, close personal contact | • **Waterborne**<br>• Young adults |
| **Incubation** | 2–6 weeks | 4–26 weeks | 2–26 weeks | 4–7 weeks in superinfection | 2–8 weeks |
| **Carrier state** | **None** | 1% blood donors | 1% | 1–10% in drug addicts | Unknown |
| **Progression to chronic hepatitis** | None | 5–10% acute infections, 90% in infants | **>80%** | • <5% in coinfection*<br>• 80% superinfection† | None |
| **Increased risk of hepatocellular carcinoma** | No | **Yes** | **Yes** | **Yes**, same as for B | Unknown, although not likely |
| **Diagnosis** | IgM against HAV | • **HBcAb is the 1st antibody, HBsAg indicates current infection**<br>• **HBeAg indicates infectivity** | ELISA for HCV Abs | Ab to Delta Agent plus HBsAg | ELISA for HEV Abs |

*Coinfection: hepatitis B and delta agent acquired at the same time
†Superinfection: delta agent acquired during chronic hepatitis B infection

## SEROLOGY OF HEPATITIS B INFECTION

| Acute Hepatitis B | Chronic Hepatitis B |
|---|---|

*The window is the time between the disappearance of the HB and before antibody to the surface antigen is detected.

## BILIARY DISEASE

| Cholelithiasis (gallstones) | • 20% of women and 8% of men in U.S.; rare before age 20, but seen in 25% of persons >60 years<br>• Most stones remain in gallbladder and are asymptomatic<br>• Famous **"4 Fs": fat, female, fertile (multiparous), older than 40 years** |
|---|---|
| | **Three Types of Stones** |
| | **Cholesterol Stones** |
| | Pure cholesterol stones are radiolucent, solitary, 1–5 cm (diameter), yellow, more common in Northern Europeans |
| | **Pigment Stones** |
| | • Small, black, multiple, and radiolucent; high incidence in Asians<br>• Associated with **hemolytic disease**, e.g., hereditary spherocytosis<br>• Cholelithiasis occurs in the young; think of hereditary spherocytosis, sickle cell disease, or other chronic hemolytic process |
| | **Mixed Stones** |
| | • 80% of all stones and **associated with chronic cholecystitis**<br>• Composed of cholesterol and calcium bilirubinate |
| Carcinoma of gallbladder | • Disease asymptomatic until late<br>• *Symptoms:* dull abdominal pain, mass, weight loss, anorexia<br>• *Pathology:* typically involves fundus and neck; 90% differentiated or undifferentiated adenocarcinomas<br>• Poor prognosis, with 3% 5-year survival rate<br>• *Risk factors:* cholelithiasis and cholecystitis (in up to 90% of patients), porcelain gallbladder (due to calcium deposition in gallbladder wall); occurs predominantly in elderly |
| Carcinoma of bile ducts (cholangiocarcinoma) | • Not associated with gallstones<br>• Men are affected more frequently; usually elderly<br>• *Symptoms:* obstructive jaundice<br>• *Risk factors:* chronic inflammation, infections, (e.g., liver flukes), ulcerative colitis |

# GASTROINTESTINAL MICROBIOLOGY

## MICROBIAL DIARRHEA: ORGANISMS CAUSING INFLAMMATORY DIARRHEA/DYSENTERY
### (Invasive Organisms Eliciting Blood, Pus In Stool, Fever)

| Most Common Sources | Common Age Group Infected | Incubation Period | Pathogenesis/ Vignette Clues | Organism | Diagnosis | Treatment |
|---|---|---|---|---|---|---|
| **Poultry, domestic animals, water** | All | 3–5 days | **Invades epithelium**, RBC and WBC in stools (most common bacterial diarrhea in U.S.) | *Campylobacter jejuni* | Oxidase $\oplus$, gram $\ominus$, curved rod, seagull-wings shape; grows at 42°C; microaerophile | • Treatment for severe cases only<br>• Erythromycin for invasive disease |
| **Poultry, domestic animals**, water | All | 8–48 hours | Penetrates to lamina propria of ileocecal region $\rightarrow$ **PMN response and prostaglandin synthesis, which stimulates** cAMP | *Salmonella* spp. | Gram $\ominus$, motile rods; nonencapsulated, oxidase $\ominus$ | • Severe cases only<br>• Sensitivity testing required |
| Water, no animal reservoirs, fecal-oral transmission | All | 1–7 days | **Shallow mucosal ulcerations and dysentery; septicemia rare** | *Shigella* spp. | Gram $\ominus$ rod; nonlactose fermenting; nonmotile | • Severe cases only<br>• Fluoroquinolones, trimethoprim-sulfamethoxazole |
| Milk, wild and **domestic animals**, fecal-oral | All | 2–7 days | Cold-climate **pseudoappendicitis**; heat-stable enterotoxin; arthritis may occur | *Yersinia enterocolitica* | Gram $\ominus$, motile rod; nonencapsulated, oxidase $\ominus$; urease $\oplus$; bipolar staining; best growth at 25°C | • Severe cases only<br>• Aminoglycosides, trimethoprim-sulfamethoxazole |
| Associated with **antibiotic use** | Pt. on antibiotics | NA | Pt. on antibiotic (clindamycin) | *Clostridium difficile* | Gram $\oplus$ rod; anaerobic spore former | Switch antibiotic; metronidazole |
| Food, water, fecal-oral | Adults | 2–3 days | Similar to *Shigella* | **Enteroinvasive E. coli** | Gram $\ominus$ rod; motile, lactose fermenter; serotyping compares O, H, K antigens | Sensitivity testing required |
| Food, water, fecal-oral | All | 2–4 weeks | Trophozoites invade colon; **flask-like lesions, extraintestinal abscesses (liver)**; travelers to Mexico | *Entamoeba histolytica* | Motile trophozoites or quadrinucleate cysts | Metronidazole |

*Definition of abbreviation:* Pt., patient.

ORGAN SYSTEMS

GASTROINTESTINAL

| MICROBIAL DIARRHEA: ORGANISMS CAUSING NONINFLAMMATORY DIARRHEA | | | | | | |
|---|---|---|---|---|---|---|
| (Noninvasive Organisms: No Blood, Pus In Stool) | | | | | | |
| Most Common Sources | Common Age Group Infected | Incubation Period | Pathogenesis/ Vignette Clues | Organism | Diagnosis | Treatment |
| Day care, water, fecal-oral | **Infants** and toddlers | 1–3 days | Microvilli of small intestine blunted; dehydration | **Rotaviruses** | Diagnosis by exclusion: dsRNA naked, double-shelled, icosahedral (Reovirus family) | Supportive |
| Water, food, fecal-oral | **Older kids and adults** | 18–48 hours | Blunting of microvilli; "cruise ship" diarrhea | **Norwalk virus** Norovirus (Norwalk-like) | Diagnosis by exclusion: ⊕ ssRNA, naked, icosahedral (Calicivirus family) | Supportive |
| Nosocomial | Young kids, immuno-compromised | 7–8 days | Death of enteric cells causes diarrhea | **Adenovirus 40/41** | Diagnosis by exclusion: naked, dsDNA, icosahedral | No specific therapy |
| **Beef, poultry, gravies,** Mexican food | All | 8–24 hours | **Enterotoxin** | *Clostridium perfringens* | Anaerobic, gram ⊕ rods, spore-forming, Nagler reaction | Not indicated |
| Water, food, fecal-oral | All ages | 9–72 hours | • Toxin stimulates adenylate cyclase<br>• Rice water stools | *Vibrio cholerae* | Curved, gram ⊖ rod; oxidase ⊕; "shooting-star" motility | Oral rehydration therapy; tetra-cycline shortens symptoms |
| Raw or **under-cooked shellfish** | Anyone eating raw shellfish | 5–92 hours | Self-limited gastroenteritis mimicking cholera | *Vibrio parahaemo-lyticus* | Curved, gram ⊖ rod; oxidase ⊕; "shooting-star" mobility | Not indicated |
| Water, uncooked fruits and vegetables | All ages | 12–72 hours | **Heat labile toxin (LT) stimulates adenylate cycla-se**; stable toxin stimulates guany-late cyclase | **Enterotoxigenic *E. coli* (ETEC)** | Gram ⊖ rod; motile; lactose fermenter; sero-typing compares O, H, K antigens | Sensitivity test-ing required |
| Food, water, fecal-oral | Infants in developing countries | 2–6 days | **Adherence to enterocytes through pili → damage to adjoining microvilli** | **Enteropathogenic *E. coli* (EPEC)** | Gram ⊖ rod; motile; lactose fermenter; sero-typing compares O, H, K antigens | Sensitivity testing required |
| Food, fecal-oral (**hamburger**) | 50% <10 years, all | 3–5 days | **Verotoxin, which inhibits 60S ribosomal subunit, causes bloody diarrhea, no fever** | **Enterohemorrhagic *E. coli* (EHEC)** | • Gram ⊖ rod; motile; lactose fermenter; serotyping compares O, H, K antigens<br>• O157H7 most common<br>• Does not fer-ment sorbitol | Antibiotics may increase risk of hemolytic-uremic syndrome |

*(Continued)*

## MICROBIAL DIARRHEA: ORGANISMS CAUSING NONINFLAMMATORY DIARRHEA (CONT'D)
### (Noninvasive Organisms: No Blood, Pus In Stool)

| Most Common Sources | Common Age Group Infected | Incubation Period | Pathogenesis/ Vignette Clues | Organism | Diagnosis | Treatment |
|---|---|---|---|---|---|---|
| Water, day care, camping, beavers, dogs, etc. | All, children | 5–25 days | Cysts ingested; trophozoites; **multiply and attach to small intestinal villi by sucking disk**, cause fat malabsorption → steatorrhea | *Giardia lamblia* | Flagellated binucleate trophozoites; "falling-leaf" motility; quadrinucleate cysts | Metronidazole |
| Day care, fecal-oral, animals, homosexuals | Children, AIDS patients | 2–4 weeks | Parasites intracellular in brush border | *Cryptosporidium parvum* | Acid-fast oocytes in stool | Nitazoxanide, puromycin, azithromycin in immunocompromised |

## DIARRHEA BY INTOXICATION

| Most Common Sources | Common Age Group Infected | Incubation Period | Pathogenesis | Symptoms | Organism | Diagnosis | Treatment |
|---|---|---|---|---|---|---|---|
| Ham, potato salad, cream pastries | All | **1–6 hours** | Heat-stable enterotoxin is produced in food (contamination by food handler with skin lesions); food sits at room temperature | Abdominal cramps, vomiting, diarrhea; sweating and headache may occur; no fever | *Staphylococcus aureus* | Symptoms, time of onset, food source | Recovery without treatment |
| **Fried rice** | All | **<6 hours** | Heat-stable toxin causes vomiting | Vomiting 1–6 hours; diarrhea 18 hours | *Bacillus cereus:* **emetic form** | Symptoms, time of onset, food source | Recovery without treatment |
| Meat, vegetables | All | >6 hours | Heat-labile toxin causes diarrhea (similar to *E. coli* LT) | Nausea, abdominal cramps, diarrhea | *Bacillus cereus:* diarrheal form | Symptoms, time of onset, food source | Recovery without treatment |
| Meat, vegetables | All | 18–24 hours | Enterotoxin | Nausea, abdominal cramps, diarrhea | *Clostridium perfringens* | Symptoms, time of onset, food source | Recovery without treatment |

*Definition of abbreviation:* LT, labile toxin.

ORGAN SYSTEMS

GASTROINTESTINAL

# The Endocrine System

## Chapter 6

# ENDOCRINE SYSTEM

## General Characteristics of Hormones

|  | Peptides and Proteins (Water Soluble) | Steroids and Thyroid Hormones (Lipid Soluble) |
|---|---|---|
| Receptors | Membrane surface | Cytoplasm and/or nucleus |
| Mechanism | Second messenger | mRNA transcription |
| Storage | Yes | No (except thyroid as thyroglobulin) |
| Plasma protein binding | No (except somatomedins) | Yes; acts as pool and prolongs effective half-life |
| Synthesis | Rough endoplasmic reticulum | Smooth endoplasmic reticulum |

# HYPOTHALAMUS AND PITUITARY OVERVIEW

## Hypothalamus-Anterior Pituitary System

### Hypothalamus and Anterior Pituitary Vascular System

### General Characteristics of the Pituitary

|  | Anterior Pituitary | Posterior Pituitary |
|---|---|---|
| Tissue | Glandular | Neuronal |
| Vascular | Indirect (portal via hypothalamus) | Direct |
| Control | Neurohormones | Neural |
| Hormones secreted | TSH, ACTH, LH FSH, GH, prolactin | ADH Oxytocin |

Occlusion or lesion of pituitary stalk reduces secretion of all anterior and posterior pituitary hormones, *except* prolactin, which is controlled by inhibitory effects of dopamine.

| Hypothalamus | Anterior Pituitary | Peripheral Target |
|---|---|---|
| Thyrotropin-releasing hormone (TRH) | Increases secretion of **thyroid-stimulating hormone (TSH)** | TSH stimulates synthesis and secretion of thyroid hormones; hypertrophy of thyroid gland |
| Corticotropin-releasing hormone (CRH) | Increases secretion of **adrenocorticotropic hormone (ACTH)** | ACTH stimulates synthesis and secretion of cortisol; hypertrophy of adrenal cortex |
| Gonadotropin-releasing hormone (GnRH) | Increases secretion of **luteinizing hormone (LH)** and **follicle-stimulating hormone (FSH)** | • LH stimulates gonadal steroids<br>• FSH stimulates follicular development (females) and spermatogenesis (males) |
| Growth hormone–releasing hormone (GHRH) (the dominant control of GH) | Increases secretion of **growth hormone (GH)** | GH actions: causes liver to produce somatomedins; metabolic and growth effects other tissues |
| Somatostatin (also known as growth hormone–inhibiting hormone [GHIH]) | Inhibits secretion of **GH** | — |
| Prolactin-inhibiting factor (dopamine [PIH]) | Inhibits secretion of **prolactin** | Prolactin stimulates lactation and inhibits GnRH, LH, and FSH |

| ANTERIOR PITUITARY HYPERFUNCTION | | |
|---|---|---|
| **Hyperprolactinemia** | • Elevated serum prolactin associated with prolactinoma (chromophobic); **most common pituitary tumor** <br> • Women: amenorrhea and galactorrhea; men: galactorrhea and infertility <br> • **Treatment:** dopamine agonists (e.g., pergolide, bromocriptine) | |
| **Excess GH** | **Gigantism** | • Results from excess GH secretion before fusion of growth plates <br> • Excessive skeletal growth may result in heights close to 9 feet <br> • Eosinophilic granuloma |
| | **Acromegaly** | • Results from excess GH secretion after fusion of growth plates <br> • Circumferential deposition of bones—enlargement of the hands and feet with frontal bossing <br> • Classic case—hat does not fit anymore |
| **Cushing disease** | • ACTH-secreting tumors in the anterior pituitary (compare with Cushing syndrome); rarely cause mass effect | |
| **Pathology** | • May be micro- or macroadenomas; generally, if active compound is released, lesion is noticed when small <br> • Large lesions can cause mass effect on the optic chiasm; very large masses (10 cm) may invade surrounding structures | |

| PITUITARY HYPOFUNCTION | | |
|---|---|---|
| **Anterior pituitary hypofunction** | • **Sheehan syndrome:** postpartum hemorrhagic infarction of pituitary associated with excessive bleeding; presents as failure to lactate <br> • **Empty sella syndrome:** atrophy of the pituitary; sella is enlarged on skull x-ray and may mimic neoplasm | |
| **Posterior pituitary hypofunction** | **Diabetes insipidus (DI)** | • Insufficient or absent antidiuretic hormone <br> • *Clinical:* polydipsia, polyuria, **hypotonic urine, high serum osmolality, hypernatremia** <br> • Central DI responds to exogenous ADH (desmopressin) therapy; nephrogenic DI does not |
| **Posterior pituitary hyperfunction** | • **Syndrome of inappropriate ADH secretion (SIADH):** as name suggests, inappropriate, excessive ADH secretion unrelated to serum osmolality <br> • *Causes:* May be paraneoplastic (**small cell lung cancer**), CNS damage, drugs, or infections (TB) <br> • *Clinical:* fluid retention, weight gain, and lethargy, **low serum osmolality, hypertonic urine, hyponatremia** | |

*Definition of abbreviation:* GH, growth hormone.

ORGAN SYSTEMS

ENDOCRINE

# ADRENAL GLAND

## ADRENAL HORMONES

### Adrenal Gland: Cortex and Medulla

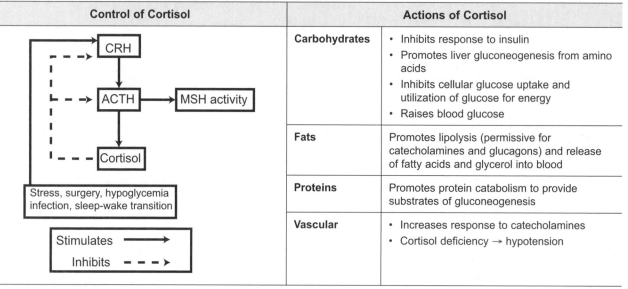

The Adrenal Gland

| Region | Hormones | Control system |
|--------|----------|----------------|
| Zona Glomerulosa | Aldosterone | Angiotensin II, $[K^+]_{plasma}$ |
| Zona Fasciculata | Cortisol | ACTH |
| Zona Reticularis | Androgens | ACTH (LH has no effect here) |

Capsule →

Medulla, produces epinephrine, controlled by sympathetic nervous system

| Control of Cortisol | Actions of Cortisol | |
|---|---|---|
| CRH → ACTH → MSH activity, ACTH → Cortisol<br><br>Stress, surgery, hypoglycemia infection, sleep-wake transition<br><br>Stimulates ——→<br>Inhibits - - -→ | **Carbohydrates** | • Inhibits response to insulin<br>• Promotes liver gluconeogenesis from amino acids<br>• Inhibits cellular glucose uptake and utilization of glucose for energy<br>• Raises blood glucose |
| | **Fats** | Promotes lipolysis (permissive for catecholamines and glucagons) and release of fatty acids and glycerol into blood |
| | **Proteins** | Promotes protein catabolism to provide substrates of gluconeogenesis |
| | **Vascular** | • Increases response to catecholamines<br>• Cortisol deficiency → hypotension |

*Note:* Fragments of ACTH precursor proopiomelanocortin (POMC) are also released and have biologic effects, notably melanocyte-stimulating hormone (MSH) activity.

## CUSHING SYNDROME

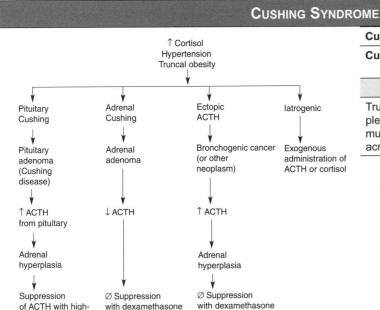

↑ Cortisol
Hypertension
Truncal obesity

**Pituitary Cushing**
↓
Pituitary adenoma (Cushing disease)
↓
↑ ACTH from pituitary
↓
Adrenal hyperplasia
↓
Suppression of ACTH with high-dose dexamethasone

**Adrenal Cushing**
↓
Adrenal adenoma
↓
↓ ACTH
↓
∅ Suppression with dexamethasone

**Ectopic ACTH**
↓
Bronchogenic cancer (or other neoplasm)
↓
↑ ACTH
↓
Adrenal hyperplasia
↓
∅ Suppression with dexamethasone

**Iatrogenic**
↓
Exogenous administration of ACTH or cortisol

| | |
|---|---|
| **Cushing (pituitary)** | ↑ cortisol   ↑ ACTH |
| **Cushing (adrenal)** | ↑ cortisol   ↓ ACTH<br>↑ aldosterone (often) |

### Clinical

Truncal obesity, buffalo hump, moon facies, facial plethora, hirsutism, menstrual disorders, hypertension, muscle weakness, back pain (osteoporosis), striae, acne, psychological disorders, bruising

## DIFFERENTIAL DIAGNOSIS OF CORTISOL EXCESS AND DEFICIENCY BASED ON FEEDBACK CONTROL

| Disorder | Plasma Cortisol | Plasma CRH | Plasma ACTH | Hyperpigmentation |
|---|---|---|---|---|
| **Primary (adrenal) excess** | ↑ | ↓ | ↓ | No |
| **Primary deficiency** | ↓ | ↑ | ↑ | Yes |
| **Secondary (pituitary) excess** | ↑ | ↓ | ↑ | Yes |
| **Secondary deficiency** | ↓ | ↑ | ↓ | No |
| **Steroid administration** (synthetics other than cortisol) | ↓<br>(but symptoms of excess) | ↓ | ↓ | No |

# ALDOSTERONE

| | Actions of Aldosterone | | Control of Aldosterone |
|---|---|---|---|

## Actions of Aldosterone

| | Renal | Effects |
|---|---|---|
| Na$^+$ | Reabsorption | ↑ total body Na$^+$ |
| K$^+$ | Secretion | ↓ plasma [K$^+$] |
| H$^+$ | Secretion | Metabolic alkalosis |
| HCO$_3^-$ | Production | Metabolic alkalosis |
| H$_2$O | Reabsorption | Volume expansion |

## Control of Aldosterone

**Aldosterone** promotes isoosmotic **reabsorption of sodium and water**. It also causes **secretion of acid** into urine and addition of bicarbonate to blood.

*Definition of abbreviations:* ACE, angiotensin-converting enzyme; CA, carbonic anhydrase; TPR, total peripheral resistance.

## LONG-TERM CONTROL OF BLOOD PRESSURE BY RENIN-ANGIOTENSIN-ALDOSTERONE

| Event | Effects | Compensation |
|---|---|---|
| **Volume expansion**<br>Saline infusion<br>Polydipsia | ↑ preload, cardiac output, and BP | • ↓ renin →↓ AII and ALD<br>• ↓ AII, ↓ ALD →↓ Na$^+$ and H$_2$O reabsorption →↑ urine flow →↓ EFV →↓ preload and cardiac output →↓ BP to normal |
| **Volume loss**<br>Hemorrhage<br>Dehydration | ↓ preload, cardiac output, and BP | ↑ renin →↑ AII and ALD →↑ Na$^+$ and H$_2$O reabsorption → ↓ urine flow →↑ EFV →↑ preload and cardiac output toward normal →↑ BP to normal |
| **Heart failure** | ↓ cardiac output and BP | ↑ renin →↑ AII and ALD → ↑ Na$^+$ and H$_2$O reabsorption →↓ urine flow →↑ EFV →↑ preload and cardiac output toward normal |

*Definition of abbreviations:* AII, angiotensin II; ALD, aldosterone; BP, blood pressure; EFV, extracellular fluid volume.

## HYPERALDOSTERONISM

| Primary hyperaldosteronism (Conn syndrome) | <ul><li>↑ aldosterone secretion</li><li>Adrenal adenoma most common cause</li><li>**Clinical:** diastolic hypertension, weakness, fatigue, polyuria, polydipsia, headache, no edema</li><li>**Lab values: hypokalemia, low renin levels, metabolic alkalosis, hypernatremia**, failure to suppress aldosterone with salt loading</li><li>**Pathology:** single well-circumscribed adenoma with lipid-laden clear cells</li></ul> |
|---|---|
| Secondary hyperaldosteronism | <ul><li>Etiologies: congestive heart failure, decreased renal blood flow (increased renin), renin-producing neoplasms, and Bartter syndrome (juxtaglomerular cell hyperplasia, hyperreninemia, hyperaldosteronism)</li><li>**Clinical:** Same as for primary, but edema may be present</li><li>**Lab values: high renin levels, hypernatremia, hypokalemia**</li></ul> |

## STEROID SYNTHETIC PATHWAYS MOST COMMONLY INVOLVED IN PATHOLOGY

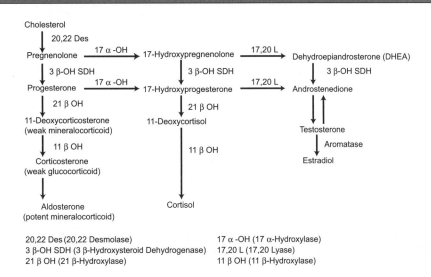

20,22 Des (20,22 Desmolase)
3 β-OH SDH (3 β-Hydroxysteroid Dehydrogenase)
21 β OH (21 β-Hydroxylase)

17 α -OH (17 α-Hydroxylase)
17,20 L (17,20 Lyase)
11 β OH (11 β-Hydroxylase)

Simplified scheme for understanding enzyme deficiencies; a vertical cut (e.g. 17 α -OH deficiency) all products to the right are deficient (cortisol, androgens) and products to the left are in excess (mineralocorticoids); a horizontal cut (e.g. 11 β OH ) all products above are excess (11-Deoxycorticosterone, 11-Deoxycortisol, androgens) and below are deficient (Aldosterone, Cortisol).

| Congenital Adrenal Hyperplasia | <ul><li>Usually due to a congenital enzyme deficiency characterized by **cortisol deficiency and enlargement of adrenal glands**</li><li>The 3 most common forms **all cause virilism** and are called **adrenogenital syndromes**:<ul><li>**Partial 21-hydroxylase deficiency:** normal aldosterone function and impaired cortisol production.</li><li>**Salt-losing syndrome: near total 21-hydroxylase deficiency** and aldosterone deficiency; infants present with vomiting, dehydration, hyponatremia, hyperkalemia</li><li>**11-hydroxylase deficiency:** leads to excessive androgen production and buildup of 11-deoxycorticosterone (a weak mineralocorticoid, which, in excess, has a strong mineralocorticoid effect), causing virilization, hypertension, hypokalemia</li></ul></li></ul> |
|---|---|

| CONGENITAL ENZYME DEFICIENCY SYNDROMES | | | | |
|---|---|---|---|---|
| **Enzyme Deficiency** | **Glucocorticoids** | **Mineralocorticoids** | **Androgens** | **Other Effects** |
| 20,22 desmolase | ↓ | ↓ | ↓ | Lethal if complete |
| 3 β-OH SDH | ↓ | ↓ | ↑ DHEA | • Masculinization of females in utero<br>• Incomplete precocious puberty (males)<br>• Adrenal hyperplasia<br>• Hyponatremia and hypovolemia |
| 21 β-OH | ↓ | ↓ | ↑ | • Masculinization of females in utero<br>• Incomplete precocious puberty (males)<br>• Adrenal hyperplasia<br>• Hyponatremia and hypovolemia |
| 11 β-OH | ↓ | ↓ aldosterone<br>↑↑↑ DOC* | ↑ | • Mineralocorticoid excess (DOC)<br>• Hypervolemia and hypernatremia<br>• Sexual effects as above |
| 17 α-OH | ↓ | ↓ aldosterone<br>↑↑↑ DOC* | ↓↓ | • DOC excess<br>• Absent secondary sexual aspects both sexes<br>• Amenorrhea |
| 17, 20 L | Normal | Normal | ↓↓ | • Absent secondary sexual aspects both sexes<br>• Amenorrhea |

*11-deoxycorticosterone, a weak mineralocorticoid that causes symptoms of mineralocorticoid overload when excessive amounts are secreted

| ADRENAL CORTICAL HYPOFUNCTION | |
|---|---|
| **Acute adrenocortical insufficiency** | • Rapid withdrawal of exogenous steroids in patients with chronic adrenal suppression<br>• Adrenal apoplexy seen in **Waterhouse-Friderichsen syndrome** (adrenal hemorrhage associated with meningococcal septicemia) |
| **Primary adrenocortical insufficiency (Addison disease)** | • Etiology: most common idiopathic; other causes: tuberculosis, other infections, iatrogenic, metastases, adrenal hemorrhage, pituitary insufficiency<br>• For clinically apparent insufficiency, 90% of the adrenal gland must be nonfunctional<br>• **Clinical:** weakness, weight loss, anorexia, nausea, vomiting, hypotension, skin pigmentation, hypoglycemia with prolonged fasting, inability to tolerate stress, abdominal pain<br>• **Lab values:** hyponatremia, hypochloremia, hyperkalemia, metabolic acidosis; ACTH levels high, cortisol and ALD levels low<br>• **Pathology:** bilateral atrophied adrenal glands<br>• ACTH and MSH share amino acid sequences; in cases of high ACTH → skin pigmentation |
| **Secondary (pituitary) adrenocortical insufficiency** | • **Etiology:** metastases, irradiation, infection, infarction, affecting the hypophysial-pituitary axis<br>• Results in decreased ACTH (less skin pigmentation) |
| **Hypoaldosteronism** | Hyponatremia, hypovolemia, hypotension, metabolic acidosis, hyperkalemia |
| **Primary**<br>**Secondary** | • ↓ aldosterone, ↑ renin and AII<br>• ↓ aldosterone, ↓ renin and AII, ↓ total peripheral resistance |

*Definition of abbreviations:* AII, angiotensin II; ACTH, adrenocorticotropic hormone; ALD, aldosterone; MSH, melanocyte-stimulating hormone.

## ADRENAL CORTICAL NEOPLASMS

| Adrenal adenomas | • Mostly asymptomatic and not steroid-producing<br>• Steroid-producing adenomas may produce Conn syndrome, Cushing syndrome, or virilization in women<br>• **Pathology:** small and unilateral nodule, yellow-orange on cut section, poorly encapsulated |
|---|---|
| Adrenal carcinomas | • Relatively rare and usually very malignant<br>• Greater than 90% are steroid-producing<br>• Pathology: tumors often large and yellow with areas of hemorrhage and necrosis |

## ADRENAL MEDULLA

| Tissue | Hormones | Control | Actions |
|---|---|---|---|
| Neural, chromaffin | Epinephrine (80%)<br>Norepinephrine (20%) | Sympathetic nervous system | Glycogenolysis, lipolysis, ↑ blood glucose, ↑ metabolic rate (requires cortisol and thyroid) |

### Disorders of Adrenal Medulla

| Pheochromocytoma | • Neoplasm of **neural crest-derived chromaffin cells** that secrete catecholamines (usually norepinephrine) → hypertension<br>• Highest incidence in children and adults age 30–50<br>• **Clinical:** paroxysmal or constant hypertension is most classic symptom; also, sweating, headache, arrhythmias, palpitations<br>• **Lab values:** elevated urinary homovanillic acid (HVA) and vanillylmandelic acid (VMA)<br>• **The Rule of 10s for pheochromocytoma:**<br>  – 10% extra-adrenal<br>  – 10% bilateral<br>  – 10% malignant<br>  – 10% affect children<br>  – 10% familial |
|---|---|
| Neuroblastoma | • **Most common malignant extracranial solid tumor of childhood**<br>• Occurs most frequently in the adrenal medulla, but may arise in sympathetic chain<br>• Amplification of the **N-*myc*** oncogene—more copies = more aggressive<br>• **Clinical:** tumors grow rapidly, metastasize widely (especially to bone); prognosis in younger patients (less than 1 year old) better than for older children<br>• **Pathology:** lobulated with areas of necrosis, hemorrhage, calcification<br>• **Microscopic appearance:** rosette pattern of small cells |

## TREATMENT FOR ADRENOCORTICAL DISEASE

| Class | Mechanism | Indications |
|---|---|---|
| **Glucocorticoids (hydrocortisone)** | Replacement therapy | For adrenocortical insufficiency (Addison disease, acute adrenal insufficiency from other causes) |
| **Mineralocorticoids (fludrocortisone)** | Replacement therapy | For chronic treatment of Addison disease in patients requiring mineralocorticoids |
| **Glucocorticoid synthesis inhibitors (aminoglutethimide metyrapone ketoconazole)** | Inhibits glucocorticoid synthesis via different mechanisms | To suppress adrenocortical steroid production in variety of disorders, e.g., Cushing disease, Cushingoid states, congenital adrenal hyperplasia |

**Normal function of antidiuretic hormone (ADH, vasopressin):** prevents changes of plasma osmolarity, restores normal blood volume and blood pressure, ↑ **permeability of renal collecting duct to water**, ↑ **reabsorption of water**, causes ↓ **urine flow**, and ↑ **urine osmolarity**

| ADH Control of Plasma Osmolarity and ECF Volume | Release of ADH from the Pituitary |
|---|---|

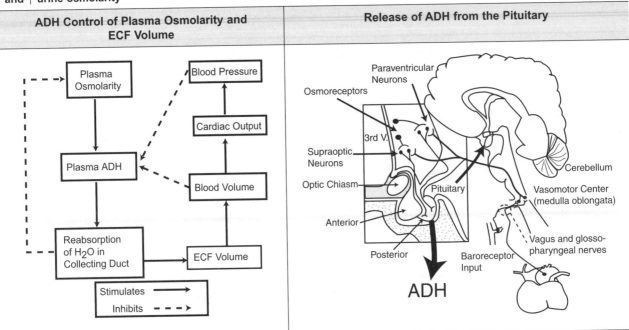

Secretion of ADH by neurons with cell bodies located in the **supraoptic and paraventricular nuclei** of the hypothalamus is **under the control of osmoreceptors and baroreceptors.** The osmoreceptors are in the AV3V region and are influenced by blood osmolarity. Atrial stretch receptors (detecting blood volume) are the largest cardiovascular influence, and arterial baroreceptors, including the carotid sinus (moderate effect) and the aortic arch (minor effect), are processed in medullary centers that regulate cardiovascular function, such as the nucleus tractus solitarius (NTS). The NTS sends efferents to the ADH-secreting neurons. The axon terminals of these neurons are in the posterior pituitary and release the hormone into the blood. Normally, osmolarity dominates control of ADH secretion; extreme changes of blood volume or cardiac output can overrride osmolarity.

## DISORDERS OF ANTIDIURETIC HORMONE (VASOPRESSIN)

| | |
|---|---|
| **Diabetes insipidus**<br>↓ ADH (central, neurogenic)<br>↓ response (nephrogenic) | • Hypovolemia, hypernatremia, metabolic alkalosis, tendency toward hypotension, large volume of dilute urine (distinguishes from dehydration)<br>• Distinguish central versus nephrogenic by testing response to ADH injection (nephrogenic → no response; central → response = concentration of urine) |
| **Dehydration (water deprived)**<br>↑ ADH to compensate | Hypovolemia, hypernatremia, metabolic alkalosis, tendency toward hypotension, small volume of concentrated urine (distinguishes from diabetes insipidus) |
| **Syndrome of inappropriate ADH (SIADH;** ↑ ADH**)** | Hypervolemia, hyponatremia, metabolic acidosis, small volume of concentrated urine (distinguishes from polydipsia) |
| **Primary polydipsia** | Hypervolemia, hyponatremia, large volume of dilute urine |

## ATRIAL NATRIURETIC PEPTIDE

| | |
|---|---|
| **Secretion** | • Secreted by **heart (right atrium)**<br>• Stimulated by **stretch (blood volume)** |
| **Actions** | • ↑ renal sodium excretion due to ↑ GFR and ↓ reabsorption of sodium (late distal tubule and collecting duct)<br>• ↓ reabsorption of water due to ↓ reabsorption of sodium<br>• Inhibits response to ADH |
| **Clinical** | • No known disorder caused by deficiency<br>• Elevated levels have clinical use as index of the severity of congestive heart failure |

# PANCREAS

<table>
<tr>
<th colspan="4" style="text-align:center">ENDOCRINE PANCREAS<br>Hormones of the Islets of Langerhans</th>
</tr>
<tr>
<th>Hormone</th>
<th>Control of Secretion</th>
<th>Target Tissues</th>
<th>Actions</th>
</tr>
<tr>
<td rowspan="3">Insulin (β cells)</td>
<td rowspan="3">
• Glucose, amino acids<br>
• Effect of glucose via ↑ ATP, closes ATP-dependent K⁺ channels, producing depolarization and exocytosis of insulin<br>
• Gastric inhibitory peptide (GIP) stimulates release
</td>
<td>Liver</td>
<td>
↑ glucose uptake (enzymatic effect)<br>
↑ glucose utilization<br>
↑ triglyceride synthesis<br>
↑ protein synthesis<br>
↑ glycogen synthesis<br>
↓ gluconeogenesis<br>
↓ glycogenolysis<br>
↓ lipolysis<br>
↓ protein catabolism<br>
↓ ureagenesis, ketogenesis<br>
↓ blood glucose concentration
</td>
</tr>
<tr>
<td>Muscle</td>
<td>
↑ glucose uptake (GLUT4 transport)<br>
↑ glucose utilization<br>
↑ protein synthesis<br>
↓ glycogenolysis<br>
↓ protein catabolism<br>
↓ blood glucose concentration
</td>
</tr>
<tr>
<td>Adipose</td>
<td>
↑ glucose uptake (GLUT4 transport)<br>
↑ triglyceride synthesis (↑ lipoprotein lipase to ↑ uptake of fatty acids)<br>
↓ lipolysis (↓ hormone-sensitive lipase)<br>
↓ blood glucose concentration
</td>
</tr>
<tr>
<td>Glucagon (α cells)</td>
<td>
• Glucose inhibits<br>
• Hypoglycemia stimulates<br>
• Amino acids stimulate
</td>
<td>Liver</td>
<td>
↑ gluconeogenesis<br>
↑ glycogenolysis<br>
↑ lipolysis<br>
↑ protein catabolism<br>
↑ ureagenesis, ketogenesis<br>
↑ blood glucose concentration
</td>
</tr>
<tr>
<td>Somatostatin (δ cells)</td>
<td>Stimulated by glucose, amino acids, fatty acids</td>
<td>Pancreas, GI tract</td>
<td>Inhibits secretion of insulin and glucagon; role is disputed</td>
</tr>
</table>

Use the fact that a carbohydrate meal increases plasma glucose as a sample application. Tracking through the feedback diagram predicts effects on carbohydrate, fat, and protein metabolism.

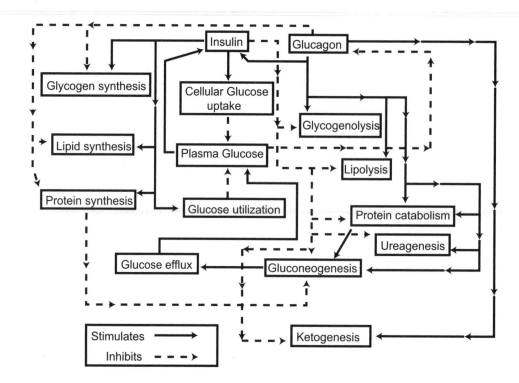

## SUMMARY OF GLUCOSE COUNTER-REGULATION

| Hormone | Stimulus | Actions |
|---|---|---|
| Glucagon | • Fasting, hypoglycemia, stress<br>• **Insulin/glucagon ratio is key to metabolism balance** | • Inhibits response to insulin (mainly in liver)<br>• Promotes catabolism, gluconeogenesis, glycogenolysis |
| Cortisol | Stress, fasting, hypoglycemia | • Inhibits response to insulin<br>• Reduces cellular glucose uptake<br>• Permissive for lipolysis<br>• Increases gluconeogenesis and protein catabolism<br>• Inhibits cellular glucose uptake |
| Epinephrine | Stress, severe hypoglycemia | • Increases glycogenolysis and lipolysis |
| Growth hormone | Fasting, sleep, stress | • Inhibits cellular uptake of glucose<br>• Stimulates lipolysis |
| Thyroid hormone | Cold, stress | • Permissive for epinephrine's effects<br>• Required for production of GH |

## INSULIN-RELATED PATHOPHYSIOLOGY

| | Glucose | Insulin | C-peptide | Ketoacidosis | Other Features |
|---|---|---|---|---|---|
| **Diabetes type 2** | ↑ | ↑ or ↔ | ↑ or ↔ | Uncommon | Familial, often obese |
| **Diabetes type 1** | ↑ | ↓ | ↓ | Yes | Often islet antibodies |
| **Insulinoma** | ↓ | ↑ | ↑ | No | Tachycardia (epinephrine) |
| **Insulin overdose** | ↓ | ↑ | ↓ | No | Tachycardia (epinephrine) |
| **Fasting hypoglycemia** | ↓ | ↑ | ↑ | No | Insulin remains at postprandial level in fasting |
| **Reactive hypoglycemia** | ↓ | ↑ | ↑ | No | Excessive secretion with oral glucose tolerance test |

## DISORDERS OF THE ENDOCRINE PANCREAS

| | |
|---|---|
| **Diabetes mellitus (DM)**<br>**Type 1** | • Often, abrupt onset with **ketoacidosis**<br>• Marked, absolute insulin deficiency, resulting from **diminished β-cell mass**<br>• Characterized by **low serum insulin** levels |
| **Type 2** | • Constitutes most cases of idiopathic diabetics, characterized by **peripheral insulin resistance**<br>• Most patients have **central obesity**; onset of disease usually after age 40<br>• These patients are **not prone to ketoacidosis** |
| **Acute metabolic complications of diabetes** | • **Diabetic ketoacidosis** (DKA) may occur in type 1 diabetics, rarely in type 2<br>• Metabolic acidosis results from accumulation of ketones<br>• High blood glucose → dehydration via an **osmotic diuresis**<br>• Treatment with insulin normalizes the metabolism of carbohydrate, protein, fat<br>• Fluids given to correct the dehydration<br>• **Hyperosmolar nonketotic coma** in patients with mild type 2; blood glucose can be elevated; treatment similar to treatment of DKA |
| **Late complications of diabetes** | • Series of long-term complications, including **atherosclerosis** (leading to strokes, myocardial infarcts, gangrene), **nephropathy, neuropathy** (distal, symmetric polyneuropathy with "stocking-glove" distribution), **retinopathy** that may lead to blindness<br>• Patients with DM are also at high-risk for:<br>  – *Klebsiella pneumoniae*<br>  – **Sinus mucormycosis**<br>  – **Malignant otitis externa (*Pseudomonas aeruginosa*)** |
| **ß-cell tumors** | • Insulinomas most commonly occur between ages of 30 and 60<br>• **Pathogenesis:** β-cell tumors produce hyperinsulinemia → hypoglycemia<br>• **Clinical features:** patients experience episodes of altered sensorium (i.e., disorientation, dizziness, diaphoresis, nausea, tremulousness, coma), which are relieved by glucose intake<br>• **Pathology:** most tumors solitary, well-encapsulated, well-differentiated adenomas of various sizes.; 10% are malignant carcinomas |
| **Zollinger-Ellison syndrome** | • Due to gastrinoma and often associated with **MEN type I**<br>• **Pathogenesis:** tumors of pancreatic islet cells secrete gastrin → gastric hypersecretion of acid<br>• **Clinical:** includes intractable peptic ulcer disease and severe diarrhea<br>• **Pathology:** 60% malignant; most tumors located in pancreas (10% in duodenum) |
| **MEN I** | • Tumors of parathyroids, adrenal cortex, pituitary gland, pancreas<br>• Associated with peptic ulcers and Zollinger-Ellison syndrome |
| **MEN IIa** | Tumors of adrenal medulla (pheochromocytoma), medullary carcinoma of thyroid, parathyroid hyperplasia or adenoma |
| **MEN IIb/III** | Medullary carcinoma of the thyroid, pheochromocytoma, and mucosal neuromas. |

ORGAN SYSTEMS

ENDOCRINE

## TREATMENT OF DIABETES

### Insulin

| Classes | Onset (hours) | Peak (hours) | Duration (hours) | Insulin Types |
|---|---|---|---|---|
| Rapid-acting | 0.25 | 0.5–1.5 | 3–5 | Lispro, aspart, glulisine |
| Short-acting | 0.5–1 | 2–4 | 5–8 | Regular |
| Intermediate-acting | 1–3 | 8 | 12–16 | NPH |
| Long-acting | 1 | No peak | 20–26 | Glargine, detemir |

### Noninsulin Antidiabetic Agents

| Drug | Mechanism | Notes |
|---|---|---|
| **Insulin secretagogues**<br>• **Sulfonylureas**<br>  – **First generation (tolbutamide, chlorpropamide)**<br>  – **Second generation (glipizide, glyburide, glimepiride)**<br>• **Meglitinides (repaglinide, nateglinide)** | • Block $K^+$ channels → depolarization of pancreatic β cells → ↑$Ca^{2+}$ influx → insulin release | • Requires functional β cells<br>• Repaglinide: faster onset and shorter duration than sulfonylureas; taken before meals to control postprandial glucose levels<br>• Side effects: hypoglycemia, weight gain |
| **Biguanides (metformin)** | May ↑ tissue sensitivity to insulin and/or ↓ hepatic gluconeogenesis | • Does not require functional β cells<br>• Will not cause hypoglycemia<br>• Most serious side effect: lactic acidosis |
| **Thiazolidinediones (rosiglitazone, pioglitazone)** | • Bind nuclear peroxisome proliferator-activated receptor-γ (PPAR-γ receptor)<br>• ↑ target tissue sensitivity to insulin, inhibits hepatic glucose output, ↑ glucose uptake | • Hypoglycemia rare<br>• Weight gain, edema |
| **α-Glucosidase inhibitors (acarbose, miglitol)** | Inhibits intestinal brush border α-glucosidase →↓ glucose absorption →↓ postprandial glucose →↓ demand for insulin | • GI distress, flatulence, diarrhea |
| **Drugs affecting glucagon-like peptide-1 (GLP-1) (exenatide\*, sitagliptin)** | • GPL-1, an incretin released from the small intestine in response to food, augments glucose-dependent insulin release, inhibits glucagon secretion, slows gastric emptying, and increases feelings of satiety<br>• Exenatide: long-acting GLP-1 receptor agonist<br>• Sitagliptin: oral DDP-4 inhibitor, prevents the breakdown of GLP-1 | • Extenatide: nausea, hypoglycemia when combined with sulfonylureas<br>• Sitagliptin: headache, URI, nasopharyngitis |
| **Pramlintide\*** | Synthetic analog of amylin, which decreases glucagon release, slows gastric emptying, and promotes satiety | • Used in type 1 and type 2 DM<br>• Hypoglycemia, GI disturbances |

### Hyperglycemic Drugs

| | | |
|---|---|---|
| **Glucagon** | ↑ hepatic glycogenolysis and gluconeogenesis, ↑ heart rate and force of contraction, relaxes smooth muscle | • Administered via intramuscular injection<br>• Major side effect: hyperglycemia<br>• Glucagon receptors stimulate adenylate cyclase and ↑ cAMP; this is basis for its use in beta-blocker overdose |

\* Exanatide and pramlintide are injectables, the rest are given orally

*Definition of abbreviations:* DDP-4, dipeptidyl peptidase 4; URI, upper respiratory infection

ORGAN SYSTEMS

ENDOCRINE

# ENDOCRINE REGULATION OF CALCIUM AND PHOSPHATE

## OVERVIEW OF HORMONAL REGULATION OF CALCIUM AND PHOSPHATE

| Hormone | Site Produced | Stimuli to Secretion or Production | Effect on Plasma Free $Ca^{2+}$ | Effect on Plasma Phosphate |
|---|---|---|---|---|
| Parathyroid Hormone (PTH) | Parathyroid gland | Low plasma $Ca^{2+}$ | ↑ | ↓ |
| 1,25-(OH)$_2$-vitamin D$_3$ | Skin → liver → kidney | Sunlight, PTH, dietary intake | ↑ | ↑ |
| Calcitonin (not essential for control) | Parafollicular cells of thyroid | High plasma $Ca^{2+}$ | ↓ | Little net effect |

## PARATHYROID HORMONE

| | |
|---|---|
| Effects on kidneys | • Calcium ↑ reabsorption<br>• Phosphate ↓ reabsorption<br>• Vitamin D ↑ production of active form 1,25 (OH)$_2$ vitamin D$_3$ from precursor 25-OH D$_3$ formed in liver |
| Effects on bone | • Receptors on osteoblasts, not on osteoclasts<br>• Rapid mobilization of $Ca^{2+}$ and phosphate from bone fluid<br>• ↑ osteoclast activity via mediators released from osteoblasts<br>• Causes bone resorption, release of $Ca^{2+}$, phosphate into plasma |
| Effects on GI tract | Indirectly stimulates $Ca^{2+}$ and phosphate absorption in small intestine through its effect to produce active form of vitamin D$_3$ |

## VITAMIN D (CALCITRIOL)

| | |
|---|---|
| Effects on kidneys | ↓ $Ca^{2+}$ and phosphate excretion (by ↑ reabsorption of both) |
| Effects on bone | ↑ resorption (with PTH); releases $Ca^{2+}$ and phosphate into plasma (but normal growth and maintenance also requires both vitamin D and PTH) |
| Effects on GI tract | ↑ $Ca^{2+}$ and phosphate absorption in intestine, ↑ both in plasma |

## CALCITONIN

| | |
|---|---|
| Effects on kidneys | ↑ phosphate excretion; ↓ $Ca^{2+}$ excretion (minor effect) |
| Effects on bone | ↓ resorption; ↑ deposition; ↓ plasma $Ca^{2+}$ (major effect) |
| Effects on GI tract | ↑ $Ca^{2+}$ and phosphate absorption in intestine (minor effect) |

ORGAN SYSTEMS

ENDOCRINE

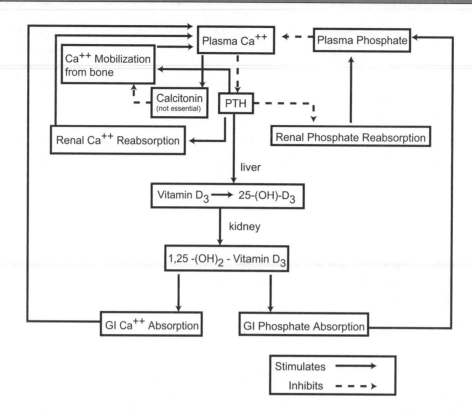

## DISORDERS OF CALCIUM AND PHOSPHATE REGULATION

| | Plasma ($Ca^{2+}$) | Plasma (Phosphate) | Effects on Bone |
|---|---|---|---|
| **Primary hyperparathyroidism** | ↑ | ↓ | Demineralization and osteopenia |
| **Primary hypoparathyroidism** | ↓ | ↑ | Malformation |
| **Deficient vitamin D (secondary hyperparathyroidism)** | ↓ | ↓ | • Osteomalacia in adults<br>• Rickets in children |
| **Excess vitamin D (secondary hypoparathyroidism)** | ↑ | ↑ | Osteoporosis |
| **Renal failure with high plasma phosphate (secondary hyperparathyroidism)** | ↓ (precipitation) | ↑ | Osteomalacia and osteosclerosis |

*Note:* Clinical presentation of hypocalcemia often includes muscle spasms and tetany; hypercalcemia presents with weakness and flaccid paralysis.

## Pathophysiology of Calcium Homeostasis

| | |
|---|---|
| **Primary hyperparathyroidism** | • Parathyroid adenoma is the most common cause; can see in MEN I and MEN IIa<br>• **Clinical:** elevated serum calcium often asymptomatic<br>• **Lab values:** ↑ **PTH and alkaline phosphatase, hypercalcemia, hypophosphatemia** |
| **Osteitis fibrosa cystica (von Recklinghausen disease of bone)** | • Occurs in **chronic primary hyperparathyroidism**<br>• Cystic changes in bone occur due to osteoclastic resorption<br>• Fibrous replacement of resorbed bone may lead to a non-neoplastic "brown tumor" |
| **Secondary hyperparathyroidism** | • Usually caused by **chronic renal failure** and decreased $Ca^{2+}$ absorption, stimulating PTH<br>• Vitamin D deficiency and malabsorption less common causes<br>• May show soft tissue calcification and osteosclerosis<br>• **Lab values:** ↑ **PTH and alkaline phosphatase, hypocalcemia, hyperphosphatemia** |
| **Hypoparathyroidism** | • Common causes are accidental removal during thyroidectomy, idiopathic, and DiGeorge syndrome<br>• **Clinical:** irritability, anxiety, tetany, intracranial and lens calcifications<br>• **Lab values: hypocalcemia, hyperphosphatemia** |
| **Pseudohypoparathyroidism** | • Autosomal recessive disorder, resulting in kidney unresponsive to circulating PTH<br>• Skeletal abnormalities: short stature, shortened fourth and fifth carpals and metacarpals |
| **Hypercalcemia** | • **Mnemonic** "MISHAP": Malignancy, Intoxication (vitamin D), Sarcoidosis, Hyperparathyroidism, Alkali syndrome (Milk-Alkali), and Paget disease<br>• **Clinical:** renal stones, abdominal pain, drowsiness, metastatic calcification |

## Drugs in Bone and Mineral Disorders

| Drug | Mechanism | Notes |
|---|---|---|
| **Bisphosphonates (alendronate, etidronate, pamidronate, risedronate)** | ↓ bone resorption | • Osteoporosis<br>• Paget disease<br>• Esophageal ulceration may occur |

# THYROID

## PHYSIOLOGIC ACTIONS OF THYROID HORMONE

| | |
|---|---|
| **Metabolic rate** | ↑ metabolic rate: high $O_2$ consumption, mitochondrial growth, ↑ $Na^+/K^+$-ATPase activity, ↑ food intake, thermogenesis, sweating, ↑ ventilation |
| **Energy substrates** | Mobilization of carbohydrates, fat and protein; ↑ ureagenesis; ↓ muscle and adipose mass |
| **Growth** | Required after birth for normal brain development and bodily growth (protein anabolic) |
| **Circulation** | ↑ cardiac output (linked to metabolism), ↑ β-adrenergic receptors on heart |

## CONTROL OF THYROID HORMONE

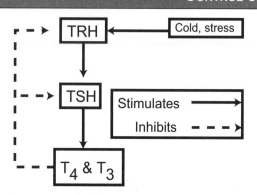

**TRH** = thyrotropin-releasing hormone (hypothalamus)

**TSH** = Thyroid-stimulating hormone (anterior pituitary); is also trophic (increases gland mass)

**$T_4$** = thyroxine (tetraiodothyronine); 90% of production, but low biologic activity

**$T_3$** = triiodothyronine; 10% of production, very potent

## SYNTHESIS AND STORAGE

| Process | Mechanism | Result |
|---|---|---|
| Uptake of $I^-$ | Active transport | ↑ follicular cell iodide |
| Oxidation | Peroxidase | Produce oxidized iodine |
| Iodination | Peroxidase | Produces MIT and DIT within thyroglobulin |
| Coupling | Peroxidase | Links MITs and DITs to form $T_4$ and $T_3$ |
| Exocytosis | Exocytosis into lumen | Storage of thyroglobulin |

*Definition of abbreviations:* DIT, diiodotyrosine; MIT, monoiodotyrosine.

| SECRETION | | |
|---|---|---|
| **Process** | **Mechanism** | **Result** |
| Transport | Endocytosis | Colloid taken up by follicular cells |
| Fusion | Lysosomes and colloid fuse | Incorporation in lysosomes |
| Proteolysis | Lysosomal enzymes | Cleave thyroglobulin into $T_3$, $T_4$, MITs, and DITs |
| Secretion | Simple diffusion | Lipid-soluble $T_3$ and $T_4$ diffuse into extracellular fluid to plasma |
| Deiodination | Deiodinase | Removes iodide from MITs and DITs to recycle it |

| REGULATION OF THYROID ACTIVITY | |
|---|---|
| **Transport** | 99% bound to thyroid binding globulin, 1% free; represents a pool to prevent rapid change of thyroid level |
| **Peripheral Conversion** | $T_4$ converted to more active $T_3$ by 5′-monodeiodinase or to inactive reverse $T_3$ by 5-monodeiodinase; occurs in most tissues giving local control of hormone action |
| **Mechanism of action** | Binding to nuclear receptors: $T_4$ has low affinity, $T_3$ has high affinity, so is responsible for most thyroid hormone effects |
| **Degradation** | Successive deiodination steps to thyronine, also sulfates and glucuronides |

| THYROID DISORDERS | | | | |
|---|---|---|---|---|
| **Disorder** | $T_4$ | **TSH** | **TRH** | **Gland Mass** |
| **Primary hypothyroidism** | ↓ | ↑ | ↑ | ↑, goiter possible |
| **Pituitary hypothyroidism** | ↓ | ↓ | ↑ | ↓, due to low TSH |
| **Hypothalamic hypothyroidism** | ↓ | ↓ | ↓ | ↓, due to low TSH |
| **Iodine deficiency** (prolonged, severe) | ↓ | ↑ | ↑ | ↑, goiter likely |
| **Pituitary hyperthyroidism** | ↑ | ↑ | ↓ | ↑, goiter possible |
| **Primary hyperthyroidism** (tumor) | ↑ | ↓ | ↓ | ↓, due to low TSH |
| **Graves disease** (autoimmune production of thyroid-stimulating immunoglobulins [TSIs]) | ↑ | ↓ | ↓ | ↑, goiter possible |

## DISORDERS OF THE THYROID GLAND

| | |
|---|---|
| **Hyperthyroidism** | • Seen most often in Graves disease, toxic multinodular goiter, toxic adenoma<br>• Clinical: tachycardia, cardiac palpitations (β-adrenergic effect), skin warm and flushed, ↑ body temperature, heat intolerance, hyperactivity, tremor, weight loss, osteoporosis, diarrhea and oligomenorrhea, eyes show a wide stare with lid lag; **exophthalmos** seen **only in Graves disease**<br>• Thyrotoxic storm: severe hypermetabolic state with 25% fatality<br>• **Lab values:** low TSH and elevated $T_4$; low TSH is most important<br>• Note: in pregnancy, ↑ in TBG secondary to high estrogen levels elevates total serum $T_4$, but not free serum $T_4$ |
| **Graves disease** | • Peaks in the third and fourth decades; more common in women; associated with other autoimmune diseases (including Hashimoto thyroiditis)<br>• Production of TSI and TGI bind and activate TSH receptors<br>• **Pathology:** diffuse, moderate, symmetric enlargement of gland<br>• **Microscopic appearance:** hypercellular with small follicles and little colloid |
| **Hypothyroidism** | • Clinical features depend on age group<br>• Lab values: elevated TSH and low $T_4$ |
| **Infants** | • Develop **cretinism**; major effects are on skeletal and CNS development; once apparent, syndrome is irreversible; neonatal screening for elevated TSH for early detection<br>• **Clinical:** protuberant abdomen, wide-set eyes, dry rough skin, broad nose, delayed epiphyseal closure |
| **Older children** | Short stature, retarded linear growth (GH deficiency caused by thyroid hormone deficiency), delayed onset of puberty |
| **Adults** | • Lethargy, weakness, fatigue, decreased appetite, weight gain, cold intolerance, constipation<br>• Myxedema: associated with severe hypothyroidism; periorbital puffiness, sparse hair, cardiac enlargement, pleural effusions, anemia |
| **Hashimoto thyroiditis** | • Chronic lymphocytic thyroiditis featuring goitrous thyroid gland enlargement<br>• Autoimmune; may be autoantibodies to the TSH receptors, $T_3$ and $T_4$; **antimicrosomal antibodies** also seen<br>• **Most common type of thyroiditis;** highest incidence in **middle aged females**<br>• **Pathology:** painless goiter, gland enlarged and firm<br>• **Microscopic appearance:** lymphocytic and plasma cell infiltrate with **Hürthle cells** (follicular cells with eosinophilic granular cytoplasm) |
| **Diffuse nontoxic goiter** | Diffuse enlargement of gland in euthyroid patients; high incidence in certain geographic areas with iodine-deficient diets |
| **de Quervain granulomatous subacute thyroiditis** | • Self-limited disease; seen more often in females in the second to fifth decades<br>• Follows **viral** syndrome, lasts several weeks with a **tender** gland<br>• May initially have mild hyperthyroidism later, usually euthyroid |
| **Riedel thyroiditis** | • Rare, chronic thyroid disease, possibly of immune origin, that causes dense fibrosis of the thyroid gland leading to hypothyroidism<br>• Presents with a hard, fixed, painless goiter<br>• May be associated with idiopathic fibrosis in other sites such as the retroperitoneum |
| **Thyroglossal duct cyst** | • May communicate with skin or base of tongue<br>• Remnant of incompletely descended midline thyroid tissue |
| **Ectopic thyroid nests** | Usually at the base of tongue; prior to removal, it must be documented that patient has other functioning thyroid tissue |

*Definition of abbreviations:* GH, growth hormone; TBG, thyroid-binding globulin; TGI, thyroid growth immunoglobulin; TSI, thyroid-stimulating immunoglobulin; TSH, thyroid-stimulating hormone.

## DRUGS FOR THYROID GLAND DISORDERS

| Class | Mechanism | Comments/Agents |
|---|---|---|
| **Hyperthyroidism Agents** | These agents are used for short-term or long-term treatment of hyperthyroid states. The most common adverse effects are related to signs and symptoms of hypothyroidism. | |
| **Thioamides** | • Inhibit synthesis of thyroid hormones<br>• They do *not* inactivate existing $T_4$ and $T_3$<br>• Propylthiouracil is able to inhibit peripheral conversion of $T_4$ to $T_3$ | • **Examples: PTU, methimazole**<br>• **Indications:** long-term hyperthyroid therapy, which may lead to disease remission and short-term treatment before thyroidectomy or radioactive iodine therapy<br>• **Side effects:** skin rash (common), hematologic effects (rare) |
| **Iodides** | • Inhibit the release of $T_4$ and $T_3$ (primary)<br>• Inhibit the biosynthesis of $T_4$ and $T_3$ and ↓ the size and vascularity of thyroid gland | • **Examples:** Lugol's solution (iodine and potassium iodide) and potassium iodide alone<br>• **Indications:** preparation for thyroid surgery; treatment of thyrotoxic crisis and thyroid blocking in radiation emergency<br>• **Note:** therapeutic effects can be seen for as long as 6 weeks |
| **Beta-Blockers** | Nonselective β-receptor blockers used for palpitations, anxiety, tremor, heat intolerance; partially inhibit peripheral conversion of $T_4$ to $T_3$ | • **Examples: nadolol, propranolol**<br>• Used to treat the signs and symptoms of hyperthyroidism |
| **Radioactive Iodine [$^{131}$I]** | Ablation of thyroid gland | • **Indications:** first-line therapy for Graves disease; treatment of choice for recurrent thyrotoxicosis in adults and elderly |
| **Hypothyroidism Agents** | These agents are used as thyroid replacement therapy. The most common adverse effects are related to signs and symptoms of hyperthyroidism. | |
| **Thyroid Hormones** | Acts by controlling DNA transcription and protein synthesis | **Examples:** synthetic $T_4$, synthetic $T_3$, or combination of synthetic $T_4$:$T_3$ in 4:1 ratio |

*Definition of abbreviation:* PTU, propylthiouracil.

## THYROID NEOPLASMS

| | |
|---|---|
| **Adenomas** | • Follicular adenoma is most common; may cause pressure symptoms, pain, and rarely thyrotoxicosis<br>• **Pathology:** usually small, well-encapsulated solitary lesions |
| **Papillary carcinoma** | • Most common thyroid carcinoma<br>• Incidence higher in women<br>• **Pathology:** papillary branching pattern; 40% have tumors containing psammoma bodies<br>• Spread to local nodes is common; **hematogenous spread rare**<br>• Resection curative in most cases |
| **Follicular carcinoma** | • More malignant than papillary cancer<br>• **Pathology:** may be encapsulated, with penetration through the capsule; colloid sparse<br>• Local invasion and pressure → dysphagia, dyspnea, hoarseness, cough<br>• **Hematogenous metastasis to lungs or bones common** |
| **Anaplastic carcinoma** | • Rapid growing, aggressive with poor prognosis; affects older patients<br>• **Pathology:** tumors usually bulky and invasive with undifferentiated anaplastic cells<br>• **Clinical:** early, widespread metastasis and death within 2 years |

# GROWTH HORMONE

## CONTROL OF GROWTH HORMONE

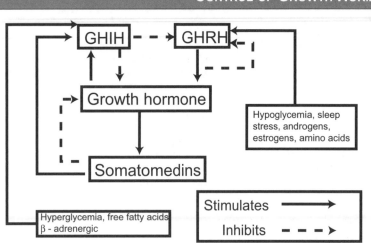

### Secretion of GH

- Pulsatile, ↑ during sleep
- Moderate in childhood
- Increases at puberty
- Lower in adults
- Secretion requires thyroid hormone
- Increased by sex steroids

## BIOLOGIC ACTIONS OF GROWTH HORMONE

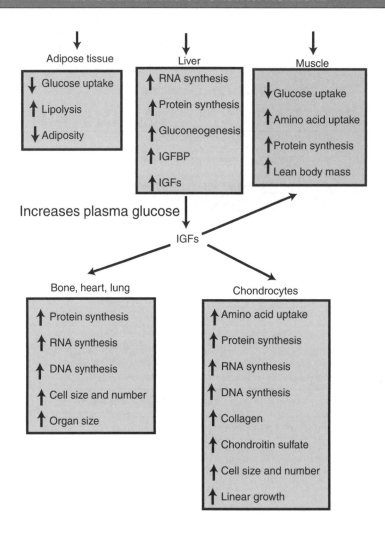

| CHILDHOOD DISORDERS | |
|---|---|
| **Dwarfism** | • Caused by:<br>  – ↓ GH or ↓ liver production of IGF (Laron syndrome)<br>  – Defective GH receptors<br>• Mental development normal<br>• Reversible with GH treatment |
| **Gigantism** | • Caused by ↑ GH prior to epiphyseal closure<br>• Increased height, increased body mass |

*Definition of abbreviation:* GH, growth hormone; IGF, insulin-like growth factor.

| ADULT DISORDERS OF GROWTH HORMONE | | |
|---|---|---|
| **Acromegaly** | ↑ GH | • Enlargement of hands and feet<br>• Protrusion of lower jaw, coarse facial features<br>• ↑ lean body mass<br>• ↓ body fat<br>• ↑ size of visceral organs<br>• Impaired cardiac function (related to mass)<br>• Abnormal glucose tolerance with tendency to hyperglycemia |
| **Deficiency** | ↓ GH | • Tendency to hypoglycemia when fasting<br>• Susceptible to insulin-induced hypoglycemia<br>• Significance of other effects disputed |

*Definition of abbreviation:* GH, growth hormone.

| TREATMENT OF GROWTH HORMONE DISORDERS | | |
|---|---|---|
| **Class** | **Mechanism** | **Comments/Agents** |
| **GH** | Stimulation of linear/skeletal growth (pediatric patients only); potentiation of cell and organ growth; enhanced protein, carbohydrate and lipid metabolism | • **Somatropin** and **somatrem** (recombinant forms of human GH)<br>• **Indications:** growth failure, Turner syndrome, cachexia, somatotropin deficiency |
| **Octreotide** | • Long-acting octapeptide that mimics somatostatin<br>• Inhibits release of GH, glucagon, gastrin, thyrotropin, insulin | • **Indications:** acromegaly, carcinoid, glucagonoma, gastrinoma, other endocrine tumors |

*Definition of abbreviation:* GH, growth hormone.

# The Reproductive System

## Chapter 7

# REPRODUCTIVE SYSTEM

## MALE AND FEMALE DEVELOPMENT

### Adult Female and Male Reproductive Structures Derived From Precursors of the Indifferent Embryo

| Adult Female | Indifferent Embryo | Adult Male |
|---|---|---|
| Ovary, follicles, rete ovarii | Gonads | Testes, seminiferous tubules, rete testes |
| Uterine tubes, uterus, cervix, and upper part of vagina | Paramesonephric ducts | Appendix of testes |
| Duct of Gartner | Mesonephric ducts | Epididymis, ductus deferens, seminal vesicle, ejaculatory duct |
| Clitoris | Phallus | Glans and body of penis |
| Labia minora | Urogenital folds | Ventral aspect of penis |
| Labia majora | Labioscrotal swellings | Scrotum |

### Congenital Reproductive Anomalies

#### Female Pseudointersexuality

- 46,XX genotype
- Have ovarian (but no testicular) tissue and masculinization of the female external genitalia
- Most common cause is **congenital adrenal hyperplasia**, a condition in which the fetus produces excess androgens

#### Male Pseudointersexuality

- 46,XY genotype
- Testicular (but no ovarian) tissue and stunted development of male external genitalia
- Most common cause is inadequate production of testosterone and müllerian-inhibiting factor (MIF) by the fetal testes; due to a 5α-reductase deficiency

| | |
|---|---|
| **5α-reductase 2 deficiency** | • Caused by a mutation in the **5α-reductase 2 gene** that renders 5α-reductase 2 enzyme underactive in catalyzing the conversion of testosterone to dihydrotestosterone |
| | • *Clinical findings:* underdevelopment of the penis and scrotum (microphallus, hypospadias, and bifid scrotum) and prostate gland; epididymis, ductus deferens, seminal vesicle, and ejaculatory duct are normal |
| | • At puberty, they undergo virilization due to an increased **T:DHT ratio** |
| **Complete androgen insensitivity (CAIS, or testicular feminization syndrome)** | • Occurs when a fetus with a 46,XY genotype develops testes and female external genitalia with a rudimentary vagina; the uterus and uterine tubes are generally absent |
| | • Testes may be found in the labia majora and are surgically removed to circumvent malignant tumor formation |
| | • Individuals present as normal-appearing females, and their psychosocial orientation is female despite their genotype |
| | • Most common cause is a mutation in the **androgen receptor (AR) gene** that renders the AR inactive |

# MALE AND FEMALE REPRODUCTIVE ANATOMY

## Male

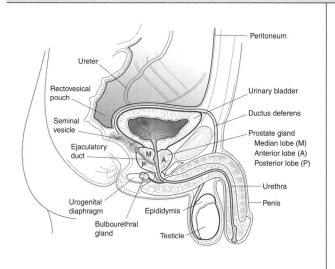

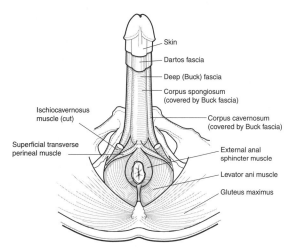

## Female

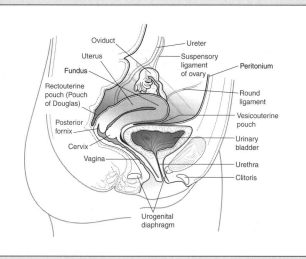

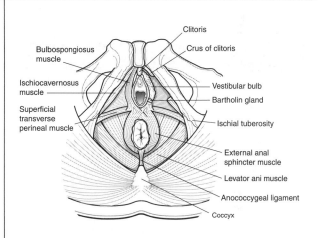

## Pelvic Floor and Perineum

- The floor of the pelvis is formed by the **pelvic diaphragm** (two layers of fascia with a middle layer of skeletal muscle).
- The muscles forming the middle layer are the **levator ani** and **coccygeus**. The levator ani acts as a muscular sling for the rectum and marks the boundary between the rectum and anal canal.
- The region below the pelvic diaphragm is the **perineum**, which contains the **ischioanal fossa**, the fat-filled region below the pelvic diaphragm surrounding the anal canal.
- The **urogenital diaphragm** is in the perineum and extends between the two ischiopubic rami. The urogenital diaphragm (like the pelvic diaphragm) is composed of two layers of fascia with a middle layer of skeletal muscle.

*(Continued)*

### Perineal Pouches

| | |
|---|---|
| **Deep perineal pouch (space)** | The deep perineal pouch is the middle (muscle) layer of the urogenital diaphragm. It contains:<br>• Sphincter urethrae muscle—serves as external sphincter of the urethra<br>• Deep transverse perineal muscle<br>• Bulbourethral (Cowper) gland (in the male only)—duct enters bulbar urethra |
| **Superficial perineal pouch (space)** | The superficial perineal pouch is the region below the urogenital diaphragm and is enclosed by the superficial perineal (Colles) fascia. It contains:<br>• Crura of penis or clitoris—erectile tissue<br>• Bulb of penis (in the male)—erectile tissue; contains urethra<br>• Bulbs of vestibule (in the female)—erectile tissue; in lateral walls of vestibule<br>• Ischiocavernosus muscle—skeletal muscle that covers crura of penis or clitoris<br>• Bulbospongiosus muscle—skeletal muscle that covers bulb of penis or bulbs of vestibule<br>• Greater vestibular (Bartholin) gland (in female only)—homologous to Cowper gland |

### Pelvic Innervation

The **pudendal nerve (S2, S3, S4 ventral rami) and its branches** innervate the skeletal muscles in the pelvic and urogenital diaphragms, the external anal sphincter and the sphincter urethrae, skeletal muscles in both perineal pouches, and the skin that overlies the perineum.

# MALE REPRODUCTIVE SYSTEM

## MALE REPRODUCTIVE PHYSIOLOGY

### Penile Erection

Erection occurs in response to **parasympathetic** stimulation (pelvic splanchnic nerves). **Nitric oxide** is released, causing relaxation of the corpus cavernosum and corpus spongiosum, which allows blood to accumulate in the trabeculae of erectile tissue.

### Ejaculation

• **Sympathetic** nervous system stimulation (lumbar splanchnic nerves) mediates movement of mature spermatozoa from the epididymis and vas deferens into the ejaculatory duct.

• Accessory glands, such as the bulbourethral (Cowper) glands, prostate, and seminal vesicles, secrete fluids that aid in sperm survival and fertility.

• **Somatic motor efferents** (pudendal nerve) that innervate the bulbospongiosus and ischiocavernous muscles at the base of the penis stimulate the rapid ejection of semen out the urethra during ejaculation. Peristaltic waves in the vas deferens aid in a more complete ejection of semen through the urethra.

### Clinical Correlation

• Injury to the bulb of the penis may result in extravasation of urine from the urethra into the superficial perineal space. From this space, urine may pass into the scrotum, into the penis, and onto the anterior abdominal wall.

• Accumulation of fluid in the scrotum, penis, and anterolateral abdominal wall is indicative of a laceration of either the membranous or penile urethra (deep to Scarpa fascia). This can be caused by trauma to the perineal region (saddle injury) or laceration of the urethra during catheterization.

## AGENTS FOR ERECTILE DYSFUNCTION

| Drug | Mechanism | Comments |
|------|-----------|----------|
| Selective phosphodiesterase (PDE) 5 inhibitors<br><br>**(sildenafil, vardenafil, tadalafil)** | Inhibits the enzyme phosphodiesterase (PDE) 5, which inactivates cGMP, leading to ↑ cGMP → vasodilation, more inflow of blood → better erection | PDE 5 inhibitors + **nitrates** (which ↑ cGMP production) → **severe hypotension** |
| Synthetic prostaglandin $E_1$ ($PGE_1$) agents<br><br>**(alprostadil)** | ↑ cAMP (via adenylate cyclase) → smooth muscle relaxation | Administered via transurethral or intracavernosal injection<br><br>*Contraindications:* intercourse with pregnant women (can stimulate uterine contractions unless used with a condom); conditions that might predispose a patient to priapism (e.g., sickle cell anemia, multiple myeloma, leukemia) |
| **Testosterone** | Replacement/supplementation for males whose serum androgen concentrations are below normal | Used if diminished libido is a significant patient complaint |

## DISEASES OF THE PENIS AND PROSTATE

### Noninfectious Disorders of the Penis

| | |
|---|---|
| **Hypospadias and epispadias** | With hypospadias, urethra opens onto the ventral surface of penis<br>Often associated with a poorly developed penis that curves ventrally, known as **chordee**<br>With epispadias, urethra opens onto dorsal surface; often associated with exstrophy of bladder<br>Either of these malformations may cause infertility |
| **Phimosis** | Prepuce orifice too small to be retracted normally<br>Interferes with hygiene; can also predispose to bacterial infections; if foreskin retracted over the glans, it may lead to urethral constriction → paraphimosis<br>*Treatment:* circumcision |
| **Penile carcinoma** | |
|     **Bowen disease** | Carcinoma in situ; can be associated with visceral malignancy<br>Men >35 years; tends to involve shaft of the penis and scrotum<br>*Gross:* thick, ulcerated plaque<br>*Micro:* squamous cell carcinoma in situ |
|     **Squamous cell carcinoma** | 1% of cancers in men in the United States, usually age 40–70.<br>Usually slow growing and non-painful; patients often delay seeking medical attention.<br>Circumcision decreases the incidence.<br>Human Papilloma virus (types 16 and 18) infection is closely associated.<br>Gross: Plaque progressing to an ulcerated papule or fungating growth.<br>Metastases can go to local lymph nodes. |
| **Peyronie disease** | Curved penis due to fibrosis of the tunica albuginea |

*(Continued)*

ORGAN SYSTEMS

REPRODUCTIVE

## Diseases of the Prostate

| | |
|---|---|
| **Prostatic carcinoma** | • Most common cancer in men; usually occurs after age 50, and the incidence increases with age<br>• Associated with race (more common in African Americans than in Caucasians, relatively rare in Asians)<br>• May present with urinary problems or a palpable mass on rectal examination<br>• Prostate cancer more common than lung cancer, but lung cancer is bigger killer<br>• Metastases may occur via the lymphatic or hematogenous route<br>• Bone commonly involved with osteoblastic metastases, typically in the pelvis and lower vertebrae<br>• Elevated PSA, together with an enlarged prostate on digital rectal exam, highly suggestive of carcinoma<br>• Most patients present with advanced disease and have a 10-year survival rate of <30%<br>• *Treatment:* surgery, radiation, and hormonal modalities (orchiectomy and androgen blockade). |
| **Benign prostatic hyperplasia** | • Formation of large nodules in the periurethral region (median lobe) of the prostate<br>• May narrow the urethral canal to produce varying degrees of urinary obstruction and difficulty urinating<br>• It is increasingly common after age 45; incidence increases steadily with age<br>• Can follow an asymptomatic pattern, or can result in urinary symptoms and urinary retention |
| **Prostatitis**<br><br>**Acute**<br><br><br><br><br><br>**Chronic** | <br><br>• Results from a bacterial infection of the prostate<br>• Pathogens are often organisms that cause urinary tract infection<br>• *Escherichia coli* most common<br>• Bacteria spread by direct extension from the posterior urethra or the bladder; lymphatic or hematogenous spread can also occur<br>• Common cause of recurrent urinary tract infections in men<br>• Two types: bacterial and nonbacterial<br>• Both forms may be asymptomatic or may present with lower back pain and urinary symptoms |

## ANTIANDROGENS

| Drug | Mechanism | Clinical Uses |
|---|---|---|
| **Flutamide** | Androgen receptor antagonist | Prostate cancer |
| **Spironolactone** | Androgen receptor antagonist (also a potassium-sparing diuretic) | Hirsutism (also used for primary hyperaldosteronism, edema, hypertension) |
| **Leuprolide** | GnRH analog | Depot form is used for prostate cancer |
| **Finasteride** | 5α-reductase inhibitor (prevents conversion of testosterone to DHT) | Benign prostatic hypertrophy (BPH), male pattern baldness |
| **Ketoconazole** | Inhibits steroid synthesis (also an antifungal agent) | Androgen receptor–positive prostate cancer |

*Definition of abbreviation:* DHT, dihydrotestosterone.

## THE TESTES

### Descent of the Testes

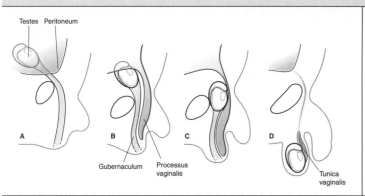

The **processus vaginalis** is an evagination of parietal peritoneum that descends through the inguinal canal during fetal life. The **tunica vaginalis** is a patent remnant of the processus vaginalis that covers the anterior and lateral parts of the testis.

A **hydrocele** is an accumulation of serous fluid in the tunica vaginalis or in a persistent part of the processus vaginalis in the cord.

(Continued)

ORGAN SYSTEMS

REPRODUCTIVE

## Normal Anatomy and Anatomic Abnormalities

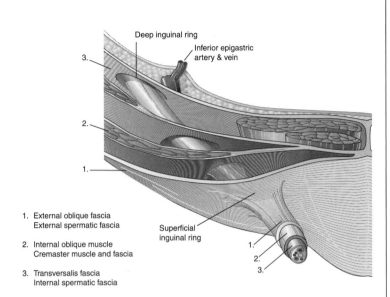

Deep inguinal ring
Inferior epigastric artery & vein
Superficial inguinal ring

1. External oblique fascia
   External spermatic fascia

2. Internal oblique muscle
   Cremaster muscle and fascia

3. Transversalis fascia
   Internal spermatic fascia

The **inguinal canal** is formed by four of the eight tissue layers of the anterior abdominal wall; outpocketings of three of these layers give rise to **spermatic fasciae**, which cover the testis and structures in the **spermatic cord**.

The spermatic cord contains the:

- **Ductus deferens**, which conveys sperm from the epididymis to the ejaculatory duct in the male pelvis
- **Testicular artery**, which arises from the abdominal aorta between the L2 and the L3 vertebrae
- **Artery to the ductus deferens**, which arises from a branch of the internal iliac artery
- **Pampiniform plexus of the testicular vein**
- **Right testicular vein**, which drains into the inferior vena cava
- **Left testicular vein**, which drains into the left renal vein.
- **Lymphatic vessels** that drain the testis. Testicular lymphatic vessels pass through the inguinal canal and drain directly to **lumbar nodes** in the posterior abdominal wall.

## Cremasteric Reflex

The **cremasteric reflex** utilizes sensory and motor fibers in the ventral ramus of the L1 spinal nerve. Stroking the skin of the superior and medial thigh stimulates sensory fibers of the **ilioinguinal nerve**. **Motor fibers** from the genital branch of the **genitofemoral nerve** cause the cremaster muscle to contract, elevating the testis.

## Abnormalities

| | |
|---|---|
| **Cryptorchidism** | <ul><li>Failure of normal descent of intra-abdominal testes into the scrotum</li><li>Most common location of a cryptorchid testis is in the inguinal canal</li><li>Unilateral or bilateral, more often on right side</li><li>Bilateral cryptorchidism can cause infertility</li><li>Maldescended testes are associated with a greatly increased incidence of testicular cancer, even once repositioned within scrotum</li></ul> |
| **Torsion** | <ul><li>Precipitated by sudden movement, trauma, and congenital anomalies</li><li>Twisting of spermatic cord may compromise both arterial supply and venous drainage</li><li>Sudden onset of testicular pain and a loss of the cremasteric reflex are characteristic</li><li>If not surgically corrected early, may result in testicular infarction</li></ul> |
| **Hydrocele** | <ul><li>Congenital hydrocele occurs when a small patency of the processus vaginalis remains so that peritoneal fluid can flow into the processus vaginalis; may occur later in life, often inflammatory causes (e.g., epididymitis)</li><li>Results in fluid-filled cyst near testes</li></ul> |
| **Varicocele** | <ul><li>Results from dilatations of tributaries of the testicular vein in the pampiniform plexus</li><li>Varicosities of the pampiniform plexus are observed when the patient is standing and disappear when the patient is lying down</li></ul> |
| **Spermatocele** | <ul><li>Retension cyst containing sperm in the rete testes or head of the epididymis</li></ul> |

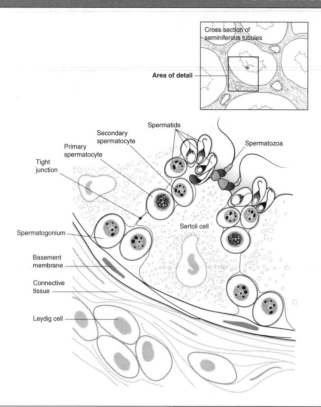

Spermatogenesis occurs in the seminiferous tubules between the **Sertoli cells**, which extend from the seminiferous tubule basement membrane to the lumen and are separated by tight junctions (blood–testis barrier) and germ cells in varying stages of spermatogenesis. The **blood–testis barrier** protects the spermatocytes and spermatids from the immune system

### Three Stages of Spermatogenesis

1. **Spermatocytogenesis** begins at puberty adjacent to the basement membrane of the Sertoli cell. Spermatogonia first undergo spermatocytogenesis, during which mitosis divides the spermatogonia into spermatocytes.

2. **Meiosis** reduces the diploid spermatocytes into haploid spermatids.

3. **Spermiogenesis** is the maturation of spermatids into mature spermatozoa.

### Spermiogenesis

During **spermiogenesis**, the spermatids undergo chromatin condensation and nuclear elongation, which forms the head of the spermatozoa.

The **acrosome**, a hydrolytic enzyme-containing region on the sperm cell head, also forms during this time.

The midpiece of the sperm has as a mitochondrial sheath that contains much of the ATP necessary for sperm movement. The **flagellum** contains an array of **9 + 2 microtubular pairs** linked by **dynein** for sperm motility. Patients with defective or absent dynein in **Kartagener syndrome** have reduced sperm motility, as well as reduced mucus clearance in the respiratory pathways, leading to bronchiectasis.

Once formed, spermatozoa detach from the Sertoli cells and combine with a fluid that aids in the movement of spermatozoa into the epididymis. In the epididymis, the fluid is reabsorbed, thereby concentrating sperm, and sperm interact with **forward motility factor**, a protein that aids in sperm motility. Ejaculated sperm must undergo **capacitation** in the uterus before fertilization can occur.

### Fertilization

**Fertilization** is a three-step process:

1. **Acrosome reaction:** Sperm close to the corona radiata release hyaluronidase, which dissolves material between corona radiata cells, allowing sperm to reach the zona pellucida.
2. **Zonal reaction:** Sperm bind to a glycoprotein of the zona and release acrosin, which facilitates penetration of the zona by the sperm head.
3. **Cortical reaction:** The first sperm to penetrate the zona fuses with the plasma membrane of the ovum and induces a calcium-dependent release of cortical granules that prevents polyspermy.

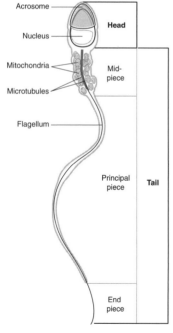

**Spermatozoon**

## HORMONAL CONTROL OF STEROIDOGENESIS AND SPERMATOGENESIS

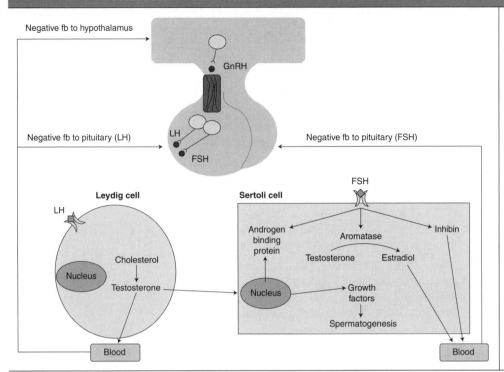

**GnRH** is synthesized in the **preoptic nucleus** and is released in a pulsatile manner into the hypophysial portal system. Binding of GnRH to its receptor on the anterior pituitary stimulates the release of LH and FSH.

*Note:* If the gonadotrophs are subjected to constant GnRH stimulation, the receptors will undergo downregulation.

- **LH** binds to the **Leydig cell** and stimulates the conversion of cholesterol into testosterone. Testosterone diffuses into blood and feeds back to inhibit hypothalamic GnRH and pituitary LH. Testosterone diffuses into the Sertoli cell and increases transcription of androgen-binding protein and growth factors that mediate spermatogenesis.

- **FSH** binds to the **Sertoli cell** and stimulates transcription of androgen-binding protein, the conversion of testosterone to estradiol, and the secretion of inhibin. Inhibin feeds back to inhibit further production of pituitary FSH.

- Sertoli cell-derived **androgen binding protein** provides an important reserve of testosterone in the testes. Because spermatogenesis is dependent on intratesticular testosterone rather than systemic testosterone, these reserves are important to normal spermatogenesis.

| INFLAMMATORY LESIONS | |
|---|---|
| **Mumps** | • Orchitis develops in approximately 25% of patients over age 10, but is less common in patients under 10<br>• Rarely leads to sterility |
| **Gonorrhea** | • Neglected urethral gonococcal infection may spread to prostate, seminal vesicles, and epididymis, but rarely to testes |
| **Syphilis** | • Acquired or congenital syphilis may involve the testes<br>• Two forms: gummas or a diffuse interstitial/lymphocytic plasma cell infiltrate<br>• Can lead to sterility |
| **Tuberculosis** | • TB usually spreads from epididymis; this is almost always associated with foci of TB elsewhere |

## TESTICULAR NEOPLASMS

### Germ Cell Tumors
Most common malignancy in men 15 to 34 years of age

| | |
|---|---|
| **Seminoma** | • Rare in infants, incidence increases to a peak in the fourth decade<br>• 10% are anaplastic seminomas; show nuclear atypia<br>• *Prognosis:* with treatment; 5-year survival rate exceeds 90%<br>• Highly radiosensitive; metastases rare |
| **Embryonal carcinoma** | • Most commonly in the 20–30-year-age group<br>• Aggressive, present with testicular enlargement<br>• 30% metastatic disease at time of diagnosis<br>• Serum AFP: elevated<br>• 5-year mortality rate 65%<br>• Less radiosensitive than seminomas<br>• Often metastasize to nodes, lungs, and liver<br>• May require orchiectomy and chemotherapy |
| **Choriocarcinoma** | • Most common in men 15–25 years of age, highly malignant<br>• May have gynecomastia or testicular enlargement<br>• Elevated serum and urine hCG levels<br>• Tends to disseminate hematogenously, invading lungs, liver, and brain<br>• Treated with orchiectomy and chemotherapy |
| **Yolk sac tumor** | • Most common in children and infants, although rare overall<br>• Elevated alpha fetoprotein (AFP)<br>• Very aggressive; exhibiting a 50% 5-year mortality rate<br>• May be considered a variant form of embryonal carcinoma |
| **Teratoma** | • Can occur at any age, but are most common in infants and children<br>• Appears as a testicular mass<br>• Exhibit a variety of tissues, such as nerve, muscle, cartilage, and hair<br>• Benign behavior during childhood, variable in adults<br>• 2-year mortality is 30%<br>• *Treatment:* orchiectomy, followed by chemotherapy and radiation |

### Non–Germ Cell Tumors

| | |
|---|---|
| **Leydig cell tumor** | • Usually unilateral<br>• Can produce androgens or estrogens<br>• *Children:* present with masculinization or feminization; *adults:* gynecomastia<br>• Usually benign and only 10% are invasive; surgery may be curative |
| **Sertoli cell** | • Usually unilateral<br>• Can produce small amounts of androgens or estrogens, usually not enough to cause endocrinologic changes<br>• Present with testicular enlargement<br>• Over 90% are benign |
| **Lymphoma** | • Lymphomas are the most common testicular cancer in elderly men<br>• The tumors are rarely confined to the testes (often disseminated) |

*Note:* Testicular neoplasms tend to metastasize to the **lumbar nodes**, whereas scrotal disease affects **superficial inguinal nodes**.

## HORMONAL CONTROL OF STEROIDOGENESIS

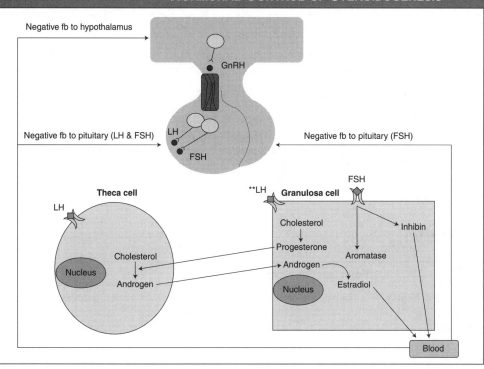

**GnRH** is synthesized in the **preoptic nucleus** and is released in a **pulsatile** manner into the hypophysial portal system. Binding of GnRH to its receptor on the anterior pituitary stimulates the release of LH and FSH.

*Note:* If the gonadotrophs are subjected to constant GnRH stimulation, the receptors will undergo downregulation.

- **LH** binds receptors on **theca cells**, resulting in production of androstenedione or testosterone. Androgens produced by the theca cells enter the granulosa cells to be converted into estrogens.

- **LH** also binds receptors on **granulosa cells** during the luteal phase and stimulates production of progesterone, which enters the theca cells. During the luteal phase, progesterone is required to maintain pregnancy if fertilization/implantation occur.

- **FSH** binds receptors on **granulosa cells**, resulting in aromatization of androgens to estradiol and synthesis of new LH receptors on the granulosa cells. Estradiol can be released into the blood or can act locally to increase granulosa cell proliferation and sensitivity to FSH.

- **FSH** also stimulates the production of **inhibin**, which negatively feeds back to inhibit further FSH secretion.

- **Estradiol** secreted into the blood negatively feeds back to inhibit hypothalamic and pituitary secretion of GnRH, and LH and FSH, respectively. This action does not occur near the ovulatory period.

*Definition of abbreviations:* LH, luteinizing hormone; FSH, follicle-stimulating hormone; GnRH, gonadotropin-releasing hormone.

ORGAN SYSTEMS

REPRODUCTIVE

# Folliculogenesis and Ovulation

| Follicular Development | Graafian follicle |
|---|---|

14 days →

Primordial follicle, Primary follicle, Developing follicles, Secondary oocyte, Mature (graafian) follicle, Secondary oocyte arrested in metaphase of meiosis II, Ruptured follicle, Early corpus luteum, Mature corpus luteum, Corpus albicans

1. Theca externa
2. Theca interna
3. Cumulus oophorus
4. Zona pellucida
5. Corona radiata
6. Follicular antrum
7. Granulosa cells

## Follicular Development

- At puberty, there are about 400,000 follicles present in the ovarian stroma, but only about 450 of these will develop (remaining follicles undergo atresia).
- The immature or **primordial follicle** (an oocyte surrounded by pregranulosa cells) is **arrested in prophase I of meiosis** until maturation.
- Starting at puberty, during each cycle, a primordial follicle becomes the **primary follicle** when the oocyte enlarges and the granulosa cells mature and proliferate. The granulosa cells secrete mucopolysaccharides, creating the **zona pellucida**, which protects the oocyte and provides an avenue for the oocyte to receive nutrients and chemical signals from the granulosa cells.
- As the follicle matures, additional granulosa cell layers are added and a layer of androgen-producing theca cells known as the **theca interna** surround the now **secondary follicle**. The secondary follicle continues to grow, and a fibrous theca externa surrounds the follicle. A follicular cavity (**antrum**) forms from granulosa cell secretions.
- The mature follicle, the **graafian follicle**, is now ready for ovulation. At the time of the LH surge, the oocyte resumes meiosis, **completes the first meiotic division, and is arrested in metaphase of meiosis II prior to ovulation**. Meiosis produces a nonfunctional first polar body, which degenerates, and a larger secondary haploid oocyte.
- If it is fertilized, the secondary oocyte completes meiosis II to form a **mature oocyte** and **polar body**.

## Ovulation

- As the antral fluid increases, the pressure becomes greater until the follicle ruptures and the oocyte is extruded.
- Following ovulation, the theca cells enlarge and begin secreting estrogen and the granulosa cells enlarge and secrete progesterone. This new endocrine organ is called the **corpus luteum** and reaches maximal development about 7 days after ovulation.
- If fertilization does not occur, the corpus luteum degenerates.
- If fertilization does occur, the corpus luteum continues to grow for about 3 months and is maintained by **human chorionic gonadotropin (hCG)** from the embryo. Once the placenta is functional, the corpus luteum is no longer necessary to maintain pregnancy.

ORGAN SYSTEMS

REPRODUCTIVE

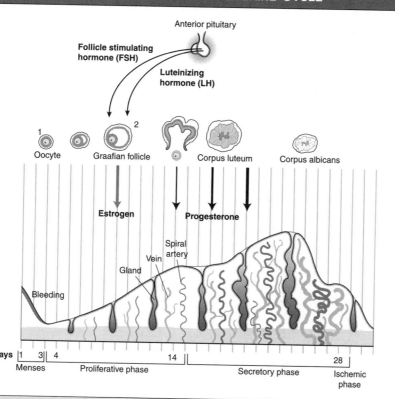

The **uterine cycle** can be divided into four phases:

- **menstruation**
- **proliferative phase**
- **secretory phase**
- **premenstruation**

As with the menstrual cycle, Day 1 of the uterine cycle begins at the onset of menses. This time period corresponds with the degeneration of the corpus luteum.

ORGAN SYSTEMS

REPRODUCTIVE

## Proliferative Phase

- The **proliferative phase** follows menses, corresponding to the latter portion of the follicular phase of the menstrual cycle and ending near ovulation.
- During this time, elevated estrogen levels stimulate the **proliferation of endometrial cells**, an **increase in length and number of endometrial glands**, and **increased blood flow** to the uterus.
- The endometrium increases in thickness sixfold and becomes contractile. Estrogen also stimulates a marked increase in progesterone receptors in the endometrium to prepare it for fertilization. **Edema** develops in the uterus toward the end of the proliferative phase and continues to develop during the secretory phase.

## Secretory Phase

- The **secretory phase** corresponds with the luteal phase of the menstrual cycle and is characterized by **endometrial cell hypertrophy, increased vascularity, and edema**.
- **Progesterone levels are elevated** during this phase and lead to a thick secretion consisting of glycoprotein, sugars, and amino acids. Like estrogen, progesterone increases cell proliferation and vascularization, but unlike estrogen, progesterone depresses uterine contractility.

## Premenstrual Phase

- The **premenstrual phase** consists of constriction of arteries, causing ischemia and anoxia. The **superficial layer of the endometrium degenerates**, and blood and tissue appear in the uterine lumen.

## MENSTRUAL CYCLE

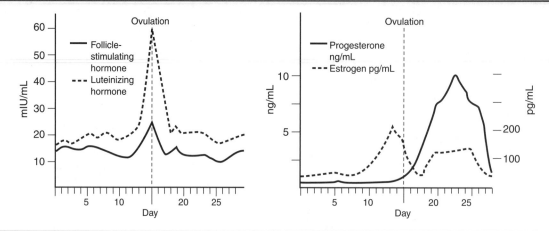

### Overview

- There are **four phases** in the menstrual cycle: **menses**, **follicular phase**, **ovulation**, and **luteal phase**.
- The **average cycle length** is **28 days**, but can vary widely. The period from ovulation to the onset of menses is always 14 days, so any variation from 28 days occurs during the **follicular** phase.

### Menses

- The onset of menses marks **Day 1** of the menstrual cycle and is triggered by a **decrease in estrogen** (decreased estrogen synthesis by granulosa cells and decreased LH) and **progesterone**. The decrease in estrogen and progesterone support for the endometrium results in tissue necrosis and arterial rupture, leading to sloughing of the superficial layer of the endometrium and bleeding.
- The elevated levels of progesterone in the luteal phase act to negatively feed back and decrease LH production. Also, luteal cells become less responsive to LH about 1 week following ovulation.

### Follicular Phase

- The **follicular phase** begins on about **Day 5** of the menstrual cycle and lasts an average of 9 days.
- When progesterone and estrogen levels decrease, the negative feedback on the hypothalamus and pituitary is removed, allowing an **increase in the frequency of GnRH pulses**. This, in turn, **stimulates FSH secretion**, thereby stimulating follicular growth (and estrogen production from proliferating granulosa cells).
- One follicle will secrete more estradiol than the others and will become the **dominant follicle** while the others undergo atresia. **Estrogen** levels continue to increase until they reach a critical point, at which estrogen changes from **negative to positive feedback** to increase GnRH pulse frequency and LH and FSH secretion. This rapid rise in GnRH pulse frequency results in a surge of both LH and FSH.

### Ovulation

- The **LH surge** and **high estrogen levels trigger ovulation** on about **Day 14** of the cycle.
- The **follicle ruptures about 24 to 36 hours after the LH surge**, during which the oocyte resumes meiosis and the first polar body is extruded.

### Luteal Phase

- The **luteal phase** begins after ovulation around Day 14 and extends to about Day 28.
- During this time the follicular cells form the **corpus luteum** and secrete **high levels of progesterone** and a lower level of estrogen (even without LH stimulation). Progesterone negatively feeds back to slow the frequency of GnRH pulses, so LH and FSH levels remain low.
- In the absence of fertilization, the corpus luteum undergoes luteolysis, causing progesterone and estrogen levels to decrease until the hormonal support for the endometrial lining declines and the cells undergo apoptosis. Menses occurs and the cycle is back at the beginning.

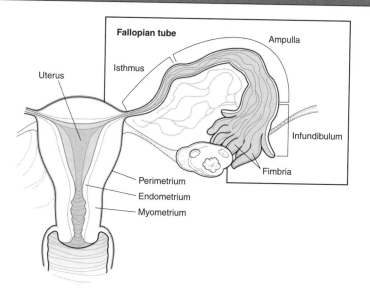

The ovulated oocyte is picked up from the intraperitoneal cavity by fimbria of the fallopian tube. Peristaltic contractions of the fallopian tube move the oocyte into the ampulla, where fertilization usually occurs 8 to 25 hours after ovulation.

- Semen ejaculated into the vagina quickly coagulates and **neutralizes** the **acidic vaginal fluids** to permit sperm survival. About 100,000 of the approximately 60 million sperm that enter the vagina will make it through the cervix. **Elevated estrogen** before ovulation **thins the cervical mucus**, allowing for easier transit of sperm to the uterus.

- Uterine fluid solubilizes the glycoproteins coating the sperm in a process called **capacitation**. Capacitation aids in fertilization by increasing energy metabolism, enhancing motility, and allowing the **acrosome reaction** that occurs at the zona pellucida. Sperm movement through the uterus is primarily accomplished by contraction of the female reproductive tract, primarily the uterus.

- Sperm are capable of fertilizing for as long as 72 hours after ejaculation. Once sperm reach the oocyte, they **bind to the zona pellucida** and **undergo the acrosome reaction**. This reaction releases hydrolytic enzymes stored in the acrosome cap, which dissolve the zona pellucida. Sperm motility is important to push the sperm head toward the oocyte. When the sperm reach the oocyte, the two membranes fuse and the contents of the sperm cell enter the oocyte. At this point, a **cortical reaction** occurs, during which the zona pellucida hardens and prevents additional sperm from entering the oocyte.

- Prior to fusing of the male and female pronucleus, the oocyte undergoes a second meiotic division, producing the second polar body and the female pronucleus. **The contents of the sperm form the male pronucleus, which fuses with the female pronucleus, forming the embryo.**

- The embryo remains in the ampulla several days, during which time rising levels of progesterone relax the uterine and fallopian tube musculature, making it easier for the embryo to pass into the uterus.

- The **embryo** usually **arrives in the uterus** by about the **third day following fertilization**, but **does not implant in the uterus for about 3 more days.** During the latter 3 days, the embryo develops a vascular system that aids in taking up nutrients it receives from uterine secretions.

ORGAN SYSTEMS

REPRODUCTIVE

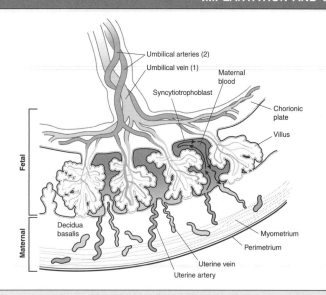

## Implantation

At the time of implantation, the trophectoderm cells of the embryo contact the maternal epithelium, resulting in increased vascular permeability in the embryo, edema in the intracellular matrix, swelling of the stromal cells with addition of glycogen granules, and sprouting and ingrowth of capillaries. This reaction is called **decidualization** and prepares the decidua for the embryo. Within about 12 days after fertilization, the embryo is completely embedded in the decidua.

Between 8 to 12 days after fertilization, **human chorionic gonadotropin (hCG) is synthesized by the blastocyst** and is structurally and functionally similar to LH. It acts on the ovary to stimulate luteal growth and to suppress luteolysis.

## Placenta

- The **placenta** allows for the exchange of nutrients and waste products between the maternal and fetal circulations. By about 5 weeks postfertilization, the placenta is developed and functional, although not fully mature.
- The placenta consists of **villi** from cell columns of chorionic **syncytiotrophoblast**, which have fetal blood vessels throughout. The villi branch and penetrate the maternal stroma, forming a mass of terminal villi that is separated from fetal capillaries by the thin layer of the villi.

## Lactation

- During pregnancy, **estrogen and progesterone** stimulate the development of the mammary glands for **lactation** while preventing milk production.
- Following delivery, estrogen and progesterone levels decline and milk production is permitted.
- The production of milk requires **prolactin**, a hormone produced by the anterior pituitary. Prolactin is normally inhibited by hypothalamic dopamine, but suckling decreases dopamine release.
- The ejection of milk requires **oxytocin**, a hormone produced in the hypothalamus and released from the posterior pituitary. **Oxytocin is released in response to suckling or baby crying** and acts on the myoepithelial cells to stimulate contraction (milk let-down). Milk is then ejected from the nipple.

ORGAN SYSTEMS

REPRODUCTIVE

## DISEASES OF PREGNANCY

### Pregnancy-induced Hypertension

| | |
|---|---|
| **Preeclampsia and eclampsia** | **Preeclampsia:** Hypertension, proteinuria, and edema |
| | Symptoms can include headache, blurred vision, mental changes, facial and extremity edema, and abdominal pain |
| | Preeclampsia is common (>5% of pregnancies) from 20 weeks' gestation onward |
| | Can cause Hemolysis, Elevated Liver function tests, and Low Platelets (HELLP syndrome) |
| | Best treatment is delivery of fetus if possible; or manage with bed rest, salt restriction, IV magnesium sulfate, antihypertensives, and diazepam if needed for treatment and/or prevention of seizures. |
| | **Eclampsia** = Preeclampsia and **seizures** |
| | Rare because of aggressive management of preeclampsia |

### Placental Abnormalities

| | |
|---|---|
| **Abruptio placentae** | Placenta detaches prematurely from the endometrium, with risk of death for the fetus and DIC in the mother |
| **Placenta previa** | Placenta overlies the cervical os; the baby must be delivered by Caesarian section to prevent life-threatening maternal or fetal hemorrhage due to tearing of the placenta during delivery |
| **Placenta accreta** | Placenta implants directly in the myometrium rather than the endometrium; following delivery, hysterectomy is usually performed to be sure all of the placenta was removed |

### Amniotic Fluid Abnormalities

| | |
|---|---|
| **Polyhydramnios** | Very large amount of amniotic fluid; usually due to severe abnormalities in the fetus such as anencephaly, esophageal atresia, or duodenal atresia |
| **Oligohydramnios** | Very small amount of amniotic fluid; usually due to severe abnormalities in the fetus such as bilateral renal agenesis or posterior urethral valves (males) that prevent urination |

### Miscellaneous

| | |
|---|---|
| **Ectopic pregnancy** | Embryo lodges in an abnormal site (most commonly in a fallopian tube, but can also be on pelvic organs or in the abdomen) |
| | Typically because of fallopian tube pathology that prevents the egg from reaching the uterine cavity |
| | Risk of potentially fatal hemorrhage to the mother |

## INFECTOUS AGENTS THAT CROSS THE PLACENTA

| **(Mnemonic: TORCH)** | Miscellaneous: |
|---|---|
| *Toxoplasma* | *Listeria monocytogenes* |
| **O**ther (Syphilis) | Parvovirus B19 |
| **R**ubella | Coxsackie B |
| **C**MV | Polio |
| **H**erpes and **H**IV | |

## FEMALE REPRODUCTIVE PHARMACOLOGY

| Class | Mechanism | Comments/Agents |
|-------|-----------|-----------------|

### Contraception

The most common methods of reversible contraception include oral contraceptives, long-acting injectable or implantable progestins, condoms, spermicides, withdrawal, diaphragm and intrauterine devices, and timely abstinence.

| Class | Mechanism | Comments/Agents |
|-------|-----------|-----------------|
| **Estrogens and progestins** | Suppresses production of FSH and LH, which leads to inhibition of ovulation and alteration of cervical mucus and the endometrium. | • Commonly used estrogens: ethinyl estradiol and mestranol<br>• Commonly used progestins: norgestrel, norethindrone, and medroxyprogesterone<br>• Are available orally as monophasic, biphasic, and triphasic combinations; also available as progestin-only preparations<br>• Are available in many other forms, including transdermal patches, vaginal rings, IUDs, and long-acting injections<br>• Can cause nausea, breast tenderness, headache, depression, thromboembolism, and weight gain<br>• Absolute contraindications include thrombophlebitis, thromboembolic disorders, cerebral vascular disease, coronary occlusion, known or suspected pregnancy, smokers over the age of 35; dramatically impaired liver function, and suspected breast cancer<br>• Other uses: female hypogonadism, HRT, dysmenorrhea, uterine bleeding, and acne |
| **Postcoital contraceptives** | Prevents pregnancy if used within 72 hours of unprotected intercourse | Different types include estrogens alone, progestins alone, combination pills, mifepristone (RU486) |
| **Intrauterine devices (IUD)** | "Devices" that create a hostile environment in the endometrium through low-grade intrauterine inflammation and increased prostaglandin formation; therefore interfere with the implantation of the fertilized ovum | Examples: Copper-T 380 (IUD) and Progesterone T (IUD) |

### Hormone Replacement Therapy (HRT)

- Used in the treatment of menopause, which is defined as a permanent cessation of menstruation secondary to a loss of ovarian follicular activity. HRT is used to prevent hot flashes, atrophic changes in the urogenital tract, and osteoporosis.
- When ERT is administered alone, it may induce endometrial growth and cancer; concomitant progesterone use prevents this. HRT has been associated with an increased breast cancer and stroke risk and is no longer as widely used.

*(Continued)*

## FEMALE REPRODUCTIVE PHARMACOLOGY (CONT'D.)

| Class | Mechanism | Comments/Agents |
|-------|-----------|-----------------|
| **Selective Estrogen Receptor Modulator (SERM)** <br> These drugs act as estrogen agonists, partial agonists, or antagonists, depending on the target tissue. | | |
| **Tamoxifen** | • Estrogen antagonist in breast <br> • Estrogen agonist in endometrium <br> • Estrogen agonist in bone | • Used in hormone-responsive breast CA; reduces risk of breast CA in very high risk women <br> • Increases risk of endometrial CA <br> • Prevents osteoporosis in woman using it for breast CA <br> • Causes hot flashes and increases risk of venous thrombosis |
| **Raloxifene** | • Partial estrogen agonist in bone <br> • Estrogen antagonist in breast <br> • Estrogen antagonist in uterus | • Prevents osteoporosis in postmenopausal women <br> • Reduces risk of breast CA in very high risk women <br> • No increased endometrial CA risk <br> • Causes hot flashes and increases risk of venous thrombosis |
| **Miscellaneous Agents** | | |
| **Clomiphene** | Fertility agent; nonsteroidal agent that selectively blocks estrogen receptors in the pituitary, reducing negative feedback mechanism and thereby increasing FSH and LH and stimulation of ovulation | Most common side effect: multiple birth pregnancy |
| **Danazol** | Inhibits ovarian steroid synthesis | Used in endometriosis and fibrocystic breast disease |
| **Anastrozole Exemestane** | Aromatase inhibitor (decrease in estrogen synthesis) | Used in breast CA in postmenopausal women |
| **Mifepristone (RU 486)** | Progesterone and glucocorticoid antagonist | Used as postcoital contraceptive and abortifacient |
| **Dinoprostone** | $PGE_2$ analog | Used to induce labor, causes cervical ripening and uterine contractions; also an abortifacient |
| **Ritodrine Terbutaline** | $\beta_2$ agonists | Relax uterus, have been used to suppress premature labor |

*Definition of abbreviations:* CA, cancer; ERT, estrogen replacement therapy; FSH, follicle-stimulating hormone; HRT, hormone-replacement therapy; LH, luteinizing hormone.

ORGAN SYSTEMS

REPRODUCTIVE

# FEMALE REPRODUCTIVE SYSTEM PATHOLOGY

## DISEASES OF THE VULVA

| Disease | Description | Distribution | Etiology/Comments |
|---|---|---|---|
| Condyloma acuminatum | Verrucous, wartlike lesions Koilocytosis, acanthosis, hyperkeratosis, and parakeratosis | Vulva, perineum, vagina, and cervix | Associated with human papillomavirus (HPV) serotypes 6 and 11 Greatly increased risk of cervical carcinoma |
| Papillary hidradenoma | Benign tumor similar to an intraductal papilloma of the breast | Occur along the milk line | |
| Extramammary Paget disease of the vulva | Erythematous, crusted rash Intraepidermal malignant cells with pagetoid spread | Labia majora | Not associated with underlying tumor |
| *Candida* vulvovaginitis | Erythema, thick white discharge | Vulva and vagina | Extremely common, especially in diabetics and after antibiotic use |

*Note:* See also Sexually Transmitted Diseases, pages 359–361.

## DISEASES OF THE VAGINA

### Vaginal Adenosis and Clear Cell Adenocarcinoma

- Rare in the general population, but greatly increased risk in females exposed to diethylstilbestrol (DES) in utero (1940–1970)
- Vaginal adenosis—benign condition thought to be a precursor of clear cell carcinoma

### Embryonal Rhabdomyosarcoma (Sarcoma Botryoides)

- Rare tumor affecting female infants and young children (age <4)
- Polypoid, "grapelike," soft tissue mass protruding from the vagina
- Spindle-cell tumor, may show cross-striations, positive for desmin, indicating skeletal muscle origin

## DISEASES OF THE CERVIX/FALLOPIAN TUBES

| Disease | Description | Etiologies | Disease Manifestations | Clinical |
|---|---|---|---|---|
| Pelvic inflammatory disease | Ascending infection from cervix to endometrium, fallopian tubes, and pelvic cavity | ***Neisseria gonorrhoeae*** (Gram ⊖ diplococcus) ***Chlamydia trachomatis*** (intracytoplasmic inclusions in mucosal cells) | Cervicitis, endometritis, salpingitis, peritonitis, pelvic abscess, perihepatitis (Fitz-Hugh-Curtis syndrome), chandelier sign *Complications:* tubo-ovarian abscess, tubal scarring, infertility, ectopic pregnancy, intestinal obstruction | - Vaginal discharge/ bleeding<br>- Midline abdominal pain, bilateral lower abdominal and pelvic pain<br>- Abdominal tenderness and peritoneal signs<br>- Fever |
| Cervical carcinoma | Third most common malignant tumor of the female genital tract in United States; peak incidence in the 40s | Associated with early first intercourse, multiple sexual partners, infection by **HPV types 16, 18**, 31 and 33, smoking, and immunosuppression | **Begins as cervical intraepithelial neoplasia (CIN)** → carcinoma in situ → invasive squamous cell cancer | May be asymptomatic, or may have postcoital bleeding, dyspareunia, discharge Early detection possible with **Papanicolaou (Pap) smear – koilocytic cells** |

| Disease | Description | Location | Pathology | Clinical |
|---|---|---|---|---|
| Endometritis | Ascending infection from the cervix | Endometrium and decidua | *Ureaplasma, Peptostreptococcus, Gardnerella, Bacteroides*, Group B *Streptococcus, Chlamydia trachomatis, Actinomyces* (yellow, granular filaments on IUD) | Associated with pregnancy or abortions (acute)<br><br>Associated with PID and intrauterine devices (IUDs) (chronic) |
| Endometriosis | • Presence of endometrial glands and stroma outside the uterus<br>• Most commonly affects women of reproductive age | Ovary<br>Ovarian and uterine ligaments<br>Pouch of Douglas<br>Serosa of bowel and bladder<br>Peritoneal cavity | Red-brown serosal nodules (**"powder burns"**)<br>Endometrioma: ovarian **"chocolate" cyst**<br>Adenomyosis = endometrial glands in the myometrium | Chronic pelvic pain linked to menses<br>Dysmenorrhea and dyspareunia<br>Rectal pain and constipation<br>Infertility |
| Leiomyoma | • **Benign smooth muscle tumor that grows in response to estrogen.**<br>• Higher incidence in African Americans<br>Malignant variant: leiomyosarcoma | May occur in subserosal, intramural, or submucosal locations in the myometrium | Well-circumscribed, rubbery, white-tan "whorled" masses<br><br>Often multiple | Menorrhagia<br>Abdominal mass<br>Pelvic pain, back pain, or suprapubic discomfort<br>Infertility |
| Leiomyosarcoma | Smooth muscle sarcoma of the uterus | Myometrium | **Gross:** Bulky tumor with necrosis and hemorrhage<br><br>**Micro:** Malignant smooth muscle cells, often with nuclear pleomorphism and increased mitotic rate | Increased incidence in blacks<br>Aggressive tumor that tends to recur<br>May present with cervical bleeding |
| Endometrial adenocarcinoma | Most common malignant tumor of the female genital tract<br><br>Most commonly affects postmenopausal women | Begins in endometrium and may invade myometrium | **Gross:**<br>Tan polypoid endometrial mass<br>Invasion of myometrium is prognostically important<br><br>**Micro:** endometrioid adenocarcinoma (most common type) | Postmenopausal vaginal bleeding<br>**RISK FACTORS:**<br>**Early menarche and late menopause**<br>**Nulliparity**<br>Hypertension and diabetes<br>Obesity<br>**Chronic anovulation**<br>**Estrogen-producing ovarian tumors, estrogen replacement therapy and tamoxifen**<br>Endometrial hyperplasia<br>Lynch syndrome (colon, endometrial, and ovarian cancers = HNPCC) |

*Definition of abbreviations:* HNPCC, hereditary nonpolyposis colorectal cancer.

ORGAN SYSTEMS

REPRODUCTIVE

## DISEASES OF THE OVARY

| Disease | Presentation | Laboratory/Pathology | Etiology | Treatment |
|---------|-------------|---------------------|----------|-----------|
| Polycystic ovary disease (Stein-Leventhal syndrome) | • Young, **obese, hirsute** females of reproductive age<br>• Oligomenorrhea or secondary amenorrhea<br>• **Infertility** | • **Elevated luteinizing hormone** (LH)<br>• Low follicle stimulating hormone (FSH)<br>• **Elevated testosterone**<br><br>Bilaterally enlarged ovaries with multiple follicular cysts | Increased LH stimulation leads to increased androgen synthesis and anovulatory cycles | Oral contraceptives or medroxyprogesterone, surgical wedge resection |
| **Epithelial Tumors** | | | | |
| Cystadenoma | Most common benign ovarian tumor<br>Pathology: Unilocular cyst with simple serous or mucinous lining | | | |
| Cystadeno-carcinoma | Most common malignant ovarian tumor.<br><br>Often asymptomatic until far advanced (presenting symptoms may be increased abdominal girth due to ascites, bowel or bladder problems)<br><br>Can produce **pseudomyxoma peritonei** | CA-125- marker for cystadenocarcinoma of ovary. Used to monitor recurrence, measure response to therapy.<br><br>Complex multiloculated cyst with solid areas<br>• Serous (serous cystadenocarcinoma) or mucinous (mucinous cystadenocarcinoma) lining with tufting, papillary structures with **psammoma bodies**<br>• Spreads by seeding pelvic cavity | **Genetic risk factors:**<br>• BRCA-1: breast and ovarian cancers<br>• Lynch syndrome | Surgery, antineoplastic drugs |
| Borderline tumor | Tumors of low malignant potential | | | |
| Brenner tumor | Rare tumor that resembles transitional carcinoma; can be benign or malignant | | | |
| Less common tumors | • Yolk sac tumor: may have structures resembling primitive glomeruli<br>• Choriocarcinoma (see table below) and embryonal carcinoma: very aggressive tumors | | | |
| **Germ Cell Tumors** | | | | |
| Teratoma | • Most are benign<br>• Occur in younger women<br>• Contain elements from **all three germ layers (ectoderm, mesoderm, endoderm)**<br>• **Immature teratoma-** contains primitive cells – **higher malignant potential** | Ovarian cyst containing hair, teeth, and sebaceous material | May be due to abnormal differentiation of fetal germ cells that arise from the fetal yolk sac | Surgical |
| Dysgerminoma | • Malignant<br>• Affects mainly young adults | Similar to seminoma in appearance | **Risk factors:**<br>Turner syndrome, pseudohermaphroditism | Radiosensitive, so good prognosis |

*(Continued)*

## DISEASES OF THE OVARY (*CONT'D.*)

### Sex Cord-Stromal Tumors

| | |
|---|---|
| Ovarian fibroma | Common tumor. Associated with Meigs syndrome = fibroma + ascites + pleural effusion |
| Granulosa cell tumor | Potentially malignant, **produces estrogen** and can produce precocious puberty, irregular menses, or dysfunctional uterine bleeding.<br>Microscopic: made of polygonal tumor cells with formation of follicle-like structures **(Call-Exner bodies)** Complications: endometrial hyperplasia and cancer |
| Sertoli-Leydig cell tumor (androblastoma) | • Androgen producing tumor, presents with virilization |

## GESTATIONAL TROPHOBLASTIC DISEASE

### Hydatidiform Mole (Molar Pregnancy)—tumor of placental trophoblast

| | |
|---|---|
| **Incidence** | 1:1,000 pregnancies |
| **Clinical** | "Size greater than dates," vaginal bleeding, passage of edematous, grape-like tissue, elevated β-hCG, invasive moles invade myometrium |
| **Treatment** | Curettage, follow β-hCG levels |

### Types

| | | |
|---|---|---|
| **Complete mole** | Results from fertilization of an ovum that lost all its chromosomal material; all chromosomal material is derived from sperm | 90% 46,XX; 10% contain a Y chromosome |
| **Partial mole** | Results from fertilization of an ovum by two sperm, one 23,X and one 23,Y | Partial moles are triploid = 69, XXY (23,X [maternal] + 23X [one sperm] +23Y [the other sperm]) |
| **Choriocarcinoma** | • **Malignant** germ cell tumor derived from trophoblast<br>• Gross: necrotic and hemorrhagic mass<br>• Micro: proliferation of cytotrophoblasts, intermediate trophoblasts, and syncytiotrophoblasts<br>• Hematogenous spread to lungs, brain, liver, etc.<br>• Responsive to chemotherapy | |

## PARTIAL MOLES VERSUS COMPLETE MOLES

| Properties | Partial Mole | Complete Mole |
|---|---|---|
| Ploidy | Triploid | Diploid |
| Number of chromosomes | 69 | 46 (All paternal) |
| β-hCG | Elevated (+) | Elevated (+++) |
| Chorionic villi | Some are hydropic | All are hydropic |
| Trophoblast proliferation | Focal | Marked |
| Fetal tissue | Present | Absent |
| Invasive mole | 10% | 10% |
| Choriocarcinoma | Rare | 2% |

# BREAST PATHOLOGY

## FIBROCYSTIC DISEASE

- Most common breast disorder, affecting approximately 10% of women; may be mistaken for CA
- Develops during reproductive life, distortion of the normal breast changes associated with the menstrual cycle
- Patients often have lumpy, tender breasts
- *Pathogenesis:* possibly due to high estrogen levels, coupled with progesterone deficiency
- *Pathology:* several morphologic patterns recognized

| | |
|---|---|
| **Fibrosis** | • Women 35 to 49 years of age; not premalignant<br>• *Gross:* dense, rubbery mass; usually unilateral, most often in the upper outer quadrant<br>• *Histology:* increase in stromal connective tissue; cysts are rare |
| **Cystic disease** | • Women 45 to 55 years of age; may predispose to malignancy<br>• *Gross:* serous cysts, firm to palpation, may be hemorrhagic; usually multifocal, often bilateral<br>• *Histology:* cysts lined by cuboidal epithelium, may have papillary projections<br>• May be an accompanying stromal lymphocytic infiltrate (chronic cystic mastitis) |
| **Sclerosing adenosis** | • Women 35 to 45 years of age; probably does not predispose to CA<br>• *Gross:* palpable, ill-defined, firm area most often in upper outer quadrant; usually unilateral.<br>• *Histology:* glandular patterns of cells in a fibrous stroma; may be difficult to distinguish from cancer |
| **Epithelial hyperplasia** | • Women over 30 years of age, increased CA risk<br>• *Gross:* variable with ill-defined masses<br>• *Histology:* ductal epithelium is multilayered and produces glandular or papillary configurations |

## TUMORS

| | |
|---|---|
| **Fibroadenoma** | • Most common benign breast tumor<br>• Single movable breast nodule, often in the upper outer quadrant; not fixed to skin<br>• Occurs in reproductive years, generally before age 30, possibly related to increased estrogen sensitivity<br>• May show menstrual variation and increased growth during pregnancy; postmenopausal regression usual<br>• *Gross:* round and encapsulated with a gray-white cut surface<br>• *Histology:* glandular epithelial-lined spaces with a fibroblastic stroma<br>• Surgery required for definitive diagnosis |
| **Cystosarcoma phyllodes** | • Fibroadenoma-like tumors that have become large, cystic, and lobulated<br>• Distinguished by the nature of the stromal component<br>• Malignant fibrous, cartilaginous; bony elements may be present<br>• *Gross:* irregular mass; often fungating or ulcerated<br>• *Histology:* myxoid stroma with increased cellularity, anaplasia, and increased mitoses<br>• Tumor initially localized but may spread later, usually to distant sites but not to local lymph nodes |
| **Intraductal papilloma** | • Most common in women 20–50 years of age; solitary lesion within a duct<br>• May present with nipple discharge (serous or bloody), nipple retraction, or small subareolar mass<br>• *Gross:* small, sessile or pedunculated, usually close to the nipple in major ducts<br>• *Histology:* multiple papillae<br>• Single intraductal papillomas may be benign, but multiple papillomas associated with an increased risk of CA |

## CARCINOMA OF THE BREAST

| | |
|---|---|
| **General features** | <ul><li>Most common cause of CA in women</li><li>Lung CA causes more deaths</li><li>Rare in women under age 25</li><li>Lifetime risk of breast CA for the average woman with no family history: 8 to 10%</li></ul> |
| **Risk factors** | <ul><li>Increasing age (40+ years)</li><li>Nulliparity</li><li>Family history</li><li>Early menarche</li><li>Late menopause</li></ul> <ul><li>Fibrocystic disease</li><li>Previous history of breast cancer</li><li>Obesity</li><li>High-fat diet</li></ul> |
| **Clinical features** | <ul><li>50% in the upper outer quadrant</li><li>Ninety percent arise in ductal epithelium</li><li>Slightly more common in the left breast; bilateral or sequential in 4% of cases</li><li>Breast mass usually discovered after self-examination or on routine physical</li></ul> |
| **Tumor suppressor genes: *BRCA1* and *BRCA2*** | Mutated *BRCA1*— <ul><li>Almost 100% lifetime risk for breast CA, often in the third and fourth decades of life</li><li>Also at increased risk for ovarian CA (men may be at increased risk for prostate CA)</li></ul> Mutated *BRCA2*— <ul><li>Increased incidence of breast CA in both women and men</li><li>Does not increase the incidence of ovarian CA in women</li></ul> |
| **Invasion** | <ul><li>May grow into the thoracic fascia to become fixed to the chest wall</li><li>May extend into the skin, causing dimpling and retraction</li><li>May cause obstruction of subcutaneous lymphatics, causing an orange-peel consistency to skin called "peau d'orange"</li><li>May invade Cooper ligaments within ducts to cause nipple retraction</li></ul> |
| **Metastases** | <ul><li>Most breast CAs disseminate via lymphatic or hematogenous routes</li><li>Involve axillary, supraclavicular, and internal thoracic nodes</li><li>Can also involve nodes of the contralateral breast</li></ul> |

ORGAN SYSTEMS

REPRODUCTIVE

## BREAST CARCINOMA TYPES

| | |
|---|---|
| **Infiltrating ductal carcinoma** | • Most common breast CA<br>• *Gross:* rock hard, cartilaginous consistency, usually 2 to 5 cm in diameter, foci of necrosis and calcification common (may be seen on mammography)<br>• *Histology:* anaplastic duct epithelial cells appear in masses, invading the stroma.<br>• Fibrous reaction responsible for the hard, palpable mass |
| **Paget disease of the breast** | • Older women; poor prognosis<br>• Form of intraductal carcinoma involving areolar skin and nipple<br>• *Gross:* skin of the nipple and areola ulcerated and oozing<br>• *Histology:* ductal carcinoma, as well as large, anaplastic, hyperchromatic "Paget cells" |
| **Noninfiltrating intraductal carcinoma** | • *Gross:* focus of increased consistency in breast tissue<br>• *Histology:* typical duct epithelial cells proliferate and fill ducts, leading to ductal dilatation<br>• Often called "comedocarcinomas" because cheesy, necrotic tumor tissue may be expressed from ducts.<br>• Rarely have a papillary pattern |
| **Medullary carcinoma with lymphoid infiltration** | • Better prognosis than infiltrating ductal carcinoma<br>• *Gross:* fleshy masses, often 5 to 10 cm in diameter, little fibrous tissue, although foci of hemorrhage and necrosis common<br>• *Histology:* sheets of large, pleomorphic cells with increased mitotic activity and a lymphocytic infiltrate |
| **Colloid (mucinous) carcinoma** | • Older women, slow growing, has a better prognosis than infiltrating ductal carcinoma<br>• *Gross:* soft, large, gelatinous tumors<br>• *Histology:* islands of tumor cells with copious mucin |
| **Lobular carcinoma** | • Multicentric; usually have estrogen receptors, arise from terminal ductules<br>• *Gross:* rubbery and ill-defined (result of their multicentric nature)<br>• *Histology:* tumor cells small and may be arranged in rings |

## FIBROCYSTIC DISEASE VERSUS BREAST CANCER

| Fibrocystic Disease | Breast Cancer |
|---|---|
| • Often bilateral<br>• May have multiple nodules<br>• Menstrual variation<br>• Cyclic pain and engorgement<br>• May regress during pregnancy | • Often unilateral<br>• Usually single nodule<br>• No menstrual variation<br>• No cyclic pain and engorgement<br>• Does not regress during pregnancy |

## MISCELLANEOUS BREAST CONDITIONS

| | |
|---|---|
| **Acute mastitis** | • Fissures in nipples during early nursing predispose to bacterial infection; usually unilateral with pus in ducts; necrosis may occur<br>• Usual pathogens: *Staphylococcus aureus* and *Streptococcus*<br>• Antibiotics and surgical drainage may be adequate therapy |
| **Mammary duct ectasia (plasma cell mastitis)** | • Occurs in fifth decade in multiparous women<br>• Presents with pain, redness, and induration around the areola with thick secretions; usually unilateral<br>• Skin fixation, nipple retraction, and axillary lymphadenopathy may occur—must be distinguished from malignancy |
| **Gynecomastia** | • Enlargement of the male breasts; most often unilateral, but may be bilateral<br>• Secondary to Klinefelter syndrome, testicular tumors, puberty, or old age<br>• Associated with hepatic cirrhosis (cirrhotic liver cannot degrade estrogens)<br>• May be important signal that patient has high-estrogen state |

# GENITOURINARY SYSTEM DISEASE

## INFECTIONS AND SEXUALLY TRANSMITTED DISEASES (STDs)

| Type Infection | Case Vignette/ Key Clues | Most Common Causative Agent(s) | Pathogenesis | Diagnosis | Treatment |
|---|---|---|---|---|---|
| **Urethritis** | Gram ⊖ diplococci in PMNs in urethral exudate | *Neisseria gonorrhoeae* | Invasive; pili assist adherence; have antigenic variation; are antiphagocytic; IgA protease | Gram ⊖ diplococci in PMNs, growth on Thayer-Martin agar, DNA probes | Ceftriaxone |
| | Culture ⊖, inclusion bodies | *Chlamydia trachomatis* | Obligate intracellular in epithelial cells; CMI and DTH cause scarring | Tissue culture; glycogen-containing inclusion bodies in cytoplasm | Tetracyclines, macrolides |
| | Urease ⊕, no cell wall | *Ureaplasma urealyticum* | Urease raises pH of urine → struvite stones | Not gram staining; diagnosed by exclusion, urinary pH | Tetracyclines, macrolides |
| | Flagellated protozoan with corkscrew motility | *Trichomonas vaginalis* | Unknown, PMN filtrate | Flagellated protozoan, corkscrew motility | Metronidazole |
| **Cystitis** | Painful urination, hematuria, fever, | *E. coli #1,* other gram ⊖ enterics | Pili, adhesins, motility, many are β hemolytic | Culture of urine ≥$10^5$ CFU/ml of gram ⊖ rods in urine | Fluoroquinolones, sulfonamide |
| | As above, in young, newly-sexually active female (honeymoon cystitis) | *Staphylococcus saprophyticus* | Sexual intercourse introduces normal flora organisms into urethra | Culture of urine, gram ⊕ cocci | Fluoroquinolones |
| | As above with increased urinary pH | *Proteus spp.* | Urease raises urinary pH, predisposes to struvite stones | Culture of urine, lactose non-fermenting gram ⊖ bacilli with swarming motility | Fluoroquinolones, TMP-SMX |
| **Pyelonephritis** | As above with flank pain and fever | *E. coli, Staphylococcus* | Strictures, urinary stasis allow colonization | Culture of urine | Fluoroquinolones, 3rd gen cephalosporin, ampicillin-sulbactam |
| **Cervicitis** | Friable, inflamed cervix with mucopurulent discharge | *Neisseria gonorrhoeae* | Invades mucosa, PMN infiltration, pili, IgA protease | Gram ⊖ diplococci, Thayer-Martin agar | Ceftriaxone |
| | | *Chlamydia trachomatis* | Obligate intracellular, CMI and DTH → scarring | Tissue culture, cytoplasmic inclusions | Tetracyclines, macrolides |
| | | Herpes simplex virus | Vesicular lesions, painful | dsDNA, nuclear envelope, icosahedral; Tzanck smear, intranuclear inclusions | Acyclovir, valacyclovir, famciclovir |

*(Continued)*

ORGAN SYSTEMS

REPRODUCTIVE

| Type Infection | Case Vignette/ Key Clues | Most Common Causative Agent(s) | Pathogenesis | Diagnosis | Treatment |
|---|---|---|---|---|---|
| **Vulvovaginitis** | Adherent yellowish discharge, pH >5, fishy amine odor in KOH, clue cells, gram ⊖ cells dominate | Bacterial vaginosis | Overgrowth of *Gardnerella vaginalis*, anaerobes | Clue cells, gram ⊖ rods | Metronidazole |
| | Vulvovaginitis, pruritus, erythema, discharge with consistency of cottage cheese | *Candida* spp. | Antibiotic use → overgrowth, immunocompromised | Germ tube test, gram ⊕ yeasts in vaginal fluids | Nystatin, miconazole |
| | "Strawberry cervix," foamy, purulent discharge; many PMNs and motile trophozoites microscopically (corkscrew motility) | *Trichomonas vaginalis* | Vaginitis with discharge | Pear-shaped trophozoites with corkscrew motility | Metronidazole |
| **Pelvic inflammatory disease** | Adnexal tenderness, bleeding, dyspareunia, vaginal discharge, fever, chandelier sign, onset often follows menses | *Neisseria gonorrhoeae* | Pili and IgA protease production | Gram ⊖ diplococci in PMNs or culture on Thayer-Martin | Ceftriaxone + doxycycline (doxycycline given for presumed coinfection with *Chlamydia*) |
| | | *Chlamydia trachomatis* | Intracellular in mucosal epithelia; causes type IV hypersensitivity damage | Tissue culture, intracytoplasmic inclusions in mucosal cells | Doxycycline, macrolides |
| **Condyloma acuminatum (genital warts)** | Lesions are papillary/wart-like, may be sessile or pedunculated, koilocytotic atypia is present, anogenital | Human papilloma virus (HPV; most common U.S. STD) | HPV proteins E6 and E7 inactivate cellular antioncogene<br><br>Associated with cervical CA | dsDNA, naked, icosahedral, intranuclear inclusion bodies | Podophyllin, imiquimod |
| **Genital herpes** | Multiple, painful, vesicular, coalescing, recurring | Herpes simplex | Latent virus in sensory ganglia reactivates | Virus culture, intranuclear inclusions, syncytia (Tzanck smear), dsDNA enveloped (nuclear), icosahedral | Acyclovir, valacyclovir, famciclovir |

*(Continued)*

ORGAN SYSTEMS

REPRODUCTIVE

| Type Infection | Case Vignette/ Key Clues | Most Common Causative Agent(s) | Pathogenesis | Diagnosis | Treatment |
|---|---|---|---|---|---|
| **Syphilis Primary** | Painless chancre forms on glans, penis (or vulva/ cervix) and heals within 1 to 3 months | *Treponema pallidum* | 3-week incubation during which spirochetes spread throughout the body | Biopsy/scraping viewed with dark-field microscopy shows spirillar organisms | Penicillin, doxycycline is an alternative |
| **Secondary** | Local or generalized rash lasting 1 to 3 months, can involve the palms and soles | | Develops 1 to 2 months after primary stage | Serology—VDRL ⊕ (nonspecific); FTA-ABS (specific) | |
| **Tertiary** | Affects central nervous system, heart, and skin; characteristic lesion is gumma, may be single or multiple; most common in the liver, testes, and bone | | Develops in one-third of untreated patients; *neurosyphilis:* including meningovascular, tabes dorsalis, and general paresis; obliterative endarteritis of vasa vasorum of the aorta can lead thoracic aneurysm | Serology – FTA-Abs, non-specific tests may be negative | |
| **Chancroid** | Nonindurated, painful ulcer, suppurative with adenopathy; slow to heal | *Haemophilus ducreyi* | Unknown | Gram ⊖ rods, chocolate agar (requires NAD and hemin) | Cefotaxime, ceftriaxone |
| **Lymphogranuloma venereum** | Soft, painless papule heals, lymph nodes enlarge and develop fistulas, genital elephantiasis may develop | *Chlamydia trachomatis* serotypes L1–3 | Obligate intracellular | Cell culture, glycogen-containing inclusions | Tetracyclines, erythromycin |

*Definition of abbreviations:* CA, cancer; CMI, cell-mediated immunity; ds, double-stranded; DTH, delayed type hypersensitivity; PMNs, polymorphonuclear leukocytes.

ORGAN SYSTEMS

REPRODUCTIVE

# The Musculoskeletal System, Skin, and Connective Tissue

## Chapter 8

## Structure, Function, and Pharmacology of Muscle

## Head and Neck Embryology and Anatomy

## Upper Extremities and Back

## Musculoskeletal Disorders

## Skin

# STRUCTURE, FUNCTION, AND PHARMACOLOGY OF MUSCLE

## FEATURES OF SKELETAL, CARDIAC, AND SMOOTH MUSCLE

| Characteristics | Skeletal | Cardiac | Smooth |
|---|---|---|---|
| **Appearance** | Striated, unbranched fibers | Striated, branched fibers | Nonstriated, fusiform fibers |
| | Z lines | Z lines | No Z lines; have dense bodies |
| | Multinucleated | Single nucleus | Single nucleus |
| **T tubules** | Form triadic contacts with SR at A-I junction | Form dyadic contacts with SR near Z line | Absent; have limited SR |
| **Cell junctions** | Absent | Junctional complexes between fibers (intercalated discs), including gap junctions | Gap junctions |
| **Innervation** | Each fiber innervated | Electrical syncytium | Electrical syncytium |
| **Action potential**<br>  **Upstroke** | Inward $Na^+$ current | • Inward $Ca^{2+}$ current (SA node)<br>• Inward $Na^+$ current (atria, ventricles, Purkinje fibers) | Inward $Na^+$ current |
|   **Plateau** | No plateau | • No plateau (SA node)<br>• Plateau present (atria, ventricles, Purkinje fibers) | No plateau |
| **Excitation-contraction coupling** | AP → T tubules → $Ca^{2+}$ released from SR | Inward $Ca^{2+}$ current during plateau → $Ca^{2+}$ release from SR | AP → opens voltage-gated $Ca^{2+}$ channels in sarcolemma; hormones and neurotransmitters → open $IP_3$-gated $Ca^{2+}$ channels in SR |
| **Calcium binding** | Troponin | Troponin | Calmodulin |

*Definition of abbreviations:* AP, action potential; $IP_3$, inositol triphosphate; SR, sarcoplasmic reticulum.

# SKELETAL MUSCLE FIBER MORPHOLOGY AND FUNCTION

Skeletal muscle connective tissue (*see* right):

**Epimysium:** dense connective tissue that surrounds the entire muscles

**Perimysium:** thin septa of connective tissue that extends inward from the epimysium and surrounds a bundle (fascicle) of muscle fibers

**Endomysium:** delicate connective tissue that surrounds each muscle fiber

Subcellular components (*see* below):

**Myofibrils:** long, cylindrical bundles that fill the sarcoplasm of each fiber

**Myofilaments: actin** and **myosin**; are within each myofibril and organize into units called **sarcomeres**

During contraction:

| | |
|---|---|
| **A band:** no change | **I band:** shortens |
| **H band:** shortens | **Z lines:** move closer together |

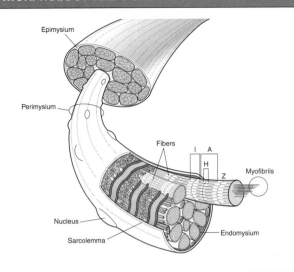

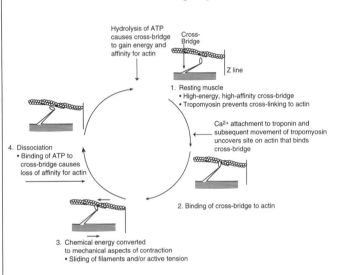

## The Crossbridge Cycle

Hydrolysis of ATP causes cross-bridge to gain energy and affinity for actin

1. Resting muscle
   - High-energy, high-affinity cross-bridge
   - Tropomyosin prevents cross-linking to actin

$Ca^{2+}$ attachment to troponin and subsequent movement of tropomyosin uncovers site on actin that binds cross-bridge

2. Binding of cross-bridge to actin

3. Chemical energy converted to mechanical aspects of contraction
   - Sliding of filaments and/or active tension

4. Dissociation
   - Binding of ATP to cross-bridge causes loss of affinity for actin

---

# RED VERSUS WHITE SKELETAL MUSCLE FIBERS

| Red Fibers (Type I) | White Fibers (Type II) |
|---|---|
| Slow contraction | Fast contraction |
| ↓ ATPase activity | ↑ ATPase activity |
| ↑ Capacity for aerobic metabolism | ↑ Capacity for anaerobic glycolysis |
| ↑ Mitochondrial content | ↓ Mitochondrial content |
| ↑ Myoglobin (imparts red color) | ↓ Myoglobin |
| Best for slow, posture-maintaining muscles, e.g., back (think chicken drumstick/thigh) | Best for fast, short-termed, skilled motions, e.g., extraocular muscles of eye, sprinter's legs, hands (think chicken breast meat and wings) |

# SMOOTH MUSCLE FUNCTION

## Types of Smooth Muscle

**Multiunit**
- Acts as individual motor unit
- Little or no electrical coupling
- Is densely innervated; contraction controlled by autonomic nervous system
- In iris, ciliary muscle of lens, and vas deferens

**Unitary (single unit)**
- Extensive electrical coupling, allowing coordinated contraction
- Has a resting tone; spontaneously active (slow waves), has pacemaker activity; activity is modulated by neurotransmitters and neurohormones
- Found mainly in the walls of hollow viscera, e.g., GI tract, uterus, bladder, ureters

**Vascular**
- Has properties of both multiunit and single-unit smooth muscle

## Smooth Muscle Contraction

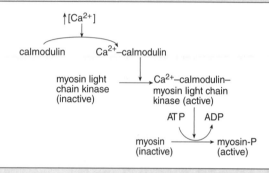

1. ↑ intracellular $Ca^{2+}$
2. $Ca^{2+}$ binds calmodulin
3. $Ca^{2+}$-calmodulin binds to and activates **myosin light chain kinase (MLCK)**
4. Myosin is phosphorylated
5. Myosin-P binds actin and shortening occurs
6. Dephosphorylation of myosin → relaxation

## Bridge to Pharmacology

**$\alpha_1$ and $M_3$ stimulation:** ↑ $IP_3$ → ↑ intracellular $Ca^{2+}$ → smooth muscle contraction

**$\beta_2$ stimulation:** ↑ cAMP → inhibits MLCK → smooth muscle relaxation

# HEAD AND NECK EMBRYOLOGY AND ANATOMY

## SKELETAL MUSCLES INNERVATED BY CRANIAL NERVES

| Muscles Derived from a Pharyngeal Arch | Cranial Nerve | Muscles | Skeletal Elements (from neural crest) |
|---|---|---|---|
| First arch—mandibular<br><br>(Mandibular hyperplasia is seen in **Treacher Collins syndrome** and in the **Robin sequence**. Both involve neural crest cells.) | **Trigeminal mandibular nerve (V3)** | Four muscles of mastication:<br>• Masseter<br>• Temporalis<br>• Lateral pterygoid<br>• Medial pterygoid<br>Plus:<br>• Digastric (anterior belly)<br>• Mylohyoid<br>• Tensor tympani<br>• Tensor veli palatini | Mandibular process<br>Maxillary process<br><br><br><br>Malleus<br>Incus |
| Second arch—hyoid | **Facial (VII)** | Muscles of facial expression:<br>• Orbicularis oculi<br>• Orbicularis oris<br>• Buccinator and others<br>Plus:<br>• Digastric (posterior belly)<br>• Stylohyoid<br>• Stapedius | Hyoid (superior part)<br>Styloid process<br>Stapes |
| Third arch | **Glossopharyngeal (IX)** | Stylopharyngeus | Hyoid (inferior part) |
| Fourth arch | **Vagus (X) superior laryngeal (external branch)**<br><br>**Vagus (X) pharyngeal branches** | Cricothyroid<br><br><br>Levator veli palatini<br>Uvular muscle<br>Pharyngeal constrictors<br>Salpingopharyngeus<br>Palatoglossus<br>Palatopharyngeus | Thyroid cartilage |
| Fifth arch | **Lost** | — | — |
| Sixth arch | **Vagus (X) recurrent laryngeal** | Lateral cricoarytenoid<br>Posterior cricoarytenoid<br>Transverse arytenoid<br>Oblique arytenoid<br>Thyroarytenoid (vocalis) | Cricoid, arytenoid, corniculate, cuneiform cartilages |
| **Muscles of myotome origin** | **Accessory (XI)** | Trapezius<br>Sternocleidomastoid | |
| | **Hypoglossal (XII)** | Genioglossus<br>Hyoglossus<br>Styloglossus | |
| | **Oculomotor (III)** | Superior, inferior, and medial rectus; inferior oblique, levator palpebrae superioris | |
| | **Trochlear (IV)** | Superior oblique | |
| | **Abducens (VI)** | Lateral rectus | |

ORGAN SYSTEMS

MUSCULOSKELETAL/SKIN

# PHARYNGEAL POUCHES

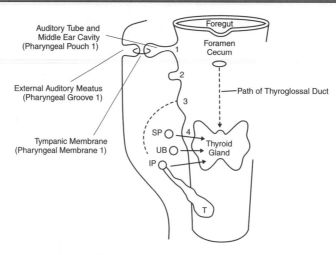

| Adult Structures Derived from the Fetal Pharyngeal Pouches | | |
|---|---|---|
| **Pouch** | **Adult Derivatives** | **Clinical Correlate** |
| 1 | Epithelial lining of auditory tube and middle ear cavity | The **DiGeorge sequence** occurs when pharyngeal pouches 3 and 4 fail to differentiate into the parathyroid glands and thymus. Patients have immunologic problems, hypocalcemia, and may have cardiovascular defects (persistent truncus arteriosus), abnormal ears, and micrognathia. |
| 2 | Epithelial lining of crypts of palatine tonsil | |
| 3 | Inferior parathyroid gland (IP) | |
| | Thymus (T) | |
| 4 | Superior parathyroid gland (SP) | |
| | Ultimobranchial body (UB) | |

The thyroid gland does not develop in a pharyngeal pouch; it develops from midline endoderm of the oropharynx and migrates inferiorly along the path of thyroglossal duct. Neural crest cells migrate into the UB to form parafollicular C cells of the thyroid.

The external auditory meatus is the only postnatal remnant of a pharyngeal groove or cleft.

# PALATE AND FACE DEVELOPMENT

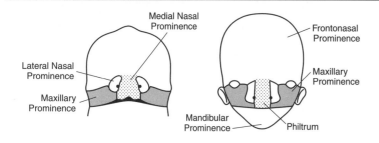

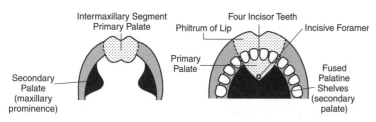

The **face** develops from the frontonasal prominence, the pair of maxillary prominences, and the pair of mandibular prominences.

The **intermaxillary segment** forms when the two medial nasal prominences fuse together at the midline and → the **philtrum of the lip**, **four incisor teeth**, and the **primary palate** of the adult.

The **secondary palate** forms from palatine shelves, which fuse in the midline, posterior to the incisive foramen.

The primary and secondary palates fuse at the **incisive foramen** to form the definitive palate.

## Clinical Correlation

**Cleft lip** occurs when the maxillary prominence fails to fuse with the medial nasal prominence.

**Cleft palate** occurs when the palatine shelves fail to fuse with each other or the primary palate.

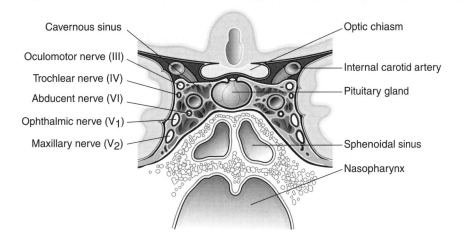

The cavernous sinuses are located on either side of the body of the sphenoid bone. Each sinus receives blood from some of the cerebral veins, ophthalmic veins, and the sphenoparietal sinus. Each cavernous sinus drains into a transverse sinus via the superior petrosal sinus and into the internal jugular vein via the inferior petrosal sinus.

## Cavernous Sinus Thrombosis

Infection can spread from veins of the face into the cavernous sinuses, producing a thrombosis that may involve the cranial nerves that course through the cavernous sinuses. Cranial nerves III, IV, and VI and the ophthalmic and maxillary divisions of CN V, as well as the internal carotid artery and its periarterial plexus of postganglionic sympathetic fibers, traverse the cavernous sinuses. All of these cranial nerves course in the lateral wall of each sinus, except for CN VI, which courses through the middle of the sinus. Initially, patients have an internal strabismus. Later, all eye movements are affected, along with with altered sensation in skin of the upper face and scalp.

ORGAN SYSTEMS

MUSCULOSKELETAL / SKIN

## BRACHIAL PLEXUS

The **brachial plexus** is formed by an intermingling of ventral rami from the C5 through T1 spinal nerves.

The ventral rami of the brachial plexus exhibit a proximal to distal gradient of innervation. Nerves that contain fibers from the superior rami of the plexus (C5 and C6) innervate proximal muscles in the upper limb (shoulder muscles). Nerves that contain fibers from the inferior rami of the plexus (C8 and T1) innervate distal muscles (hand muscles).

Five major nerves arise from the brachial plexus: the **musculocutaneous, median**, and **ulnar** nerves contain anterior division fibers and innervate muscles in the anterior arm, anterior forearm, and hand that act mainly as flexors. The **axillary** and **radial** nerves contain posterior division fibers, and innervate muscles in the posterior arm and posterior forearm that act mainly as extensors.

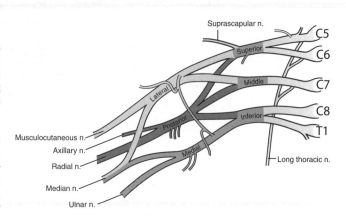

| LESIONS OF ROOTS OF THE BRACHIAL PLEXUS | | | | |
|---|---|---|---|---|
| **Lesioned Root** | **C5** | **C6** | **C7** | **C8** | **T1** |
| **Dermatome paresthesia** | Lateral border of upper arm | Lateral forearm to thumb | Over triceps, midforearm, middle finger | Medial forearm to little finger | Medial arm to elbow |
| **Muscles affected** | Deltoid Rotator cuff Serratus anterior Biceps Brachioradialis | Biceps Brachioradialis Brachialis Supinator | Latissimus dorsi Pectoralis major Triceps Wrist extensors | Finger flexors Wrist flexors Hand muscles | Hand muscles |
| **Reflex test** | — | Biceps tendon | Triceps tendon | — | — |
| **Causes of lesions** | Upper trunk compression | Upper trunk compression | Cervical spondylosis Herniation of C6/C7 disk | Lower trunk compression | Lower trunk compression |

ORGAN SYSTEMS

MUSCULOSKELETAL/SKIN

## UPPER AND LOWER BRACHIAL PLEXUS LESIONS

### Upper (C5 and C6) Brachial Plexus Lesion:  Erb-Duchenne Palsy

- Usually occurs when the head and shoulder are forcibly separated (e.g., accident, birth injury, or herniation of disk)
- Trauma will damage **C5** and **C6** roots of the upper trunk
- Primarily affects the **axillary, suprascapular,** and **musculocutaneous nerves** with loss of function of the intrinsic muscles of the shoulder and muscles of the anterior arm
- Arm is medially rotated and adducted at the shoulder: loss of **axillary** and **suprascapular** nerves. The unopposed latissimus dorsi and pectoralis muscles pull the limb into adduction at the shoulder
- The forearm is extended and pronated: loss of **musculocutaneous** nerve
- **Sign is "waiter's tip"**
- Sensory loss on lateral forearm to base of thumb: loss of musculocutaneous nerve

### Lower (C8 and T1) Brachial Plexus Lesion: Klumpke's Paralysis

- Usually occurs when the upper limb is forcefully abducted above the head (e.g., grabbing an object when falling, thoracic outlet syndrome, or birth injury)
- Trauma will injure the **C8** and **T1** spinal nerve roots of the inferior trunk
- Primarily affects the ulnar nerve and the intrinsic muscles of the hand with weakness of the median-innervated muscles of the hand
- Sign is combination of **"claw hand" (ulnar nerve)** and **"ape hand" (median nerve)**.
- May include a Horner syndrome
- Sensory loss on medial forearm and medial 1½ digits

## LESIONS OF NERVES OF THE BRACHIAL PLEXUS

### Radial Nerve (C5, C6, C7, C8)

| Axilla: (Saturday night palsy or using crutches) | Mid-shaft of humerus at radial groove or lateral elbow (lateral epicondyle) | Wrist: (laceration) |
|---|---|---|
| • Loss of extension at the elbow, wrist and MP joints<br>• Weakened supination<br>• Sensory loss on posterior arm, forearm, and dorsum of thumb<br>• Distal sign is **"wrist drop"** | • Loss of forearm extensors of the wrist and MP joints<br>• Weakened supination<br>• Sensory loss on the posterior forearm and dorsum of thumb<br>• Distal sign is **"wrist drop"** | • No **motor loss**<br>• Sensory loss only on dorsal aspect of thumb (first dorsal web space) |

### Median Nerve (C6, C7, C8, T1)

| Elbow: (Supracondylar fracture of humerus) | Wrist: (carpal tunnel or laceration) |
|---|---|
| • Weakened wrist flexion (with ulnar deviation)<br>• Loss of pronation<br>• Loss of flexion of lateral 3 digits, resulting in the inability to make a complete fist; sign is **"hand of benediction"**<br>• Loss of thumb opposition (opponens pollicis muscle); sign is **ape (simian) hand**<br>• Loss of first two lumbricals<br>• Thenar atrophy<br>• Sensory loss on palmar surface of the lateral hand and the palmar surfaces of the lateral 3½ digits<br><br>*Note:* **A lesion of median nerve at the elbow results in the "hand of benediction" and "ape hand."** | • Loss of thumb opposition (opponens pollicis muscle); sign is **ape or simian hand**<br>• Loss of first two lumbricals<br>• Thenar atrophy<br>• Sensory loss on the palmar surfaces of lateral 3½ digits. Note sensation on lateral palm may be spared.<br><br>*Note:* **Lesions of median nerve at the wrist present without hand of benediction and with normal wrist flexion, digital flexion, and pronation.** |

*(Continued)*

## LESIONS OF NERVES OF THE BRACHIAL PLEXUS (*CONT'D.*)

### Ulnar Nerve (C8, T1)

#### Elbow (medial epicondyle), wrist (lacerations), fracture of hook of hamate, midshaft clavicle fracture

- Loss of hypothenar muscles, third and fourth lumbricals, all interossei and adductor pollicis
- With elbow lesion, there is minimal weakening of wrist flexion with radial deviation
- Loss of **abduction** and **adduction of digits 2–5** (interosseus muscles)
- Weakened IP extension of digits 2–5 (more pronounced in digits 4 and 5)
- Loss of thumb adduction
- Atrophy of the hypothenar eminence
- Sign is **"claw hand"** (note that clawing is greater with a wrist lesion)
- Sensory loss on medial 1½ digits

### Axillary Nerve (C5, C6)

#### Fracture of the surgical neck of the humerus or inferior dislocation of the shoulder

- Loss of abduction of the arm to the horizon
- Sensory loss over the deltoid muscle

### Musculocutaneus Nerve (C5, C6, C7)

- Loss of elbow flexion and weakness in supination
- Loss of sensation on lateral aspect of the forearm

### Long Thoracic Nerve (C5, C6, C7)

- Often damaged during a radical mastectomy or a stab wound to the lateral chest (nerve lies on superficial surface of serratus anterior muscle)
- Loss of abduction of the arm above the horizon to above the head
- Sign of **"winged scapula"**; patient unable to hold the scapula against the posterior thoracic wall

### Suprascapular Nerve (C5, C6)

- Loss of shoulder abduction between 0 and 15 degrees (supraspinatus muscle)
- Weakness of lateral rotation of shoulder (infraspinatus muscle)

| BACK MUSCLES | | |
|---|---|---|
| **Action** | **Muscles Involved** | **Innervation** |
| Extend/Rotate vertebrae | 1. Splenius capitis, splenius cervicis | Dorsal rami of spinal nerves |
| | 2. Erector spinae:<br>• Iliocostalis<br>• Longissimus<br>• Spinalis | Dorsal rami of spinal nerves |
| | 3. Transversospinalis:<br>• Semispinalis<br>• Multifidus<br>• Rotatores | Dorsal rami of spinal nerves |

The **lumbosacral plexus** is formed by an intermingling of the ventral rami of the L2 through S3 spinal nerves. The ventral rami of the lumbosacral plexus exhibit a proximal to distal gradient of innervation. Nerves that contain fibers from the superior rami of the plexus (L2 through L4) innervate muscles in the anterior and medial thigh that act at the hip and knee joints. Nerves that contain fibers from the inferior rami of the plexus (S1 through S3) innervate muscles of the leg that act at the joints of the ankle and foot.

**Four** major nerves arise from the lumbosacral plexus:

The **obturator** and **tibial** nerves contain anterior division fibers and innervate muscles in the medial and posterior compartments of the thigh, the posterior compartment of the leg, and in the sole of the foot.

The **femoral** and **common fibular** nerves contain posterior division fibers and innervate muscles in the anterior compartment of the thigh, in the anterior and lateral compartments of the leg, and in the dorsum of the foot.

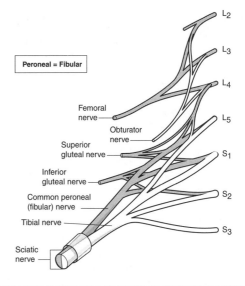

| Lesioned Root | L3 | L4 | L5 | S1 |
|---|---|---|---|---|
| Dermatome paresthesia | Anterior thigh | Medial leg | Anterior leg, dorsum of foot | Lateral foot, sole |
| Reflex test | — | Patellar tendon | — | Achilles tendon |
| Muscles affected | Hip flexors<br>Hip adductors | Knee extensors<br>Hip adductors | Dorsiflexors<br>Toe extensors | Plantar flexors<br>Toe flexors |
| Causes of lesions | Osteoarthritis | Osteoarthritis | Herniation of L4/L5 disc | Herniation of L5/S1 disc |
| **Lesioned Nerve** | **Obturator<br>(L2–L4)** | **Femoral<br>(L2–L4)** | **Common Fibular<br>(L4, L5, S1, S2)** | **Tibial<br>(L4, L5, S1–S3)** |
| Altered sensation | Medial thigh | Anterior thigh, medial leg to medial malleolus | Anterior leg, dorsum of foot | Posterior leg, sole, and lateral border of foot |
| Reflex test | — | Patellar tendon | — | Achilles tendon |
| Motor weakness | Adduction of thigh | Extension of knee | Dorsiflexion, eversion of the foot | Plantar flexion<br>Toe flexion |
| Common sign of lesion | — | — | Footdrop | — |
| Causes of lesions | Pelvic neoplasm<br>Pregnancy | Diabetes<br>Posterior abdominal neoplasm<br>Psoas abscess | Compression at fibula neck<br>Hip fracture/dislocation<br>Misplaced gluteal injection<br>Piriformis syndrome | Hip fracture/dislocation<br>Penetrating trauma to buttock |

ORGAN SYSTEMS

MUSCULOSKELETAL / SKIN

# MUSCULOSKELETAL DISORDERS

## Skeletal Disorders

### Achondroplasia

- Autosomal dominant form of dwarfism; mutation of the fibroblast growth factor receptor 3 (FGFR3)
- Abnormal cartilage synthesis
- Decreased epiphyseal bone formation
- Short limbs, proportionately large body and head (disease spares the cranium and vertebral bones), "saddle nose"

### Enchondromatosis

- Cartilaginous masses within the medullary cavity of bone
- **Ollier disease:** nonhereditary, multiple, most commonly hands and feet
- Patients present with pain and fractures; may undergo malignant transformation
- **Maffucci syndrome:** Familial; enchondromas and hemangiomas of the skin

### Fibrous dysplasia

- Focal fibrous replacement of bone
- Incidence higher in male teenagers
- Usually monostotic; often asymptomatic or may lead to pathologic fracture
- Affects long bones, ribs, skull, and facial bones
- Fibrosis starts within the medullary cavity and remains encased in cortical bone
- **McCune-Albright syndrome:** Association of polyostotic fibrous dysplasia, café-au-lait spots, and sexual precocity in women

### Hyperparathyroidism (osteitis fibrosa cystica)

- Osteoclasts resorb bone
- Kidney wastes calcium
- Osteitis fibrosa cystica more common in primary hyperparathyroidism
- Bone pain and fractures
- Fibrous replacement of marrow, causing cystic spaces in bone and "brown tumors"

### Hypertrophic osteoarthropathy

- Idiopathic painful swelling of wrists, fingers, ankles, knees, or elbows
- Periosteal inflammation, new bone forms at the ends of long bones, metacarpals, and metatarsals
- Arthritis commonly seen, often with digital clubbing
- Etiology: Intrathoracic carcinoma, cyanotic congenital heart disease, and inflammatory bowel disease
- Regresses when underlying disease treated

### Osteochondromatosis

- Bony metaphyseal projections capped with cartilage
- Gardner syndrome: Exostoses and colonic polyps—may become carcinomas

### Osteogenesis imperfecta

Defect in type I collagen characterized by fragile bones, blue sclera, and lax ligaments
- *Type I:* autosomal dominant mild-to-moderate disease
- *Type II:* autosomal recessive stillborn infant; generalized crumpled bones
- *Type III:* autosomal recessive progressive severe deformity; white sclera
- *Type IV:* autosomal dominant variable severity; normal sclera

*(Continued)*

### Osteomalacia and rickets

- **Vitamin D deficiency** due to chronic renal insufficiency, intestinal malabsorption, or dietary deficiency; osteoid produced in normal amounts but not calcified properly (diffuse radiolucency on bone films); low calcium and phosphorus and high alkaline phosphatase
- *Rickets:* children, prior to closure of the epiphyses. Bone deformities, "rachitic rosary" (deformity of the chest wall), bowing of legs, and fractures
- *Osteomalacia:* impaired mineralization of normal osteoid matrix; fractures, deformities

### Osteomyelitis

- Spread by direct inoculation of bone or hematogenous seeding
- *Staphylococcus aureus, Streptococcus, Haemophilus influenzae*
- *Salmonella* (sickle cell disease); *Pseudomonas* (intravenous drug users and diabetics)
- *Mycobacterium tuberculosis* (Pott disease): tuberculous osteomyelitis of spine
- Patients present with fever, localized pain, erythema, and swelling
- X-ray may be normal for up to 2 weeks, then may show periosteal elevation
- **Specific findings** include:
  - Sequestrum, a necrotic bone fragment
  - Involucrum, new bone that surrounds the area of inflammation
  - Brodie abscess, localized abscess formation in the bone

### Osteopetrosis

- Osteoclasts unable to resorb bone
- Increased density of cortex with narrowing of erythropoietic medullary cavities
- Brittle bones, anemia, blindness, deafness, hydrocephalus, cranial nerve palsies
- *Autosomal recessive:* affects children, causing early death due to anemia and infections (no bone marrow)
- *Autosomal dominant:* adults—fractures

### Osteoporosis

- Decrease in bone mass; postmenopausal women
- Estrogen deficiency, low density of original bone, lack of exercise
- Bone formed normally but in decreased amounts (thinned cortical bone, enlarged medullary cavity)
- All bones are affected; x-ray shows generalized radiolucency
- Weight-bearing bones predisposed to fractures

### Paget disease

- Excessive bone resorption with replacement by soft, poorly mineralized matrix (woven appearance microscopically); x-ray: enlarged, radiolucent bones
- Patients present with pain, deformity, fractures
- Laboratory tests: extremely elevated alkaline phosphatase
- Polyostotic: skull, pelvis, femur, and vertebrae
- Progresses from an osteolytic to an osteoblastic phase
- May cause bone hypervascularity with increased warmth of the overlying skin

ORGAN SYSTEMS

MUSCULOSKELETAL/SKIN

## MICROBIOLOGY OF OSTEOMYELITIS

| Type Infection | Case Vignette/Key | Most Common Causative Agent | Mechanism of Pathogenesis | Diagnosis | Treatment |
|---|---|---|---|---|---|
| Fever, bone pain with erythema and swelling; some patients (particularly those with diabetes) may have associated cellulitis | Adults, children, and infants without major trauma or special conditions | *Staphylococcus aureus* | Hematogenous spread → lytic bone lesions, lytic toxins | Blood culture or bone biopsy | Nafcillin, 3rd gen cephalosporin, IV vancomycin |
| | Sickle cell anemia | *Salmonella* spp. | HbS patients are functionally asplenic and cannot kill bloodborne pathogens | Gram ⊖, oxidase ⊖, nonlactose fermenting | 3rd gen cephalosporin, fluoroquinolones, chloramphenicol |
| | Trauma | *Pseudomonas aeruginosa* | Capsule protects against phagocytosis | Gram ⊖, oxidase ⊕, blue-green pigments; grape odor | Antipseudomonal beta-lactam + aminoglycoside, or carbapenem + antipseudomonal fluoroquinilone + aminoglycoside |
| | Spine, hip, knee, hands. Immigrants—Indian subcontinents | *Mycobacterium tuberculosis* | Tuberculous granuloma erodes into bone | Acid-fast bacilli or auramine stain | Multiple drug therapy |

| MUSCULOSKELETAL TUMORS |||
|---|---|
| **Osteoblastic Tumors** |||
| Osteoblastoma | Similar to an osteoid osteoma, but is large and painless; often involves vertebrae; may be malignant |
| Osteoid osteoma | Benign; affects diaphysis of long bones; often tibia or femur<br>Causes pain that is worse at night and relieved by aspirin<br>X-ray findings—central radiolucency surrounded by a sclerotic rim<br>Pathology: brown nodule surrounded by dense sclerotic cortical bone |
| Osteoma | Benign; frequently involves skull<br>*Hyperostosis frontalis interna*: osteoma that extends into the orbit or sinuses<br>Pathology: dense normal bone |
| Osteosarcoma | Malignant; produces osteoid and bone<br>**Most common bone tumor**<br>Men are affected more often than women; usually second and third decade of life<br>Associated with Paget disease in older patients<br>Present with localized pain and swelling, weight loss, and anemia<br>Classic x-ray findings—Codman triangle (periosteal elevation) and bone destruction<br>Pathology: large, necrotic, and hemorrhagic mass<br>Poor prognosis; patients are treated with amputation and chemotherapy<br>Metastasis to the lungs common |
| **Chondromatous Tumors** |||
| Chondromyxoid fibroma | Benign, rare; affects young men<br>Firm mass within the metaphyseal marrow cavity of the tibia or femur<br>Contains fibrous and myxomatous tissue; must be differentiated from a malignant lesion |
| Chondrosarcoma | Malignant tumor; age range 30–60; men affected more than women<br>May arise de novo or secondarily from pre-existing enchondroma<br>Slower growing than osteosarcomas<br>Typically presents with pain and swelling<br>Involves the spine, pelvic bones, and upper extremities |
| Enchondroma | Solitary cartilaginous growth within the spongiosa of bone<br>Solitary growths are similar to those in the multiple form (Ollier disease) |
| Osteochondroma | Benign metaphyseal growth; may be solitary; lesions identical to those in multiple form |
| **Miscellaneous Tumors** |||
| Ewing sarcoma | Malignant, rare; usually affects adolescents; often males<br>Arises from mesenchymal cells<br>Presents as pain, tenderness, and early widespread dissemination<br>Commonly affects the pelvis and metaphysis of long tubular bones |
| Giant cell tumor | Malignant, uncommon; affects ages 20–50; arises in the epiphyseal region of long bones<br>Presents as a bulky mass with pain and tenderness<br>X-ray findings—expanding area of radiolucency without a sclerotic rim |
| Lipoma | Very common, soft, yellow, benign fatty tumor<br>Often found subcutaneously; simple excision is curative |
| Liposarcoma | Malignant tumor of fatty tissue typically seen in middle-aged or older adults<br>Typically found in deep subcutaneous tissues, deep fatty tissue of legs, or retroperitoneal areas |

| JOINT PATHOLOGY | |
|---|---|
| **Ankylosing spondylitis** | Occurs predominantly in young men with HLA-B27<br>Also associated with inflammatory bowel disease<br>Involves the sacroiliac joints and spine |
| **Felty syndrome** | Polyarticular rheumatoid arthritis associated with HLA-B27<br>Splenomegaly and leukopenia |
| **Gout** | **Hyperuricemia** leads to deposition of monosodium urate crystals (**needle-shaped and negatively birefringent**) in joints, leading to recurrent bouts of acute arthritis<br>• Caused by overproduction of uric acid (under 10%) or underexcretion of uric acid (over 90%)<br>• Joints are affected asymmetrically; **great toe** (first metatarsal joint) is classically affected (podagra)<br>• Later stages → chronic arthritis and **tophi** in affected joints<br>• Uric acid kidney stones develop in up to 25% of patients<br>**Primary gout** (90% of cases): due to inborn error of purine metabolism, usually from an unknown enzyme deficiency (Lesch-Nyhan syndrome is a rare cause due to HGPRT deficiency)<br>**Secondary gout:** hyperuricemia unrelated to purine metabolism |
| **Juvenile rheumatoid arthritis (Still disease)** | Peak incidence from 1–3 years; girls affected more frequently<br>Often preceded by acute febrile illness<br>Periarticular swelling, lymphadenopathy, hepatosplenomegaly, and absence of rheumatoid factor<br>Variable course; resolution may occur |
| **Osteoarthritis (degenerative joint disease)** | Incidence ↑ with age; women more affected than men<br>Affects 80% of people over 70 years old in at least one joint<br>Aging or wear and tear (biomechanical) most important mechanism<br>Insidious onset with joint stiffness, ↓ range of motion, and effusions<br>X-ray findings—narrowing of the joint space due to loss of cartilage and osteosclerosis<br>Joint fluid—few cells and normal mucin<br>Most commonly affected joints—vertebrae, hips, knees, and distal interphalangeal (DIP) joints of fingers |
| **Pseudogout (chondrocalcinosis)** | Calcium pyrophosphate crystal deposition<br>Associated with multiple diseases (e.g., Wilson disease, hypothyroidism, diabetes mellitus) |
| **Psoriatic arthritis** | Similar to rheumatoid arthritis, but absence of rheumatoid factor<br>Associated with HLA-B27 |
| **Rheumatoid arthritis** | Progressive arthritis<br>More common in women, ages 20–60 years<br>Autoimmune reaction with the formation of circulating antibodies (rheumatoid factor)<br>Symptoms—low-grade fever, malaise, fatigue, and morning stiffness<br>Physical examination—joint swelling, redness, and warmth<br>Synovial fluid—increased cells (usually neutrophils) and poor mucin<br>Elevated sedimentation rate and hypergammaglobulinemia<br>X-ray findings—erosions and osteoporosis<br>Starts in the small joints of the hands and feet but may involve any joint; usually symmetric involvement |
| **Suppurative arthritis** | Tender, red, swollen joint (e.g., "a hot knee")<br>Monoarticular; high neutrophil count in joint fluid<br>Due to *Staphylococcus*, *Streptococcus*, and gonococci<br>**Reiter syndrome:** arthritis, uveitis, and conjunctivitis—possibly due to *Chlamydia* |

| | | INFECTIOUS ARTHRITIS | | | |
|---|---|---|---|---|---|
| **Presentation** | **Case Vignette/ Key Clues** | **Most Common Causative Agent** | **Mechanism of Pathogenesis** | **Diagnosis** | **Treatment** |
| Pain, redness, low-grade fever, tenderness, swelling, reduced joint mobility | #1 overall, except in the 15–40 age group, where gonococcal is more prevalent | *Staphylococcus aureus* | Coagulase inhibits phagocytosis | Gram ⊕, coagulase ⊕ cocci, catalase ⊕ | Nafcillin, 3rd gen cephalosporin, IV vancomycin |
| | 15–40 years; mono- or polyarticular | *Neisseria gonorrhoeae* | Pili mediate adherence and inhibit phagocytosis | Gram ⊖ diplococcus; ferments glucose but not maltose | e.g., ceftriaxone |
| | Prosthetic joint | Coagulase-negative staphylococci | Biofilm allows adherence to Teflon® | Gram ⊕, catalase ⊕ cocci | Nafcillin, 3rd gen cephalosporin |
| | Viral | Rubella and hepatitis B, parvovirus | Immune complex mediated (type III hypersensitivity) | Detect immune complexes | Immunosuppressive therapy |
| | Chronic onset, monoarticular, weightbearing joints | *M. tuberculosis* or fungal | Granulomas erode into bone | Acid-fast bacillus or auramine stain, fungus stain | Multiple drug therapy |

MUSCULOSKELETAL/SKIN

# RHEUMATOID ARTHRITIS DRUGS

The rheumatoid arthritis (RA) **medications** can be divided into **three major classes**: anti-inflammatory drugs, bridging therapy, and disease-modifying antirheumatic drugs (DMARDs). Pharmacologic goals of therapy are to decrease pain, maintain "normal" functional status, reduce inflammation, decrease disease progression, and facilitate healing.

| Drug | Mechanism/Other Uses | Adverse Effects |
|---|---|---|
| **Anti-inflammatory Drugs** | | |
| Salicylates (aspirin) | **Irreversibly** inhibit COX-1 and -2, decreasing PG synthesis <br>• Low dose: ↓ platelet aggregation <br>• Intermediate dose: antipyretic, analgesic <br>• High dose: anti-inflammatory | • Chronic use associated with gastric ulcers, upper GI bleeding, acute renal failure, and interstitial nephritis <br>• Large doses can produce tinnitus, vertigo, respiratory alkalosis <br>• Overdose → metabolic acidosis, hyperthermia, dehydration, coma, death |
| NSAIDs (ibuprofen, naproxen, diclofenac, ketoprofen, indomethacin) | **Reversibly** inhibit COX-1 and -2, leading to decreased production of PGs <br>Anti-inflammatory, analgesic, antipyretic; indomethacin used to close PDA | • Abdominal distress, bleeding, ulceration <br>• Renal damage (especially in patients with renal disease) due to clearance by kidney |
| COX-2 inhibitors (celecoxib) | Selectively inhibit COX-2 <br>**COX-1 pathway:** produces PGs that protect the GI lining, maintain renal blood flow, and aid in blood clotting <br>**COX-2 pathway:** produces PGs involved in inflammation and pain | • Beneficial because of reduced GI side effects <br>• This drug class is under scrutiny due to ↑ incidence of stroke and MI. At this time, rofecoxib and valdecoxib have been taken off the market. |
| **DMARDs** | • May slow or reverse joint damage <br>• Indicated for the treatment of RA when anti-inflammatory therapy insufficient to control patient's symptomatology <br>• DMARDs usually do not show benefit for 6–8 weeks or longer; so, **bridging therapy** (corticosteroids) may be used until a full therapeutic effect is obtained. <br>• DMARDs have severe and potentially fatal side effects. | |
| Hydroxychloroquine | • Stabilizes lysosomes, ↓ chemotaxis <br>• Also an antimalarial | Ophthalmic abnormalities, dermatologic reactions, hematotoxicity, GI reactions |
| Methotrexate | • Inhibits dihydrofolate reductase, immunosuppressant <br>• Also an antineoplastic | Hemotoxicity, ulcerative stomatitis, renal toxicity, elevated LFTs |
| Sulfasalazine | • Metabolized to 5-aminosalicylic acid (5-ASA) and sulfapyridine; parent drug and/or metabolites have anti-inflammatory and/or immunomodulatory properties <br>• Used in inflammatory bowel disease | Rash, GI distress, headache, hematotoxicity |
| Gold compounds | • ↓ macrophage and lysosomal functions | Dermatitis, hematotoxicity, nephrotoxicity |
| Azathioprine | • ↓ purine metabolism and nucleic acid synthesis; immunosuppressant | Hematologic, GI disturbance, secondary infection, increased risk of neoplasia |
| Penicillamine | • ↓ T-cell activity and rheumatoid factor <br>• Also a chelating agent | GI disturbances, proteinuria, bone marrow suppression, neurotoxicity |
| Etanercept | Binds TNF | Injection site reactions |
| Leflunomide | Inhibits cell proliferation and antiinflammatory | Hepatotoxicity, immunosuppression, GI disturbance, alopecia, rash, teratogen |
| Infliximab | • Monoclonal antibody to TNF-α <br>• Also used in inflammatory bowel disease | Infusion reactions, infections, activation of latent TB |

*Definition of abbreviations:* COX, cyclooxygenases; DMARDs, disease-modifying, slow-acting antirheumatic drugs; LFTs, liver function tests; PGs, prostaglandins; TNF, tumor necrosis factor; TB, tuberculosis.

There are **three** primary ways of treating gout: *1*) decreasing inflammation in acute attacks (NSAIDs, colchicine, intra-articular steroids), *2*) using uricosuric drugs to increase renal acceleration of uric acid, and *3*) decreasing conversion of purines to uric acid by inhibiting xanthine oxidase (allopurinol).

| Agents | Mechanism | Comments |
|---|---|---|
| **Acute treatment of gout** | Acute treatment measures include NSAIDs (primarily indomethacin), colchicine, and corticosteroids (used only in resistant cases). | |
| **NSAIDs** | (*See* Rheumatoid Arthritis Drugs table.) | **Indomethacin** is drug of choice for acute gouty arthritis, although other NSAIDs also effective |
| **Colchicine** | **Binds tubulin and prevents microtubule assembly** Reduces the inflammatory response by decreasing leukocyte migration and phagocytosis | Previously considered drug of choice for gouty arthritis; however, its side effect profile limits its usage **Adverse effects:** severe diarrhea and abdominal distress, hematologic (bone marrow depression, aplastic anemia, or thrombocytopenia), renal failure, hepatic failure, peripheral neuropathy, alopecia |
| **Chronic/prophylactic treatment of gout** | These agents are used for the treatment and/or prevention of hyperuricemia with gout and gouty arthritis. | |
| **Uricosuric agents** (probenecid, sulfinpyrazone) | **Inhibits reabsorption of uric acid**, thus ↑ its excretion | Inhibits the secretion of many weak acids (e.g., penicillin, methotrexate) **Adverse reactions:** may precipitate acute gouty arthritis, which can be prevented by concurrent NSAIDs; cross-allergenicity with other sulfonamides |
| **Allopurinol** | **Inhibits xanthine oxidase**, the enzyme responsible for conversion of hypoxanthine and xanthine to uric acid | Also used as an adjunct to cancer chemotherapy Inhibits metabolism of 6-mercaptopurine and azathioprine (which are metabolized by xanthine oxidase) **Adverse reactions:** GI distress, rash |

| | |
|---|---|
| **Malignant fibrous histiocytoma** | Relatively common, affecting adult men > women Arise in soft tissue or bones Lower extremities > upper; also abdominal cavity |
| **Pigmented villonodular synovitis** | Villous proliferation of synovium colored brown by hemosiderin deposition Probably a reactive response to recurrent trauma or possibly a neoplastic process that does not metastasize |
| **Synoviosarcoma** | Rare tumor, early adulthood; affects males and females equally Slow growing, painless masses Aggressive, early metastases to the lung and pleura Two-thirds occur in lower extremities and one-third in upper extremities Arise from synovial lining cells of bursae and tendon sheaths |

ORGAN SYSTEMS

MUSCULOSKELETAL/SKIN

## MUSCLE DISORDERS

### Muscular Dystrophies

| | |
|---|---|
| **Becker muscular dystrophy** | X-linked recessive inheritance or spontaneous<br>Milder; patients may walk until age 20 or 25<br>Cardiac lesions are mild |
| **Duchenne muscular dystrophy** | Severe, **X-linked**, abnormal **dystrophin** protein, loss of muscle cell membrane stability<br>Elevation of creatine kinase and histologic degeneration precedes clinical features<br>Pelvic girdle weakness and ataxia<br>Course is progressive; children unable to walk by the age of 10<br>Pseudohypertrophy of the calves characteristic<br>Myocardial muscle involvement accompanies other muscle degeneration; may cause death<br>Heterozygous female carriers have subclinical degeneration of muscle fibers |
| **Facioscapulohumeral muscular dystrophy** | Autosomal dominant, but spontaneous mutation relatively common<br>Usually involves the face, neck, and shoulder muscles; pelvic muscles in later stages |
| **Limb-girdle muscular dystrophy** | Autosomal recessive<br>Weakness begins in pelvic or shoulder girdle; may retain ambulation for 25 years |
| **Myotonic dystrophy** | Autosomal dominant pattern or spontaneous mutations<br>Trinucleotide repeat (CTG) in a protein kinase<br>Clinically unique: weakness, atrophy, and myotonia (tonic contractions)<br>Head and neck muscles frequently weak and atrophic |

### Additional Muscular Disorders

| | |
|---|---|
| **Myasthenia gravis** | **Autoimmune** disease; antibodies against **neuromuscular junction acetylcholine receptors** (nicotinic AChR)<br>Typically affects young women with **fluctuating weakness** but **no sensory** abnormalities; worsens with increased use of muscles<br>Diagnosis—decremental response on EMG or improvement with **edrophonium**<br>May have **thymic abnormalities**, including thymoma (10–20%) or thymic hyperplasia (70–80%) |
| **Lambert-Eaton myasthenic syndrome** | • Closely related to myasthenia gravis with similar symptoms<br>• Autoantibodies are directed against NMJ $Ca^{2+}$ channels<br>• May occur in a paraneoplastic setting |
| **Myositides** | **Polymyositis** and **dermatomyositis**; autoimmune or collagen vascular diseases<br>Polymyositis more common in females<br>Neck and proximal limb muscle weakness, dysphagia, and muscle pain<br>Dermatomyositis: purple discoloration of the eyelids (heliotrope rash) and ↑ risk of internal malignancies |
| **Myositis ossificans** | Ossification at the site of traumatic hemorrhage<br>Pain, swelling, and tenderness |
| **Rhabdomyosarcoma** | Most common soft tissue sarcoma in children<br>40% have metastases at the time of diagnosis<br>**Embryonal rhabdomyosarcoma:**<br>• Most often located in head and neck tissues<br>• Sarcoma botryoides: embryonal rhabdomyosarcoma with a grape-like, soft, polypoid appearance usually located in the genitourinary or upper respiratory tract |

*Definition of abbreviation:* EMG, electromyogram; NMJ, neuromuscular junction.

ORGAN SYSTEMS

MUSCULOSKELETAL/SKIN

# SKIN

## SKIN AND SKIN APPENDAGES

The integument consists of the skin (epidermis and dermis) and associated appendages (sweat and sebaceous glands, hairs, and nails). The epidermis is devoid of blood vessels and contains a stratified squamous epithelium derived primarily from ectoderm.

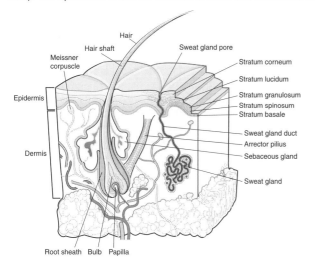

The **epidermis** is composed of five layers in thick skin:

- **Stratum basale:** a proliferative layer of columnar/cuboidal cells

- **Stratum spinosum:** a multilaminar layer of cuboidal/polygonal cells

- **Stratum granulosum:** has more flattened polygonal cells containing basophilic granules

- **Stratum lucidum:** a thin, eosinophilic layer of squamous cells

- **Stratum corneum:** a thick layer containing anucleate keratinized cells

- The **epidermis** contains four cell types: **keratinocytes**, which produce keratin; **melanocytes** (derived from neural crest) that produce melanin; **Langerhans cells**, which are antigen-presenting cells; and **Merkel cells**, associated with nerve fibers.
- The **dermis** is a connective tissue layer mainly of mesodermal origin.
- **Sweat glands** may be eccrine or apocrine.
- **Sebaceous glands** are branched, holocrine acinar glands that discharge their secretions onto hair shafts within hair follicles. They are absent in the palms and soles.
- **Hair** is composed of keratinized epidermal cells. Hair follicles and the associated sebaceous glands are known as pilosebaceous units.

## SKIN PATHOLOGY

| | |
|---|---|
| **Acanthosis nigricans** | Epidermal hyperplasia producing velvety hyperpigmentation of body folds in areas such as axilla, neck, and groin<br>Can be associated with hyperlipidemia, diabetes, and visceral malignancies. |
| **Actinic keratosis** | Premalignant and may develop into squamous cell carcinoma<br>Fair-skinned people of middle age associated with chronic sun exposure |
| **Atopic dermatitis (eczema)** | Itchy eruption that often preferentially involves the flexural areas<br>Typically diagnosed at about 6 months of age — often a lifetime illness with a remitting/flaring course; thought to be due to an immediate hypersensitivity (Type I) reaction with elevated serum IgE<br>May be associated with asthma, allergic rhinitis, and food allergy |
| **Basal cell carcinoma** | Rough, crusty, red papules up to 1 cm in diameter<br>Invasive, but rarely metastasizes<br>Occurs on sun-exposed areas in middle-aged or elderly individuals with fair complexions<br>Complete excision is usually curative; 50% recurrence rate |
| **Bullous pemphigoid** | Autoantibodies to dermoepidermal junction antigens<br>Pemphigus vulgaris is due to autoantibodies to keratinocyte intercellular junction antigens |
| **Capillary hemangiomas** | Arise within the first weeks of life and usually resolve spontaneously; starting at 1–3 years of age; most completely gone by age 5<br>Soft, red, lobulated mass, 1–6 cm in diameter, composed of thick-walled capillaries |

*(Continued)*

| | |
|---|---|
| **Contact dermatitis** | Localized skin rash caused by contact with a foreign substance<br>Rash is typically bright red, sometimes with blisters, wheals, or urticaria; may have intense itchiness and burning sensation<br>Can be due to chemical irritation (with or without light exposure), true allergic reaction, or physical irritation<br>Often resolves spontaneously; treated with oral antihistamines or hydrocortisone cream; systemic corticosteroids can be used in severe, persistent cases |
| **Dermatitis herpetiformis** | Vesicular, pruritic disease often associated with celiac sprue<br>IgA is found at the dermoepidermal junction |
| **Erythema multiforme** | Hypersensitivity reaction to drugs<br>Stevens-Johnson syndrome is the severe form. |
| **Erythema nodosum** | Hypersensitivity reaction that causes inflammatory nodules in adipose tissue (panniculitis), typically on the anterior shins<br>Peak age in the 20s to 30s; female predominance<br>Can be associated with diseases that stimulate the immune system, including tuberculosis, coccidiomycosis, histoplasmosis, leprosy, sarcoidosis, and streptococcal infections |
| **Kaposi sarcoma** | Malignant mesenchymal tumor characterized by an aggressive course in patients with AIDS and by a slower course in elderly men without HIV<br>Caused by human herpes virus type 8 (HHV8) |
| **Lichen planus** | Small, itchy, purple, polygonal papules of the skin and oral mucosa<br>Dense infiltrate of lymphocytes at the dermal epidermal junction accompanied by irregular, "saw-tooth" extensions of the dermis into the epidermis |
| **Malignant melanoma** | Peaks by ages 40–60<br>**Lentigo maligna** melanoma grows horizontally first (radial growth), followed by vertical dermal invasion (nodular growth) and forms a large, brown-black patch<br>Best prognosis of all forms of melanoma<br>**Nodular** melanoma shows extensive dermal invasion and rapid growth<br>Raised brown-black lesions may be found anywhere on skin or mucosa<br>Worst prognosis of the melanomas<br>Prognosis related to **depth of invasion** |
| **Melasma** | Hyperpigmentation occurring in pregnancy, sometimes called "mask of pregnancy" because it often involves the face |
| **Nevocellular nevus** | Common benign mole containing nevocytes derived from melanocytes<br>• Junctional nevus: nevocytes are just at the dermoepidermal junction<br>• Dermal nevus: nevocytes just in the dermis<br>• Compound nevus: nevocytes are both at the junction and in the dermis |
| **Nevus flammeus (port wine stain)** | Common congenital lesion; composed of telangiectatic vessels<br>Usually located on the neck or face as a large, flat, irregular pink patch that tends to resolve spontaneously |
| **Pemphigus vulgaris** | Potentially life-threatening blistering disease of skin and mucous membranes<br>Autoimmune etiology involving antibodies directed against desmoglein 3<br>Blisters form within the epidermis |
| **Pityriasis rosea** | Self-limited skin eruption that characteristically starts with a single, isolated lesion called the "herald patch" and then 1 or 2 weeks later progresses to a generalized rash with large numbers of large, flaky, reddish skin lesions |
| **Psoriasis** | Silvery, scaly plaque that primarily affects knees, elbows, and the scalp |
| **Seborrheic keratosis** | Common benign (but often biopsied) skin lesion of elderly people - flat, greasy papules that appear "stuck on" on the head, trunk, and extremities<br>Microscopically shows a thickened, benign epidermis composed of basaloid cells with horn cyst formation within the epidermis |

*(Continued)*

ORGAN SYSTEMS

MUSCULOSKELETAL/SKIN

## Skin Pathology (cont'd.)

| Squamous cell carcinoma | Malignant tumor; most frequently in sun-exposed areas with peak at 60 years of age<br>Preponderance among women<br>When on sun-exposed regions, rarely metastasizes<br>When on unexposed skin, up to 50% metastasize |
|---|---|
| Toxic epidermal necrolysis (TENS; Lyell's syndrome) | Life-threatening dermatologic condition in which the epidermis detaches from the dermis all over the body, particularly involving the mucous membranes<br>Considered to be a very severe form of Stevens-Johnson syndrome<br>Typically occurs as a severe reaction to medications, notably including sulfonamides, non-steroidal anti-inflammatory drugs, allopurinol, anti-HIV drugs, corticosteroids, and anticonvulsants<br>Patients are treated similarly to those with severe burns |
| Urticaria | Urticaria (hives) due to localized areas of allergic-based mast cell degranulation leading to dermal edema with intense itchiness |
| Vitiligo | Vitiligo is an acquired pigmentation disorder characterized by localized areas of complete skin depigmentation |

## Infectious Diseases of the Skin, Mucous Membranes, and Underlying Tissues

| Case Vignette/ Key Clues | Common Causative Agents | Mechanism of Pathogenesis | Diagnosis | Treatment |
|---|---|---|---|---|
| **Furuncles, carbuncles** | | | | |
| Neck, face, axillae, buttocks | *Staphylococcus aureus* | Coagulase breaks fibrin clot<br>Neutrophils + bacteria → pus | Catalase ⊕, coagulase ⊕, gram ⊕ cocci in grape-like clusters | Nafcillin for methicillin-sensitive *S. aureus* (MSSA); vancomycin for methicillin-resistant *S. aureus* (MRSA) |
| Inflamed follicles from neck down | *Pseudomonas aeruginosa* (hot tub folliculitis) | Capsule inhibits phagocytosis | Oxidase ⊕, gram ⊖ rod, blue-green pigment, grape odor | Antipseudomonal beta-lactam + aminoglycoside |
| **Acne vulgaris** | | | | |
| Inflammation of follicles and sebaceous glands; adolescent | *Propionibacterium acnes* | Fatty acids and peptides produced from sebum cause inflammation | Gram ⊕ rod, identified by clinical clues | Tetracycline, macrolide |
| **Cutaneous Lesions (scratching mosquito bites, cat scratches, etc.)** | | | | |
| Initially vesicular; skin erosion; honey-crusted lesions | *Streptococcus pyogenes* | Streptokinase A and B DNAse, hyaluronidase | Catalase ⊖, gram ⊕ cocci, bacitracin sensitive | Penicillin, macrolide |
| Initially vesicular but with longer-lasting bullae | *Staphylococcus aureus* | Exfoliatins produce bullae | Catalase ⊕, coagulase ⊕, gram ⊕ cocci, in clusters | Nafcillin for MSSA; vancomycin for MRSA |
| **Red, raised, butterfly-wing facial rash** | | | | |
| Dermal pain, edema, rapid spread | *Streptococcus pyrogenes* (erysipelas) | M protein inhibits phagocytosis, erythrogenic exotoxins, hyaluronidase | Catalase ⊖, gram ⊕ cocci, bacitracin-sensitive | Penicillin, macrolide |

*(Continued)*

| Case Vignette/ Key Clues | Common Causative Agents | Mechanism of Pathogenesis | Diagnosis | Treatment |
|---|---|---|---|---|
| **Jaw area swelling with pain, sinus tract formation, yellow granules in exudate** | | | | |
| Carious teeth, dental extraction or trauma | *Actinomyces israelii*; "lumpy jaw"; actinomycosis | Unknown | Gram ⊕, anaerobic, filamentous branching rods, non-acid fast | Penicillin |
| **Vesicular lesions** | | | | |
| Sometimes preceded by neurologic pain | Herpes | Virus-rich vesicles ulcerate dsDNA, enveloped (nuclear membranes) | Cell culture, intranuclear inclusion, multinucleated cells | Acyclovir, valacyclovir, famciclovir |
| Sometimes large | *Staphylococcus aureus* | Exfolatins produce bullae | Catalase ⊕, coagulase ⊕, gram ⊕ cocci, in clusters | Nafcillin for MSSA; vancomycin for MRSA |
| **Subcutaneous granulomas/ulcers/cellulitis** | | | | |
| Tropical fish enthusiasts; granulomatous lesion (most commonly freshwater) | *Mycobacterium marinum* | Trauma + water exposure → granulomas form | Biopsy, slow growing acid-fast bacilli | Clarithromycin initially, then antimycobacterial therapy |
| Cellulitis following contact with saltwater or oysters | *Vibrio vulnificus* | Cytolytic compounds, antiphagocytic polysaccharides | Green colonies on TCBS agar (alkaline), gram ⊖ rod, oxidase ⊕ | Tetracycline, aminoglycosides |
| Solitary or lymphocutaneous lesions; rose gardeners or florists; sphagnum moss | *Sporothrix schenckii* (rose gardener's disease) | Ulceration or abscess | Cigar-shaped yeast in pus | Potassium iodide, ketoconazole |
| Subcutaneous swelling (extremities, shoulders), sinus tract formation, granules (mycetoma) | *Actinomyces, Nocardia* | Unknown; granules are microcolonies | *Actinomyces*— Gram ⊕, anaerobic, filamentous branching non-acid fast rods *Nocardia*—partially acid-fast, branching filaments, aerobic | *Actinomyces*— penicillin, doxycycline, clindamycin *Nocardia*—sulfonamide, sulfa antibiotics; carbapenem for resistant cases |
| **Malignant pustule** | | | | |
| Pustule → dark-red, fluid-filled, tumor-like lesion → necrosis → black eschar surrounded by red margin; postal worker or wool handler/ importer | *Bacillus anthracis* | Poly-D-glutamate capsule, exotoxin causes edema, cell death Three-component toxin | Gram ⊕, spore-forming, encapsulated rods | Ciprofloxacin, penicillin |
| As above, with pseudomonal septicemia | *Pseudomonas aeruginosa*, (**ecthyma gangrenosum**) | Endotoxin | Blood culture, gram ⊖, oxidase ⊕, produces blue-green pigments, fruity odor | Susceptibility testing necessary |

*(Continued)*

| Case Vignette/ Key Clues | Common Causative Agents | Mechanism of Pathogenesis | Diagnosis | Treatment |
|---|---|---|---|---|
| **Burns, cellulitis** | | | | |
| Blue-green pus; grape-like odor | *Pseudomonas aeruginosa* | Capsule inhibits phagocytosis | Oxidase ⊕, gram ⊖ rod, blue-green pigments, grape odor | Antipseudomonal beta-lactam + aminoglycoside |
| **Wounds** | | | | |
| Surgical wounds (clean) | *Staphylococcus aureus* | Same as above for *S. aureus* | Same as above for *S. aureus* | Nafcillin for MSSA, vancomycin for MRSA |
| Surgical wounds (dirty) | Enterobacteriaceae, anaerobes | Contamination from fecal flora | Gram ⊖ facultative anaerobes | 3rd gen cephalosporin |
| Trauma with damage to blood supply | *Clostridium perfringens* and others | Alpha toxin (lecithinase) gas production, edema, cytotoxicity | Nagler reaction, anaerobic, gram ⊕ rod, spore forming | Debridement, clindamycin, chloramphenicol, tetracycline |
| Animal bites (various) | *Pasteurella multocida* | Capsule | Gram ⊖ rods (bite wounds are not generally cultured) | Amoxicillin/clavulanate |
| Human bites, fist fights | *Eikenella corrodens* | Pili, phase variation | Gram ⊖ oral floral | 3rd generation cephalosporins, fluoroquinolones |
| Dog bites | *Capnocytophaga canimorsus* | Sialidase allows adherence to host cells | Gram ⊖ fusiform | As above |
| Rat bites | *Streptobacillus moniliformis and Spirillum minus* | Endotoxin | Gram ⊖ pleomorphic rod | Penicillin G or V |
| Cat scratches, resulting in lymphadenopathy with stellate granulomas | *Bartonella henselae* | Obligate intracellular | Gram ⊖ envelope | Various antibiotics (rifampin, ciprofloxacin, gentamicin, TMP-sulfamethoxazole) |
| Shallow puncture wound through tennis shoe sole | *Pseudomonas aeruginosa* | Capsule inhibits phagocytosis | Oxidase ⊕, gram ⊖ rod, blue-green pigments | Antipseudomonal beta-lactam + aminoglycoside |
| **Leprosy** | | | | |
| Blotchy, red lesions with anesthesia; facial and cooler areas of skin | *Mycobacterium leprae* (tuberculoid form) | Cell-mediated immunity kills intracellular organisms, damages nerves | Acid-fast, intracellular bacilli in punch biopsy, ⊕ lepromin test | Dapsone, clofazimine +/- rifampin |
| Numerous nodular lesions; leonine facies | *Mycobacterium leprae* (lepromatous form) | Humoral immunity elicited does not stop growth of organisms | Acid-fast, intracellular bacilli in punch biopsy, ⊖ lepromin test | Dapsone, clofazimine +/- rifampin |

*(Continued)*

| Case Vignette/ Key Clues | Common Causative Agents | Mechanism of Pathogenesis | Diagnosis | Treatment |
|---|---|---|---|---|
| **Keratinized area of skin (ringworm)** | | | | |
| Reddened skin lesion in growing ring shape, raised margin; infection nail bed or hair shaft | *Trichophyton* spp. (skin, hair, nails) *Epidermophyton* spp. (skin, nails) *Microsporum* spp. (skin, hair) | Fungi germinate in moist areas, invade | Wood's lamp (fluoresce), skin scraping and KOH; arthroconidia | Topical miconazole or oral imidazoles if hair shaft or nails infected |
| **Dermatitis** | | | | |
| Itching skin rash after swimming in fresh water lakes (swimmer's itch) | Bird schistosomes | Skin penetration by cercariae → death in skin → hypersensitivity | Clinical signs and history | Topical anti-inflammatory |
| Snake-like tracks on bare skin exposed to dog/cat feces (plumber's itch, cutaneous larva migrans) | Dog and cat hookworms (*Ancylostoma* spp.) | Skin penetration by larvae → death in skin → hypersensitivity (type 1) | Clinical signs and history | Topical anti-inflammatory, thiabendazole |
| **Warts** | | | | |
| Plantar surfaces | HPV 1 (dsDNA, naked icosahedral) | Virus infects basal layers of skin, stimulates cells to divide | Intranuclear inclusion bodies | Cryotherapy |
| Common warts | HPV serotypes 2, 4 | | | |
| Umbilicated warts; wrestling teams; may be anogenital | *Molluscum contagiosum* (pox family, dsDNA, enveloped complex) | Infects epidermal cells to form fleshy lesion | Intracytoplasmic inclusions | Cryotherapy |
| Anogenital warts | HPV 6 and 11 (most common) HPV 16 and 18 (premalignant) | Virus stimulates cell division Cervical intraepithelial neoplasia Tumor suppressor gene inactivation | Intranuclear inclusion bodies | Imiquimod, interferon-$\alpha$, cidofovir |
| **Mucocutaneous erosive lesions** | | | | |
| Foreign immigrant or military stationed in the Middle East, ulcers; chronic facial disfiguration; sandfly vector | *Leishmania* spp. | Amastigotes intracellular in macrophages, proliferate and spread | Finding amastigotes with flagellar pocket inside phagocytic cells in biopsy | Antimonials pentamidine |

ORGAN SYSTEMS

MUSCULOSKELETAL/SKIN

| Type of Rash | Progression | Other Symptoms | Causative Agent(s) | Pathogenesis | Diagnosis | Treatment |
|---|---|---|---|---|---|---|
| **Scarlet fever** | | | | | | |
| Erythematous maculopapular (sandpaper-like) | Trunk and neck → extremities (spares palms and soles) | Sore throat, fever, nausea | *Streptococcus pyogenes* | Exotoxins A–C (superantigens) | Gram ⊕, catalase ⊖ cocci | Penicillin, clindamycin |
| **Toxic shock syndrome** | | | | | | |
| Diffuse, erythematous, macular sunburn-like | Trunk and neck → extremities with desquamation on palms and soles | Acute onset, fever >102 F, myalgia, pharyngitis, vomiting, diarrhea; hypotension leading to multiorgan failure | *Staphylococcus aureus* | TSST-1 (superantigen) | Gram ⊕, catalase ⊕, coagulase ⊕ cocci | Nafcillin, oxacillin; vancomycin in penicillin allergic patients |
| **Staphylococcal skin disease: scalded skin disease and scarlatina** | | | | | | |
| Perioral erythema, bullae, vesicles, desquamation | Trunk and neck → extremities, except tongue and palate; large bullae and vesicles precede exfoliation | Abscess or some site of infection | *Staphylococcus aureus* | Endotoxin | Gram ⊕, catalase ⊕, coagulase ⊕ cocci | Nafcillin, oxacillin; vancomycin in penicillin allergic patients |
| **Lyme disease** | | | | | | |
| Erythematous concentric rings (Bull's eye) | Originates at site of tick bite | Fever, headache, myalgia, Bell's palsy | *Borrelia burgdorferi* (#1 vector-borne disease in U.S.) | Invades skin and spreads to involve heart, joints and CNS. Arthritis is type III hypersensitivity | Serology | Doxycycline, ceftriaxone |
| **Epidemic typhus** | | | | | | |
| Petechiae → purpura | Trunk → extremities; spares palms, soles, and face | Fever, rash, headache, myalgias, and respiratory symptoms | *Rickettsia prowazekii* | Endotoxin | Serology, Weil-Felix | Doxycycline, chloramphenicol |
| **Rocky Mountain spotted fever (most common on East Coast)** | | | | | | |
| Petechiae | Ankles and wrists → generalized with palms and soles | Fever, rash, headache, myalgias, and respiratory symptoms | *Rickettsia rickettsii* | Endotoxin (overproduces outer membrane fragments) | Serology, Weil-Felix | Doxycycline, chloramphenicol |
| **Early meningococcemia** | | | | | | |
| Petechiae → purpura | Generalized | Abrupt onset, fever, chills, malaise, prostration, exanthem → shock | *Neisseria meningitidis* | Endotoxin | Gram ⊖ diplococcus on chocolate agar; LPA for capsular antigens | Ceftriaxone |

*(Continued)*

ORGAN SYSTEMS

MUSCULOSKELETAL/SKIN

| Type of Rash | Progression | Other Symptoms | Causative Agent(s) | Pathogenesis | Diagnosis | Treatment |
|---|---|---|---|---|---|---|
| **Secondary syphilis** | | | | | | |
| Skin: maculopapular; mucous membrane: condylomata lata | Generalized bronze rash involving the palms and soles | Fever, lymphadenopathy, malaise, sore throat, splenomegaly, headache, arthralgias | *Treponema pallidum* | Endotoxin | Serology: VDRL (nonspecific), FTA-ABS (specific) | Penicillin, doxycycline, erythromycin |
| **Measles** | | | | | | |
| Confluent, erythematous, maculopapular rash, unvaccinated child | Head → entire body Koplik's spots | Cough, coryza, conjunctivitis, and fever (prodrome); oral lesions, exanthem, bronchopneumonia, ear infections (unvaccinated individual) | Rubeola virus; negative sense RNA virus, non-segmented = Paramyxovirus | T-cell destruction of virus-infected cells in capillaries causes rash | Virus cultures, serology | Supportive |
| **Chickenpox/ Shingles** | | | | | | |
| Asynchronous rash, unvaccinated child | Generalized with involvement of mucous membranes | Fever, pharyngitis, malaise, rhinitis, exanthem | Varicella zoster virus (Herpesviridae, dsDNA) | Virus replicates in mucosa and is latent in dorsal root ganglia | Tzanck smear (find syncytia), Cowdry type A intranuclear inclusions, PCR | Supportive, avoid aspirin due to Reye syndrome |
| Unilateral vesicular rash following a dermatome, 50-60 year old patient | Restricted to one dermatome | Fever, severe nerve pain, pruritus | Varicella zoster virus (Herpesviridae, dsDNA) | Reactivation of latent infection | Tzanck smear (find syncytia), Cowdry type A intranuclear inclusions, PCR | Acyclovir, famciclovir, valacyclovir |

ORGAN SYSTEMS

MUSCULOSKELETAL/SKIN

# The Hematologic and Lymphoreticular System

# HEMATOPOIESIS

All of the different blood cells are derived from stem cells in the bone marrow, as shown below.

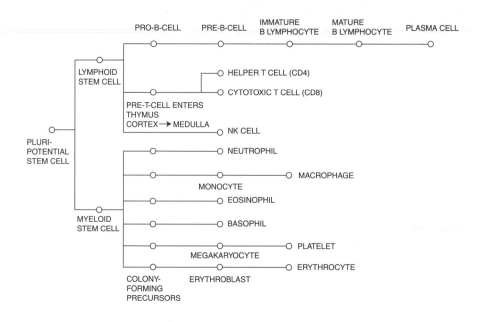

# HEMOSTASIS

Hemostasis is the sequence of events leading to the cessation of bleeding by the formation of a stable fibrin-platelet plug. It involves the vascular wall, platelets, and the coagulation system.

## Platelet Function and Dysfunction

**Platelets** are anuclear, membrane-bound cellular fragments derived from megakaryocytes in the bone marrow. They have a short lifespan of approximately 10 days. There are normally 150,000–400,000 platelets per $mm^3$ of blood. Platelet activity is measured by **template bleeding time**. Clinically, dysfunction is seen as **petechiae**. The platelet reaction consists of three steps. Dysfunction of each step is associated with different diseases:

- Adhesion (e.g., von Willebrand disease, Bernard-Soulier syndrome)
- Primary aggregation (e.g., thrombasthenia)
- Secondary aggregation and release (e.g., aspirin, storage pool disease)

| FORMATION OF THE PLATELET PLUG | |
|---|---|
| **Vascular wall injury** | • Injury causes exposure of subendothelial extracellular collagen<br>• Arteriolar contraction due to reflex neurogenic mechanisms, and the local release of **endothelin** occurs |
| **Adhesion** | • **von Willebrand factor (vWF)** binds exposed collagen fibers in the basement membrane<br>• Platelets adhere to vWF via **glycoprotein Ib** and become **activated** (shape change, degranulation, synthesis of **thromboxane $A_2$, $TxA_2$**)<br>• Deficiency of vWF → **von Willebrand disease**; deficiency of glycoprotein Ib receptor → **Bernard-Soulier syndrome** |
| **Release reaction** | • Release contents of platelet dense bodies (e.g., **ADP**, **calcium**, serotonin, histamine, epinephrine) and alpha granules (fibrinogen, fibronectin, factor V, vWF, platelet-derived growth factor)<br>• Membrane expression of phospholipid complexes (important for coagulation cascade) |
| **Aggregation** | • **ADP** and **thromboxane $A_2$ ($TxA_2$)** is released by **platelets** and **promote aggregation** ($TXA_2$ production is inhibited by **aspirin**)<br>• Cross-linking of platelets by **fibrinogen** requires the **GpIIb/IIIa receptor**, which is deficient in **Glanzmann thrombasthenia**<br>• Decreased endothelial synthesis of antithrombogenic substances (e.g., prostacyclin, nitric oxide, tissue plasminogen activator, thrombomodulin) |

| DISORDERS OF PLATELET NUMBERS | |
|---|---|
| **Thrombocytopenia** | • **Decrease** in the platelet count (normal = 150,000–400,000/mm$^3$)<br>• **Clinical features:** bleeding from small vessels, often skin, GI/GU tracts; **petechiae** and **purpura** are seen<br>• **Classification:** decreased production (aplastic anemia, drugs, vitamin $B_{12}$ or folate deficiency); increased destruction, (e.g., DIC, TTP, ITP, drugs, malignancy); abnormal sequestration |
| **Idiopathic thrombocytopenic purpura (ITP)** | • Spleen makes antibodies against platelet antigens (e.g., GpIIb–IIIa, GpIb–IX); platelets destroyed in the spleen by macrophages<br>• Acute form (children): self-limited, postviral<br>• Chronic form (adults): ITP may be primary or secondary to another disorder (e.g., HIV, SLE)<br>• Smear shows enlarged, immature platelets; normal PT and PTT<br>• Treatment: corticosteroids, immunoglobulin therapy, splenectomy |
| **Thrombotic thrombocytopenic purpura (TTP)** | • **Clinical features:** pentad (thrombocytopenic purpura, fever, renal failure, neurologic changes, microangiopathic hemolytic anemia); usually in young women<br>• Smear shows few platelets, schistocytes, and helmet cells<br>• **Hemolytic uremic syndrome (HUS):** mostly in children after gastroenteritis with bloody diarrhea; organism: verotoxin-producing *E. coli* O157:H7; similar clinical triad |
| **Thrombocytosis (reactive)** | Increase in count due to bleeding, hemolysis, inflammation, malignancy, iron deficiency, stress, or postsplenectomy |
| **Essential thrombocythemia** | Increase in count due to primary myeloproliferative disorder |

| DISORDERS OF PLATELET FUNCTION LEADING TO INCREASED BLEEDING | |
|---|---|
| **Bernard-Soulier disease** | Defective platelet plug formation secondary to decreased Gp1b, which causes impaired platelet-to-platelet aggregation |
| **Glanzmann thrombasthenia** | Defective platelet plug formation secondary to decreased GpIIb/IIIa, which causes impaired platelet-to-platelet aggregation |
| **von Willebrand disease** | Defective platelet plug formation due to an autosomal dominant defect in quantity or quality of von Willebrand factor (vWF); increased bleeding time and increased PTT (because vWF stabilizes factor VIII) |

ORGAN SYSTEMS

HEME/LYMPH

# COAGULATION

Coagulation begins anywhere from a few seconds to 1–2 minutes after an injury.

## Intrinsic Pathway

- **Factor XII** (Hageman factor) is activated on contact with the collagen
- "a" indicates activated form

## Extrinsic Pathway

Initiated by exposure to tissue thromboplastin

## Common Pathway

Factors IXa, VIIa, VIIIa, platelet phospholipids, and calcium activate factor X

### Thrombin (IIa):

- Able to catalyze own activation
- Increases platelet aggregation
- Activates **factor XIII** (fibrin-stabilizing factor) and potentiates binding of factors V and VIII to phospholipid/Ca$^{2+}$ complex

### Fibrinogen (I):

- Split into self-polymerizing fibrin monomers
- Initially bind via loose hydrogen and hydrophobic bonds
- **Factor XIII** catalyzes formation of strong covalent bonds

## Vitamin K–Dependent Factors

Factors II (prothrombin), VII, IX, X, protein C, and protein S

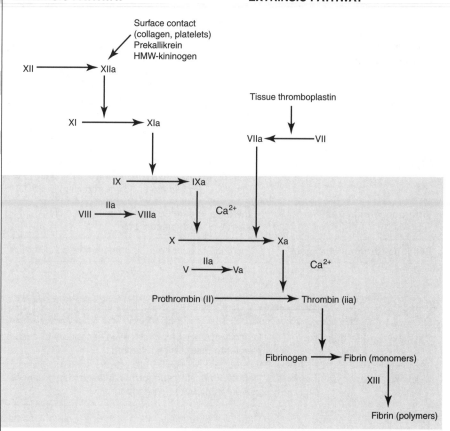

# FINAL STEP: CLOT RETRACTION AND DISSOLUTION

- After the clot is formed, it begins to shrink.
- Edges of small wounds are pulled together by platelet actinomyosin.
- Fibrinolysis (dissolution) requires activation of plasminogen.
- Clot releases plasminogen activator, which converts plasminogen to plasmin, which in turn proteolyses fibrinogen and fibrin.
- Urokinase and streptokinase are exogenous sources of plasminogen activation. Tissue plasminogen activator (t-PA) is endogenously produced, but can also be administered as a drug in the setting of acute myocardial infarction.

# ERYTHROPOIESIS

**Erythropoiesis** is the process of RBC formation. Bone marrow stem cells (colony-forming units, CFUs) differentiate into proerythroblasts under the influence of the glycoprotein **erythropoietin**, which is produced by the kidney.

**Proerythroblasts** → **basophilic erythroblasts** → **normoblasts (nucleus extruded)** → **reticulocyte (still contains some ribosomes)** → **erythrocyte** (remain in the circulation approximately 120 days and are then recycled by the spleen, liver, and bone marrow)

# DISORDERS OF RED BLOOD CELLS

| POLYCYTHEMIA (INCREASE IN RED BLOOD CELL MASS) | |
| --- | --- |
| Polycythemia vera (primary) | • Myeloproliferative syndrome<br>• Males age 40–60<br>• Vessels distended with viscous blood, congestive hepatosplenomegaly, and diffuse hemorrhages<br>• Management is generally with therapeutic phlebotomy |
| Secondary polycythemia | • Increased erythropoietin levels<br>• Etiologies: high altitude, cigarette smoking, respiratory, renal and cardiac disease and malignancies (e.g., renal cell carcinoma, hepatoma, leiomyoma, adrenal adenoma, cerebellar hemangioblastoma) |
| Relative polycythemia | Fluid loss with stable RBC mass (vomiting, diarrhea, burns) |

# ANEMIA

Secondary to decreased production, increased destruction, sometimes both
**Symptoms:** palpitations, high-output heart failure, pallor, fatigue, dizziness, syncope, and angina

| Decreased Production (Low Reticulocyte Count) | |
|---|---|
| **Decreased production** (low reticulocyte count) **Iron deficiency** (smear: hypochromic, microcytic) | • An important differential feature between the thalassemia traits and iron deficiency is that thalassemia traits result in an elevated number of microcytes, whereas iron deficiency results in a decreased number of microcytes. <br> • Serum iron, total iron-binding capacity (TIBC), and ferritin confirm the diagnosis. |
| **Megaloblastic—B$_{12}$/folate** (smear: macrocytic, hypersegmented neutrophils) | • Impaired DNA synthesis <br> • Vitamin B$_{12}$ deficiency neurologic (subacute combined degeneration) and hematologic sequelae <br> • **Vitamin B$_{12}$:** copious body stores, years to develop deficiency <br> *Causes:* dietary deficiency, malabsorption, tapeworm, bacterial overgrowth, deficiency of intrinsic factor (pernicious anemia) <br> • **Folate:** deficiency develops much more quickly (months) <br> *Causes:* deficient intake (poor diet, alcoholism, malabsorption), increased need (pregnancy, malignancy, increased hematopoiesis), or impaired use (antimetabolite drugs) <br> • Must treat patient with both folate and B$_{12}$. Folate may reverse anemia in a B$_{12}$ deficiency but not neurologic complications |
| **Aplastic** | • Pancytopenia <br> • *Multiple etiologies:* idiopathic, drugs, including alkylating agents, chloramphenicol, radiation, infections, and congenital anomalies (i.e., Fanconi anemia) <br> • Prognosis is poor <br> • Bone marrow transplant may be curative |
| **Myelophthisic** | Displacement of hematopoietic bone marrow by infiltrating tumor |
| **Myeloid metaplasia with myelofibrosis** | • Chronic myeloproliferative disorder with small numbers of neoplastic myeloid stem cells <br> • Resultant bone marrow fibrosis leads to pancytopenia |

| Thalassemias | | |
|---|---|---|
| **Types** | **Key Points** | **Clinical Picture** |
| **ALPHA** | Secondary to gene deletion: **four** genes can be deleted: <br><br> **1 deleted:** silent carrier    **3 deleted:** HbH disease <br><br> **2 deleted:** trait           **4 deleted:** hydrops fetalis, Bart Hb | • Variable clinical severity <br> • Non α-chain aggregates less toxic <br> • Mild hemolysis and anemia tend to be milder; Bart's in the neonate leads to anoxia and intrauterine death |
| **BETA** | • Defects in mRNA processing. <br> • Homozygous: β-thalassemia major <br> • Heterozygotes: β-thalassemia minor | • Mediterranean countries, Africa, and Southeast Asia <br> • Relative excess of α chains; Hb aggregates and becomes insoluble <br> • Intra- and extramedullary hemolysis <br> • Extramedullary hematopoiesis <br> • Secondary hemochromatosis |
| **HB ELECTROPHORESIS** | • α-Thalassemia: normal HbA$_2$ and HbF <br> • β-Thalassemia minor (trait): elevated HbA$_2$, HbF | |

| Increased Destruction (Normal–High Reticulocyte Count) | |
|---|---|
| **Blood loss** | Loss rather than destruction |
| | Clinical features depend on rate and severity of blood loss |
| | Chronic loss better tolerated, regenerate by increasing erythropoiesis |
| | Acute blood loss: possible hypovolemia may lead to shock and death |
| | Hematocrit may be initially normal because of equal plasma and RBC loss; will decrease as interstitial fluid equilibrates |
| | *Extravascular*—premature RBC destruction, hemoglobin (Hb) breakdown, and a compensatory increase in erythropoiesis |
| | *Intravascular*—elevated serum and urinary Hb, jaundice, urinary hemosiderin, and decreased circulating haptoglobin. Bile pigment gallstones arise from chronic, not acute hemolysis |
| **Warm hemolytic anemia** | IgG |
| | Secondary to drugs, malignancy, and SLE |
| **Cold hemolytic anemia** | IgM |
| | Functions below body temperature in the periphery |
| | Associated with mononucleosis, *Mycoplasma* infection, idiopathic hemolytic anemia, and hemolytic anemia associated with lymphoma |
| **Paroxysmal hemolytic anemia** | IgG |
| | Functions in the periphery |
| **Hereditary spherocytosis**<br><br>*Presplenectomy smear:* spherical cells lacking central pallor and reticulocytosis<br><br>*Postsplenectomy smear:* more spherocytes and Howell-Jolly bodies | Autosomal dominant defect in spectrin |
| | Less pliable; vulnerable to destruction in the spleen |
| | Anemia, jaundice, splenomegaly, cholelithiasis |
| | Exhibit characteristically increased osmotic fragility |
| | Treatment: splenectomy |
| **G6PD deficiency**<br><br>*Smear:* reticulocytosis and Heinz bodies (Hb degradation products) | X-linked deficiency of the enzyme (hexose monophosphate shunt) |
| | Decreased regeneration of NADPH, therefore glutathione |
| | Older cells unable to tolerate oxidative stress |
| | Associated with drugs (e.g., sulfa, quinine, nitrofurantoin), infections (particularly viral), or certain foods (fava beans) |
| **Paroxysmal nocturnal hemoglobinuria** | Acquired deficiency of a membrane glycoprotein |
| | Chronic intravascular hemolysis |
| | Predisposes to stem cell disorders (e.g., aplastic anemia, acute leukemia) |
| | Most frequently die of infection or venous thrombosis |

* See **Appendix D** for Abnormal Erythryocytes on Peripheral Smear

ORGAN SYSTEMS

HEME/LYMPH

## Sickle Cell Disease

| Incidence | Key Points | Clinical Picture |
|---|---|---|
| • 0.2% of the U.S. African-American population has disease<br>• 8% carry trait | • Substitution of valine for glutamic acid at position 6 of the beta chain<br>• Sickle trait: 40% HbS-sickle in extreme conditions<br>• "Sickle prep" is a blood sample treated with a reducing agent, such as metabisulfite; sickled cells may be seen<br>• Definitive diagnosis made by Hb electrophoresis<br>• HbS aggregates at low oxygen tension; leads to sickling<br>• Heterozygote is protected from *Plasmodium falciparum* malaria | • Microvascular occlusion and hemolysis<br>• Recurrent splenic thrombosis and infarction; autosplenectomy usually by age 5<br>• Also affects liver, brain, kidney, bones, penis (painful prolonged erection—priapism)<br>• Vaso-occlusive crises ("painful crises") may be triggered by infection, dehydration, acidosis<br>• Aplastic crises: Parvovirus<br>• Functional asplenia: vulnerable to *Salmonella* osteomyelitis and infections with encapsulated organisms, such as *Pneumococcus*<br>• Most patients die before age 30 |

## Agents Used to Treat Anemia

| Class | Mechanism | Indications |
|---|---|---|
| Iron | Needed to form heme, the oxygen-carrying component of hemoglobin | Iron deficiency (microcytic hypochromic) anemia |
| Vitamin $B_{12}$ (cyanocobalamin, hydroxocobalamin) | Required for DNA synthesis, RBC production, and nervous system function | Pernicious anemia and anemia resulting from gastric resection |
| Folate | Essential for DNA synthesis and maintenance of normal erythropoiesis | Folic acid deficiency secondary to malabsorption syndrome and dietary insufficiency; macrocytic/ megaloblastic anemias |
| Hydroxyurea (HU) | An antimetabolite that inhibits ribonucleotide reductase<br><br>HU reactivates HbF synthesis and increases the number of reticulocytes containing HbF in sickle cell patients | Sickle cell anemia, polycythemia vera, and chronic myelogenous leukemia |
| Erythropoietin (EPO)<br><br>Darbepoetin alpha | EPO is normally produced by the kidney<br><br>Stimulates RBC production | Used for a variety of anemias, including anemia of renal failure<br><br>Hypertension a common and severe side effect<br><br>Erythropoiesis-stimulating agents increase the risk of tumor progression or recurrence; severe caution when used in patients with cancer |

# WHITE BLOOD CELLS

Leukocytes can be divided into **granulocytes** and **agranulocytes** based on the presence of cytoplasmic granules.

| GRANULOCYTES | | | |
|---|---|---|---|
| **Granulocyte Type** | **Features** | **Functional Role** | **Relative Abundance** |
| **Neutrophils** | • 3–5 nuclear lobes<br>• Contain **azurophilic granules** (lysosomes)<br>• Specific granules contain bactericidal enzymes (e.g., lysozyme) | First cells in **acute inflammation** | 54–62% of leukocytes<br>Normal value: 1800–7800/μl |
| **Eosinophils** | • Bilobed nucleus<br>• Acidophilic granules contain hydrolytic enzymes and peroxidase | More numerous in the blood during **parasitic infections and allergic diseases** | 1–3% of leukocytes<br>Normal value: 0–450/μl |
| **Basophils** | Large basophilic and metachromatic granules, which contain proteoglycans, heparin, and histamine. Note that **mast cells are essentially tissue basophils.** | Degranulate in **type I hypersensitivity**, releasing granule contents and producing slow-reacting substance (SRS-A) = leukotrienes $LTC_4$, $LTD_4$, $LTE_4$ | 1% of leukocytes<br>Normal value: 0–200/μl |

# GRANULOPOIESIS

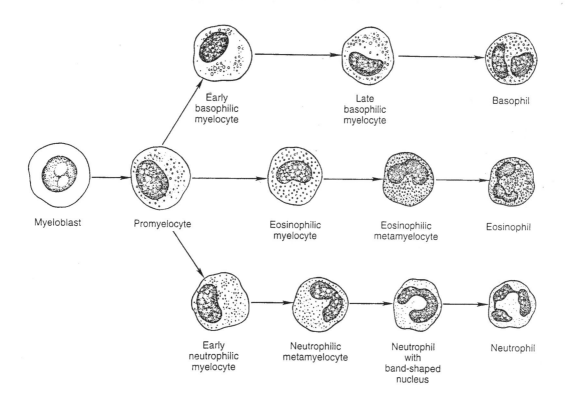

Early basophilic myelocyte — Late basophilic myelocyte — Basophil

Myeloblast — Promyelocyte — Eosinophilic myelocyte — Eosinophilic metamyelocyte — Eosinophil

Early neutrophilic myelocyte — Neutrophilic metamyelocyte — Neutrophil with band-shaped nucleus — Neutrophil

## AGRANULOCYTES

| Agranulocyte Type | Features | Functional Role | Relative Abundance |
|---|---|---|---|
| **Lymphocytes** | Dark blue, round nuclei; scant cytoplasm | T cells, B cells, null cells in immune system | 25–33% of leukocytes Normal value: 1000–4000/µl |
| T cells | Differentiate in thymus | Helper and suppressor cells modulate the immune response | — |
| B cells | Differentiate in bone marrow | Humoral immunity—antibodies produced by plasma cells | — |
| NK (Natural Killer) cell | Produced in bone marrow | Destroy some tumor cells and some virus-infected cells on which MHC class I antigens are not expressed | 10% of total lymphocyte count |
| **Monocytes/macrophages** | • Largest peripheral blood cells<br>• Kidney-shaped nuclei, stain lighter than lymphocytes | Monocytes are precursors of tissue macrophages (histiocytes), osteoclasts, alveolar macrophages, and Kupffer cells of the liver | 3–7% of leukocytes Normal value: 0–900/µl |

# DISORDERS OF LEUKOCYTES

## NONNEOPLASTIC WHITE BLOOD CELL DISORDERS

| | | |
|---|---|---|
| **Neutropenias: decreased production** (most common) | • Megaloblastic anemia<br>• Aplastic anemia<br>• Leukemia/lymphoma<br>• Autoimmune destruction of stem cells | • Lack of innate immune defense<br>• Constitutional symptoms and a high susceptibility to infection, particularly gram-negative septicemia<br>• Poor prognosis: death from overwhelming infection<br>• Infected, necrotic ulcers may occur in mucosa (oral cavity, skin, vagina, anus, gastrointestinal tract)<br>• Granulocyte-macrophage colony-stimulating factor (GM-CSF) and granulocyte-stimulating factor (GSF) are now used to treat postchemotherapy neutropenias |
| **Neutropenias: increased destruction** | Splenic sequestration, often immune-mediated (e.g., Felty syndrome) | |
| **Drug-induced neutropenia** | Alkylating agents, chloramphenicol, sulfonamides, chlorpromazine, and phenylbutazone | • Usually reversible<br>• Chloramphenicol: dose-related marrow suppression in all patients; aplastic anemia in rare individuals |
| **Polymorphonuclear leukocytosis** (most common) | • Acute bacterial infection, tissue necrosis, and "stress"<br>• Increased bands and left shift | • Döhle bodies (round, blue, cytoplasmic inclusions, product of rough endoplasmic reticulum)<br>• Toxic granulations: coarse, dark, granules (lysosomes) |
| **Monocytosis** | Tuberculosis, endocarditis, malaria, brucellosis, rickettsiosis | |
| **Lymphocytosis** | Tuberculosis, brucellosis, pertussis, viral hepatitis, cytomegalovirus infections, infectious mononucleosis | |
| **Mononucleosis** | • Increase in mononuclear cells: lymphocytes and monocytes<br>• Viral infections, EBV, CMV | |
| **Eosinophilic leukocytosis** | Neoplasms, allergy, asthma, collagen vascular diseases, parasitic infections, skin rashes | |

## HEMATOPOIETIC GROWTH FACTORS

| | | |
|---|---|---|
| Granulocyte colony-stimulating factor (G-CSF; filgrastim) | A glycoprotein that stimulates the bone marrow to produce granulocytes while promoting their survival and differentiation | Accelerates neutrophil recovery following chemotherapy; used for primary and secondary neutropenia |
| Granulocyte-macrophage colony-stimulating factor (GM-CSF, sargramostim) | A glycoprotein growth factor for erythroid megakaryocyte and eosinophil precursors. It also enhances the survival and function of circulating granulocytes, monocytes, and eosinophils | |

## NONNEOPLASTIC LYMPH NODE DISORDERS

| | | |
|---|---|---|
| Nonspecific lymphadenitis | Drugs, toxins, or infection | • In neck following dental or tonsillar infection<br>• In axillary/inguinal regions after infections of the extremities<br>• Enlarged abdominal lymph nodes (mesenteric adenitis) may cause abdominal pain resembling acute appendicitis |
| Generalized lymphadenopathy | Systemic viral or bacterial infections | • May be a precursor to AIDS<br>• Associated with hyperglobulinemia and normal CD4 lymphocyte counts |
| Acute lymphadenopathy | • Swollen, red-gray nodes with prominent lymphoid follicles<br>• Older patients have fewer germinal centers than children | |
| Chronic lymphadenopathy | Most common in axillary and inguinal nodes; nodes large and nontender | |
| **Microscopic Findings: Three Basic Patterns** | | |
| Follicular hyperplasia<br><br>B-cell antibody response | • Large germinal centers, containing mostly B cells, helper T cells, and histiocytes<br>• Seen in bacterial infections or with exposure to new antigens | |
| Paracortical hyperplasia<br><br>T-cell reaction | • Reactive changes in cortex<br>• Seen with phenytoin use, viral infections, or secondary immune responses | |
| Sinus histiocytosis | • Lymphatic sinusoids prominent and distended with macrophages<br>• Seen in nodes draining carcinomas or any chronic inflammation | |

## Hodgkin Disease

- Contiguous spread (from one node to the next) with spleen involved before liver
- High cure rate, rarely has leukemic component
- **Reed-Sternberg (RS)** cells (large, containing large "owl-eyed" nucleoli with a clear halo; abundant cytoplasm) are necessary, but not sufficient, to make diagnosis
- Bimodal age distribution (high peak: 15–35; low peak: 50+) in both men and women
- Clinical: painless cervical adenopathy +/− constitutional symptoms

### Four Variants of Hodgkin Disease

| | |
|---|---|
| **Lymphocyte predominance** | Sea of lymphocytes, few RS cells, variable number of histiocytes, little fibrosis, and no necrosis |
| **Nodular sclerosis** | • More common in women<br>• Mediastinal, supraclavicular, and lower cervical nodes<br>• Mixture of lymphocytes, histiocytes, a few eosinophils, plasma cells, and RS cells. Collagen bands create nodular pattern; RS cells called lacunar cells |
| **Mixed cellularity** | • Mixture of neutrophils, lymphocytes, eosinophils, plasma cells, and histiocytes<br>• Large number of RS cells |
| **Lymphocyte depletion** | • Rare lymphocytes, many RS cells with variable eosinophils, plasma cells, and histiocytes<br>• Diffuse fibrosis may be seen |

*Worsening Prognosis*

ORGAN SYSTEMS

HEME / LYMPH

## NON-HODGKIN LYMPHOMAS (NHL)

- Lymphadenopathy and hepatosplenomegaly. In 30% of cases, initial involvement extranodal
- Usually discovered in only one chain of nodes—usually cervical, axillary, inguinal, femoral, iliac, or mediastinal
- Patients present with local or generalized lymphadenopathy, abdominal or pharyngeal mass, abdominal pain, or GI bleeding
- Involve lymph nodes or lymphoid tissue in the gut, oropharynx, liver, spleen, and thymus
- **Do not produce RS cells**, do not spread in contiguity, and frequently have a leukemic or blood-borne phase
- Occur in late 50s (rare and more aggressive in children and young adults)
- Weight loss common sign of disseminated disease
- Common in immunosuppressed patients

Two main categories: **nodular** (better prognosis) and **diffuse**

Staging similar to Hodgkin disease but staging less clinically significant in NHL because prognosis is more affected by histology, and the disease is often disseminated at time of diagnosis

| Disease | Characteristics | Pathology |
|---|---|---|
| Follicular lymphoma | Median age 60–65; median survival 8–10 years<br>Painless adenopathy<br>t(14;18) translocation brings bcl-2 close to heavy chain immunoglobulin gene<br>May be associated with immunodeficiency states | Follicular or nodular pattern of growth with areas resembling germinal centers but lacking normal germinal center architecture |
| Well-differentiated lymphocytic lymphoma (diffuse) | Older patients<br>Generalized lymphadenopathy, hepatosplenomegaly<br>Often seeds the blood late in the disease similar to CLL<br>Bone marrow almost always involved<br>Survival: 5–7 years | Lymph nodes replaced by small round lymphocytes with scant cytoplasm, dark nuclei, and rare mitoses |
| Poorly differentiated lymphocytic lymphoma (PDLL) (nodular or diffuse) | Middle-aged or older<br>Lymphadenopathy, infiltration of bone marrow, liver, and spleen at the time of diagnosis<br>Prognosis is fair: nodular PDLL > diffuse PDLL | Atypical lymphocytes<br>Nuclei are irregular and indented with coarse chromatin<br>Mitoses are rare<br>Leukemic phase less common |
| Histiocytic lymphoma (B cells) (diffuse >> nodular) | Nodal or extranodal involvement (skin, bone, gastrointestinal tract, brain); rarely, liver and spleen involvement; leukemic phase rare<br>Prognosis poor unless treated with combination chemotherapy | Large cells with vesicular nuclei and prominent nucleoli; may be pleomorphic |
| Mixed lymphocytic-histiocytic lymphoma (nodular) | Prognosis fair; remission may be achieved with combination chemotherapy | Cells with atypical lymphocytes and large histiocytes |
| Lymphoblastic lymphoma (diffuse) Cells similar to ALL | Bimodal—high peak: adolescents/young adults, low peak: 70s; male:female ratio, 2.5:1<br>Associated with a mediastinal mass, particularly in boys<br>Often express T-cell markers<br>Prognosis uniformly poor; T-cell lymphomas worse | Uniform size, scant cytoplasm, delicate chromatin, and absent nucleoli<br>Nuclear membrane is loculated or convoluted<br>Frequent mitoses |
| Burkitt undifferentiated lymphoma | Endemic in Africa (mandible or maxilla) and sporadic in the United States (abdomen)<br>Children or young adults<br>Tied to **Epstein-Barr virus (EBV),** especially the African form<br>Leukemic phase is rare; prognosis is fair<br>African Burkitt: translocations (8;14, 2;8, or 8;22) bring c-myc gene close to enhancers of heavy or light chain synthesis in B cells | Sea of moderately large lymphocytes with lipid-containing vacuoles interspersed with macrophages to produce **"starry sky pattern."** |
| Undifferentiated non-Burkitt lymphoma | Rare, usually adults, not associated with EBV<br>Cells more variable than in Burkitt; may be multinucleate, have a single nucleolus and pale, scant cytoplasm | Cell markers show both B- and T-cell neoplasms<br>Aggressive, as are all diffuse, large-cell lymphomas |
| Mantle cell lymphoma | Median age 60; median survival 3 years<br>t(11;14) translocation links immunoglobin heavy chain to bcl-1<br>Can present with lymphadenopathy, fever, night sweats, massive splenomegaly, or hepatomegaly | Expansion of the mantle zone surrounding germinal centers with small to medium atypical lymphocytes |

## Cutaneous T-Cell Lymphomas

| Mycosis fungoides | Three phases of skin lesions: inflammation, plaque, and tumor. Epidermal and dermal infiltrates by neoplastic T (CD4) cells with cerebriform nuclei. Nodules and fungating tumors may develop later in the disease. Nodal and visceral dissemination can occur. |
|---|---|
| Sézary syndrome | Rare chronic disease with progressive, pruritic erythroderma, exfoliation, and lymphadenopathy. "Sézary cells," T cells with cerebriform nuclei (similar to those seen in mycosis fungoides) infiltrate the peripheral blood. May be considered a preterminal phase of mycosis fungoides. |

## Leukemias

| Disease | Characteristics | Pathology |
|---|---|---|
| Acute lymphocytic leukemia (ALL) | • 60–70% of cases occur in childhood; peak age 4; rare over 50<br>• Half the children are cured; prognosis for adults is very poor<br>• Fatigue, fever, epistaxis, gingival petechiae, ecchymoses 2° to thrombocytopenia; may have subarachnoid or cerebral hemorrhage<br>• Present with lymphadenopathy, bone pain, hepatosplenomegaly<br>• Most likely leukemia to involve CNS<br>• Prognosis: death often from infection or bleed<br>• Most cells pre-B cells; T-cell variants occur, usually affecting boys and causing a thymic mass that may compress the trachea | Smear: lymphoblasts are prominent; mature WBCs rare<br><br>**CD10 (CALLA)** is the diagnostic surface marker; terminal deoxynucleotidyl transferase (TDT) positive in both B-cell and T-cell ALL and negative in AML |
| Acute myelogenous leukemia (AML) | 20% of acute leukemia in children, most common acute leukemia in adults<br>Signs and symptoms resemble ALL, except usually also present with lymphadenopathy or splenomegaly<br>AML: t(15;17); acute promyelocytic leukemia: t(1;12) | Primary cell type variable; see the French, American, and British (FAB) Classification of Myelogenous Leukemias, page 405. |
| Chronic myelogenous leukemia (CML) | • Middle age but may occur in children/young adults<br>• Fatigue, fever, night sweats, and weight loss<br>• Splenomegaly (up to 5 kg) giving abdominal discomfort<br>• Variable remission period, may develop blast crisis<br>• Two-thirds convert to AML; one-third to B-cell ALL<br>• **Philadelphia chromosome (Ph1), t(9;22): *bcr:abl* translocation** is pathognomonic; present in 95% of cases<br>• Prognosis in CML is worse in Ph1-negative patients | • Marked leukocytosis<br>• Low-to-absent leukocyte alkaline phosphatase<br>• Elevated serum vitamin $B_{12}$ and vitamin $B_{12}$–binding proteins<br>• High uric acid levels (due to rapid cell turnover) |
| Chronic lymphocytic leukemia (CLL) | • Over 60 years of age<br>• Asymptomatic or fatigue and weight loss; lymphadenopathy and hepatosplenomegaly later findings<br>• Higher incidence of visceral malignancy<br>• Median survival with treatment is 5 years but varies widely; prognostic factor is extent of disease | Lymph node histology indistinguishable from diffuse, well-differentiated lymphocytic lymphoma<br>Classic cell: CD5 B cell<br>Cells do not undergo apoptosis |
| Hairy cell leukemia | • Rare disease; cells express tartrate-resistant acid phosphatase<br>• Present with hepatosplenomegaly; pancytopenia common<br>• Prognosis: may now be cured with 2-chloro-deoxyadenosine (2CdA), an apoptosis inducer | Leukemic cells have "hair-like" cytoplasmic projections visible on phase-contrast microscopy<br>Cells express some B-cell antigens |
| Adult T-cell leukemia/lymphoma (CD4 T cell) | • Endemic in Japan<br>• Lymphadenopathy, hepatosplenomegaly, skin involvement, and hypercalcemia<br>• Poor prognosis; however, many infected patients do not progress to disease | Caused by human T-cell leukemia/lymphoma virus (HTLV1); exposure to the virus may be decades earlier |
| Myelodysplastic syndromes | Proliferative stem cell disorders—maturation defect<br>Gray zone between benign proliferation and frank acute leukemias<br>One-third of these patients later develop frank acute myelocytic leukemia | Presents as pancytopenia in elderly patients |

\* See **Appendix D** for Abnormalities of White Blood Cells and Platelets on Peripheral Smear

## Leukemia Clues

| | |
|---|---|
| Children | ALL |
| Myeloblasts | AML |
| Auer rods | AML, promyelocytic |
| DIC | Promyelocytic |
| Elderly | CLL |
| Splenomegaly | CML |
| Philadelphia chromosome | CML |
| Tartrate-resistant acid phosphatase | Hairy cell |
| HTLV-1 | Adult T cell |

## THE FRENCH, AMERICAN, AND BRITISH (FAB) CLASSIFICATION OF MYELOGENOUS LEUKEMIAS

| | | |
|---|---|---|
| M0 | Undifferentiated | — |
| M1 | Myeloblasts without maturation | Myeloblasts have round-oval nuclei<br>Auer rods |
| M2 | Granulocyte maturation | — |
| M3 | Promyelocytic | Auer rods<br>DIC |
| M4 | Mixed myeloid and monocytic | Features of both myelocytes and monocytes |
| M5 | Monoblastic or monocytic | — |
| M6 | Erythroid differentiation | Di Guglielmo disease<br>Atypical multinucleated RBC precursors<br>Usually converts to AML |
| M7 | Megakaryocytic differentiation | — |

## PLASMA CELL DYSCRASIAS

| | |
|---|---|
| **Polyclonal hypergammaglobulinemia** | 1–2 weeks after an antigen stimulus (e.g., bacterial infection); also associated with granulomatous disease, connective tissue disorders, and liver failure<br>Elevated serum globulins, elevated ESR<br>Polyclonal Bence-Jones proteins in serum or urine<br>Hyperviscosity of blood may lead to sludging and rouleaux formation with subsequent thrombosis, hemorrhage, renal impairment, and right-sided congestive heart failure |
| **Waldenström macroglobulinemia** | Age 60–70 years in both men and women<br>Monoclonal IgM resembles lymphocytic lymphoma with M-protein spike on serum protein electrophoresis<br>Symptoms due to hypergammaglobulinemia and tumorous infiltration<br>Hepatosplenomegaly, lymphadenopathy, bone pain, and hyperviscosity<br>Blindness and priapism due to hyperviscosity may be seen<br>2–5-year survival rate with chemotherapy |
| **Monoclonal gammopathy of undetermined significance (MGUS)** | Asymptomatic M-protein spike on serum electrophoresis<br>Prognosis: initially thought benign, but approximately 2% may later develop myeloma, lymphoma, amyloidosis, or Waldenström macroglobulinemia |
| **Multiple myeloma** | Peak incidence is 50–60 years old; male = female<br>Multifocal plasma cell neoplasms in the bone marrow, occasionally soft tissues<br>Monoclonal immunoglobulin (IgG)<br>Signs and symptoms result from excess abnormal immunoglobulins (causing hyperviscosity) and from infiltration of various organs by neoplastic plasma cells<br>Proteinuria may contribute to progressive renal failure<br>Infiltration of bone with plasma cell neoplasms may lead to bone pain and hypercalcemia<br>Over 99% of patients have elevated levels of serum immunoglobulins or urine Bence-Jones proteins, or both<br>Serum protein electrophoresis (SPEP) shows homogeneous peak or "spike"<br>Marrow is infiltrated with plasma cells (usually over 30%) in various stages of maturation, called "myeloma cells"; contain cytoplasmic inclusions (acidophilic aggregates of immunoglobulin) called Russell bodies<br>Multiple osteolytic lesions throughout the skeleton; appear as "punched-out" defects on x-ray<br>Kidney: protein casts in distal tubules<br>Prognosis: less than 2-year survival without therapy; death usually results from infection, bleeding, or renal failure (**Bence-Jones proteins**) |

# HEMATOLOGIC CHANGES ASSOCIATED WITH INFECTIOUS DISEASE

## CHANGES IN BLOOD CELLS

| Signs and Symptoms | Case Vignette/ Key Clues | Most Common Causative Agents | Pathogenesis | Diagnosis | Treatment |
|---|---|---|---|---|---|
| Anemia | Megaloblastic Ingestion of raw fish | *Diphyllobothrium latum* | Parasite absorbs $B_{12}$ | Operculated eggs in stool | Niclosamide |
| | Normocytic | Chronic infections | Bacteria chelate iron | Culture, Gram stain | Depends on agent |
| | Microcytic and hypochromic (iron-deficiency anemia) | *Ancylostoma, Necator Trichuris* | Hookworms suck blood; trichuris damages mucosa | Golden brown, oval eggs; eggs with bipolar plugs | Mebendazole |
| Patient with cyclic or irregular fever, ↓ hemoglobin and hematocrit | Travel to tropics, parasites in RBCs | *Plasmodium* spp. | Parasite lyses RBC<br><br>Autoimmune RBC destruction | Rings/trophozoites in blood film | Chloroquine, etc. (considerable drug resistance), followed by primaquine if *P. vivax* or *P. ovale* |
| ↓ CD4 cell count | Lymphadenopathy Opportunistic infections | HIV | Virus infects and destroys CD4 ⊕ T cells, and macrophages | ELISA, Western blot | NRTIs, NNRTIs, protease inhibitors, fusion inhibitors, CCR5 antagonists, integrase inhibitors |
| ↑ PMNs (neutrophilia) | — | Generally found in many extracellular bacterial infections | *N*-formyl methionyl peptides are chemotactic for PMNs | Culture, Gram stain | Depends on agent |
| ↑ eosinophils (eosinophilia) | — | Allergy | ECF-A released by mast cells attracts eosinophils | Skin testing: wheal and flare | Antihistamines |
| | | Helminths during migrations | Parasites release allergens | Depends on agent | Depends on agent |
| ↑ monocytes and/or lymphocytes | — | Intracellular organisms: viruses, *Listeria, Legionella, Leishmania, Toxoplasma* | Intracellular organisms elicit TH1 cells and CMI | Depends on agent | Depends on agent |
| Above plus fever, fatigue, lymphadenopathy, myalgia, headache | Infectious mononucleosis<br><br>Heterophile ⊕, Downey type II cells (reactive T cells), sore throat, lymphadenopathy, young adult | Epstein-Barr virus | Virus infects B lymphocytes via CD21; CTLs respond to kill virus-infected cells | Monospot ⊕ Complete blood count | Supportive |
| | Heterophile ⊖ | CMV | Virus infects fibroblasts; CTLs respond to kill virus-infected cells | Monospot ⊖ Virus culture | Ganciclovir (severe cases) |
| Lymphocytosis with hacking cough | Unvaccinated child, hypoglycemic | *Bordetella pertussis* | Tracheal cytotoxin, fimbrial antigen, endotoxin, ↓ chemokine receptors | Gram ⊖ rod Culture Bordet-Gengou agar or serology | Erythromycin, antitoxin |

# Dental Anatomy, Occlusion, and Histology

# Contents

## DEFINITIONS

| General | Exfoliation | Process of shedding or losing deciduous teeth |
|---|---|---|
| | Mixed dentition | Containing a combination of both primary and permanent teeth |

| Arrangement | Maxilla | Stationary, upper jaw |
|---|---|---|
| | Mandible | Lower, moveable jaw |
| | Arch trait | Characteristics of the teeth of 1 arch (3 roots in a maxillary molar versus 2 in a mandibular molar) |
| | Type trait | Differences between the arch components of each class that make them easily identifiable (difference between manibular central incisor and mandibular lateral incisor) |
| | Set trait | Characteristic that identifies what dentition the tooth belongs to |

| Types of Teeth | Deciduous | Primary teeth<br>20 teeth in all<br>Must be exfoliated |
|---|---|---|
| | Permanent | Adult dentition<br>32 teeth in all<br>Usually erupt between 6–18 years |
| | Succedaneous | Take the place of the exfoliated primary teeth |

## ANATOMY OF A TOOTH

| Crown | Surface portion that erupts through the gingiva Composed of enamel, dentin, and pulp |
|---|---|
| Root | Anchoring portion of the tooth Composed of cementum, dentin, and pulp |
| Clinical crown | Portion visible in the oral cavity |
| Gingiva | Soft tissue surrounding crown and boundary between clinical crown and root |
| Alveolus | Bony socket anchoring tooth |
| Cervical line | Boundary between anatomic crown and root (cementoenamel junction) |

## Root Structure

**Single-rooted** teeth: all anteriors, maxillary second premolar, mandibular first and second premolars)

**Bi**furcation—**2** terminal roots (maxillary first premolar, mandibular molars)

**Tri**furcation—**3** terminal roots (maxillary molars)

**Root trunk**—common part of the tooth root before the root separates

**Cervical line**—boundary between the enamel of the anatomical crown and the cementum of the anatomical root (cementoenamel junction)

Each root usually has one canal, *except:**

| | |
|---|---|
| Maxillary | second premolar (occasionally) |
| | molars (mesiobuccal can have 2) |
| Mandibular | central (occasionally) |
| | lateral (occasionally) |
| | canine (occasionally) |
| | first premolar (occasionally) |
| | second premolar (occasionally) |
| | molars (mesial root has 2 canals; distal may have 2) |

*Note that there are rare exceptions to rules about roots.

## Pulp Cavity

**Pulp chambers** and **pulp canals** make up the pulp cavity.

The **pulp chamber** is generally in the crown portion of the mouth. It is a singular chamber in all teeth and extends into the root trunk, generally 1–2 mm below the cervical line. The chamber outline follows the outline of the tooth.

**Pulp horns** are projections of the pulp chamber into the major cusps of the teeth. They are also found in mammelons of the maxillary incisors when teeth are young.

## Tissue

| | Composition | Characteristics | Function | Location | Strength |
|---|---|---|---|---|---|
| **Enamel** | 96–98% inorganic material (mineral) | Hard, translucent<br>Cannot repair itself<br>Complete at time of eruption | Protects biting surface of tooth | Covers anatomic crown | Hardest substance in body |
| **Cementum** | 50% organic<br>50% inorganic | 2 types: cellular, acellular<br>Blood supply through the cementum (nourishment from outside tooth) | Provides anchoring mechanism to tooth (periodontal ligament between cementum and alveolar bone) | Covers surface of anatomic root | Less dense than enamel |
| **Dentin** | 22% organic*<br>65% inorganic*<br>13% water*<br>Composed of tubules (extension of nerve tissue from pulp extend into these tubules) | Makes up bulk of tooth<br><br>**2 types:** primary (produced during development) and secondary (formed to protect the pulp) | Provides elasticity to tooth | Beneath the enamel and cementum | Softer and less brittle than enamel |
| **Pulp** | Nerves, blood vessels, lymph | Formative (will produce dentin throughout life)<br>Contains odontoblasts | Provides nutrients to tooth<br>Sensory (pain from heat, cold, decay, etc.) | Innermost portion of the tooth | Soft tissue |

*Values vary in some texts; it has been stated that as much as 60–65% of dentin may be inorganic.

## CHARACTERISTICS OF CLASSES

| Class | Number per Quadrant | Characteristics | Function | Position |
|-------|---------------------|-----------------|----------|----------|
| Incisors (I) | 2 | Front teeth, single rooted<br>Straight incisal edge | Cutting, aesthetics, phonetics, biting | Central—closest to midline<br>Lateral—2nd position from midline |
| Canines (C) | 1 | Canine prominence of tooth seen at corner of mouth<br>Long rooted | Cutting, shearing, tearing | 3rd position from midline |
| Premolars (PM) | 2 | Single roots, except for maxillary first premolar (2 roots) | Mastication | 4th and 5th position from midline |
| Molars (M) | 3 | Grinding, chewing<br>4 cusps or more<br>Wide masticating surface | Mastication | 6th, 7th, and 8th position from midline |

## ANATOMIC DIVISIONS AND ORIENTATIONS

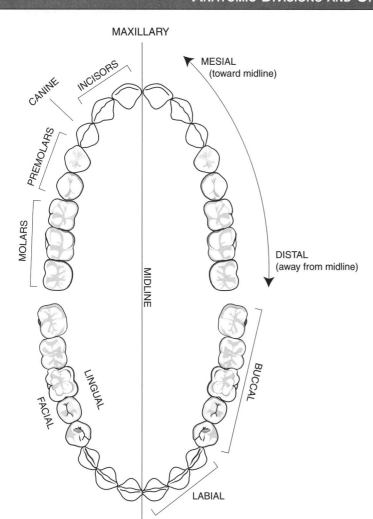

### Surfaces

**Occlusal**—biting surface of posterior teeth

**Incisal**—biting surface of anterior teeth

**Gingival/Cervical**—area near gingiva

**Contact area**—area that contacts an adjacent tooth on the proximal surface of the tooth

### Definitions

**Mesial**—closer to midline

**Distal**—away from midline

**Proximal**—area between two teeth

**Lingual**—surface facing the tongue also **palatal** in maxilla)

**Facial**—outer surface facing toward cheek

**Labial**—surface facing check in anterior teeth

**Buccal**—surface facing check in posterior teeth

## Imaginary Thirds

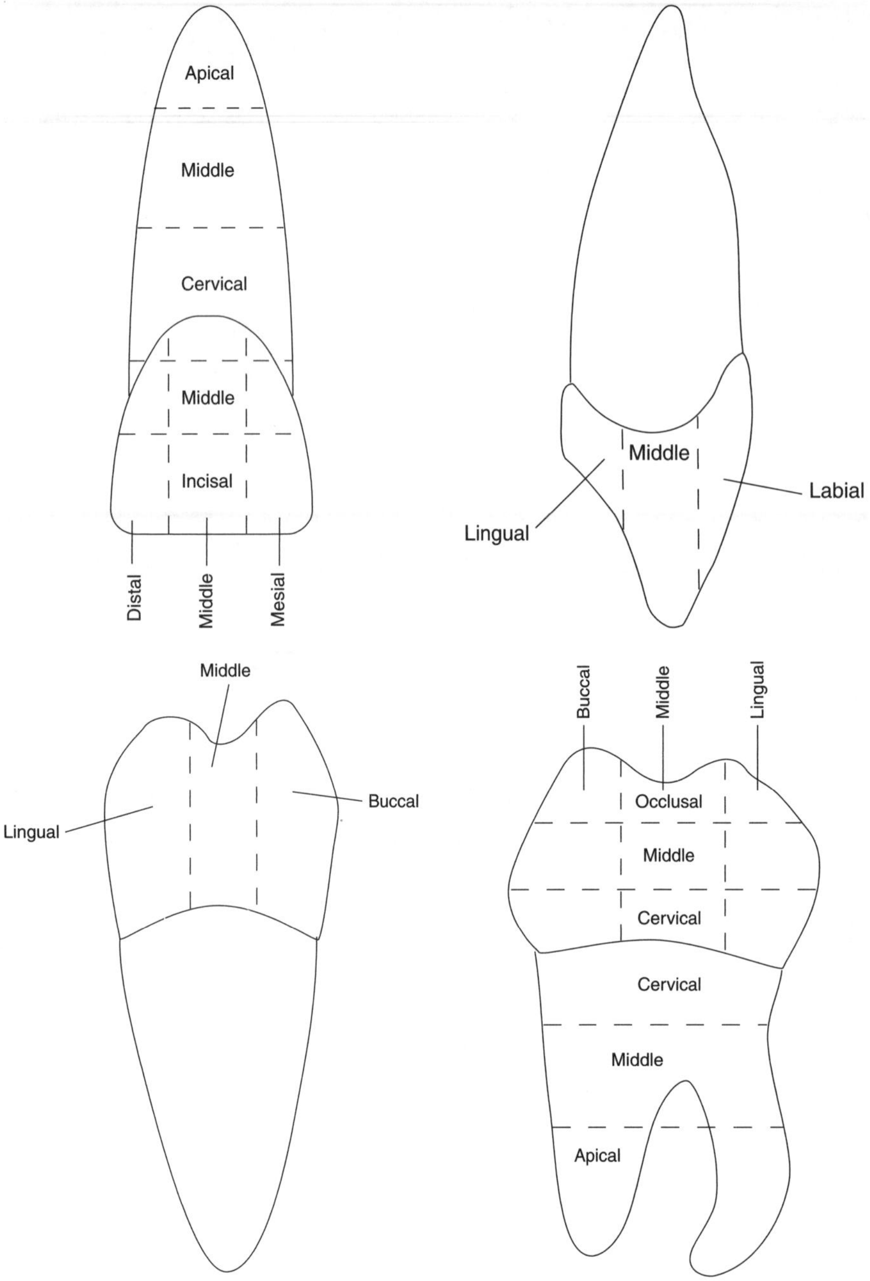
Apical
Middle
Cervical
Middle
Incisal
Distal
Middle
Mesial
Middle
Lingual
Labial
Middle
Lingual
Buccal
Buccal
Middle
Lingual
Occlusal
Middle
Cervical
Cervical
Middle
Apical

### Examples

**Incisal Third**

Horizontal third closest to the working surface

**Cervical Third**

Horizontal third closest to the neck of the tooth and gingiva

**Middle Third**

Middle of the crown

| NOMENCLATURE | |
|---|---|
| **Shorthand** | |
| **Permanent Dentition** | |
| **UNIVERSAL SYSTEM** | **FDI (FEDERATION DENTAIRE INTERNATIONALE)** |
| Teeth are numbered from 1–32 starting with the permanent maxillary right third molar, i.e., perm/max/right/central incisor = #8. | Uses quadrant system |

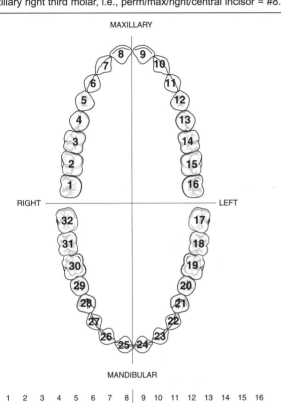

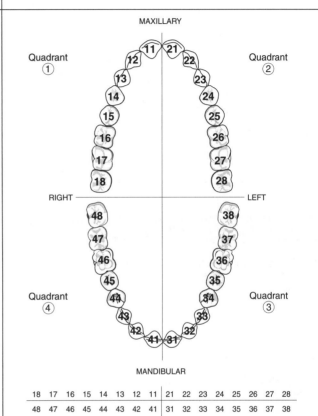

| | | | | | | | | | | | | | | | | | | | | | | | | | | | | | | | | |
|---|---|---|---|---|---|---|---|---|---|---|---|---|---|---|---|---|---|---|---|---|---|---|---|---|---|---|---|---|---|---|---|
| 1 | 2 | 3 | 4 | 5 | 6 | 7 | 8 | 9 | 10 | 11 | 12 | 13 | 14 | 15 | 16 | | 18 | 17 | 16 | 15 | 14 | 13 | 12 | 11 | 21 | 22 | 23 | 24 | 25 | 26 | 27 | 28 |
| 32 | 31 | 30 | 29 | 28 | 27 | 26 | 25 | 24 | 23 | 22 | 21 | 20 | 19 | 18 | 17 | | 48 | 47 | 46 | 45 | 44 | 43 | 42 | 41 | 31 | 32 | 33 | 34 | 35 | 36 | 37 | 38 |

| **Primary Dentition** | |
|---|---|
| **UNIVERSAL SYSTEM** | **FDI (FEDERATION DENTAIRE INTERNATIONALE)** |
| Teeth are numbered from A–T starting with the primary maxillary right second molar, i.e., perm/max/right/central incisor = E. | Uses quadrant system |

| | | | | | | | | | | | | | | | | | | | | |
|---|---|---|---|---|---|---|---|---|---|---|---|---|---|---|---|---|---|---|---|---|
| A | B | C | D | E | F | G | H | I | J | | 55 | 54 | 53 | 52 | 51 | 61 | 62 | 63 | 64 | 65 |
| T | S | R | Q | P | O | N | M | L | K | | 85 | 84 | 83 | 82 | 81 | 71 | 72 | 73 | 74 | 75 |

## Dental Formula

The number of teeth in each class constitutes the dental formula. The number of teeth on one quadrant of the upper jaw is indicated over the number of the same class on the lower jaw. You must multiply the sum by two to get the total number of teeth.

**Anterior teeth — incisors and canines**
**Posterior teeth — premolar and molars**

### Permanent Teeth

$$\text{I } \tfrac{2}{2} + \text{C } \tfrac{1}{1} + \text{PM } \tfrac{2}{2} + \text{M } \tfrac{3}{3} = 16 \times 2 = 32$$

### Primary Teeth (No Premolars)

$$\text{I } \tfrac{2}{2} + \text{C } \tfrac{1}{1} + \text{M } \tfrac{2}{2} = 10 \times 2 = 20$$

| Naming Teeth |
| --- |

| Standard order: | 1. Set |
| --- | --- |
|  | 2. Arch |
|  | 3. Quadrant |
|  | 4. Type and class |

i.e., "permanent/mandibular/right/first molar"

## DEVELOPMENT OF CUSPS AND LOBES

**Tooth germs (or tooth buds)** are small groupings of cells that develop during the eighth week of embryonic development. **Calcification**, the hardening of tooth tissues by the deposition of minerals found within, begins at the fourth to fifth month of fetal life. Calcification begins in permanent teeth just after birth.

## Lobes

All anterior teeth develop from **four major growth centers** called **lobes**, i.e., **mammelons** and **cingula**.

The posterior teeth develop from four to five lobes. Cusps develop from the lobes, and the coalescence of lobes is marked by developmental grooves.

**Lobes**

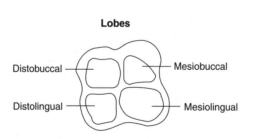

Distobuccal — Mesiobuccal
Distolingual — Mesiolingual

**Mammelons**

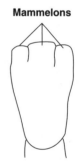

The lobes of a tooth act as the major center of the formation of enamel. In the fully developed tooth, these lobes give rise to the formation of **cusps, mammelons, and cingula**. The coalescence of the lobes is marked by the formation of developmental depressions (anterior teeth) and developmental grooves (posterior teeth).

Anterior teeth (incisors and canines) have four facial lobes: distolabial, middlelabial, mesiolabial, and one lingual lobe, cementum.

Premolars have four lobes: distobuccal, middlebuccal, mesiobuccal, and one lingual lobe, lingual cusp.

**Molars** have **four lobes:** distolingual, distobuccal, and mesiolingual, mesiobuccal. The maxillary first molar has the cusp of Carabelli (a small fifth cusp), and the mandibular first molar has a fifth cusp (distal cusp).

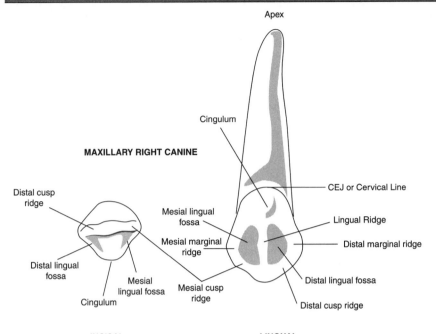

MAXILLARY RIGHT CANINE

INCISAL

LINGUAL

**Fossa:** irregular rounded depression on surface of crown

**Lingual fossa:** broad shallow depression on lingual surface of anterior teeth

**Central fossa:** deep depression in central portion of anterior or posterior

**Triangular fossa:** triangular fossa located in the marginal ridges of the posterior teeth

**Cusp:** elevation on the crown portion of tooth; forms the bulk of the occlusal surface

**Cingulum:** rounded eminence or bulge on lingual side of anterior teeth

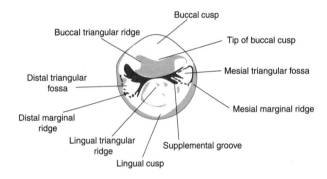

MAXILLARY RIGHT SECOND PREMOLAR

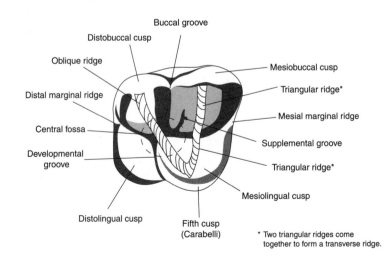

* Two triangular ridges come together to form a transverse ridge.

[[[[[]] represents triangle formed by the major ridges of the maxillary first molar.

MAXILLARY RIGHT FIRST MOLAR

**Ridge:** any linear elevation on surface of tooth; named according to location

**Marginal ridge:** rounded borders of enamel; form mesial and distal margins of occlusal surfaces of premolars and molars; form mesial and distal margins of lingual surfaces of incisors and canines

**Triangular ridge:** prominent elevation, triangular in cross-section

**Transverse ridge:** union of two triangular ridges crossing the occlusal surface of posterior tooth

**Incisal ridge:** found on newly erupted anterior teeth (mammelons)

**Oblique ridge (maxillary molars only):** transverse ridge that runs from distal buccal to mesial lingual cusp

DENTAL REVIEW

Although there are general rules for cusp and root numbers, numerous anomalies exist.

All teeth are wider faciolingually than mesiodistally, except for:

- maxillary central and lateral incisors
- mandibular first, second, and third molars.

Smallest tooth—mandibular central incisor
Longest tooth—maxillary canine

|  | **Maxillary** | **Mandibular** |
|---|---|---|
| **Anterior** | Wider, less symmetrical crown | Long, narrow symmetric crown |
| **Molars** | Wider in a faciolingual direction | Wider in a mesiodistal direction |
|  | 3 roots—2 facial, 1 lingual (palatal) | 2 roots—1 mesial, 1 distal |
| **Premolars** | First premolar has 2 roots; others are single roots | All single roots |
| **Posteriors** |  |  |
| **Occlusal tables** | More centered in a faciolingual direction<br>Centered over root trunk | Somewhat lingually placed |
| **Buccal cusps** | Displaced from midline in faciolingual direction; height of contour low | Buccal cusp more toward middle of tooth in the faciolingual direction |
| **Lingual cusps** | Displaced from midline in faciolingual direction | Lingual almost in line with lingual profile of root |
| **Occlusal view** | Equal amounts of buccal and lingual surfaces seen | More buccal (up to 1/3) than lingual surface seen |
| **Contours** | Buccal height is low; lingual heights relatively high on crown | Buccal height of contour very low, near cervical |

## FUNDAMENTAL GEOMETRIC SHAPES OF CROWNS

### Axial Views

| Facial or Lingual View of All Teeth | Mesial or Distal View of Anterior Teeth | Mesial or Distal View of Maxillary Posterior Teeth | Mesial or Distal View of Mandibular Posterior Teeth |
|---|---|---|---|
| | | | |
| **All teeth** are fundamentally **trapezoidal** when viewed **facially or lingually**. The long side of the trapezoid is the occlusal or incisal, and the short side is the cervical. | **Incisors and canines**, when viewed from **mesial** or **distal**, are **triangular** in shape. | **Maxillary posteriors**, when viewed from **mesial** or **distal**, are fundamentally **trapezoidal**. The long side is the cervical. | **Mandibular posteriors**, when viewed from **mesial** or **distal**, are **rhomboidal**. The lingual occlusal and the buccocervical angles are acute. |

DENTAL REVIEW

The **height of contour, or the crest of curvature,** is the greatest elevation of the tooth. The contact areas are also considered the location of the height of contour on the proximal surfaces.

Knowing the heights of contour helps to understand contact relationships.

- Generally, the **mesial height of contour** is more incisal or occlusal than is the distal, except for the mandibular central incisor, premolars, and possibly molars.
- The **lingual height of contour** of the mandibular posteriors is much more occlusal than that of the maxillary posteriors.
- The **facial height of contour** of the maxillary posteriors is generally more occlusal than that of the mandibular posteriors.
- The **facial and lingual heights of contour** generally have a convexity of approximately 0.5 mm, except for the lingual of the mandibular posteriors, where it may measure up to 1 mm.

| Maxillary Heights of Contours/Contacts | | | | |
|---|---|---|---|---|
| | Lingual | Facial | Mesial Contact | Distal Contact |
| **Central incisor** | Cervical 1/3 | Cervical 1/3 | Incisal 1/3 | Junction of middle and incisal 1/3 |
| **Lateral incisor** | Cervical 1/3 | Cervical 1/3 | Junction of middle and incisal 1/3 | Middle 1/3 |
| **Canine** | Cervical 1/3 | Cervical 1/3 | Junction of middle of incisal 1/3 | Middle 1/3 |
| **First premolar** | Middle 1/3 | Cervical 1/3 | Middle 1/3 | Middle 1/3 |
| **Second premolar** | Middle 1/3 | Cervical 1/3 | Middle 1/3 | Middle 1/3 |
| **First molar** | Middle 1/3 | Cervical 1/3 | Middle 1/3 | Middle 1/3 |
| **Second molar** | Middle 1/3 | Cervical 1/3 | Middle 1/3 | Middle 1/3 |
| **Third molar** | Middle 1/3 | Cervical 1/3 | Middle 1/3 | No distal contact |

| Mandibular Heights of Contours/Contacts | | | | |
|---|---|---|---|---|
| | Lingual | Facial | Mesial Contact | Distal Contact |
| **Central incisor** | Cervical 1/3 | Cervical 1/3 | Incisal 1/3 | Incisal 1/3 |
| **Lateral incisor** | Cervical 1/3 | Cervical 1/3 | Incisal 1/3 | Incisal 1/3 |
| **Canine** | Cervical 1/3 | Cervical 1/3 | Incisal 1/3 | Middle 1/3 |
| **First premolar** | Junction of cervical and middle 1/3 | Cervical 1/3 | Middle 1/3 | Middle 1/3 |
| **Second premolar** | Middle 1/3 | Cervical 1/3 | Junction of middle and occlusal 1/3 | Junction of middle and occlusal 1/3 |
| **First molar** | Middle 1/3 | Cervical 1/3 | Junction of middle and occlusal 1/3 | Middle 1/3 |
| **Second molar** | Middle 1/3 | Cervical 1/3 | Middle 1/3 | Middle 1/3 |

Contact areas are influenced by the **size**, **form**, and **alignment** of the teeth. They are located at the **widest portion of a tooth** and correspond to the height of the contour. They function to:

- Stabilize the arch
- Prevent food impaction
- Protect the interproximal gingival tissue

Interproximal caries typically form immediately apical to the contact area.

Contact areas are described by **two coordinates: incisocervical** (occlusocervical) and **faciolingual.**

| Incisocervical (occlusocervically) | Faciolingual | |
|---|---|---|
| At the mesial and distal heights of contour<br><br>Mesial contact area is more occlusal or incisal than the distal (except for mandibular central incisors, premolars, possibly molars. | Anterior teeth centered faciolingually<br><br>Posterior teeth placement may be more facial in the buccal third. | <br>Faciolingual<br><br>Occlusocervical |

| DEJ (Dentinoenamel) | CEJ (Cementoenamel) | CDJ (Cementodentinal) |
|---|---|---|
| Dentin meeting enamel | Between cementum and enamel; border of anatomic crown | Cementum meets dentin |
| Found only in crown | Mesial curvature greater than on distal of same tooth<br>Curvature becomes less distinct as you move toward posterior<br>Molar's CEJ relatively straight<br>Greatest mesial CEJ curvature of all teeth on maxillary central incisor (~3.5 mm; mesial surface) | Found only in root |

The greatest curvature of cervical line is on the mesial surface.

**Line angle**—where two surfaces come together to form a line, e.g., anterior teeth: mesiolabial, distolabial

**Point angle**—where three surfaces come together to form a point; takes name of surfaces involved, i.e., posterior teeth: mesiolingual/occlusal, mesiobuccal/occlusal

| Definition | Gap between two adjacent teeth, as teeth curve away from contact area<br>Form is dependent upon size, shape, and form of teeth<br>Four embrasures per contact area: lingual, facial, incisal/occlusal, gingival |
|---|---|
| Functions | Act as spillways for food from occlusal surfaces<br>Make teeth more self-cleansing |
| **Characteristics**<br>**Maxillary anteriors**<br>**Mandibular anteriors**<br>**Posteriors**<br>**Incisals** | Lingual is greater than facial<br>Facial is greater than lingual<br>Lingual is generally greater than the facial (except maxillary molars)<br>Incisal/occlusal is smaller than the gingival<br>Incisal may be missing between the mandibular central incisors because of high placement of mesial contact areas |

# INCISORS

## General

Incisors are involved with all of the main functions: **mastication, aesthetics, and phonetics.**

There are **8** permanent incisors (2 per quadrant). The central incisors are at the midline with the lateral incisors distal to the centrals.

Incisors are the **first succedaneous teeth to erupt.**

All incisors except the mandibular central have rounder distoincisal angles than mesioincisal angles (mandibular central is symmetric).

**Smallest tooth**—mandibular central incisor
**Bilaterally symmetric**—mandibular central incisor
**Most distinct lingual anatomy**—maxillary lateral incisor
**Incisal edge not perpendicular to labiolingual bisecting line**—mandibular lateral incisor

| Maxillary | Mandibular |
|---|---|
| Larger | Smaller |
| Wider mesiodistal diameter **(arch trait)** | Wider labiolingual diameter |
| More distinct lingual anatomy | Less distinct lingual anatomy |
| May have lingual pits | Does not have lingual pits |
| Incisal edge is centered labiolingually | Incisal edge is lingual to labiolingual midpoint |
| Heights of contour more toward middle/incisal | Heights of contour more incisal |
| Lingual embrasure is greater than facial | Facial embrasure is greater than lingual |
| Contacts more cervically located | Contacts near incisors |
| More rounded distoincisal angles | Labial surface is straighter and flatter |

## SUMMARY OF LATERAL VERSUS CENTRAL MAXILLARY INCISORS

| | Maxillary Central Incisor | Maxillary Lateral Incisor |
|---|---|---|
| **Crown** | Not as rounded as lateral | Characterized by roundness; slightly more round on mesioincisal (distinctly so on distoincisal angles) |
| **Root Cross-Section** | Round | Ovoid |
| **Other Features** | Distinct lingual anatomy | More distinct lingual anatomy |
| | Distinct mammelons on incisal edge | Mammelons may be present only on newly erupted tooth |

## SUMMARY OF LATERAL VERSUS CENTRAL MANDIBULAR INCISORS

| Mandibular Central Incisor | Mandibular Lateral Incisor |
|---|---|
| Smallest tooth | Not as small as central |
| Bilaterally symmetric | Not symmetric |
| Mirror mesial and distal axial surfaces | Distoincisal angle more round |
| Incisal edge perpendicular to a labiolingual bisecting line | Incisal edge not perpendicular to a labiolingual bisecting line |

| Position | | |
|---|---|---|
| | Right | Left |
| Universal | 8 | 9 |
| International | 11 | 21 |

| Developmental Data | |
|---|---|
| First evidence of calcification | 3–4 months after birth |
| Enamel completed | 4–5 years |
| Eruption | 7–8 years |
| Root completed | 10 years |
| Number of roots | 1 |
| Number of pulp horns | 3 |
| Developmental lobes | 4 |

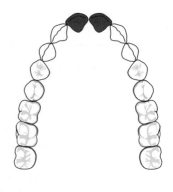

## Maxillary Right Central Incisor

| Labial | Lingual | Mesial | Distal | Incisal |
|---|---|---|---|---|
| Surface convex in both directions | Slightly more narrow than labial | Triangular (wedge-shaped) | Similar to mesial | Triangular |
| Developmental depressions, lobulated appearance | Trapezoid | Apex of root toward labial | Wedge-shaped, more rounded | Incisal edge centered, straight, three mammelons |
| Mammelons at time of eruption | Lingual fossa scoop-like | Crest of curvature in cervical third | | Cingulum toward distal |
| Trapezoid | Tendency for lingual fossa and cingulum to have central pit | Greatest cervical line curvature | | Cross section at the cervical line is roundish |
| Incisal outline straight | Distinct mesial and distal marginal ridges and lingual fossa | Contour relatively straight | | |
| Root cone-shaped | | | | |
| Imbrication lines (faint curved lines parallel to CEJ) | | | | |

## Variations on the Central Incisor

- Microdontia
- Macrodontia
- Hypercementosis—excessive amount of cementum
- Gemination (split)—
  Partial (1 pulp, 1 large tooth)
  Complete (results in twin teeth)

- Fusion—two teeth fused together along cementum; each tooth has own pulp
- Dilaceration—sharp angle of the root of tooth
- Plexion—sharp bend

The maxillary lateral incisor is the **most variable** of teeth, ranging from absent to peg-shaped to normal incisor shape. Its lingual surface can be flat, bulbous, or deeply pitted. It is characterized also by the **roundness of its distoincisal and mesioincisal angles** and is the incisor **most likely to need a lingual restoration**.

The lateral incisors complement the central incisors. They are **smaller** in dimension, **except in root length**, and the **features** of the **lateral** are more **prominent**.

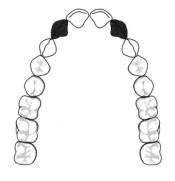

### Position

| | Right | Left |
|---|---|---|
| **Universal** | 7 | 10 |
| **International** | 12 | 22 |

### Developmental Data

| | |
|---|---|
| **First evidence of calcification** | 1 year |
| **Enamel completed** | 4–5 years |
| **Eruption** | 8–9 years |
| **Root completed** | 11 years |
| **Number of roots** | 1 |
| **Number of pulp horns** | 1–3 |
| **Developmental lobes** | 4 |

| | |
|---|---|
| **Width** | Wider mesiodistally than labiolingually |
| **Root** | Conical in shape |
| **Angle** | Distoincisal angle more rounded than the mesioincisal |

### Variations on the Lateral Incisor

- Missing altogether—partial anodontia
- Extra lateral incisor—supernumerary (accessory tooth between two maxillary central incisors called **mesiodens**)
- Incomplete development of mesial and distal lobe—"peg lateral"
- Lingual surface—deep pit, dens en dente

### Maxillary Right Lateral Incisor

| Labial | Lingual | Mesial | Distal | Incisal |
|---|---|---|---|---|
| Surface has more curvature than central / Distal outline more rounded / Root surface length greater in proportion to crown than in central | Smaller than central / Distinct anatomy: **mesial** and **distal marginal ridges, cingulum, lingual fossa, central pit** / Incisal edge well developed / Lingual fossa more concave / Tendency to have pit / Cingulum appears more prominent / Surface may be lobulated and slightly convex | Crest of curvature in cervical third / Cervical line deeper than on distal | Cervical line not as deep as in mesial | More ovoid in shape / Mesiolabial and distolabial line angle more rounded / Evidence of lobes seen |

DENTAL REVIEW

The mandibular central incisor is the **narrowest** and **most symmetric** of all teeth. **Mesial and distal profiles mirror one another.**

| Position | | |
|---|---|---|
| | **Right** | **Left** |
| **Universal** | 25 | 24 |
| **International** | 41 | 31 |

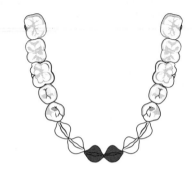

| Developmental Data | |
|---|---|
| **First evidence of calcification** | 3–4 months after birth |
| **Enamel completed** | 4–5 years |
| **Eruption** | 6–7 years |
| **Root completed** | 9 years |
| **Number of roots** | 1 |
| **Number of pulp horns** | 1–3 |
| **Developmental lobes** | 4 |

| | |
|---|---|
| **Width** | Narrowest of all teeth |
| **Root** | Ovoid on cross section; wider labiolingually than mesiodistally; symmetry |
| **Angles** | Mesioincisal and distoincisal angles very sharp |

| Mandibular Right Central Incisor | | | | |
|---|---|---|---|---|
| **Labial** | **Lingual** | **Mesial** | **Distal** | **Incisal** |
| Root relatively long and straight

Cervical line more rounded than on lingual

Smooth surfaces (no marginal ridge)

Almost perfectly symmetrical crown | Indistinct lingual anatomy

Root relatively long and straight

Small cingulum

Almost perfectly symmetrical crown | Roots are wide faciolingually with depressions on both sides

Incisal edge on or lingual to root axis | Distal surface of crown and root very similar to mesial view

Distal contact area more toward cervical than mesial contact | Symmetry between mesial and distal

Incisal edge toward lingual |

Mandibular lateral incisors are similar to mandibular central, except for the following:

- Lingual anatomy is indistinct.
- Mesial contour is straight with a height of contour at incisal edge.
- Incisal edge is **lingual to the labiolingual midpoint of the crown**, but the edge itself is not at right angles to a line bisecting the crown. However, it does follow arch curvature, making the distal end more lingually placed. The incisal edge appears to be rotated on the root.
- The root itself is very ovoid, being wider labiolingually than mesiodistally and may have mesial and distal depressions.

| Position | | |
|---|---|---|
| | **Right** | **Left** |
| **Universal** | 26 | 23 |
| **International** | 42 | 32 |

| Developmental Data | |
|---|---|
| **First evidence of calcification** | 3–4 months after birth |
| **Enamel completed** | 4–5 years |
| **Eruption** | 7–8 years |
| **Root completed** | 10 years |
| **Number of roots** | 1 |
| **Number of pulp horns** | 1–3 |
| **Developmental lobes** | 4 |

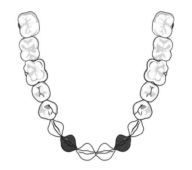

| Width |
|---|
| Wider mesiodistally than central incisor |

| Mandibular Right Lateral Incisor | | | | |
|---|---|---|---|---|
| **Labial** | **Lingual** | **Mesial** | **Distal** | **Incisal** |
| Asymmetric crown | Anatomy indistinct<br><br>Cingulum distal to the long axis of tooth | Greater height of curvature of the CEJ<br><br>From mesial, more of the lingual is visible (distal tilt) | Distal portion of incisal edge has a lingual turn | Incisal edge not straight mesiodistally and curves toward lingual on distal edge<br><br>Cingulum is slightly toward distal<br><br>Marginal ridge longer on mesial than distal side |

DENTAL REVIEW

There is only **one canine per quadrant** in the human. They are only teeth with a **single cusp**. The canines are the **longest** and **most stable teeth** in the adult permanent dentition and have an **oversized root**.

| Maxillary | Mandibular |
|---|---|
| Wider mesiodistally | Narrower mesiodistally |
| Distinct lingual anatomy (lingual cingulum) | Less distinct anatomy on lingual (cingulum less pronounced) |
| Contact point more cervical | Contact areas and heights of contour higher; contact points more incisal |
| Anomalies rare (maybe tubercle between cusp tip and lingual ridge); very stable | One anomaly is a bifurcated root |
| Longest tooth in mouth | Anatomic crown longer |
| Incisal edge centered labiolingually | Incisal edge lingual to the labiolingual midpoint |
| Buccal tip centered in the long axis of the tooth | Cusp tip distally displaced |
| Wider mesiodistally | Narrower mesiodistally |
| Longer total length | Shorter total length |
| Distinct lingual anatomy; may have lingual pit | Lingual anatomy less distinct |
| Crown generally in line with root and is shorter, fatter | Longer, slimmer crown that appears distally bent |
| Incisal edge in labiolingual midpoint | Incisal edge lingual to labiolingual midpoint |
| Prominent distal and mesial marginal ridge | Less prominent marginal ridges |
| Lingual ridge from cusp to cingulum | Less prominent lingual ridge |
| Labial surface has prominent middle lobe running from cusp tip to cervical line | |
| Buccal surface marked by three-lobed appearance | |

The maxillary canine is pointed and the **longest tooth in the mouth**.

| Position | | |
|---|---|---|
| | **Right** | **Left** |
| **Universal** | 6 | 11 |
| **International (FDI)** | 13 | 23 |

| Developmental Data | |
|---|---|
| **First evidence of calcification** | 4–5 months after birth |
| **Enamel completed** | 6–7 years |
| **Eruption** | 11 to 12 years |
| **Root completed** | 14 to 15 years |
| **Number of roots** | 1 |
| **Number of pulp horns** | 1–3 |
| **Developmental lobes** | 4 |

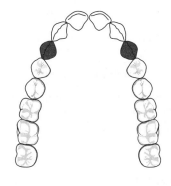

| Maxillary Right Canine | | | | |
|---|---|---|---|---|
| **Labial** | **Lingual** | **Mesial** | **Distal** | **Incisal** |
| Root is long and tapers evenly<br><br>Mesial ridge longer than distal<br><br>Mesial incisal angle sharp<br><br>One-cusp tip | Outline similar to facial<br><br>Pronounced cingulum<br><br>Marginal ridges<br><br>Lingual fossae (mesial and distal)<br><br>Possible lingual pit | Root is straight (wider labial lingually than mesial distally)<br><br>Mesial cervical line more curved than distal | Distal contour is very bulbous or convex | **Triangular**<br><br>Cusp tip is facial and mesial in placement<br><br>Cingulum is slightly distal<br><br>Pulp cavity centered in root<br><br>Root is wider faciolingually than mesiodistally |

| Anomalies |
|---|
| One anomaly associated with the mandibular canine is a bifurcated root. |

The mandibular canine is also a long, pointed tooth in which the total length is less than the maxillary canine, but the crown is longer. It has a **trilobed buccal surface**.

| Position | | |
|---|---|---|
| | **Right** | **Left** |
| **Universal** | 27 | 22 |
| **International (FDI)** | 43 | 33 |

| Developmental Data | |
|---|---|
| **First evidence of calcification** | 4–5 months after birth |
| **Enamel completed** | 6–7 years |
| **Eruption** | 9–10 years |
| **Root completed** | 12–14 years |
| **Number of roots** | 1 |
| **Number of pulp horns** | 1–3 |
| **Developmental lobes** | 4 |

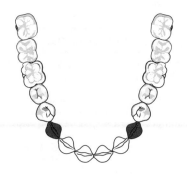

| Manibular Right Canine | | | | |
|---|---|---|---|---|
| **Labial** | **Lingual** | **Mesial** | **Distal** | **Incisal** |
| Mesial cusp ridge is shorter than distal | Anatomy is less distinct than maxillary canine<br><br>Lingual pit is rare | Profile straight<br><br>Possible root concavity<br><br>Mesial cervical line more curved than distal | Similar to mesial view | Occlusal outline<br><br>Crown is distally inclined with cusp tip slightly distally displaced<br><br>Incisal edge is lingual to labiolingual midpoint<br><br>Cingulum is distally positioned<br><br>More symmetric than maxillary canine |

# PREMOLARS

## General

There are two premolars per quadrant. The buccal cusp is more predominant than the lingual, and each premolar has **two cusps**. Premolars are also known as bicuspids.

Maxillary and mandibular premolars are **approximately the same size mesiodistally and in total length**.

Know the premolars well. A surprisingly large number of dental anatomy questions involve these teeth.

| Maxillary | Mandibular |
|---|---|
| Greater faciolingual diameter | Smaller faciolingual diameter |
| More distinct lingual cusps | Less distinct lingual cusps |
| Occlusal table centered faciolingually | Occlusal table lingually displaced |
| Two roots (buccal and lingual) | Buccal cusps more toward faciolingual midpoint |
| Buccal surface is straighter from height of contour to cusp tip | Buccal surface more convex |
| Prominent mesial root concavities | Rounder roots on cross-section |

| Comparison of Developmental Data of Premolars | | | | |
|---|---|---|---|---|
| | **Maxillary First** | **Maxillary Second** | **Mandibular First** | **Mandibular Second** |
| **First evidence of calcification** | 1½–1¾ years | 1–2½ years | 1¾–2 years | 2¼–2½ years |
| **Enamel completed** | 5–6 years | 6–7 years | 5–6 years | 6–7 years |
| **Eruption** | 10–11 years | 10–12 years | 10–12 years | 11–12 years |
| **Root completed** | 12–13 years | 12–14 years | 12–13 years | 13–14 years |
| **Number of lobes** | 4 | 4 | 4 | 4–5 |
| **Number of roots** | 2 | 1 | 1 | 1 |

| Comparison of the Premolars | | | | |
|---|---|---|---|---|
| | **Maxillary First** | **Maxillary Second** | **Mandibular First** | **Mandibular Second** |
| **Root** | 2 roots | 1 root | 1 root<br><br>Relatively round and conical | 1 root<br><br>Roundest and conical root on cross section |
| **Cusps** | Distally displaced buccal cusp and mesially displaced lingual cusp | Buccal and lingual cusps equal and centered mesiodistally | Large buccal cusp dominates | **2 to 3 cusps**<br><br>If 3, 2 are lingual, with mesiolingual larger than distolingual<br><br>"Y" occlusal pattern for 3 cusps; "H" occlusal pattern for 2 cusps |
| **Occlusal table** | Trapezoidal | Rectangular | **Lingually inclined** | Square-shaped<br><br>Less inclined than first premolar |
| **Occlusal outlines** | Hexagonal | Ovoid | Diamond | Square |
| **Grooves** | Mesial intraradicular groove<br><br>Mesial marginal developmental groove | Short central groove<br><br>Numerous supplemental grooves | **Mesiolingual developmental groove** | Lingual groove with 2 lingual cusps (3-cusp type) |
| **Ridges** | Lingual convergence<br><br>Buccal cusp ridge inclines toward mesiolingual (twisted appearance) | Little lingual convergence | **Transverse ridge**<br><br>Well-developed buccal ridge<br><br>Mesial ridge less distinct than distal marginal ridge<br><br>Lingual convergence | Little lingual convergence |
| **Other distinguishing features** | "Broad-shouldered"<br><br>Prominent mesial concavity<br><br>Prominent buccal lobes | "Narrow shouldered"<br><br>Less prominent mesial axial concavity than maxillary first | Most resembles **canine**<br><br>**Lingual cusp that resembles a cingulum**<br><br>Transitional tooth<br><br>Greatest discrepancy in size of buccal and lingual cusps and width (buccal dominant)<br><br>Mesial/distal fossae with pits<br><br>Prominent mesial bulge | Central pit<br><br>Equal buccal and lingual surfaces |

The maxillary first premolar has a **prominent buccal ridge**, and its buccal surface is wider than the lingual surface. It is the **only premolar that has two roots** (one buccal and one lingual) and **two cusps**.

The maxillary first premolar and its **intraradicular groove** is important to know for the **NBDE Part I**. Root planing of the mesial side and adapting a matrix band on the mesial side can both be difficult because of this groove.

| Position | | |
|---|---|---|
| | **Right** | **Left** |
| **Universal** | 5 | 12 |
| **International (FDI)** | 14 | 24 |

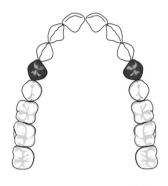

| Maxillary First Right Premolar | | | | |
|---|---|---|---|---|
| **Buccal** | **Lingual** | **Mesial** | **Distal** | **Occlusal** |
| Rounded, long cusp<br><br>Prominent buccal ridge running axially and bordered by depressions that give the surface a 3-lobed appearance<br><br>Surface wider than lingual surface ("broad-shouldered") | Lingual cusp smaller<br><br>Lingual cusp slightly mesial to midpoint and smaller than buccal cusp<br><br>Surface rounded | Marked mesial concavity runs onto mesial root surface (**mesial interradicular groove**)<br><br>**Mesial marginal developmental groove** (extension of central groove) interrupts mesial marginal ridge and progresses down mesial surface | Buccal cusp distally placed and larger than lingual cusp<br><br>Also has developmental depression | **Hexagonal crown profile** (mesial and distal surfaces converge toward lingual)<br><br>**Trapezoidal occlusal table**<br><br>2 cusps that are well defined: buccal is larger, and lingual is shifted mesially |

| Variants and Anomalies |
|---|

- Single root
- Occasionally 3 rooted

The maxillary second premolar is a **"narrow-shouldered"** tooth from the buccal and is **slightly smaller** than the first premolar. It has **indistinct lobes**; a slight mesial concavity or even convexity may be seen on the mesial surface. **The mesial marginal ridge is not interrupted by a groove. Cusps** are more of an **equal height and lengths**, and the **tips are centered** on the tooth in a mesiodistal direction.

| Position | | |
|---|---|---|
| | Right | Left |
| Universal | 4 | 13 |
| International (FDI) | 15 | 25 |

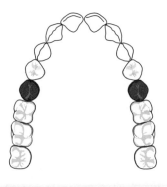

| Maxillary Second Right Premolar | | | | |
|---|---|---|---|---|
| **Buccal** | **Lingual** | **Mesial** | **Distal** | **Occlusal** |
| | | | | D · · · M |
| **Indistinct lobes**<br><br>Buccal cusp is **shorter and rounder** than first premolar | Lingual cusp almost as big as buccal cusp<br><br>Lingual cusp tip shifted mesially<br><br>Smallest and most indistinct | Surface round<br><br>Mesial marginal ridge is **not** interrupted by groove | Surface round | **Ovoid to round** shape<br><br>**Rectangular** occlusal table<br><br>Little lingual convergence |

| Variants and Anomalies |
|---|
| More variability than in first maxillary premolar |

The mandibular first premolar may be viewed as a **transitional tooth, resembling a canine**. Its buccal cusp is much larger than is the lingual cusp, which may resemble a cingulum. It is the **only posterior tooth with a lingually inclined occlusal table.**

| Position | | |
|---|---|---|
| | **Right** | **Left** |
| **Universal** | 28 | 21 |
| **International (FDI)** | 44 | 34 |

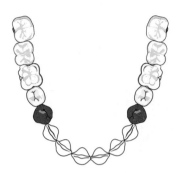

| Mandibular First Right Premolar | | | | |
|---|---|---|---|---|
| **Buccal** | **Lingual** | **Mesial** | **Distal** | **Occlusal** |
| Outline is almost bilaterally symmetrical<br><br>Large pointed buccal cusp<br><br>Well-developed buccal ridge | **Smallest and indistinct cusp of all premolars**<br><br>Lingual cusp may resemble a cingulum<br><br>**Mesiolingual developmental groove** produces slight concavity at about the mesiolingual line angle | Prominent mesial bulge<br><br>Very large buccal cusp tip centered over root tip<br><br>Reduced lingual cusp<br><br>Mesial/distal fossae with pits<br><br>Marginal ridges well developed | Very large buccal cusp tip centered over root tip<br><br>Reduced lingual cusp<br><br>Mesial/distal fossae with pits<br><br>Marginal ridges well developed | **Diamond shaped**, with convergence to the lingual<br><br>Marginal ridges well developed<br><br>Mesial and distal fossae with pits<br><br>Mesiolingual developmental groove |

| Variants and Anomalies |
|---|
| • Grooved or bifurcated roots<br>• Crown and root may be variable |

DENTAL REVIEW

The mandibular second premolar is generally larger than the mandibular first premolar. It is distinguished by its **two variations of the lingual cusp.** If the mandibular second premolar has three cusps (more common) instead of two, the two appear on the lingual view and the mesiolingual is much larger than the distolingual. The mesiolingual cusp is also separated by a lingual groove extending from the central pit.

| Position | | |
|---|---|---|
| | **Right** | **Left** |
| **Universal** | 29 | 20 |
| **International (FDI)** | 45 | 35 |

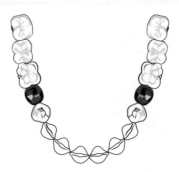

| Manibular Second First Premolar | | | | |
|---|---|---|---|---|
| **Buccal** | **Lingual** | **Mesial** | **Distal** | **Occlusal** |
| Buccal width nearly equal with lingual; buccal cusp size more equal with lingual cusp size | Lingual width nearly equal with buccal; lingual cusp size more equal with buccal cusp size<br><br>If 3 cusps, 2 are lingual, with mesiolingual larger than distolingual<br><br>Mesiolingual and distolingual cusp separated by lingual groove extending from central pit<br><br>Little occlusal surface seen from the lingual<br><br>In the single lingual cusp variant, its tip is shifted mesially | Buccal cusp is slightly shorter than first mandibular premolar<br><br>Buccal cusp slightly longer than lingual cusp | | Square in outline<br><br>Central pit<br><br>Variant groove patterns:<br><br>• Y (3 cusps with central pit)<br><br>• H (2 cusps with single developmental groove crossing transverse ridge from mesial to distal) |

### Variants and Anomalies

• One or two lingual cusps
• Missing altogether

## General

The molar is derived from *mola*, Latin for "millstone." The main function of molars is to grind food, thus explaining their **large occlusal surfaces**. The most complicated of the adult human dentition, they can have from **three to five cusps** and **two to three roots**.

Questions on NBDE part I concerning molar anatomy will usually focus more on the first molar. This is because of increasing variation in the second and third molars.

| Maxillary Molar | Mandibular Molar |
|---|---|
| 3 roots | 2 roots |
| 4 pulp horns | 2 pulp horns |
| 4 cusps and extra variable Carabelli cusp (trait) | 5 cusps |
| Buccal cusps unequal | Buccal cusps equal |
| Lingual cusps unequal; cusp of Carabelli mostly present | Lingual cusps equal; cusp of Carabelli absent |
| Oblique ridge diagonal | Oblique ridge not found on mandibular molars |
| Occlusal table centered labiolingually | Occlusal table lingually placed |
| Equal amounts of buccal and lingual surfaces may be seen from occlusal | More buccal surface than lingual surface may be seen from occlusal |
| Lingual height of contour in middle third just above junction of middle and cervical thirds | Lingual height of contour in middle third just below the junction of the middle and occlusal thirds |
| Wider faciolingually than mesiodistally | Wider mesiodistally than faciolingually |
| Distolingual groove | Buccal pit |

| Developmental Data | | | | | | |
|---|---|---|---|---|---|---|
| | **Maxillary** | | | **Mandibular** | | |
| | **First** | **Second** | **Third** | **First** | **Second** | **Third** |
| **First evidence of calcification** | Birth | 2 ½ years | 7–9 years | Birth | 2½–3 years | 8–10 years |
| **Enamel completed** | 3–4 years | 7–8 years | 12–16 years | 2½–3 years | 7–8 years | 12–16 years |
| **Eruption** | 6 years | 12–13 years | 17–21 years | 6–7 years | 11–13 years | 17–21 years |
| **Root completed** | 9–10 years | 14–16 years | 18–25 years | 9–10 years | 14–15 years | 18–25 years |
| **Number of lobes** | 5 | 4 | 4 | 5 | 4 | 4 |
| **Number of roots** | 3 | 3 | 3 (may be fused into 1; highly variable) | 2 | 2 | 2 (may be fused into 1; may be 3; highly variable) |

DENTAL REVIEW

## Comparison of the Maxillary Molars

| | Maxillary First | Maxillary Second | Maxillary Third |
|---|---|---|---|
| **Root** | **3 roots** (2 buccal, 1 lingual)<br>Buccal roots look like "pliers handles"; distobuccal smallest<br>Large lingual root longest, "banana shaped" (almost straight) and centered between buccal roots<br>30% have fourth canal found in mesiobuccal root | **3 roots** (2 buccal, 1 lingual)<br>Buccal roots distally inclined<br>Roots are within crown profiles when seen from all angles | **3 roots** (2 buccal, 1 lingual)<br>Often short<br>Very distally inclined<br>Tend to fuse (lingual to buccal) |
| **Cusps** | **4 major** (2 buccal, 2 lingual)<br>**Fifth** minor cusp: **Carabelli**<br>ML and MB cusps very large<br>DB cusp large; DL cusp smaller<br>4 pulp horns (1 per major cusp) | **4 major**<br>No Carabelli trait<br>ML and MB cusps smaller than first<br>DB cusp smaller; DL cusp even smaller (may be missing)<br>4 pulp horns (1 per major cusp) | **Usually 3**<br>No Carabelli trait<br>ML and MB cusps smaller than second<br>DB cusp much smaller; DL cusp usually missing |
| **Occlusal outlines** | Rhomboidal | Rhomboidal or heart-shaped | Heart-shaped or triangular |
| **Grooves** | Lingual groove separates lingual cusps<br>Buccal groove runs between buccal cusps<br>Distal groove extends from central pit distolingually toward oblique ridge | Usually a short buccal groove; no buccal pit<br>Similar to first molar | Variable pattern |
| **Ridges** | Oblique ridge most prominent, connects distobuccal cusp to mesiolingual cusp<br>Mesial marginal ridge longer and more distinct than distal marginal ridge | Oblique ridge from distobuccal to mesiolingual<br>Similar to first molar | Oblique ridges may be missing<br>Variable pattern |
| **Other distinguishing features** | Looks like two premolars stuck together<br>Distal and central fossa<br>Distal triangular fossa contains distal pit<br>Mesiolingual > mesiobuccal > distobuccal > distolingual | More exaggerated difference in cusp size: mesiolingual > mesiobuccal > distobuccal > distolingual | More variable morphology than any other tooth<br>May be the most often congenitally missing |

## Comparison of the Mandibular Molars

| | Mandibular First | Mandibular Second | Mandibular Third |
|---|---|---|---|
| **Root** (for more details, see individual tooth) | 2 roots<br>Rounded apex<br>Mesial root largest<br>Roots less distally inclined than in second molar | 2 roots<br>More distinctly distally inclined<br>Pointed apex<br>Proximal root concavities not usually seen | 2 roots<br>Extremely distally inclined<br>Short, often fused |
| **Cusps** | 5 cusps | 4 cusps | 4 cusps (highly variable) |
| **Occlusal outlines** | Pentagonal | Rectangular | Ovoid |
| **Grooves** | 2 buccal grooves (MB and DB)<br>Mesial and distal marginal grooves | Single buccal groove<br>No marginal grooves | Single buccal groove<br>No marginal grooves |
| **Ridges** | Two transverse ridges, no oblique ridge | Two transverse ridges, no oblique ridge | Two transverse ridges, no oblique ridge |
| **Other distinguishing features** | Prove to misshapen enamel defect: mulberry molar<br>Largest of the mandibular teeth | Most symmetric of the molars<br>No distal cusp | Often has variable morphology<br>May be the most often congenitally missing<br>Common tooth to have enamel pearls |

The **Carabelli trait** is the most distinguishing feature of the maxillary first molar, and is highly variable, from being a full cusp to being barely visible.

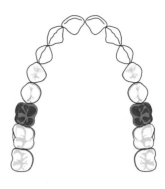

| Position | | |
|---|---|---|
| | **Right** | **Left** |
| **Universal** | 3 | 14 |
| **International (FDI)** | 16 | 26 |

| Maxillary First Right Molar | | | | |
|---|---|---|---|---|
| **Buccal** | **Lingual** | **Mesial** | **Distal** | **Occlusal** |

D     M

| Buccal | Lingual | Mesial | Distal | Occlusal |
|---|---|---|---|---|
| Larger mesiobuccal cusp<br><br>Cervical line straight<br><br>Mesiobuccal and distobuccal dominate<br><br>Buccal developmental groove<br><br>**Roots:** Buccal roots joined in common root trunk (extends 2.5–3.5 mm from cervical line)<br><br>Root trunk may have deep developmental groove<br><br>All roots can be seen from buccal view, with lingual root in between | Lingual surface convex throughout<br><br>Lingual developmental groove (extension of distolingual groove)<br><br>Larger mesiolingual cusp sometimes has Carabelli trait<br><br>**Root:** Lingual is largest root (greatest diameter in mesiodistal direction)<br><br>Massive root trunk<br><br>Vertical depression on its lingual surface extending from cervical line<br><br>Mesiobuccal has a mesial contour; distobuccal has distal contour | Flat to concave surface<br><br>Cusp of Carabelli seen<br><br>**Roots:** From mesial view, only mesiobuccal and lingual roots seen (distobuccal blocked by mesiobuccal) | Convex surface throughout, except for concave-to-flat area immediately above distobuccal root<br><br>Distal marginal ridge shorter than mesial | **Rhomboid** shape<br><br>**Angles:** Mesiobuccal and distolingual **acute**; distobuccal and mesiolingual **obtuse**<br><br>4 major cusps<br><br>Cusp of Carabelli on mesiolingual cusp<br><br>Lingual groove separates lingual cusps<br><br>**Oblique ridge** (mesiolingual to distobuccal cusps)<br><br>**Major** fossae: distal and central<br><br>**Minor** fossa: mesial triangular, distal triangular<br><br>**Distal pit**<br><br>Largest crown of all maxillary molars |

The maxillary second molar is very similar to the first molar, with the following exceptions: *1)* **the distobuccal cusp is relatively smaller or absent,** *2)* **the absence of the cusp of Carabelli,** *3)* the mesiobuccal and distolingual angles are more acute, whereas the mesiolingual and distobuccal angles are more obtuse, and *4)* there are **more supplemental grooves** on the occlusal surface.

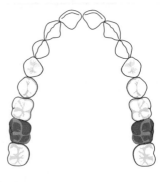

| Position | | |
|---|---|---|
| | **Right** | **Left** |
| **Universal** | 2 | 15 |
| **International (FDI)** | 17 | 27 |

| Maxillary Second Right Molar | | | | |
|---|---|---|---|---|
| **Buccal** | **Lingual** | **Mesial** | **Distal** | **Occlusal** |
| Crown is shorter occlusocervically and is narrower mesiodistally<br><br>Distobuccal cusp is smaller<br><br>**Root:** Mesiobuccal and distobuccal root are inclined distally and are more parallel and usually the same length | Distolingual cusp smaller<br><br>No Carabelli cusp<br><br>**Root:** Lingual root may be distally inclined (no "pliers handles") | Crown is shorter than first molar<br><br>Roots confine themselves to width of crown | | **Rhomboidal** (large distolingual cusp) or **heart-shaped** (smaller distolingual cusp)<br><br>Distobuccal cusp smaller and less defined than first molar<br><br>Oblique ridge less dominant<br><br>Differences in cusp size is more exaggerated than on first molar |

| Variants and Anomalies |
|---|
| • Distolingual cusp absent<br>• Occlusal shape rhomboidal or heart-shaped<br>• Fused root |

DENTAL REVIEW

The maxillary third molar, as well as the maxillary lateral incisor, is known for **extreme variability of form.** Pointed, peg-like maxillary third molars are not uncommon. The sometimes fused, pointed roots can make extraction of these teeth easier than expected.

| Position | | |
|---|---|---|
| | **Right** | **Left** |
| **Universal** | 1 | 16 |
| **International (FDI)** | 18 | 28 |

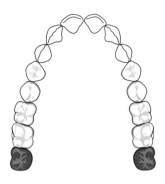

### Maxillary Third Right Molar

| Buccal | Lingual | Mesial | Distal | Occlusal |
|---|---|---|---|---|
| Distobuccal cusp smaller than mesiobuccal (sometimes missing)<br><br>**Roots:** Buccal roots most often fused | Distolingual cusp often absent (mostly one large lingual cusp)<br><br>**Root:** Lingual root often fused to buccal cusps | Crown outline rounded, bulbous | **No contact point** on distal surface<br><br>Crown outline also rounded, bulbous | **Heart-shaped or triangular**<br><br>Oblique ridge may be small or missing<br><br>Smallest crown of the maxillary molars<br><br>Mesiolingual cusp is largest; distobuccal is smallest (or distolingual, if present) |

#### Variants and Anomalies

- Impaction common
- Many cusps and grooves possible
- Distobuccal cusp small
- Distolingual cusp missing

DENTAL REVIEW

The mandibular first molar has a **distinctive pentagonal ("home plate") occlusal outline**, and two buccal and one lingual groove form the pattern distinctive to this tooth. The **buccal half is divided into three cusps, and the lingual is divided into two.**

| Position | | |
|---|---|---|
| | **Right** | **Left** |
| **Universal** | 30 | 19 |
| **International (FDI)** | 46 | 36 |

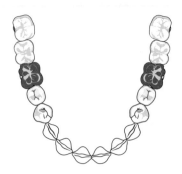

| Mandibular First Right Molar | | | | |
|---|---|---|---|---|
| **Buccal** | **Lingual** | **Mesial** | **Distal** | **Occlusal** |
| 3 cusps seen | 3 cusps seen | Rhomboid (tilted lingually) | 3 cusps seen (distobuccal, distal, distolingual) | **Pentagonal** ("home plate") shape |
| 2 developmental grooves (mesiobuccal and distobuccal) | Developmental groove separates 2 lingual cusps | Lingual surface straighter than convex buccal surface | Tooth tapers toward distal | **5** functional cusps |
| Mesiobuccal groove ends in **buccal pit** on buccal surface | Prominent cervical ridge height | Mesial marginal groove notches mesial marginal groove | Distal marginal ridge notched by distal marginal groove | **3 fossae, each with pit:** central, mesial, and distal |
| Trapezoidal shape (wider at occlusal) | **Roots:** 2 visible | Buccal cervical ridge | **Root:** Curves distally; blunt, distal smaller than mesial; may have shallow proximal root concavity; joined with mesial at common root trunk | Buccal outline divided into 3 (mesiobuccal and distobuccal grooves) |
| Distal outline more rounded | | **Root:** Mesial root is the broadest root in the arch in a buccolingual direction; curves distally; distinct proximal root concavity on mesial surface; blunt; joined with distal at common root trunk | | Lingual outline divided into 2 (lingual groove) |
| Mesiobuccal cusp widest; distobuccal smallest | | | | Distal marginal ridge smaller than mesial marginal ridge (both ridges cut through by developmental grooves) |
| **Roots:** 2 clearly seen; distal root is less curved than mesial | | | | |

| Variants and Anomalies | |
|---|---|
| • Distal cusp absent | • Sixth cusp rare |
| • Occasionally 2 mesial roots | |

The mandibular second molar is similar to the first molar except that it is *1)* smaller, *2)* the **distal cusp is missing**, *3)* the lingual and buccal surfaces are similar in length, *4)* there is **only one buccal groove**; *5)* the crown is also shorter, and *6)* there are **no developmental grooves interrupting the marginal ridges.** Finally, *7)* roots are more distally inclined than the first molar and have a more pointed apex.

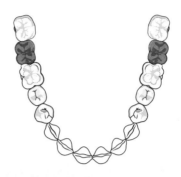

| Position | | |
|---|---|---|
| | **Right** | **Left** |
| **Universal** | 31 | 18 |
| **International** | 47 | 37 |

| Mandibular Second Right Molar | | | | |
|---|---|---|---|---|
| **Buccal** | **Lingual** | **Mesial** | **Distal** | **Occlusal** |
| Buccal groove separates mesiobuccal from distobuccal cusps<br><br>Trapezoidal shape<br><br>No distal cusp (4 cusps)<br><br>**Roots:** Closer together than first mandibular molar and are distally inclined | Trapezoidal shape<br><br>Lingual groove<br><br>**Roots:** Closer together than first mandibular molar and are distally inclined | Looks similar to first molar<br><br>Cusps of equal height | Cusps of equal height<br><br>Distal marginal ridge helps form profile<br><br>Cervical line flat | **Rectangular**<br><br>4 cusps<br><br>3 grooves (buccal, lingual, central)<br><br>3 fossae, each with pit (central, medial, distal)<br><br>Two transverse ridges |

### Variants and Anomalies

- 2 root canals for each root
- Five cusps (rare)

DENTAL REVIEW

Third molars vary in shape and **do not have a standard form**. They are usually smaller than the second molar.

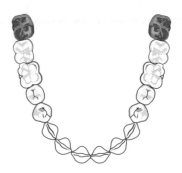

| Position | | |
|---|---|---|
| | **Right** | **Left** |
| **Universal** | 32 | 17 |
| **International (FDI)** | 48 | 38 |

| Mandibular Third Right Molar | | | | |
|---|---|---|---|---|
| **Buccal** | **Lingual** | **Mesial** | **Distal** | **Occlusal** |
| Crown short and bulbous<br><br>**Roots:** distally inclined; poorly developed | | Resembles first and second molars, but shorter crown | | **Ovoid to round**<br><br>4–5 cusps<br><br>May have indistinct grooves |

### Variants and Anomalies

- Most commonly missing permanent teeth
- Often under- or oversized
- Supernumerary (fourth molars)
- May be partially erupted (susceptible to periodontal infections)
- Occlusal surface may be crenulated (numerous grooves)
- Often fail to erupt

## GENERAL

The deciduous dentition (also called "primary" or "baby" teeth) helps permanent teeth develop proper alignment, spacing, and occlusion. As stated in the first few pages of the General Characteristics section, there are 20 primary teeth in all (10 maxillary and 10 mandibular).

**MAXILLARY**

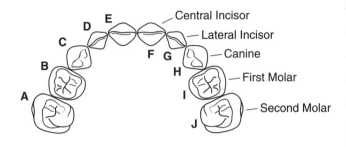

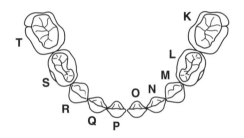

**MANDIBULAR**

| Maxillary | Eruption* (months) | Shedding (years) |
|---|---|---|
| Central incisor | 8–12 | 6–7 |
| Lateral incisor | 9–13 | 7–8 |
| Canine (cuspid) | 16–22 | 10–12 |
| First molar | 13–19 | 9–11 |
| Second molar | 25–33 | 10–12 |
| Mandibular | | |
| Central incisor | 6–10 | 6–7 |
| Lateral incisor | 10–16 | 7–8 |
| Canine (cuspid) | 17–23 | 9–12 |
| First molar | 14–18 | 9–11 |
| Second molar | 23–31 | 10–12 |

*Note that teeth tend to erupt in pairs.

Also, eruption and shedding patterns are seen earlier in girls.

| Maxillary | Calcification (weeks in utero) | Root Formation Complete (months) |
|---|---|---|
| Central incisor | 14 | 10 |
| Lateral incisor | 16 | 11 |
| Canine (cuspid) | 17 | 19 |
| First molar | 15 | 16 |
| Second molar | 19 | 26 |
| Mandibular | | |
| Central incisor | 14 | 8 |
| Lateral incisor | 16 | 13 |
| Canine (cuspid) | 17 | 20 |
| First molar | 15½ | 16 |
| Second molar | 18 | 27 |

### Primary Teeth Characteristics as Differing from Permanent Teeth

In general, the fewer primary teeth are **smaller and whiter** than permanent teeth and generally resemble the teeth that replace them, **except for the first molars**, which resemble nothing in the permanent dentition. **Primary molars** are replaced by **permanent premolars**.

### Development of Primary Teeth

- Development begins at 6 weeks in utero
- Calcification begins at 18 weeks in utero (approx 4–6 months)
- By the age of 3, apices are completely formed

| Features | Comparison with Permanent Teeth |
|----------|--------------------------------|
| Crowns | Crown-to-root ratio is smaller<br>Shorter and fatter<br>Rounded |
| Roots | Marked bowing and flaring<br>Molars: long and slender with little or no trunk<br>Incisors and canines: longer and slender |
| Enamel | Thinner |
| Surfaces | Lingual and facial cervical bulges<br>Facial and lingual surfaces are flatter<br>No mammelons on anterior teeth |
| Arch | More circular |
| Ridges | Cervical ridges more prominent |

## ANTERIOR TEETH

The primary incisors and canines resemble the permanent ones, **except for traits listed in the following table.** A notable trademark of the anteriors is **cervical constricture**.

| Tooth | Position (Right/Left) | Replaced by | Differences from Permanent Replacement |
|-------|----------------------|-------------|----------------------------------------|
| Maxillary primary central incisor* | E/F<br>51/61 | Maxillary permanent central incisor | Smooth labial surface<br>No mammelons<br>Cingulum may be prominent<br>Cervical constricture: facial and lingual cervical bulges<br>Height of crown smaller than mesiodistal diameter |
| Maxillary primary lateral incisor* | D/G<br>52/62 | Maxillary permanent lateral incisor | Labial surface smoother than permanent<br>No mammelons<br>More distinct lingual anatomy<br>Cervical constricture |
| Maxillary primary canine | C/H<br>53/63 | Maxillary permanent canine | Diamond-shaped crown from facial<br>Labial surface smoother<br>Prominent cingulum (cusped appearance)<br>Mesial and distal contacts are at same level<br>Longer mesial incisal slope than distal incisal slope<br>Height of crown less than mesiodistal diameter |
| Mandibular primary central | P/O<br>81/71 | Mandibular permanent central incisor | Labial surface smooth, unmarked, flat<br>Prominent cingulum on lingual<br>Often, developmental groove or depression on distal of root<br>Cervical contricture |
| Mandibular primary lateral | Q/N<br>82/72 | Mandibular permanent lateral incisor | Prominent cingulum on lingual<br>Cervical constricture |
| Mandibular primary canine | R/M<br>83/73 | Mandibular permanent canine | Arrow-shaped from facial<br>Smooth labial surface<br>Longer distal incisal ridge than mesial incisal ridge |

*These teeth are most damaged by baby bottle tooth decay (BBTD).

The primary first molar resembles nothing in the adult dentition. In general, **upper molars** have **3 roots**, whereas the **lower molars** have only **2**. First molars are also distinguished by a bulge on the buccal surface (cervical bulge).

| Tooth | Position | Replaced by | Traits |
|---|---|---|---|
| **Maxillary primary first molar** | B/I 54/64 | Maxillary permanent first premolar | Resembles nothing in permanent dentition<br>Two-cusped (mesiobuccal and mesiolingual)<br>**Nodule resembling small cusp** may be present on mesial ridge of the mesiobuccal cusp<br>**Occlusal table outline is rectangular** with deep prominent **buccal developmental groove** (terminates in central pit)<br>Frequently, **oblique ridge** from mesiolingual cusp to distobuccal cusp area<br>Heights of contour low and prominent<br>**Three roots very divergent, without trunk root;** looks like "elephant charging" when viewed from lingual and inverted |
| **Maxillary primary secondary molar** | A/J 55/65 | Second maxillary premolar | Closely resembles maxillary permanent first molar (4 cusps, Carabelli trait), except:<br>• Squatter and more bulbous<br>• More prominent cervical bulges<br>• Very little root trunk |
| **Mandibular primary first molar** | S/L 84/74 | Mandibular permanent first premolar | Resembles nothing in permanent dentition<br>**Looks more like a molar than maxillary primary first molar**<br>4 cusps (2 buccal, 2 lingual); mesiobuccal and mesiolingual largest<br>**Transverse ridge** between mesiobuccal and mesiolingual (largest) cusps<br>Mesial/distal profiles: highly convex<br>Occlusal **outline rhomboidal** because of buccal cervical ridge<br>Occlusal **table rectangular**<br>Buccal profile: **low, prominent buccal cervical ridge** (unique; gives "pregnant" appearance)<br>Deep buccal groove, shallow lingual groove; may have mesial marginal groove<br>**2 roots: mesial larger**<br>Central pit radiating a central groove (goes to mesial pit and buccal and lingual grooves) |
| **Mandibular primary second molar** | T/K 85/75 | Mandibular permanent second premolar | Closely resembles mandibular permanent second molar, except:<br>• 2 roots more divergent and without root trunk<br>• Cervical bulges<br>• All 3 buccal cusps equal in size (distal cusps smallest in permanent first molar) |

### Isomorphy of Primary Second and Permanent First Molars

In summary, there is remarkable resemblance between the maxillary and mandibular second primary molars and their first permanent molar counterparts, even down to the smallest detail.

This information about primary teeth is important to know for the NBDE Part I exam:

- The maxillary first primary molar somewhat resembles a premolar.
- The mandibular first primary molar has the most unique buccal cervical bulge or ridge.
- The mandibular first primary molar has prominent transverse ridge.
- The mandibular first and maxillary first primary molars resemble nothing in permanent dentition.
- The mandibular second and maxillary second primary molars resemble the mandibular first and maxillary first permanent molars, respectively.

# OCCLUSION

Occlusion is the general contact relationship between the occlusal surfaces of the maxillary and mandibular arches and individual teeth.

## ARCH-TO-ARCH RELATIONSHIPS

When the two arches come together, each tooth opposes two teeth in the opposite arch, with the exception of the **mandibular central incisor** and **the maxillary third molar**, each of which only opposes one tooth. Knowing the general relationships described below are critical when answering most occlusion questions.

| The Maxillary Arch |
| --- |
| Each tooth in the maxillary arch opposes two teeth in the mandibular arch—its counterpart in the mandibular arch, plus the tooth distal to its counterpart, except the maxillary third molar. |

| Example |
| --- |
| The first maxillary premolar opposes the first mandibular premolar and second mandibular premolar. |

| The Mandibular Arch |
| --- |
| Each tooth in the mandibular arch opposes two teeth in the maxillary arch—its counterpart in the maxillary arch, plus the tooth mesial to its counterpart, except the mandibular central incisor. |

| Example |
| --- |
| The first mandibular molar opposes the first maxillary molar (its counterpart), plus the second maxillary premolar (tooth mesial to its counterpart). |

*Note:* The tip of the maxillary canine is placed in the labial embrasure.

The arch form of the maxillae is larger compared with the mandibular arch, providing an overlapping of the maxillary teeth over the mandibular teeth. The **horizontal overlap** is referred to as **overjet,** and the **vertical overlap** is referred to as **overbite.** This overhanging provides a protective feature during opening and closing movements of the jaws. Soft tissues are displaced during the act of closure until the teeth have come together in occlusal contact. Therefore, the cheeks, lips, and tongue are less likely to be caught and injured during mandibular movements.

## CONCEPTS AND DEFINITIONS

The numbers in the first column of the table correspond with the figure.

| | Area | Definition | Examples |
| --- | --- | --- | --- |
| 1 | Guiding cusp | Cusp of tooth **not in contact in occlusion** but **outside** occluding area<br><br>Opposing embrasures or grooves in the opposing dentition | Buccal cusps of maxillary posteriors and lingual cusps of mandibular posteriors |
| 2 | Supporting (holding) cusp | Cusp of tooth that **contacts the opposing arch on marginal ridges or central fossa area**<br><br>Responsible for **supporting the forces of occlusion** | Buccal cusps of mandibular posteriors and lingual cusps of maxillary posteriors |
| 3 | Occlusal slope | | |
| 4 | Guiding incline | Inclines or slopes of the guiding cusps from the guiding cusp tip toward the center of tooth | Lingual inclines of buccal cusps of maxillary posteriors and buccal inclines of lingual cusps of mandibular posterior |
| 5 | Functional outer aspect (FOA) | The outside 1–2 mm of supporting cusp<br><br>Makes contact with guiding inclines of guiding cusps of opposing dentition when in occlusion | 1–2 mm wide strip from buccal cusp tips of mandibular posteriors on buccal surface, and 1–2 mm wide strip from lingual cusp tips of maxillary posteriors on lingual surface |

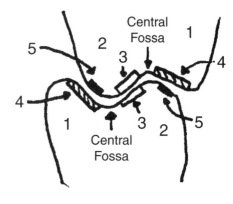

The **buccal cusps of the mandibular posteriors** and **the lingual cusps of the maxillary posteriors** are the holding, supporting, or occluding cusps, and they contact marginal ridges and central fossae in the opposing arch.

The **buccal cusps of the maxillary posteriors** and the **lingual cusps of the mandibular posteriors** are the guiding cusps and oppose the embrasures and grooves of the opposing dentition.

Therefore, on each posterior tooth, we should expect **3 areas of contact** during occlusion:

1. The FOA of the holding cusp contacting the guiding incline(s) of the guiding cusp in the opposing dentition
2. The occlusal slope of the holding cusp contacting the occlusal slope of the opposing holding cusp
3. The guiding incline(s) of the guiding cusp contacting the FOA of the holding cusp of the opposing dentition

## SUMMARY OF OCCLUSAL CONTACTS

### Tooth Contacts in a Class I Normal Occlusion*

| Maxillary Teeth | Mandibular Occlusal Contact | Mandibular Teeth | Maxillary Occlusal Contact |
|---|---|---|---|
| Central incisor | Central and lateral | Central incisor | Maxillary central incisor |
| Lateral incisor | Lateral incisor and canine | Lateral incisor | Central and lateral incisors |
| Canine | Canine and first premolar | Canine | Lateral incisor and canine |
| First premolar | First and second premolars | First premolar | Canine and first molar |
| Second premolar | Second and first molars | Second premolar | First and second premolar |
| First molar | First and second molars | First molar | Second premolar and first molar |
| Second molar | Second and third molars | Second molar | First and second molar |
| Third molar | Third molar | Third molar | Second and third molar |

*The **mandibular central incisor** is the **only anterior tooth** that occludes with only one tooth.
The **maxillary third molar** is the only **posterior tooth** that occludes with only one tooth.

### Tooth Guidance in Mandibular Movements

| | |
|---|---|
| Canine guided | The maxillary and mandibular canine contact during working side mandibular movement, causing all posterior teeth to disocclude. |
| Group function | The maxillary canine and buccal cusps of the posterior teeth contact during working side mandibular movement, causing the disocclusion of the posterior teeth on the nonworking side. |
| Anterior guidance | Contact between the lingual surface of the maxillary teeth and the facial surfaces of the mandibular teeth during protrusive movement of the mandible disocclude all the posterior teeth. |

Detailed information on angle classification is not needed until the NBDE Part II. Know the classes as described here.

## Class I

In reality, the class I type of occlusion described by Angle is a **malocclusion**. Even though it has a normal cusp-groove relationship, there may be anterior crowding. Normal occlusion is not classified by Angle's system.

The mesiobuccal cusp of the first maxillary molar is **opposite** the mesiobuccal groove of the mandibular first molar. The maxillary canine is **in the labial embrasure** between the mandibular canine and the mandibular first premolar.

Class I occlusion is often called **neutroclusion.**

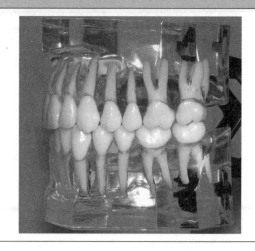

## Class II

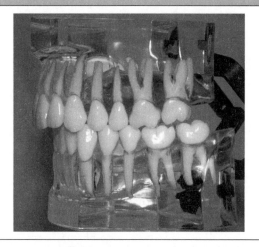

In class II occlusion, the mandible is small or **micrognathic**.

The mesiobuccal cusp of the first maxillary molar is **anterior** to the mesiobuccal groove of the mandibular first molar. The maxillary canine is **anterior** to the **labial embrasure** of the mandibular canine and the mandibular first premolar (often called **distoclusion**).

The lower arch is mesial to the upper arch.

## Class III

In class III occlusion, the mandible is large or **prognathic**.

The mesiobuccal cusp of the first maxillary molar is **posterior** to the mesiobuccal groove of the mandibular first molar. The maxillary canine is **posterior** to the labial embrasure of the mandibular canine and the mandibular first premolar (often called **mesioclusion**).

The lower teeth are mesial to the upper teeth.

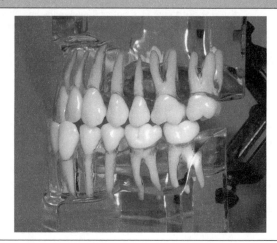

DENTAL REVIEW

| Curves | |
|---|---|
| **CURVE OF SPREE** | **CURVE OF WILSON** |
| The anterior–posterior relation of the teeth viewed from the lateral, i.e., from the side. | The tilting of the mandibular posteriors lingually when the arches are viewed from the front (the maxillary posteriors tilt facially or buccally). |
| • The ma**x**illary arch is conve**x**.<br>• The **mandibular** arch is **concave**. | • The ma**x**illary arch is conve**x**.<br>• The **mandibular** arch is **concave** |

| Root Angulation | |
|---|---|
| **Roots** | **Angles** |
| Mandibular | Anterior teeth angled distally<br>Posterior teeth angled facially |
| Maxillary | Anterior teeth angled distally<br>Posterior teeth angled lingually, except distobuccal root of first maxillary molar (inclined buccally) |

## TEMPOROMANDIBULAR JOINT (TMJ)

The temporomandibular joint is both a **ginglymoarthrodial** joint **(hinge and gliding)** and a **diarthrosis** joint **(capable of free movement)**. It is located between the mandibular (glenoid) fossa of the temporal bone and the condylar head of the mandible.

The **mandibular condyle** is an oblong process wider mediolaterally than anteroposteriorly with a rounded posterior aspect and concave anterior aspect **(fovea pterygoidea)**. Its articulating surface, the **superior anterior aspect**, is slightly convex. The condyle, as well as the articular tubercle, is covered by a rather thick layer of fibrous avascular tissue (fibrous connective tissue). The **articular eminence** is located anterior to the rather thin-boned articular fossa of the temporal bone.

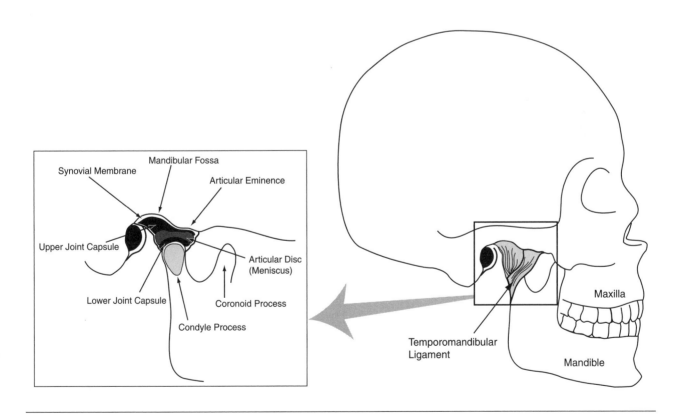

DENTAL REVIEW

| Breakdown of Structures | | |
|---|---|---|
| **Bone** | **Condyle** | **Cancellous (spongy)** bone covered by a thin layer of compact bone<br><br>Marrow is red, except in older persons, where it may be replaced by fatty marrow |
| | **Glenoid (mandibular) fossa** | Roof of fossa consists of thin layer of compact bone |
| | **Articular tubercle** | Consists of spongy bone covered with a thin layer of compact bone |
| **Joint components** | **Articular disc** | Dense, fibrous tissue with a few elastic fibers<br><br>Center is very dense connective tissue; no blood vessels |
| | **Articular space** | Divided into two compartments:<br>• **Lower**—between condyle and disc (hinge movement, rotation)<br>• **Upper**—between disc and temporal bone (sliding movement, translation) |
| **Ligaments** | **Temporomandibular (lateral)** | Consists of two short, fibrous bands attached to: *(1)* the lateral surface of zygomatic arch and to the tubercle on its inferior border superiorly, and *(2)* the lateral surface and posterior border of the neck of the mandible inferiorly. |
| | **Sphenomandibular** | Thin band attached to spine of sphenoid bone and descends to the lingula of the mandibular foramen; gives support to mandible and helps limit the maximum opening of the jaw |
| | **Stylomandibular** | Extends from near the apex of the styloid process of temporal bone to the angle and posterior border of the ramus of the mandible; relaxed when the mouth is closed and when in extreme protrusion becomes tense |
| | **Capsular ligament (fibrous capsule)** | Surrounds entire joint; composed of fibrous tissue reinforced by accessory ligaments; restricts movement of mandibular condyle on wide opening |
| | **Lateral ligament** | Provides strong reinforcement of anterior lateral wall of capsule and helps prevent excess lateral and posterior displacement of mandible |

| FUNCTIONAL CONTACTING MOVEMENTS | |
|---|---|
| **Non-Working Side (Balancing Side)** | **Working Side** |
| When the mandible is moved left or right, it is the side to which the mandible is moved. | When the mandible is moved to the left or right, it is the side to which the mandible is moved. |

| MASTICATORY MUSCLE FUNCTION | |
|---|---|
| Closing (elevating the mandible) | Masseter, medial pterygoid, temporalis |
| Opening (depressing the mandible) | Lateral pterygoid, mylohyoid, digastric, geniohyoid |
| Protruding | Lateral pterygoid |
| Lateral motion | Lateral pterygoid<br>• **Right lateral pterygoid** moves the mandible to the **left**<br>• **Left lateral pterygoid** moves the mandible to the **right** |
| Retruding | Temporalis, especially the posterior fibers |

| | Movement of the Mandible | Working Side Condyle | Non-Working Side Condyle |
|---|---|---|---|
| **Protrusive** | Mandible moves directly forward | Both condyles move simultaneously **forward and downward** along the articular eminence | |
| **Lateral** | Mandible moves to right or left without moving forward | Condyle **rotates** | Condyle moves **forward and downward** |
| **Lateral protrusive** | Combination of lateral and protrusive movements | Condyle **rotates** and moves **forward and down** | Condyle moves **anteriorly, downward, and medially** |
| **Retrusive** | Mandible moves directly backward | Both condyles move **upward and back** into mandibular fossa | |

### Mandibular Contacting Movement

When interpreting mandibular contacting movement, remember that the **maxillary teeth** are stationary and the **mandible** moves. If given a diagram of the maxillary arch with mandibular cusp pathways shown, the movement indicated would be the true movement of the mandible. If a diagram of mandibular teeth was shown, and maxillary cusps were illustrated, the movement of the maxillary cusps would be opposite the movement of the mandible.

The balancing side or nonworking side should not contact during the lateral contacting movements because of the mandibular condyles moving downward on the articular eminence.

The figures illustrate contacting movement.

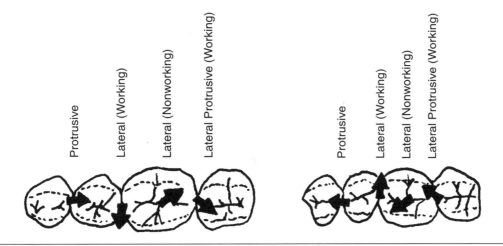

DENTAL REVIEW

Expect at least one question on the Posselt envelope of motion. Remember that the outline is the extreme position of all movements. The mandible can take any position within this outline.

## Posselt Envelope of Motion

The **Posselt envelope of motion** defines the border movements of the mandible. To arrive at this diagram, one could place a tracer in the mandible between the two central incisors and record the position of the tracer when the mandible moves. The tracing records the **anterior–posterior** and **inferior–superior** positions. Remember that this is a recording of mandibular motion **viewed from the lateral**.

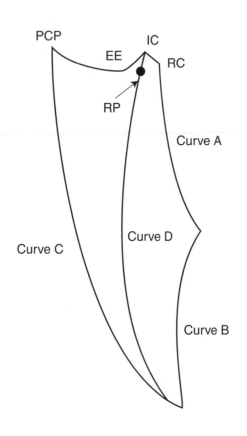

**Sagittal View**

### Intercuspal (IC) Position

The **intercuspal (IC)** position is the **highest position of the mandible** and is seen when the teeth are in maximum intercuspation. Also known as **centric occlusion.**

### Retruded Contract (RC) Position

**Retruded contact (RC)** is the most retruded position of the mandible (retruded contacting position, centric relation). In 90% of the population, the IC (or centric occlusion) is approximately 1.25 mm anterior to the **centric relation,** and in the other 10%, IC corresponds to RC. When going to this RC position, the mandible must move downward and posteriorly from its height in the intercuspal position. This is because of the holding cusps of the mandibular teeth sliding on the mesial inclines of maxillary cusps located posterior to them.

### Opening Movements

The **mandibular condyles** are capable of two types of **opening** movement when in retruded contacting position:

- **Pure rotational movement (*curve A* in figure)**—The rotatory movement accounts for the first 20 or so millimeters of mandibular opening, and then ligaments become taut. For further opening, the ligaments must be loosened, and this is achieved by the mandibular condyles moving down the articular eminence.

- **Translational movement (*curve B* in figure)**—The mandible opens further (translational movement) to its maximal opening (40–50 mm separation of the anterior teeth).

The line that connects the position of maximal opening to protruded contact position (*curve C* in figure) is the **protrusive opening path**. This line describes the curve made if the mandible were placed as far forward as possible and then opened as far as possible.

*Curve D* represents normal chewing movement.

## Protruded Contact Position (PCP)

**The protruded contact position (*PCP*)** describes the most protruded or anterior position of the mandible. If the jaw is in this position, the incisors would not be in an edge-to-edge relationship, but instead the mandibular incisors would be more anterior than the maxillary incisors.

## Edge to Edge (EE)

From PCP, remaining in tooth contact, the mandible is pulled backward until the incisors are edge to edge **(position EE, or "edge to edge").** The mandible must move down so that the incisors can come edge to edge.

Moving from EE to IC, the mandibular cusps slide up the distal inclines of the maxillary cusps anterior to them. ***Curve D*** in the figure on the previous page illustrates the mandibular path when opening to the position of maximum opening. This curve is not pure rotatory motion, but rather **translational movement.** It is not a border movement because it occurs within the envelope of motion.

## Normal Rest Position (RP)

**Point RP** is the normal **rest position** of the mandible. At rest, the teeth are not contacting. This position is also known as the **postural position** or **physiologic rest position.** The distance from RP to IC is called **freeway space.** That is, it represents the space between the teeth when the mandible is in the postural position (2–3 mm).

Rest position is determined primarily by musculature.

| Frontal View | |
|---|---|
| 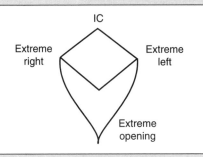 | This figure represents the same movement as above, but here, in the lateral contacting positions, the mandible is opened to its maximum. <br><br> The **chewing stroke**, or **masticatory stroke**, when seen from the anterior on the lateral, is well within the borders of the mandibular movement. It is described as a pear- or tear-shaped movement. When chewing, the chewing is usually unilateral, favoring a particular side. This accounts for the displacement towards one side of the inferior portion of this movement. |

| Horizontal View | |
|---|---|
| 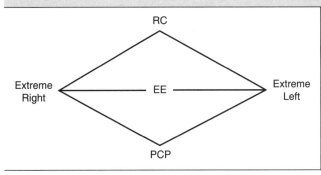 | This diamond-shaped figure is a tracing of the mandible when starting in the RC position and then moving to the extreme right (right lateral contacting position), then moving to PCP (protruded contact position), then to the extreme left (left lateral contacting position), and finally back again to RC. |

# ORAL MUCOSA

The oral cavity is lined throughout with **oral epithelium (stratified, squamous epithelium)** and the underlying **lamina propria (connective tissue layer)**. Under the oral mucosa is the submucosa, which also differs from place to place, depending on the function of the particular area.

The surface epithelium may be categorized as **keratinized** or **nonkeratinized**. A full keratinized potential does not present in mucosal cells under normal conditions, except in the masticatory mucosa, although it may be expressed in any area under irritation. Because the keratinized potential does not present in the majority of mucosal cells, the stratum granulosum and the corneum are not seen.

## LAYERS OF THE EPITHELIUM

| Layer | Characteristics |
|---|---|
| Stratum basal layer (stratum germinativum) | Single layer of cuboidal to low columnar cells<br>Basal layer provides new cells for the other epithelial layers<br>Mitosis or cell division occurs at this level |
| Stratum spinosum (prickle cell layer) | A multilayer of polyhedral-like cells bound together by means of numerous desmosomal junctions<br>Toward the surface, these cells flatten and widen considerably<br>**No further changes occur in the nonkeratinizing epithelium** |
| Stratum granulosum | Flattened polygonal cells filled with basophilic keratohyalin granules<br>This layer not seen in nonkeratinized epithelium |
| Stratum lucidum | Transitional zone<br>This layer appears in the epidermis of thick shin (palms, soles) and not seen in oral |
| Stratum corneum | Anucleated (cells have lost their nuclei)<br>Flat cells filled with keratin |

The **lamina propria** is a dense layer of connective tissue. Its papillae indent the epithelium and carry both blood vessels and nerves. Between the connective tissue papillae are the epithelial rete pegs.

## TYPES OF STRATIFIED SQUAMOUS EPITHELIUM

Three types of stratified squamous epithelium are found in the oral cavity.

| Type | Location | Characteristics | Appearance |
|---|---|---|---|
| **Nonkeratinized (nonmasticatory)** | Buccal mucosa<br>Cheeks<br>Floor of the mouth<br>Lips<br>Soft palate<br>Ventral surface of the tongue<br>Alveolar mucosa | Basal cell, prickle cell, and outer most nonkeratinized layers | It appears as a soft, moist surface |
| **Orthokeratinized (masticatory)** | Gingival<br>Dorsal surface of the tongue<br>Hard palate | Basal cell, prickle cell, granular, and outer most keratinized layers | Coral-pink in color and highly vascular |
| **Parakeratinized** | Dorsum of the tongue<br>Attached gingiva | Basal cell, prickle cell, and keratinized layers | Associated with lingual papillae of the tongue<br>Taste buds present in this tissue |

| DIFFERENCE BETWEEN SKIN OF LIP AND MUCOUS MEMBRANE | |
|---|---|
| **The Skin of the Lip** | **The Transition Zone (Vermilion Border)** |
| Keratinized epithelium—moderate thickness | Keratinized tissue ends in this area |
| Papillae of connective tissue—few and short | Long papillae carrying large capillary loops close to the surface |
| Sebaceous glands in association with hair | Few sebaceous glands |
| Sweat glands | |

| IMPORTANT CELLS OF THE EPITHELIUM | |
|---|---|
| **Keratinocytes** | Responsible for the production of keratin |
| | Not found in oral mucosa |
| **Melanocytes** | Derivatives of neural crest ectoderm |
| | Responsible for production of pigment |
| **Langerhans cells** | Immune system cells |
| | Antigen-presenting cells |
| **Merkel cells** | Function in concert with nerve fibers |
| | Sensory cells |

## PERIODONTIUM

The **gingival unit** consists of the **free gingiva, attached gingiva**, and **alveolar mucosa.** The gingival unit has a lining epithelium of either **masticatory mucosa**, which is thick keratinized epithelium with a dense collagenous connective tissue corium, or **lining mucosa**, which is thin, nonkeratinized epithelium with loose connective tissue corium containing elastic, and sometimes muscle, fibers.

Masticatory mucosa is found in the free and the attached gingiva, hard palate, and dorsum of the tongue, and lining mucosa is found elsewhere in the oral cavity.

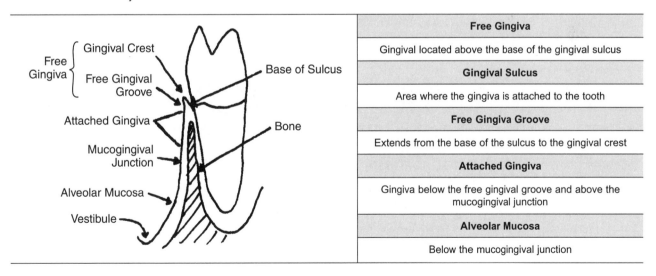

| Free Gingiva |
|---|
| Gingival located above the base of the gingival sulcus |
| **Gingival Sulcus** |
| Area where the gingiva is attached to the tooth |
| **Free Gingiva Groove** |
| Extends from the base of the sulcus to the gingival crest |
| **Attached Gingiva** |
| Gingiva below the free gingival groove and above the mucogingival junction |
| **Alveolar Mucosa** |
| Below the mucogingival junction |

DENTAL REVIEW

## ATTACHMENT APPARATUS

The attachment apparatus consists of the cementum, periodontal ligament, and alveolar bone. The periodontal ligament surrounds the tooth and connects to the bone, acting like a hammock. The attachment apparatus provides proprioceptive information to stimuli like pressure and pain. The bone and cementum can be resorbed when under controlled pressure, allowing for orthodontic movement of the teeth.

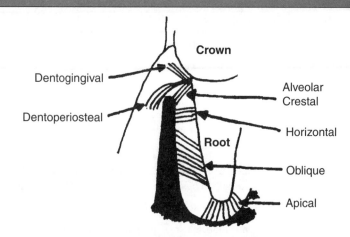

### Principal Fiber Group

The principal fiber group comprises collagen fibers, which **do not attach to alveolar bone**.

| | |
|---|---|
| **Dentogingival** | Runs from the cementum into the free gingiva |
| **Dentoperiosteal** | Runs from the cementum apically, over the alveolar crest of the bone, into the periosteum of the attached gingiva |
| **Transseptal** | Runs from the cementum of one tooth, over the alveolar crest bone, to the cementum of an adjacent tooth |
| **Circular** | Not attached to cementum; runs in the free gingiva around the tooth in a circular manner |

### Periodontal Fiber Group

The periodontal fiber group comprises collagen fibers, which **run from cementum to alveolar bone**.

| | |
|---|---|
| **Alveolar crestal** | Runs from supra-alveolar cementum down to the alveolar crest |
| **Horizontal** | Runs from the cementum directly across to the alveolar bone |
| **Oblique** | Largest group of fibers<br>Runs from the cementum, from the root to the bone, in a diagonal coronal direction |
| **Apical** | Runs from apex of root to alveolar bone in base of alveolus |

## THE PERIODONTAL LIGAMENT (PDL)

The periodontal ligament (PDL) is the connective tissue that surrounds the root of the tooth and attaches the root of the tooth to the bony alveolus.

| | |
|---|---|
| **Functions** | **Formative:** cementoblasts, fibroblasts, and osteoblasts are derived from cells in the PDL<br>**Supportive:** maintains the tooth in its position<br>**Sensory:** extremely good innervation in PDL<br>**Nutritive:** extremely good blood supply in the PDL |
| **Blood supply** | 1. Periosteal blood supply from alveolar bone (**major source**)<br>2. Arteries of gingiva, which anastomose with the PDL (**minor source**)<br>3. Arteries of the periapical area, which arise from the vessels entering the pulp (**minor source**) |
| **Nerve supply** | Nerves follow path of blood vessels<br>Free nerve endings are receptors for pain and proprioceptive stimuli* |
| **Lymphatics** | Follow path of blood vessels<br>Flow of lymph is from ligament toward and into alveolar bone |

*Note:* The proprioceptive information regulates the masticatory musculature and protects the tooth from sudden overload due to severe masticatory stresses.

DENTAL REVIEW

| Damage to the PDL | |
|---|---|
| **In Loss of Function** | **In Occlusal Trauma** |
| 1. The PDL narrows. | 1. Alveolar bone is reabsorbed. |
| 2. The regular arrangement of fibers is lost. | 2. PDL is widened. |
| 3. The PDL becomes a thin membrane with irregularly arranged fibers. | 3. Tooth becomes loose. |
| 4. Cementum may become thickened. | 4. When source of trauma removed, repair usually occurs. |

| INNERVATION OF IMPORTANT ORAL STRUCTURES | | |
|---|---|---|
| **TONGUE** | **Function** | **Innervation** |
| Anterior 2/3 | Sensory, nontaste | Lingual branch of the mandibular nerve (**CN V**) |
| Anterior 2/3 | Taste | Chorda tympani of the facial nerve (**CN VII**) |
| Posterior 1/3 | Taste, general sensory | Lingual branch of the glossopharyngeal nerve (**CN IX**) |
| Entire tongue | Motor innervation | Hypoglossal nerve (**CN XII**) |
| **TEETH** | **Type** | **Innervation** |
| | Lower molar and premolar | Inferior alveolar nerve of the mandibular nerve (**CN V3**) |
| | Lower incisors | Inferior alveolar nerve of the mandibular nerve (**CN V3**) incisal branch |
| | Maxillary third through first molar | Posterior superior alveolar nerve of the maxillary nerve (**CN V2**) |
| | Mesial buccal root of the maxillary first molar and the maxillary premolars | Middle superior nerve of the maxillary nerve |
| | Maxillary canines and incisors | Anterior superior alveolar nerve of the maxillary nerve |
| **SUPPORTING TISSUES** | **Tissue** | **Innervation** |
| Mandibular | Lingual gingiva and supporting tissue | Lingual nerve of the mandibular nerve (**CN V3**) |
| | Buccal molar region | Inferior alveolar nerve and the buccal nerve |
| | Anterior to molars | The mental nerve |
| Maxillary | Buccal tissues | Anterior, middle, and posterior superior alveolar nerve |
| | Posterior lingual | Greater palatine nerve |
| | Anterior lingual | Nasopalatine nerve |

*Note:* The trigeminal nerve CN V supports both the dental (teeth) and the periodontal tissues. The maxillary nerve (CN V2) innervates the maxillary structures. The mandibular nerve (CN V3) innervates the mandibular structures.

DENTAL REVIEW

# THE TONGUE

## Papillae Types

| Papillae Type | Vascular/ Nonvascular | Taste Buds? | Location |
|---|---|---|---|
| **Filiform** | Nonvascular | No | Rows, anterior to middle |
| **Fungiform** | Vascular | Yes | Anterior only |
| **Circumvallate (vallate)** | Vascular | Yes | 10 to 12 only, V-shaped row near anterior/posterior border |
| **Foliate** | Nonvascular | No | Lateral border of the tongue |

### Foramen Caecum

Remnant of thyroglossal duct; located at the apex of the "V" formed by the circumvallate

### Other Papillae

Additional taste buds can be found on the posterolateral palate, epiglottis, and the pharynx

## Tongue Innervation and Development

| Anterior two thirds | General sensation CN V (trigeminal) Taste by CN VII (facial) |
|---|---|
| **Posterior third (including the circumvallate)** | CN IX (glossopharyngeal) |
| **Most posterior (valleculae and minor taste buds)** | CN X (vagus) |
| **Development of the tongue** | Branchial arches 1–4 Lingual buds (bilateral swellings) Tuberculum impar Copula |
| **Branchial arch and associated cranial nerve** | Arch 1—CN V Arch 2—CN VII Arch 3—CN IX Arch 4—CN X |